NEW CONCEPTS IN CRANIOMANDIBULAR AND CHRONIC PAIN MANAGEMENT

Edited by

Harold Gelb, DMD

*Adjunct Clinical Professor,
Tufts University School of Dental Medicine*

*Formerly Clinical Professor,
Department of Restorative Dentistry,
University of Medicine and Dentistry of New Jersey*

*Formerly Director of Temporomandibular Joint Clinic,
Department of Otolaryngology,
New York Eye and Ear Infirmary*

*Founder of the Harold Gelb Craniomandibular
Pain Center, Tufts University
School of Dental Medicine*

M Mosby-Wolfe

Exclusive distribution worldwide,
except Spain:

Mosby-Wolfe

Times Mirror International Publishers Ltd.

Lynton House
7-12 Tavistock Square
LONDON - WC1H 9LB
England

ISBN: 0.7234.2041.6

A CIP catalogue record for this book is available from the British Library

© Espaxs, S.A. Publicaciones Médicas, 1994
Rosselló, 132
08036 - Barcelona
(Spain)

All rights reserved. No part of this publication may be reproduced
or transmitted by any means, electronic, mechanical, or otherwise,
including photocopying and recording, or by any information
storage or retrieval system, without permission-in writing-from
the publishers.

Printed in Spain

ACKNOWLEDGEMENTS

It has been fifteen years since I first edited a book dealing with a multidisciplinary approach to the diagnosis and treatment of craniomandibular (TM) disorders. Once again, I am fortunate and grateful to have been able to assemble such a fine group of health care professionals as the contributors for this current book. The knowledge and experience necessary to coordinate an approach to the diagnosis, treatment, and management of the chronic pain patient that is both successful and cost effective requires the input of brilliant minds. Through the years I have had the good fortune to be exposed to the teachings and publications of many such individuals. While I cannot mention all of them in this short space, I would like to recognize several of the individuals who have contributed to my professional development in this particular area. They are: Hans Kraus, MD; Janet Travell, MD; David Simon, MD; Rene Caillet, MD; Victor Stoll, DDS; George Goodheart, DC; Willie B. May, DDS; and William Sutherland, DO.

I am grateful to my excellent office staff, as well as my personal secretary, Laura Emanuel. My professional associates Michael Gelb, DDS, MS; Richard Sousa, DDS, and Wayne Prigoff, DDS, were most supportive. I also wish to thank Aaron Weiss, DDS, for his help in translating some of the early manuscripts.

Above all, let me acknowledge the support, encouragement and patience of my wife and best friend, Sally.

Harold Gelb, DMD

NOTICE

Dentistry is an ever-changing science. As new research and clinical experience broaden our knowledge, changes in treatment are required. The editors and the publisher of this work have made every effort to ensure that the procedures herein are accurate and in accord with the standards accepted at the time of publication.

CONTRIBUTORS

Mary Mathews Brion, MSW
    Certified Alexander Teacher

Grant R. N. Bowbeer, DDS, MS
    Private Practice

Lynn E. Buono, BA
    Certified Alexander Teacher

Howard J. Dananberg, DPM
    Private Practice

Albert G. Forgione, PhD
    Associate Clinical Professor, General Dentistry; Chief Clinical Consultant, Tufts University School of Dental Medicine, Boston, Massachusetts.

Harold Gelb, DMD
    Former Clinical Professor, Department of Restorative Dentistry, University of Medicine and Dentistry of New Jersey, Newark, New Jersey; Former Associate Clinical Professor, Department of Removable Prosthodontics, Temple University College of Dentistry, New York, New York; Adjunct Clinical Professor, Department of General Dentistry; Founder, Dr. Harold Gelb Craniomandibular Pain Center, Tufts University School of Dental Medicine, Boston, Massachusetts.

Michael Gelb, DDS
    Clinical Associate Professor, Division of Basic Science, Department of Oral Medicine and Pathology; Director, Continuing Dental Education, TMJ and Craniofacial Pain Program, New York University College of Dentistry, New York, New York; Clinical Assistant Professor, Tufts University College of Dentistry, Boston, Massachusetts.

Stanley Knebelman, DMD
    Private Practice; Certified Alexander Teacher

Richard T. Koritzer, DDS, PhD
    Professor of Anatomy, Georgetown University College of Dentistry, Washington, DC.

Hans Kraus, MD
    Formerly Associate Professor of Physical Medicine, New York University, New York, New York.

Jeffery S. Mannheimer, MA, PT
    Clinical Assistant Professor and Director, Physical Therapy Tract, Continuing Education Program in Diagnosis and Treatment of Oralfacial Pain and TMJ Dysfunction, University of Medicine and Dentistry of New Jersey, Newark, New Jersey; Clinical Assistant Professor, Department of Orthopedic Surgery and Rehabilitation, Program in Physical Therapy, Hanemann University School of Medicine, Philadelphia, Pennsylvania.

Noshir Mehta, DDS, MDS, MS
    Director of the Gelb Craniomandibular Pain Center, and Associate Clinical Professor, Department of Periodontics, Tufts University School of Dental Medicine, Boston, Massachusetts.

Murad N. Padamsee, DMD
    Clinical Associate, General Dentistry and TMJ Disorders, Tufts University School of Dental Medicine, Boston, Massachusetts.

Richard Pertes, DDS
    Clinical Associate Professor and Acting Director, Center for TMJ Disorders and Orofacial Pain Management, University of Medicine and Dentistry of New Jersey, Newark, New Jersey.

Patricia Ralston-Dressler, MEd
    Certified Alexander Teacher

Lucille St. Hoyme, PhD
    Curator Emeritus, Physical Anthropology, The Smithsonian Institution, Washington, DC; Visiting Scientist, Department of Anatomy, Maryland University Dental School, Baltimore, Maryland.

Eric Paul Shaber, DDS
    Associate Professor, Oral and Maxillofacial Surgery, University of the Pacific, San Francisco, California; Attending Surgeon: Mount Sinai Medical Center; Pacific Medical Center; Veterans Administration Medical Center, San Francisco, California.

Lionel A. Walpin, MD
    Private Practice

David Walther, DC
    Private Practice

Alan Weinstein, DO
    Associate Clinical Professor; Director, Division of Thermography, Pain Center, University of Medicine and Dentistry of New Jersey, Newark, New Jersey.

Christine Gail Wheaton, MS, PT
    Private Practice, Formerly Instructor in Kinesiology, Northeastern University, Boston, Massachusetts.

George E. White, DDS, PhD
    Associate Professor and Chairman, Department of Oral Pediatrics, Tufts University College of Dentistry, Boston, Massachusetts.

CONTENTS

Preface i

Introduction v

Chapter 1 General Principles 1

Chapter 2 Posture: The Process of Body Use; Principles and Determinants 13

Chapter 3 Diagnosis and Treatment of Muscle Pain 77

Chapter 4 Scoliosis Evaluation & Documentation with
Computerized Infrared Thermography 85

Chapter 5 Prevention and Restoration of Abnormal Upper
Quarter Posture 93

Chapter 6 Mandibular Rest Position: Relationship to Occlusion,
Posture and Muscle Activity 163

Chapter 7 The Essentials of the Alexander Technique 177

Chapter 8 A Biophysical Model for Craniomandibular Management 187

Chapter 9 An Orthopedic Approach to the Diagnosis and
Treatment of Craniocervical Mandibular Disorders 215

Chapter 10 The Effect of Macroposture and Body Mechanics on
Dental Occlusion 261

Chapter 11 Craniomandibular Dysfunction in the Growing Child 271

Chapter 12 Skeletal Facial Types — "The Missing Link" 309

Chapter 13 Postural Consideration for the Orthodontic Patient 321

Chapter 14 Foot Malfunction and Its Relationship to
Craniomandibular Disorders 335

Chapter 15 Applied Kinesiology and the Stomatognathic System 349

Conclusion 369

Index 371

PREFACE

After more than forty years of active practice, with thirty-five devoted to the diagnosis and treatment of craniomandibular (TMJ) disorders, certain truths have come to seem self evident. The most obvious of these is that many, many patients suffer from chronic pain, which is probably the most frequent cause of disability, and as a consequence constitutes a major national and world health problem with monumental economic overtones. Although accurate statistics are not always readily available, it is believed that chronic pain states cost the American people over fifty billion dollars annually. Included in this figure are costs for medical, hospital, and other health services, in addition to the price of lost work productivity, compensation payments, and litigation.

The Nuprin Pain Report, conducted in 1985, provided the first broad-based systematic study of the frequency, severity, and cost of problems associated with pain. It provided estimates of the number of days people had been unable to work or engage in routine activities during the preceding year, and categorized those estimates according to the different kinds of pain involved. In total, an estimated four billion sick days were lost by all individuals over the age of 18 (approximately 23 days per person). Among members of the full-time work force, an estimated 550 million days were lost (approximately 5 days per person) in the year studied.

The breakdown of the lost millions of work days by full-time workers in the United States was as follows: headaches—156.9; backaches—88.8; muscle pains—58.2; joint pains—107.8; stomach pains—98.7; menstrual pains—24.5 and dental pains—15.1. Looking at headaches alone, we find that they are broken down into three major groups: 2% traction and inflammatory, 8% vascular, and 90% of the muscle contraction type.

Headaches unquestionably comprise the most common type of pain experienced by adult Americans. Using the Nuprin study as a guideline, we can say that approximately 3 out 4 American adults (73% in the study) suffered from one or more headaches in the last year. Among those suffering from multiple pains, the types of pain described as most troublesome (again, the statistics are from the Nuprin survey) were backaches (16% of all adults), headaches (15%), and joint pain (11%), followed by stomach pains (6%), muscle pains (5%), premenstrual or menstrual pains (3%), and dental pains (3%).

A demographic profile of pain sufferers in the study revealed striking differences in the prevalence and severity of various pains according to the following factors:

1. **Age.** Young people in the study were more apt to experience pain than older people. This held true for headaches, backaches, muscle pains, stomach pains, premenstrual and menstrual pains, and dental pains. The one exception was joint pain, which becomes more prevalent with age.
2. **Sex.** Women were more likely to experience pain than men; headaches were more likely to affect them and to do so more often; females also experienced more backaches, joint pains, and stomach pains than males.
3. **Race.** Again, according to the survey, white Americans generally experienced pain more than blacks or Hispanics; in particular they tended to suffer more frequently from backaches, muscle pains, and joint pains. Interestingly, white women experienced fewer days of premenstrual and menstrual pain than black or Hispanic women.
4. **Income.** There were no remarkable differences in the prevalence of pain between members of different income groups. Notwithstanding, those with incomes under $15,000 were shown to be somewhat more likely to experience joint pains, while

those with household incomes over $50,000 were somewhat more likely to suffer from muscle pains.
5. **Family History.** The survey found a strong familial correlation. Those individuals whose parents experienced severe pain at some point in their lives experienced more backaches, muscle pains, and joint pains.

According to the Nuprin Report, most Americans with only occasional pain (defined as pain one to five days in the last year) felt that pain has only a minimal effect on their day-to-day lives. but those with more than occasional pain (six or more days in the last year) often stated that the experience could severly upset their daily routines, causing lost work days, interrupted sleep, and eventually even incapacitation.

The Nuprin survey also investigated the relationship between stress and pain. The hypothesis that evolved was a simple one: the more stress an individual is subjected to the greater the chance that he or she will experience pain.

Most individuals sought professional advice or treatment when they experience more than just the occasional type of pain. Over half of those surveyed had seen a physician, 18% a chiropractor, and 12% a pharmacist. Only 3% of those interviewed consulted a pain specialist or nutritionist, and just 2% consulted an acupuncturist, spiritual counselor, or faith healer regarding their pain. Of interest, among headache and dental pain sufferers, 23% had seen a dentist for their pain.

The more severe the pain, the more inclined the individual was to seek professional advice. Along the same lines, the largest percentage of pain sufferers who opted not to seek professional help said that the primary reason was their pain not being severe enough. Moreover, all of those suffering unbearable pain consulted a professional health provider (82% saw a physician).

Of those with more than occasional pain who consulted a doctor, 40% said that the physician recommended prescription drugs. An additional 20% reported that their doctor recommended non-prescription drugs for the relief of their pain. Furthermore, 18% stated that their doctor recommended exercise; 10% said a change in diet was suggested; 9% mentioned the use of heat/cold treatment; and 7% said meditation or other relaxation techniques were prescribed. A minimal percentage of pain sufferers said their doctors recommended TENS, electrical stimulation, or biofeedback. None of the patients said that their doctors recommended hypnosis.

As for results, among those pain sufferers who consulted a physician, a majority (73%) said that their doctor was very or somewhat successful in relieving their pain. A similar assessment was made by roughly 70% of those who consulted a chiropractor, a nutritionist (69%), a dentist (67%), or a pain specialist (65%).

Now we turn from the Nuprin survey to a brief discussion of the back as a problem area which merits special attention. Backaches prompt more than 19 million doctor visits and strike about 8 million new victims each year, in addition to the 75 million already afflicted. Every year approximately 200,000 people undergo surgery for persistent low back pain, but surgery fails completely in about 20% of the cases, and three out of five patients continue to have symptoms despite the surgery. Lower back pain, as the major cause of activity restrictions among people under 45, cuts into the most productive time of life.

No specific "back personality" has been identified, and some experts are quick to point out that many of the emotional problems seen in back patients are more likely to be a result of the ailment rather than a cause. A Swedish back expert, Dr. Alf L. Nachemson, has shown that exercise improves the delivery of nutrition to spinal disks, perhaps delaying the deterioration that affects all backs. Disk disease is believed to account for only 5 to 10% of these cases; 80 to 85% of back pain is now attributed to muscular weakness, and the remaining 10% is judged to be a result of structural defects or disease, such as malformed vertebrae, arthritis, a tumor, or a dislocation of the facet joints between two vertebrae.

Not far behind colds as one of the nation's leading causes of time lost from work, backaches are, ironically, often caused by working conditions—the many hours white-collar workers sit in poorly designed chairs, with strained postures, and the heavy lifting common among blue collar workers. Low back pain does not seem to be primarily the result of biomechanical shortcomings, but rather of biomechanical abuse, obesity, the aging process, and that hallmark of affluence, sedentary living.

The elderly patient is treated for pain syndromes more frequently than for any other complaint. Degenerative joint disease is probably the most common cause of pain in this age group. Other causes would include trauma, metastatic bone pain, cancer pain, claudication, fibromyositis, polymyalgia rheumatica, renal colic, angina/myocardial infarction, gout, rheumatoid arthritis, shoulder syndromes, and a variety of post-surgical causes of pain. However, as can be seen in the earlier-mentioned statistics, an extremely high percentage of patients presenting with chronic pain have a strong musculo-skeletal component involved.

Renee Cailliet, in his book *Neck and Arm Pain*, states "Of all the musculo-skeletal and neuromuscular conditions causing pain and disability in man, pain and dysfunction originating in the neck, shoulders and upper extremities is exceeded only by low back pain. The musculo-skeletal system must be fully understood in its static anatomical sense and in its kinetic function before abnormality and the mechanism of pain production and dysfunction can be recognized and understood. Pathological changes can be prevented; and when a complete reversal of abnormal changes is impossible, at least the symptoms and disability caused by these changes can be ameliorated."

In keeping with the theme of this book, a clarification of the difference between neuromuscular function and dysfunction will be undertaken to thread a link between the specialty areas of medicine, dentistry, osteopathy, physical therapy, chiropractic, and the behavorial sciences. The common meeting ground for all the specialities in the health field is biology in general and function specifically. Utilization of the basic sciences such as anatomy, physiology, histology, and pathology in conjunction with clinical practice and experience are the basis for a clear understanding of what is normal and of the deviations therefrom.

Up to the present time, determined attempts to attack pain by purely medical means have impeded both innovative thinking and the development of effective treatment approaches. Since pain is traditionally perceived as a neurophysiological problem, it is initially presumed to have organic causes. If the diagnostic findings in a given case fail to yield a clear physical basis for reports of pain, the doctor usually assumes the pain is psychogenic and refers the patient to a psychiatrist. The psychiatrist, in turn failing to find clearcut evidence of mental pathology, will then refer the patient back to yet another specialist. This is not uncommon in our clinical practice and may be due to the fact that most physicians are not yet aware of the importance of craniomandibular disorders in the etiology of pain syndromes, and are certainly not sufficiently conversant with the role of postural imbalance in chronic pain states.

This book presents the views of clinicians and researchers with varied backgrounds from around the world in an attempt to provide a new look at the posture maintenance problem. It is our hope that the material presented will add to the understanding and effective treatment of the chronic pain patient.

Harold Gelb, DMD

Introduction

Pain: A Complex Perceptual Experience

Eric Paul Shaber, DDS

Pain is a complex perceptual experience, and chronic pain is the most seriously disabling psychosocial disease known to the human race. To merely consider pain as a symptom of a larger, more important organic problem is folly. Pain is a formidable disorder in and of itself, requiring the combined cooperation and expertise of various allied health care providers.

Pain can be simply categorized as acute or chronic. Acute pain is biologically valuable as a signal of tissue damage. But chronic pain involves a mix-up in the central neuronal circuitry, and is *never* a valuable experience: it is *always* malefic.[1] Pain is physiologic function of receptor specificity, central summation, central conversion, inhibition, and descending controls.[2] Pain response is a social function based on past experience, the situational meaning of the event, and one's cultural background.[3]

In an attempt to unwind the phenomenon of pain, we must begin by exploring the physiology of the pain experience.

Receptor Specificity

There are specific areas of unique nerve tufts that give rise to pain when stimulated (irritated). The particular mode of irritation may be chemical, thermal, or pressure-mediated.

There are basically three groups of nerve fibers: A, B, and C. Fibers "A" and "C" transmit pain. The "A" fibers are myelinated and transmit pain very quickly. The "C" fibers are unmyelinated and transmit their impulses rather slowly.[4] (The clinical concept of first and second pain now becomes apparent). These specific pain receptors (A and C fibers) are sensitive to changes in the ambient pH and biogenic amine levels. These receptors will respond appropriately by propagating and generating enhanced pain transmission or by decreasing the central transmission of pain impulses.

Central Summation

Pain fibers enter the central nervous system through the dorsal root and ultimately find their way to the substantia gelatinosa (laminas two and three). From the substantia gelatinosa, pain impulses are propelled to the T-cells (the pain action cells). It is this system of nerve movement which has given rise to the neurophysiologic postulate of Melzack and Wall. This hypothesis is the first truly unifying concept of pain specificity. It is known as the Gate Control Theory.

Central Convergence

Pain and temperature impulses arising from throughout the body travel via a similar spinal pathway, the lateral spinothalamic tract. It is this scientific fact of impulse transmission that allows us to better understand why physical medicine modalities (heat and vapocoolants) decrease pain and increase myofascial range of motion, when applied to the body.[5,6] The lateral spinothalamic tract, when bombarded (counterirritated) by temperature, does not readily transmit pain impulses. The course of central convergence is completed when the pain impulse is forwarded centrally through the thalamus to its ultimate conclusion in the cortex.

Inhibition

Inhibitory impulses travel via direct stat antinociceptive pathways from the thalamus to the substantia gelatinosa. Inhibitory impulses compete with other centrally transmitted nerve impulses for propagation at the substantia gelatinosa.

Descending Controls

When the body's own internal pain reduction system (the enkephalin system) is stimulated, a compound called endorphin is released. This endogenous opiate is found in close proximity to pain transmission receptors in the central nervous system. When the endorphin couples with the afferent neuron, pain transmission is blocked. The control of nociception by endogenous opiates is well documented, and now considered a physiologic fact.

Once one is armed with the basic scientific knowledge required to understand the pain experience, it becomes abundantly clear that each medical specialist should view pain in the context of a larger unifying concept. Unfortunately, the "state of the science" teaches members of each medical specialty to evaluate pain from his or her particular area of expertise and responsibility. For example, the surgeon believes that pain is an organic dilemma, while the psychotherapist views pain as an emotional crisis which has been set into motion. The disparity between these two positions is profound and untenable; further, neither position is clearly supported by known scientific information.

The contention that chronic pain is a long-term manifestation of repeated acute pain events is, for the most part, inappropriate and leads to clinical frustration. It is now felt that chronic pain is a special disease with its own neuro-pathophysiology and biochemical derangements. To treat the chronic pain patient by utilizing acute pain modalities is both purposeless and potentially dangerous.

It is incumbent upon that special clinician/practitioner who treats pain disorders to be armed with the known scientific information. The abatement of pain is the foremost responsibility of practitioners in the healing arts.

REFERENCES

1. Melazck R. *The Puzzle of Pain*. Basic Books, Inc; New York, NY: 1973.
2. Dubner R. Neurophysiology of pain. *Dent Clin North Am*. 1978;22:11-30.
3. Steinbach RA, et al. Chronic low back pain: "lowback loser." *Postgrad Med*. 1973;53:135-138.
4. Mense S, Schmidt RF. Muscle pain: which receptors are responsible for the transmission of noxious stimuli? In: *Physiological Aspects of Clinical Neurology*. Oxford. Blackwell Scientific Publications; 1977.
5. Travell J. Myofascial trigger points: clinical view. In: *Advances in Pain Research and Therapy Vol. 1*. Raven Press; New York, NY: 1976.
6. Travell J, Rinzler S. The myofascial genesis of pain. *Postgrad Med*. 1952;22:425.

Chapter 1

General Principles

Harold Gelb, DMD

Postural Considerations

In l947, the Posture Committee of the American Academy of Orthopaedic Surgery defined standard posture as a relative arrangement of body parts in a state of balance which protects supporting structures against injury or progressive deformity.

The force of gravity plays a significant role in the morphological relationships between parts of the body. The erect posture of man is aimed at musculoskeletal efficiency, and in stance this posture is maintained primarily by ligamentous support. The superincumbent curves of the spine — cervical and lumbar lordosis and dorsosacral kyphosis — can be readily observed in the evolution of the child from birth to the final point of erect posture. The body tends to be better balanced, with less expenditure of energy, if none of its parts are too far from the vertical axis. In addition, the amount of muscle contracture needed to keep the head aligned vertically above the trunk and pelvis is minimal if all the parts of the body concerned are close to the vertical center of gravity.[1]

Whereas the upright posture of man has long been considered one of his godlike qualities, it is not an unmixed blessing, having made civilized man susceptible to fallen arches, prolapses, and similar ills that flesh may be heir to. It is reasonable to assume that some of the developmental and dysfunctional problems encountered in everyday practice are in some way related to the adaptations required for the maintenance of posture.

On December l2, l973, Nikolaas Tinbergen received the Nobel Prize for Physiology and Medicine as a result of his research in the area of childhood autism. In the lecture he delivered that evening, he made observations regarding the research and findings of F.M. Alexander and W. Barlow. Tinbergen, his wife, and one of his daughters had undergone treatment with different Alexander teachers. He stated, "We discovered that the therapy is based on exceptionally sophisticated observation, not only by means of vision but also to a surprising extent by using the sense of touch. It consists in essence of no more than a very gentle, first exploratory, and then corrective manipulation of the entire muscular system. This starts with the head and neck, then very soon the shoulders and chest are involved, and finally the pelvis, legs and feet, until the whole body is under scrutiny and treatment." (What is actually done varies from patient to patient depending on what kind of misuse the diagnostic exploration has revealed).

From personal experience, Tinbergen was able to confirm some of the seemingly fantastic claims made by Alexander and his followers, namely, that many types of underperformance and even ailments, both mental and physical, can be alleviated, sometimes to a surprising extent, by teaching the body musculature to function in a different fashion. The evidence given and documented by Alexander and Barlow of the beneficial effects on a variety of vital functions no longer seemed astonishing to Tinbergen. That long list included rheumatism (including various forms of arthritis); respiratory troubles (and even potentially lethal asthma following in their wake); circulation defects which could lead to high blood pressure and also to some dangerous heart conditions; gastrointestinal disorders of many types; various gynecological conditions; sexual failures; migraines and depressive states that often lead to suicide;

in short, a very wide spectrum of diseases both somatic and mental that are not caused by identifiable organisms.

Once one knows that an empirically developed therapy has demonstrable effects, one likes to know how it could work — what its physiological explanation could be. And here some recent discoveries in the borderline field between neurophysiology and ethology can make some aspects of the Alexander therapy more understandable and more plausible than they could have been in Sherrington's time.

One of these new discoveries concerns the key concept of reference. There are many strong indications that at various levels of integration, from single muscle units up to complex behavior, the correct performance of many movements is continuously checked by the brain. It does this by comparing a feedback report that says, "orders carried out" with the feedback expectation for which, with the initiation of each movement, the brain has been altered. Only when the expected feedback and the actual feedback match does the brain stop sending out commands for corrective action.

What Alexander discovered beyond this "is that a lifelong misuse of the body muscles (such as caused by, for instance, too much sitting and too little walking) can make the entire system go wrong. As a consequence, reports that all is correct are received by the brain (or perhaps interpreted as correct) when in fact all is very wrong. A person can feel at ease, for example, when slouching in front of a television set, when in fact he is grossly abusing his body."

Another biologically interesting aspect of the Alexander therapy is that every session clearly demonstrates that the innumerable muscles of the body continuously operate as an intricately linked web. Whenever a gentle pressure is used to make a slight change in leg posture, the neck muscles react immediately; conversely, when the therapist helps one to release the neck muscles, it is amazing to see quite pronounced movements, for instance, of the toes, even when one is lying on a couch.

What have these examples in common? First, they stress the importance of open-minded observation — of "watching and wondering." This basic scientific method is still often looked down on by those blinded by the glamour of apparatus, by the prestige of tests; and by the temptation to turn to drugs. "But," as Tinbergen stated, "it is by using this old method of observation that both autism and general misuse of the body can be seen in a new light; to a much larger extent than is now realized, both could very well be due to modern stressful conditions."

"Medical science and practice meet with a growing sense of uneasiness and lack of confidence from the side of the general public. The causes of this are complex, but at least in one respect the situation could be improved; a little more open-mindedness; a little more collaboration with other biological sciences, and a little more attention to the body as a whole and to the unity of body and mind could substantially enrich the field of medical research."

Various chapters in this book will attempt to pick up on the observations and recommendations of Tinbergen, presenting to other health professionals an updated look and approach to posture and the chronic pain patient.

Feldenkrais,[2] in contrast to Tinbergen, has expounded on deep-seated patterns in emotionally evoked postures. He has stated that improper head balance is rare in young children, except in cases of structural abnormalities. But repeated emotional upheaval can cause a child to adopt attitudes and positions that "ensure" safety. As a result, contraction of the flexor muscles, inhibiting extensor tone, ensues. Newborn infants exhibit a similar response as a reaction to the fear of falling.

Repeated emotional stress experienced by children results in flexion, with concurrent inhibition of the extensors. This developed attitude in the upright erect posture becomes one of flexion at the hips and spine with forward head posture. This posture then becomes habitual and feels quite normal. As a result, the antigravity muscles work in an imbalanced posture without letup, resulting in fatigue and muscular discomfort.

The postural patterns which produce pain can be ascertained by an understanding of what is normal and then, of the deviations therefrom. In evaluating the mechanisms of pain production in static and kinetic postural relationships, the exact sites of pain production must first be determined. Once the site of the tissue eliciting the pain has been located, specific movements or positions of the skeletal as well as vertebral components that irritate those tissues can be ascertained. Travell and Rinzler,[3] and later Travell and Simons,[4] as well as Bonica[5] and Kraus,[6] have described a group of disorders characterized by the presence of a hypersensitive area, called the trigger area, together with a specific pain syndrome, muscle spasm, tenderness, stiffness, limitation of motion, or weakness.

A trigger point (trigger zone, trigger spot, trigger area) is defined as "focus of hyperirritability in a tissue that when compressed is locally tender and, if sufficiently hypersensitive, gives rise to referred pain and tenderness and sometimes to referred autonomic phenomena and distortion of proprioception. Types include myofascial, cutaneous, fascial, ligamentous and periosteal trigger points."[4] It should be emphasized that trigger points are physical signs, not symptoms, and patients are generally unaware of them. The zone of reference is defined as "the specific region of the body at a distance from the trigger point, where the phenomena (sensory, motor, autonomic) that it causes are observed."[4]

Trigger points occur on various parts of the body in various muscles. Besides triggering pain, they may also produce peripheral nerve entrapment. For example, trigger points in scalenus muscles can produce scalenus spasm and scalenus syndrome; trigger points in the piriformis muscles produce nerve compression of the sciatic nerve. Once a single muscle has been affected by trigger points, the whole system of synergists and antagonists is affected, and muscle dysfunction then leads to more episodes of spasm and tension, and then to more trigger points. Thus trigger points produced by muscular dysfunction cause pain in the jaw, neck, and shoulder girdle muscles, with radiation to extremities. Oral and facial pain will spread to occipital, cervical, and shoulder girdle muscles, causing trigger points, muscle spasm, and sometimes even scalenus syndrome. Scalenus syndrome includes peripheral nerve entrapment at the brachial plexus, frequently leading to misdiagnosis of cervical disc disease. Trigger points in the sternocleidomastoid muscle may cause vertigo, leading to an incorrect diagnosis of Meniere's disease.[6]

Travell[7] has classified the causes of myofascial trigger points into two categories: 1) precipitating and 2) predisposing factors. The factors that precipitate the condition are: sudden trauma; unusual or excessive exercise; chilling of the body; immobilization; and an acute myocardial infarction or appendicitis, with localized reflex spasm of extremities, as in popliteal thrombosis, rupture of an intervertebral disc with nerve root pressure, and acute emotional stress.

The factors that predispose to the myofascial trigger mechanism are the following: chronic muscular strain, produced by repetitive movement frequently performed over a long period of time; general fatigue; acute infectious illness, e.g., infectious mononucleosis, acute hepatitis, or an acute upper respiratory infection (post-infective myalgias); a chronic focus of infection; nutritional deficiencies; a progressive lesion of the nervous system; nervous tension; syndromes of menopause and the male climacteric, and hypometabolism with creatinuria. It is our feeling that these trigger points play an important role in many of the chronic pain states seen in clinical practice.

Travell and Simons, in their text, *Myofascial Pain and Dysfunction, The Trigger Point Manual*, state that their chapter on "perpetuating factors" is the most important in the book, because it addresses the most neglected part of the management of myofascial pain syndromes. As they state — and I must agree — the length of time that benefits from treatment last is dependent on whatever perpetuating factors remain unresolved. Recognition of these factors will not only simplify the treatment of pain for patients, but will make dental and medical audiences much more receptive to information on trigger points in general when it is delivered at various scientific meetings, seminars, and postgraduate courses. Unfortunately, today's medical and dental school curriculum does not adequately cover this material as part of the undergraduate educational program, and the tendency on the part of practitioners is to ignore or de-emphasize concepts that were not part of their earlier training.

For the purposes of this book, mechanical stress (as a cause of chronic pain) has been divided into structural inadequacies, postural stresses, and constriction of muscles.[4] A discussion of these factors follows herein, as I will attempt to present some of my own views in brief. Many of these factors are discussed in much greater detail by the various other practitioners who have contributed to this book, and one only need turn to the appropriate chapters for a wealth of detailed information.

Some of the major structural inadequacies, which cause postural or physical stress are skeletal asymmetry and disproportion. Asymmetries would include a short leg and a small hemi-pelvis, while skeletal disproportions would involve a long second metatarsal bone (a Dudley J. Morton foot) and short upper arms. Muscular stress can also be caused by misfitting furniture, poor posture, abuse of muscles, constricting pressure on muscles, and prolonged immobility, all of which occur frequently and are almost always correctable.

Leg length discrepancies occur more frequently than most of us believe. For example, a group of elementary school children showed a measurable leg length difference in 75% of the sample studied.[8] This figure increased to 92% for a group of senior high school students, using the same measurement technique. Compensations generally developed as spinal curvatures, which did not reduce the asymmetries.[9] These uncorrected differences tended to grow larger as the children got bigger. Two other studies, on the other hand, have shown that leg length differences corrected during childhood often became smaller.[10,11] In another study of 1000 soldiers with backaches,[12] leg lengths were measured radiographically, using a positioning device, and discrepancies of 0.5 cm (3/16 inch) or more were found to be significantly correlated with symptoms and disability. The authors themselves state that when repeated measurements consistently show a discrepancy of 0.5 cm (3/16 inch) or more in a patient with low back pain, the problem should be corrected. Further, Maigne has reported relief of intractable headaches by equalizing leg length with a heel lift.[13]

It is believed that the short leg imposes a strain on the musculature because the muscles attempt to correct the resulting distortions of axial alignment (functional scoliosis) in order to maintain the head and shoulders balanced over the feet. Of particular clinical interest is the fact that if the leg length difference is about 1 cm (3/8 inch) or less, the shoulder on the side opposite to the shorter leg is lower. This postural relationship is found to be associated with a C-type scoliosis.[14] In this situation, raising the left heel causes the right shoulder to be elevated.

When the leg difference is 1.3 cm (1/2 inch) or more, the shoulder on the same side as the short leg usually sags. In this case, the spine has an S-type scoliosis, and the muscle that suffers most from this axial deviation at the lumbar level is the quadratus lumborum, the most commonly overlooked source of low back pain.[15,16,17]

A tilted shoulder girdle axis requires constant compensation by neck muscles to maintain the head erect and the eyes level. This perpetuates trigger points in the scalene, levator scapulae, sternomastoid and upper trapezius muscles, of which the last two frequently cause headaches. The sternomastoid and upper trapezius muscles may also induce satellite trigger points in the masticatory muscles, in turn contributing to facial pain and headache.

Here are some helpful hints for examining the patient when a leg length problem is suspected. First, the arm on the side of the short leg tends to hang away from the body, while the arm on the other side rests against it. The narrowing of the waist and the bulge of the hip appear greater on the long-leg side. The border of the gluteal fold appears to be lower on the short side.[14,18]

The most prominent bony portion of each ilium posteriorly (posterior superior iliac spines) can be palpated and fairly accurately located with the thumbs, then compared visually for degree of levelness.[8,18,19] Variability in the levels of the iliac spines is often even more clearly revealed by having the patient bend forward 90 degrees at the hips while sighting across the sacrum, looking for any difference in elevation between the two sides.[19,20]

If the patient is asked to swing first one foot and then the other back and forth, the foot of the short leg will move much more easily. Swinging the long leg requires upward displacement of the pelvis on that side for the foot to be able to clear the floor.[13] The position of the scapulae is quite accurately determined by palpating the relative levels of their lower poles. A tilt of the shoulder girdle axis is of special importance in patients with head, neck, shoulder-arm, and upper back pain.[4]

When the patient first arrives in the office for a workup, body asymmetry may initially be observed by noting any difference in the size of the two halves of the face, any tilt or lurch to one side when the patient walks,[11] or by noting if the patient assumes a short-leg stance, standing with body weight on the short leg and the foot of the long leg forward with the knee slightly flexed or with the long leg placed diagonally to the side. In order to confirm the accuracy of the correction, a millimeter or two of lift may be added to see if the pelvis, and perhaps the shoulders, tip the other way due to over-correction. Many patients can immediately feel this unfamiliar strain.[4]

The need for correction can be convincingly impressed upon the patient by removing a correcting heel lift, then exhibiting the resultant body distortion by having them view themselves in a full-length mirror. If the lift is then transferred to the long leg (doubling the discrepancy) most patients will be distressed by the observable increase in the crookedness of the body. The lift should be quickly returned to the short side to relieve any feeling of muscle strain.

Small hemi-pelvis patients tend to sit crookedly and lean toward the small side. A study done years ago reported that 20-30% of patients examined in an orthopedic practice were found to have a small hemi-pelvis, occurring either separately or in conjunction with a short leg, usually on the same side.[21] The examination of the pelvis, back, and shoulders is basically the same as that used for a short leg, with special attention paid to scoliosis, the position of the posterior superior iliac spines,[19] the relative heights of the iliac crests, and tilting of the shoulder girdle axis.

The results of such an examination can be confusing if the pelvis happens to be twisted around the horizontal axis through the sacroiliac joints. Such an obliquity is most easily detected by placing the thumbs on the posterior superior iliac spines and resting the hands over the crests of the ilia, pointing each index finger to an anterior superior iliac spine with the finger tips at equal distances from the spines bilaterally. The patient, who is seated, then rocks the pelvis backward, and the relative heights of the anterior and superior spines are noted on each side of the pelvis. The patient is then told to rock the pelvis forward for comparison. When all the points on one side are lower than those on the other side, regardless of the position of the pelvis, that half of the pelvis is smaller. The obliquity caused by a tilted pelvis (one anterior spine dipping much lower) distorting the evaluation of a small hemi-pelvis, should be corrected as described by Bourdillion[19] and Maigne.[13]

To correct problems associated with a small hemi-pelvis, the following procedure can be used. With the patient seated on a hard surface, increments of lift beneath the ischial tuberosity on the small side are added until the spine is straightened and the pelvis leveled. This correction must then be approximately doubled for a moderately soft chair seat and tripled for a very soft sofa. A permanent correction can be made by having the patient use a "sit-pad" or "butt lift," which is nothing more than a felt pad of proper thickness sewn into the underwear or placed in a long back pants pocket, or even a small magazine tucked under the low ischium when sitting. Chairs that are used regularly may be fitted with either a divided pneumatic seat cushion that allows separate inflation of either half, or one that gives better spinal support, i.e., the TWIN-REST[*] cushion and the BOTTOMS-UP.[**]

---

[*] Fashion Able, Rocky Hill, NJ 08553
[**] Roloke Company, Medical Products Division, Culver City, CA 90230

Another problem is soft auto seats, a common source of poor support, especially for those individuals doing much driving. This can be remedied by using a product such as a WAL-PIL-O LUVS YA BACK SUPPORT which will provide a stable base with a firm support for the back. Patients should also be wary of unwittingly tilting the pelvis by sitting on the wallet in the back pocket. The BOTTOMS UP does more than offer spinal support. It improves function, successfully dealing with the problem. In addition, BOTTOMS UP accessories (wedges) are available to elevate one side in case of a small hemipelvis. The BOTTOMS UP pelvic spinal posture seat and LUVS YA BACK SUPPORT can each be used individually or together. Both products have Multiphase Surface Contour for sensory awareness, anatomical support, and function.

Long second metatarsals, generally accompanied by a short first metatarsal bone, have been labeled as a "Dudley J. Morton" or "classic Greek" foot. This condition is known to perpetuate pain in the low back, thigh, knee, leg, and dorsum of the foot with or without numbness and tingling.[22] "The patients generally complain of weak ankles, frequently turn and sprain these joints, and have difficulty learning to ice skate."

Surprisingly, the prevalence of this condition is higher than generally believed, as shown by a study of 3,619 Canadian enlisted men, unselected for symptoms.[23] It was found that 1,596 (22%) of their feet had first and second metatarsals of equal length; 2,878 (40%) had a first metatarsal shorter than the second by 0.1-1.2 cm; and 2,693 (38%) had a first metatarsal longer than the second by 0.1-1.2 cm.

This syndrome may be greatly aggravated by pressure caused by a tight shoe, one which is too small for all the toes or has a tight cap over the toes. It is also aggravated by high heels. Symptoms usually appear in the shorter leg (which receives heavier impact) even though both feet have the same disproportion of first and second metatarsal bones.[4]

Morton has recommended correcting the disproportion by the insertion into the shoe of a leather sole with a leather buildup of 0.3 cm (1/8 inch) to 0.5 cm (3/16 inch) under the head of only the first metatarsal bone.[24] The correction can be made simply by inserting one or two thicknesses of KIRO-FELT directly under the head of the first metatarsal bone.

What is most interesting about this condition is that trigger points in the lower extremity can interact with tense muscles of the head and neck, restricting the movement of the latter. Releasing tension in the lower extremity muscles (as a result of inactivation of their trigger points, especially those perpetuated by a short-first, long-second metatarsal relationship) may at once increase a trigger point; restricted inter-incisal opening of the jaws by 20 or 30%.[4]

Short upper arms (in relation to torso height) are ararely recognized, but not particularly uncommon, source of muscle strain and perpetuation of trigger points in the shoulder girdle musculature. This disparity places undue stress on the elevators of the shoulder, thereby perpetuating trigger points in the upper trapezius and the levator scapulae muscles. The practitioner must be able to recognize such shortness of the arms in patients with persistent trigger points in these muscles, and then make the seating corrections necessary. The basic problem is simple: the patient's elbows fail to reach the armrest of the usual chair. For most of us, the average armrest height from a compressed seat bottom is 22 cm (8 1/2 inches), and ranges from 18-25 cm (7-10 inches).[25] Needed elbow support can be obtained by adding to armrest height with either cellulose sponges or plastic foam pads glued beneath a writing board.

Postural stresses[4] that should be considered are generally due to misfitting furniture, poor posture, abuse of muscles, and immobility. Misfitting furniture, in which one sits for long periods, may not be designed for comfort or may be well-designed but used for the wrong purpose. In either event this will rapidly tire and strain muscles. Seating should be designed so that correct posture can be maintained by the chair and not by sustained efforts of the muscles.

Travell[26] has listed nine common faults of the chairs most of us use: "no support for your low back; armrests too low or too high; too scooped a backrest in its upper portion; backrest short, failing to support your upper back; jackknifing effect at hips and knees;

high front edge of the seat, shutting down the circulation in your legs; seat bottoms soft in the center, creating a bucket effect which places the load on the outer side of your thighs, rather than on bony points in the buttocks; an excellent chair may be the wrong size for you." As mentioned before, auto seats are among the worst offenders in all regards.

Poor posture frequently results in chronic muscular strain that perpetuates myofascial trigger points. There are many examples of poor posture that contribute to continued trigger point activity: unphysiologic positioning at a desk or work surface; head tilt resulting from poorly adjusted reading glasses; reading and copy material not placed at eye level, causing forward head tilting, placing a load on the posterior neck and upper back muscles; kyphotic, round-shouldered, posture when sitting and standing, placing the load on the more caudal back muscles as well as causing a chronic shortening of the pectoral muscles; a standing posture with the weight on the heels, which tends to shift the head forward as a counterweight, resulting in a loss of the normal cervical and lumbar lordotic curves; writing on the lap; using neck and shoulder muscles to cradle the telephone against the ear; malpositioning of working materials while typing; and certain disabilities that continuously influence posture such as unilateral deafness, unilateral blindness, and an old injury that restricts the normal range of motion.[4]

An important aspect of poor posture is to view it with respect to training, background, and childhood environment. Parental example is of major significance in the establishment of accepted normal posture. Competitive activity and examples from siblings and classmates also leave their mark on the psyche, which in turn molds postural patterns.[27]

Posture, may in fact, be viewed as a somatic depiction of inner emotions. Our posture may be said to be "organ language," a feeling expression, in fact an exteriorization of our inner feelings. The depressed, dejected person will tend to stand in a "drooped" manner with the upper back rounded and the shoulders depressed by the "weight of the world carried on his back." This posture is a picture of fatigue. The "hyperkinetic" person will portray his feelings not only in posture but in the abruptness and irregularity of his movements. This posture is represented as that of an uneasy aggressor, in combat pose, ready to leap or ready to withdraw in a defensive crouch. The tall girl may stand slumped because as a youngster she wished to be as short as her companions. She has literally learned to stoop "down to their height." The short girl may have stood on her toes "to her full height" to be taller. The full-bosomed girl, affected by teasing or fearful of lacking modesty, sat, stood and walked with rounded shoulders to decrease the apparent size of her bosom.[27]

All patterns of posture developed in childhood, whether for real or imagined reasons, become deep seated. An abnormal pattern can gradually mold tissues into somatic patterns that then remain as a structural monument to earlier psychic molding.[27]

Muscles are abused by poor body mechanics that produce needlessly stressful movements through sustained isometric contraction or muscular immobility, caused by too many repetitions of the same movement, or by excessively quick and jerky movements. Examples of such move ments might be leaning over while twisting to the side to lift an item from a shelf; leaning over the sink to brush your teeth; stooping forward to get in and out of a chair; and standing on one leg to put on a skirt or trousers rather than sitting.

Problematical sources of sustained contraction include such activities as painting a ceiling, hanging drapes or a picture, holding a chainsaw or other power tool in a fixed position, holding a rope tight on a sailboat, or merely standing still in one place or position, such as stiffly at military attention or while tensely impatient in a checkout line. Wearing high-heeled shoes or cowboy boots causes a sustained shortened position of the calf muscles.[4]

Immobility or lack of movement tends to aggravate and perpetuate myofascial trigger points, especially if the muscle is in a shortened position to begin with. This is generally observed when people sleep in a particular position that positions a muscle in its shortest length; when a muscle can not be moved through its full range of motion due to a fracture, deformity, or articular disease; when individuals are so intent on an activity such as writing or reading that they forget to change body position; when patients develop habits of guarding against certain movements due to pain; or because they have been advised against movement of a part of the body.[4]

Attention must also be paid to what occurs at night during sleep. The patient must avoid shortening the pectoralis major muscle by folding the arms across the chest. The corner of the pillow should be tucked between the head and shoulder, (not tucked under the shoulder) in order to drop the shoulder backward. Sleeping position and choice of pillows are important. Two pillows have received wide recognition over the years, the CERVIP-ILLO, designed by Ruth Jackson, M.D.,[28] and the WAL-PIL-O design by Lionel Walpin, M.D.[29] The former is a homogenous tubular-shaped pillow, while the latter is rectangular, offering four combinations of head and neck support. Head and neck support and upper extremity position are important during sleep, and this subject is covered in more detail later. There are also special pillows designed to maintain the head in normal alignment with the rest of the body while retaining a moderate cervical lordosis at the same time.

Constricting pressure on a muscle can also perpetuate trigger points. This type of problem is commonly caused by the pressure from the strap of a heavy purse hung over the shoulder, or by narrow bra straps that support heavy bosoms and groove the upper trapezius.

Dental malocclusions, bruxing, clenching, and emotional tension can interact to overload the masticatory and neck muscles, perpetuating trigger points in those areas. These factors are the underlying cause of much of the head and face pain seen with the myofascial pain dysfunction syndrome, which is covered extensively in this book.

One must be acutely aware that the mechanical factors mentioned here are extremely significant, but not the only answer to the vexing problems we face daily with our patients.

The role of nutritional inadequacies in the treatment of patients with myofascial pain disorders is also of paramount importance.[4] The role of several water-soluble vitamins such as B1, B6, B12, folic acid, vitamin C, and various elements such as calcium, magnesium, iron and potassium should not be overlooked by the practitioner. The B-complex vitamins mentioned above play an important role in normal body metabolism as a coenzyme to an apoenzyme (the latter requiring the coenzyme to perform its metabolic function), but are not necessarily synthesized by the body. The need for these as well as other vitamins may appear on three different levels: vitamin insufficiency, vitamin deficiency and vitamin dependency.

Vitamin insufficiency may be the result of inadequate ingestion of the vitamin, improper absorption, inadequate utilization, increased metabolic requirement, increased excretion, or increased destruction within the body.[30,31] The customary laboratory screening tests will identify the offending perpetuating factors: serum vitamin levels, a blood chemistry profile, a complete blood count with indices, the erythrocyte sedimentation rate, thyroid hormone levels (T3 and T4 by radioimmunoassay), and a urinalysis.

In our experience, another factor, hypoglycemia, has to be kept in mind when treating chronic-pain patients. Recurrent attacks of hypoglycemia tend to perpetuate myofascial trigger points. Two types of hypoglycemia are noted, fasting and postprandial, which occur for different reasons but present similar symptoms.[4]

Noteworthy is the increased activity of myofascial trigger points during systemic viral illnesses (especially herpes simplex) at any chronic focus of bacterial infection, and in the presence of infestation, by specific groups of parasites. Although the exact mechanism by which these diseases cause their effects is not clear, every effort must be made to control them if the patient is to get well.

Of utmost importance is the attitude of the physician or other health professionals: we should not assume that psychological factors are primary. It is exceedingly easy for us as physicians to blame a patient's psyche for our own inability to recognize all of the musculoskeletal and neurophysiological factors that may contribute to a patient's chronic pain. This wrong assumption (above) is frustrating, even devastating, for most patients, leading to depression and other negative psychological states.

Chronic Pain States

There are many reasons why chronic pain patients receive less than optimum attention and care. Whereas medical and dental students, physicians, and other health professionals learn how to manage acute pain, few schools teach the basics necessary to make a correct diagnosis and prescribe the proper treatment for a chronic pain patient.

How the clinician thinks of pain is too often dependent upon his or her training and specialty area. The neurologist views pain as a neurophysiologic abnormality, and the neurosurgeon approaches the problem surgically or with electrical implantation. The psychiatrist approaches chronic pain as an emotional response to an internal emotional conflict. The behavioral scientist carries this thinking further, viewing the "pain" as a psychosocial maladjustment with resultant manipulative response. The pharmacologist considers pain states to be biochemical aberrations amenable to treatment with medication. The orthopedist evaluates pain in the back or neck as a condition which will respond to bracing or surgical intervention. The physiatrist usually evaluates the problem with electrodiagnostic means, and treats with modalities involving heat, cold, and exercise—all of which can be greatly expanded, as will be seen in the chapters that follow. The dentist and other health professionals such as physical therapists, osteopaths, and chiropractors have their own approaches as well, based upon their training and experience. Ideally, all groups should interrelate with one another, but the fact is that chronic pain may persist in some cases to such an extent that it refutes all our theories.[27]

A recently conducted survey of nearly 500 patients with chronic back pain offers us some thought-provoking findings.[32] Long-term relief was obtained from the care provided by orthopedists and neurosurgeons in only 23% and 26% of the cases studied, respectively. Those results compare with the success rate for chiropractors of 28%. Neurologists, by contrast, proved to be least effective in providing dramatic long-term relief — "solving" only 2% of their cases. Finally, note that physiatrists proved to be the most effective practitioners in these cases, providing long term relief in 86% of their cases.

Chronic pain is probably the most serious disabling disease of humans. Pain can no longer be considered a mere symptom, but as something which can be a disease in and of itself. Knowledgeable practitioners realize that intractable pain can lead to narcotic addiction, expansive disability, disruption of family relationships, and ill-advised surgery of questionable value.

Brena[33] believes chronic pain to be a recognizable disease state involving many factors that interact with one another. He has enumerated five consequences seen in chronic pain which pain ex perts have labled the "Five D's" syndrome:

1. Drug: abuse or misuse.
2. Dysfunction: a decrease in function, performance, or even the quality of life.
3. Disuse: loss of flexibility, strength, endurance and alternate degeneration.
4. Depression: with significant loss, real or imaginary, reactive depression may result.
5. Disability: inability to perform daily living activities or pursue gainful employment.

Numerous concepts of pain relate to neurophysiologic, physiologic, behavorial, or psychiatric factors, but all may eventually need to relate to noxious irritation of soft tissues throughout the body, including those within the vertebral column.

Bonica[34] has classified chronic pain into three groups:

1. Persistent peripheral noxious stimulants including long-term medical conditions such as arthritis, herniated disc, and cancer;
2. Neuraxis pain involving the nervous system, the peripheral nerves, the cord or the brain;
3. Learned pain behavior as a result of rewards received for being sick or impaired.

Current pain concepts imply that there are neuronal pools at various levels of the CNS that act as a pain pattern-generating mechanism. These pools are influenced by peripheral impulses and also by central stimuli descending from a higher center. They comprise a pattern-generating center which contains the dorsal horns and all its internuncial connections. The influences upon the pool can be somatic, visceral, or autonomic. Either loss of input or excess input can result in overreaction of the pool. Loss of input can occur as a result of nerve damage with afferentation, whereas excess input can be produced by distant tissue irritation.[27]

If this concept were valid, it would explain the credibility of a number of therapeutic approaches such as local anesthetic nerve blocks, TENS, sympathetic nerve blocks, active exercise, and various antidepressant or tranquilizing drugs. Any one or all of these therapies could have a beneficial affect on the pool.

Apparently pain is not influenced primarily by the intensity of afferent nociceptive input, but is influenced markedly by higher central processes.[27]

REFERENCES

1. Cailliet R. *Soft Tissue Pain and Disability.* Philadelphia, Pa: F. A. Davis Company; 1986 10th Printing.
2. Feldenkrais M. *Body and Nature Behavior,* ed 3. New York, NY: International Universities Press, Inc; 1975.
3. Travell JG, Rinzler SH. Scientific exhibit: Myofascial genesis of pain. *Postgrad Med.* 1952;11:425.
4. Travell JG, Simons DG. Myofascial Pain and Dysfunction - The Trigger Point Manual. Baltimore, Md: Williams and Wilkens; 1983:103-164.
5. Bonica JJ. The Management of Pain with Special Emphasis on the Use of Analgesic Block in Diagnosis and Therapy. Philadelphia, Pa: Lea and Febiger; 1959.
6. Kraus H. Muscular Aspects of Oral Dysfunction, pp. 115-122. In: Gelb H. ed. *Clinical Management of Head, Neck and TMJ Pain and Dysfunction* 2nd ed. St. Louis, Mo: Ishiyaku EuroAmerica; 1991.
7. Travell J. Referred pain from skeletal muscle, the pectoralis major syndrome of breast pain and soreness and the sternomastoid syndrome of headaches and dizziness. *N Y J Med.* 1955;55:331.
8. Klein KK. A study of the progression of lateral pelvic asymmetry in 585 elementary, junior and senior high school boys. *Am Correct Therap J.* 1969;23:171-173.
9. Pearson WM. Early and high incidence of mechanical faults. *J Osteopathy.* 1954;61:18-23.
10. Klein KK, Redler I, Lowman CL. Asymmetries of growth in the pelvis and legs of children: a clinical and statistical study. 1964-1967. *JAOA.* 1968;68:153-156.
11. Redler I. Clinical significance of minor inequalities in leg length. *New Orleans Med Surg J.* 1952;104:308-312.
12. Rush WA, Steiner HA. A study of lower extremity length inequality. *Am J Roentgen Rod Ther.* 1946;56:616-623.
13. Maigne R. *Orthopedic Medicine, A New Approach to Vertebral Manipulation.* WT Liberson, trans. Springfield, Ill: Charles C. Thomas; 1972:192,292-390.
14. Judovich B, Bates W. *Pain Syndrome,* ed. 3. Philadelphia, Pa: FA Davis Company; 1949:46-51.
15. Hudson OC, Hettesheimer CA, Robin PA. Causalgic backache. *Am J Surg.* 1941;52:297-303.
16. Sola AE, Williams RL. Myofascial pain syndromes. *Neurology.* 1956;6:91-95.
17. Travell JG. The quadratus Lumborum muscle: an overlooked cause of low back pain. *Arch Phys Med Rehabil.* 1976;57:566.
18. Sicuranza BJ, Richards J, Tisdall LH. The short leg syndrome in obstetrics and gynecology. *Am J Obstet Gynecol.* 1970;107:217-219.
19. Bourdillion JF. *Spinal Manipulation,* ed. 2. New York, NY: Appleton-Century-Crofts; 1973:39-43.
20. Beal MC. A review of the short leg problem. *JAOA.* 1950;50:109-121.
21. Lowman CL. The sitting position in relation to pelvic stress. *Physiother Rev.* 1941;21:30-33.
22. Travell J. Low back pain and the Dudley J. Morton foot (long second toe). *Arch Phys Med Rehabil.* 1975;56:566.
23. Harris RI, Beath T. The short first metatorsal, its incidence and clinical significance. *J Bone Joint Surgery.* 1949;31-A:553-565.
24. Morton EJ. *The Human Foot.* New York, NY: Columbia University Press; 1935:156-157.
25. Diffrient N, Tilley AR, Bardagjy JC. *Humanscale.* Cambridge, Ma: M.I.T. Press; 1975:19-22.
26. Travell J. *Office Hours: Day and Night.* New York, NY: The World Publishing Company; 1968:270,284,285,301,302.
27. Calliet R. *Low Back Pain.* ed. 3. Philadelphia, Pa: FA Davis Company; 1981:24.
28. Jackson R. *The Cervical Syndrome.* ed. 4. Springfield, Ill: Charles C. Thomas; 1977:310-311.
29. Walpin LA. Bedroom posture: the critical role of a unique pillow in relieving upper spine and shoulder girdle pain. *Arch Phys Med Rehabil.* 1977;58:507.

30. Herbert V. The nutritional anemias. *Hosp Pract.* 1980;15:65-89.
31. Herbert V, Colman N, Jacob E. Folic acid and vitamin B12. In: Goodhart RS, Shils ME, eds. *Modern Nutrition in Health and Disease.* ed. 6. Philadelphia, Pa: Lea and Febiger; 1980:229-225.
32. Sobel D. Oh, your aching back. *New York Magazine.* 1986;19:42-49.
33. Brena SF. *Chronic Pain: America's Hidden Epidemic.* New York, NY: Atheneum/SMI; 1978.
34. Bonica JJ. *The Management of Pain.* Philadelphia, PA: Lea and Febiger; 1953.

Chapter 2

Posture: The Process of Body Use; Principles and Determinants

Lionel A. Walpin, MD

INTRODUCTION—AN OVERVIEW

In customary usage, the word "posture" has taken several meanings: body position, how one holds the body, stance, and pose, to name a few. These definitions, however, do not help people enhance their health, and may cause frustration in attempts to practice or improve posture. In fact, these definitions encourage attempts to be straight and stiff, which is self-defeating. Posture is not a simple matter: it is most easily understood—and taught to patients—as a functional, dynamic process which they can see, monitor and correct.

While there are many determinants of posture, alignment is probably the most important one. The goal is a stable alignment in neutral range at rest and during obvious movement of the head, neck, torso or limbs. Ease of body movement within and from neutral to nonneutral alignment is the ultimate clinical test of posture, of body use. Ease of movement must be evaluated during both dynamic and static activities. Static activities equal relative rest, and breathing, swallowing and physiologic postural sway are examples. A selectively stable alignment, in neutral range, allows movement to proceed instantly without having to shift body weight or unlock joints. The body will sacrifice mobility for stability. If (focal or regional) selective stability is not achieved, the body will lock itself up. While this provides general stability, it is nonphysiologic and movement throughout the body is lost. Movement is the benchmark of good posture, i.e., body use. Considered in this way, the understanding of what posture is, its clinical evaluation and its modification and improvement (treatment) become much easier both for the patient and the health professional.

Given its complexity, posture has been difficult even for health professionals to describe or define. Most incorrectly equate posture and alignment while they also confuse it with position. The word posture is often used incorrectly or vaguely. Again, posture is not simply a matter of alignment, but must be considered as a *process*, the process of body (somatic) use. This is a departure from traditional thinking. But it will become evident that evaluation and improvement of posture are much easier and more enjoyable, for practitioner and patient alike, if considered functionally and dynamically in terms of *movement*, not just statically in terms of alignment.

Everyone seems to agree that posture is important for overall well-being. Health professionals rarely fail to point to bad posture as an important factor in somatic disorders and somatic pain, including temporary dysfunctions such as muscle spasm, joint malalignment, and the chronic structural changes of degenerative arthritis and soft tissue contractures. Further, medical authors often advise their readers to correct a patient's posture, but rarely describe how to do so. This is unfortunate. On their own, patients end up trying to be straight and erect, only making matters worse, for they are either tall, rigid and locked up or slumped and locked when they tire of trying to be straight and erect.

Considering posture as a process based on specific principles and determinants (see Appendices 1 and 2 to this chapter) allows us to prevent, diagnose and treat dysfunctions of the somatic system in an organized and focused fashion. Using this system, patients' practical understanding of posture, and their cooperation in education and treatment, are better because the principles and determinants can be demonstrated and explained functionally. Specific activities become easier because movement is freer, more efficient, less fatiguing and less painful.

Defining posture as a process allows us to analyze the positive or negative contribution of each postural determinant in an individual patient, leading to a rational, organized, step-by-step treatment program. Sometimes treatment is simple, requiring only minor correction of one or a few determinants. With normal tissues and nonneutral alignment, loss of mobility due to being either too erect or slumped and with (or without) alignment-related pain, proper instruction alone can result in rapid improvement of alignment, body attitude and body movement and loss of pain. Development of kinesthetic awareness, organization and sequence of movement, and balanced functional strength for coordinated acceleration and deceleration of movement are all helpful over the long range.

If, however, the patient doesn't present with normal tissues, instead showing dysfunction or derangement with joint hypermobility, hypomobility, soft tissue contracture, muscle spasm, muscle weakness, muscle tension and trigger points (these are typically associated with pain, especially during dynamic movement), it is not enough to give instruction either orally or with hands-on physical cueing. In such cases with hypomobility, in addition to manual soft tissue and joint mobilization treatment techniques, specific exercises are necessary to improve tissue structure and function. With hypermobility, stabilization exercise techniques are often helpful and sclerotherapy/prolotherapy injections[18] may be indicated. Functional body supports may also be important. All of these essential topics will be covered in the following discussion, which begins with further clarification of terminology.

TERMS RELATED TO POSTURE AND THE CONCEPTS THEY IMPLY

Posture is the process of body (somatic) use: using the somatic system as a functional and structural unit. It should not be confused with alignment, body attitude or position. Structurally, the somatic system is the body's framework of skin, skeletal, arthrodial and myofascial structures and their related vascular, lymphatic and neural elements, including the autonomic nervous system.[1] Posture, the process of body use, depends on a comprehensive integration and interrelation of all factors which influence the somatic system: anatomical (structural); physiological (functional); biomechanical (both intrinsic and extrinsic, i.e., environmental); and, of course, psychological.

Because it can be seen and felt, movement is the best clinical benchmark for evaluating posture. This refers to all movements, e.g., postural sway, breathing and dynamic movements through space. Further, posture is not only "good" or "bad"; there is a clinical spectrum along which it improves or worsens (Table 2-1). Usually, as alignment improves, movement becomes qualitatively and quantitatively easier, smoother and with increased range, and thus posture (body use) is better. Good alignment, however, does not necessarily mean that the other determinants of posture, flexibility, for example, also have good quality. A person may have a tall, upright appearance but be inflexible because myofascial, ligamentous and capsular soft tissues are too tight or too stiff. That person has poor body use and thus "bad" posture.

Clinically, movement has a wide range:

a. From small amplitude involuntary postural sway movements (relatively static).
b. To involuntary and voluntary breathing.
c. Shifting to maintain body balance because of the differing contours, sizes and weights of individual body parts and regions.[47]
d. All the way to movement during full dynamic activities such as walking. (Dynamics depend largely on functional strength, power, coordination, speed and stability.)

Table 2-1. Classification of "Good" and "Bad" posture in relation to alignment and flexibility.

Type	Example	Alignment	Flexibility	Remarks
1. Good	Sitting Types I and II	Neutral	Yes	Move in and out of neutral with controlled rhythmic abdominal pelvic-hip movements.
2. Good	Bending Throwing	Neutral and Nonneutral	Yes No	A nonneutral region provides stability for a neutral region in a specific function.
3. Good	Acute pain with knee flexion Lateral shift of spine	Protected in Nonneutral	No, at the protected segment or joint	An adaptive compensatory posture, for up to 2 weeks. Beyond that, contracture can occur and motion is jeopardized.
4. Good	Standing Bending from hips	Protected in Neutral	No, at the protected segment	Dynamic Stabilization in neutral range. Capability of motion of the stabilized joint is preserved.
5. Good	Sitting with sling support	Neutral and Nonneutral	Yes, at upper spine No, at pelvis and hips	Sling support around knees and around pelvis to allow patient to participate in certain painful activities, for short duration. This is a planned, adaptive, nonphysiologic compensation. (Not healthy for routine use)
6. Bad	Chronic pain with knee flexion	Protected in Nonneutral	No	The malalignment produces its own problems including contractures. A nonadaptive compensatory posture.
7. Bad	Habitual slumped sitting	Nonneutral	No	No purpose, just a bad habit.
8. Bad	Sitting with sling support	Neutral and Nonneutral	Yes, at upper spine No, at pelvis and hips	Sling compresses hips and limits hip and spine motion. When used for ordinary or non-special sitting activities, it is planned nonadaptive nonphysiologic compensation. The lack of pelvic motion and compressed hips causes other problems at hips, pelvis and lumbar spine.

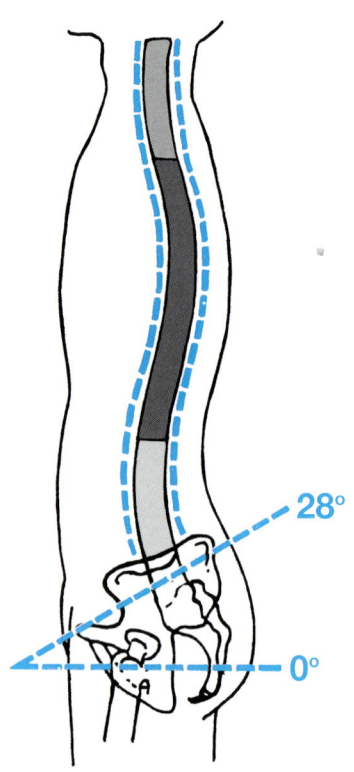

Fig. 2-1. Neutral balanced alignment (NBA), flexible and stable in three planes: sagittal, frontal and transverse. Dashed lines represent physiologic barriers, the limit of active motion and postural sway.

"On balance" alignment vertically allows NBA. Sacral angle ranges from approximately 20°-34° in both sitting and standing positions.

The clinical hallmark of good posture is the capability of instantaneous active physiologic movements (ideally painless) into any of the three cardinal planes, as well as vertically. Movement starts from "neutral balanced" and "on balance" alignments and takes place within neutral and into and then out of nonneutral ranges. (Figs. 2-1 and 2-2) All active involuntary and voluntary movements are included. There should be no need to first unlock joints or to shift body weight in one direction or another in order to move.

Movement "focuses" around and starts from neutral alignment, just as one moves the gears in an automobile transmission from neutral to park in one direction and from neutral to drive in the opposite direction. One may draw analogies between park and hyperflexion (nonneutral) and between drive and hyperextension (nonneutral). In nonneutral body alignment (park and drive), freedom of movement is restricted. In the body, neutral occupies a range between the physiologic barriers (dynamic stabilization, one of the five types of clinical alignment, takes place anywhere in the neutral range and the location can vary from activity to activity and from position to position), while in a transmission it is a single "place."

One factor in the miscommunication of ideas between patients, therapists and doctors, as well as frustration between parents

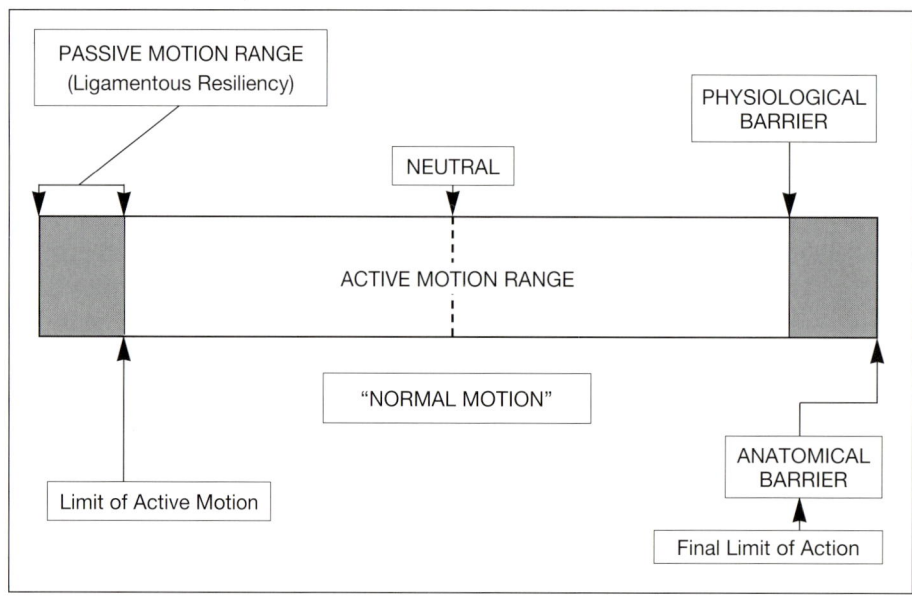

Fig. 2-2. "Normal Active Motion" limited by physiologic barriers. (Reprinted with permission of JAOA.)

and children, is the frequent misuse of "posture" interchangeably with the words alignment, position, and attitude. *Alignment* refers to the angular or geometric relationships in any or all of the three planes and vertically between two or more contiguous or noncontiguous body parts or regions. Alignment is dependent, in part, on soft tissue length and the forces acting on the joints. We will discuss five types of clinical alignment later.

Position refers to the spatial relationship of the body to the environment, e.g., sitting, lying prone or supine and standing. The differences in meaning between posture, alignment (postural alignment) and position are more important clinically than semantically. For example, in a recent lecture about atypical facial pain, the speaker stated that the pain worsens with changes in "head position" while his projected slide used the term "head posture." The speaker probably meant "alignment." It is important to know if he was really referring to the angular relationships (alignment) between the craniovertebral joints rather than to a change in the head and neck, as a unit, in space (position).

Body attitude refers to the configuration, contour, shape, and ultimately, the appearance of the body. Attitude during relatively static activity such as quiet sitting and quiet standing (there is always some movement) is called *pose*, while body attitude during an obvious dynamic activity is called *form*. Posture is often evaluated, especially by lay people, on the basis of appearance. This is an incorrect approach, but the conclusion reached, "bad posture," is often correct since slumped and slouched body contours happen to be associated with continual and widespread nonneutral alignments which interfere with movement. Unfortunately, these conclusions, coincidentally correct as they are, do not facilitate correct posture in a systematic way, since they are based on superficial observations of body attitude and not on an understanding of functional dynamics. Conclusions about good "posture" are far less likely to be coincidentally correct.

A common source of confusion and a detriment to treatment is telling someone to "stand up straight" to correct their posture. This causes confusion because there is no anatomic or kinesthetic basis for the word. We are familiar with the ordinary meaning of straight as in "straight line," thus referring to an absence of curvature. But there are no straight bones; the body is arranged as a series of curves and triangles:[10] joint surfaces are curved (specific kinesthetics result from arthrokinematics and orthokinematics of joints and bones); the collagen fibers in ligaments and joint capsules have an internal weave; fascia forms a 3-dimensional web throughout the body; the thickness of fascia varies; attachments to muscles are uneven and muscles often run at angles from origins to insertions. Thus, the brain receives few, if any, signals from truly straight structures.

Further, the spine is a series of natural curves in neutral alignment in the sagittal plane. If the spine straightens, it is in nonneutral alignment. "Normal" lordosis is a neutral alignment. Thus, except for an anatomically straight midline in the frontal plane (right/left symmetry), there is no anatomic, kinesthetic or physiologic justification for the word "straight" being applied to posture. When someone tries to be straight, it causes unnecessary muscle work, stiffness, physical strain and unhealthy holding patterns. There is discomfort because of compression on one side of a joint(s) with ligamentous tension on the other side and restricted movement.

Nevertheless, the term "straight" can be helpful when used to refer to *on balance* alignment wherein the *regional* upper weight centers (the head and rib cage) are aligned and balanced vertically (straight) over the natural bases of support, i.e., over the pelvis when sitting, and over the pelvis and feet when standing. Associated with this (vertical) on balance alignment is *neutral balanced* alignment of each spinal segment. Both of these alignments may refer to regions, individual spinal segments and to peripheral joints. Movements are preserved regionally and segmentally. These alignments will be discussed in detail shortly.

On balance alignment makes movement easy; this is very different from the typical inflexibility that occurs when someone is asked to stand or sit "straight." Clinicians typically have not evaluated posture in terms of it being a process of body use, nor monitored it by evaluating movement. Again, in the author's view, "straight" is acceptable only when it refers to either the midline in the frontal plane or to "on balance" alignment of regions, not segments. "On balance" alignment and the associated neutral balanced alignment are evaluated by the availability of active and passive movement.

Regarding extrinsic factors, products such as so-called "ergonomic" chairs are frequently disappointing. This may be due to the chair's design, but often the disappointment is also due to the user expecting to be placed or held in a "proper" position or posture (actually, postural alignment). Most importantly, the user lacks knowledge of correct body use, including not knowing how to use the pelvis as body center. These chairs, as well as lumbar supports, foot orthotics, and cervical pillows and many other devices have traditionally been incorrectly advertised as being good for posture as long as they offer some physical support or alter alignment or position. But sometimes these devices actually make alignment worse and interfere with body use. We should look at these devices more closely with regard to body use and how the body works. Further, health professionals should be actively involved in carefully selecting supportive devices and in training patients to properly use them, functionally.

To return to our discussion of terminology, *comfort* and *relaxation* are other buzz words whose presumed universal benefits have been taken for granted, incorrectly. Both factors are important, but neither is automatically nor continuously beneficial. First, comfort must refer to relative rest *and* during movement. Similarly, relaxation must include at least intermittent attention to body use to avoid disuse, misuse and abuse.

To relax, one should not habitually collapse. An individual also may remain comfortable at rest (at least for a reasonable time) by slumping progressively away from a painful somatic dysfunction. But, if one remains so slumped for too long or if the slumping away from pain is progressive, it is detrimental. One may also slump, detrimentally, away from a spinal segment(s) that has only less flexibility than others, or away from a spinal segment(s) that has a truly restrictive motion barrier.[8] In either case, the body takes the path of least physical resistance.

In the presence of a motion barrier, the body moves at the next available joint in the kinetic chain. In the presence of a joint(s) with relative inflexibility (without a true restrictive motion barrier) the body compensates and maintains an overall balance of forces by changing its alignment at a more flexible joint(s). These areas of compensation are then in nonneutral alignment and the forces around them are out of balance. Thus, if a patient with diminished hip extension either due to inflexibility or a true motion barrier stands, he would compensate by extending at the more flexible lumbar spine. The lumbar spine would probably be aligned in hyperextension (nonneutral) and, over time, would suffer microtrauma. (Clinical testing for areas of relative inflexibility and flexibility and motion barriers was described years ago by Kraus and Weber.[3]) Movement from the nonneutral alignments into other planes will be restricted, uncomfortable and even painful.

The priority often placed on using products that are comfortable at rest, without regard to restoring on balance and neutral balanced alignments and comfort during movement, is in itself a source of somatic dysfunction and mechanical pain. It would be far better to eliminate the dysfunction and restore neutral alignment and movement. One must manage comfort judiciously. It is well known, for example, that a supine person with a knee joint effusion is more comfortable holding the knee flexed. Unfortunately, this causes further flexion contracture which in turn causes damage to the knee during ambulation.

POSTURE IN THE CONTEXT OF FUNCTION

Posture requires integration of the entire body: the extent depends on the activity carried out (Table 2-2), the position and the determinants that are involved. For example, we classify sitting according to four types (Tables 2-3 and 2-4). Movement is required in the transition from one type to another, and Types I and II should not be sedentary. Correct movement, initiated at the pelvis, requires hip joint mobility and fine tuning of pelvic rotation and lateral movement by functionally strong abdominal (lower, transverse and oblique), pelvic and low back muscles. Even total relaxation involves body movement, i.e., breathing and swallowing. These functions must be performed correctly.

Despite all the exercise programs available to the public and despite all the professional therapy programs, relatively few people have been properly instructed or trained in posture. There are three major reasons for this: 1) the emphasis on "straight" alignment rather than movement (The difference between the vertical line of reference by plumb line and the gravity plumb line should be reviewed.[4,38]); 2) the importance of the pelvis in controlling alignment and initiating movement has been both unappreciated and neglected (Table 2-5); and 3) the important functional roles of the craniovertebral joints and the feet as *adaptive mechanisms* have not been appreciated.

The craniovertebral joints (occiput-C1-C2-C3) and subtalar joints of the feet are "universal" joints. It is important for these to have freedom of motion. The feet are natural mobile adaptors and the craniovertebral joints are the final adaptors for head alignment and balance. If the craniovertebral joints are not free, the important sensory organs of the head and neck cannot provide, as accurately, the important information needed for interaction with the environment. Also, if those joints are not free, the spine locks down from above and movement is compromised throughout the spine and pelvis. Patients' low back pains often increase when sitting in a car if their craniovertebral joints are compressed because their heads are too close to the roof. In the animal world, a deer's head and neck, when lowered to eat or drink, must remain mobile in order to hear, smell and see danger, e.g., a lion. This requirement for free movement of the head and neck for normal function and freedom of body movement is no different for humans.

We should release the upper body and rely on the pelvis to initiate the movement that is needed for correct upper body function in sitting and for lower extremity function in walking and running. The hip joints are the hinges for clinical (postural) movement of the pelvis in sitting, standing, and walking.

Structure and proper use of the pelvis is critical for good body use. Often there is failure to free the upper body (head, neck, shoulders and upper back) because of lack of awareness and lack of training in body centering at the pelvis to provide stability, mobility and alignment of the upper body. For example, it is not possible to correct forward head alignment without first rotating the pelvis forward into neutral pelvic alignment. This provides the correct natural base of support for on balance and neutral balanced alignments of the head and neck, allowing the craniovertebral joints and suboccipital muscles to be free, i.e., not compressed and tight.

Some *regional examples of posture* are dental occlusion[31] and sitting. The former depends on the interrelationships of all the components of the stomatognathic or masticatory system.[31] One such relationship is head and neck alignment which, in turn, depends on factors beyond the head and neck.

Pelvic alignment is critical in Types I and II sitting and very important in Type III sitting. (The author classifies sitting as Types I, II, III and IV.) Especially in Types I and II, the alignment can be dynamically controlled by muscles, while it is also responsive to the effects of gravity and the surface reactions from the seat surface. Pelvic alignment can be aided greatly, actively and passively, by a special multicontoured seat surface to be described in the section on sitting.

Sitting is usually, and incorrectly, thought of as a homogeneous and sedentary activity. However, just as running includes jogging and sprinting, there are several types of sitting functions. Sitting is often combined with such activities as reaching forward and sideways. During those movements, the pelvis must provide stability for the torso, head and neck while retaining its own stability and mobility. Suffice it to state, for now, that functional strength of the abdominal muscles, especially the lower abdominal, is necessary for fine tuning the distance and speed of forward and backward pelvic rotation. Free movement of the hip joints is necessary for pelvic rotation, then the spine follows the pelvis. The spine cannot move physiologically unless the pelvis can move and the pelvis cannot move unless the hip joints can move.

Table 2-2. Important clinical examples for correct body use and for correcting poor body use.

A. Head and Neck

1. Forward head/neck alignment (FHA), commonly referred to as forward head posture (FHP) is based on nonneutral alignments in the sagittal plane. Movement into other planes is interfered with. To correct FHA the pelvis must first be aligned in neutral range, under the upper weight centers.

2. Swallowing requires that the mid-tongue move up into the concave Donder's space on the roof of the mouth (mid-hard-palate). This allows the tongue to stabilize the head and neck in neutral alignment during swallowing.

3. Rising/sitting must be initiated at the pelvis with the functional use and support of abdominal muscles. The pelvis rotates forward. Quadriceps, hip extensors and gastrocnemius muscles are important. The body moves upward and forward on rising (not down and forward). The craniovertebral joints (OCC-C1-C2-C3) must not hyperextend when rising or moving downward to sit.

4. Ordinary breathing should be diaphragmatic. Use of accessory (neck) muscles should be avoided.

5. Gait should be heel/toe. The heel provides a fulcrum for movements of the pelvis and lumbar regions. The floor reactions from the heel provides support for those areas. Stability is from the bottom up. In contrast, a toe/heel gait causes pelvic and spinal instability. The result is cervical and lumbar hyperextension (hyperlordotic-nonneutral alignments). Stability of those areas is accomplished incorrectly, i.e., from the top downward.

B. Chest

1. Diaphragmatic breathing done properly should expand the lower chest anteriorly, laterally and posteriorly.

2. Anterior and posterior pelvic rotations must be initiated at the pelvis, not at the upper chest.

C. Lumbar

1. To help prevent hyperlordosis, shortened lumbar muscles, compressed facet joints and stretched anterior soft tissues, the abdominal muscles should be functionally strong and the lower chest should expand with diaphragmatic breathing.

2. While sitting, lengthen along two "opposing" lines in the sagittal plane to attain neutral spinal curves and release and balance of the soft tissues along the spine. The two lines extend from sacrum to suprasternal notch and from pubis to and through the thoracolumbar junction. The two lines cross at the thoracolumbar junction.[10]

D. Bending Forward

1. Flex the head, then neck flexion followed by thoracic, lumbar and hip flexion, sequentially.

2. The "opposite" technique, initiated at the hips, allows dynamic lumbar stabilization in neutral rather than allowing lumbar flexion. However, it also produces head/neck (craniovertebral) extension.

E. Reaching Forward

1. Neutral pelvic alignment is critical. Without it, shoulder flexion is greatly restricted when the pelvis rotates posteriorly, causing spinal slump.

Table 2-2. continued

F. Reaching Sideways

1. When sitting, shift laterally at the hips to maintain the upper body centers of gravity over the pelvis, on balance. The pelvis provides stability for the upper body, which remains mobile and is free to reach. If the pelvis tilts to one side instead of shifting laterally at the hips, with body weight resting on one buttock, the upper body loses its mobility, for it must participate in the stabilization process.
2. Reaching sideways can also be accomplished by bending sideways (right), but the left leg and foot must then be placed farther to the left to maintain body weight centered over the pelvis.
3. The scapular stabilizing muscles should be active during reaching movements.

G. Pelvis and Hips

1. The pelvis is the body's center. Body movement is initiated at the pelvis.
2. To be able to move the spine and pelvis normally, the hips must move normally.
3. If the hips are not aligned in neutral, the pelvis and spine cannot be in comfortable neutral alignment.

H. Sitting

1. Lumbar lordosis (neutral) should be present in all four types of sitting (I-IV).
2. Sitting slumped (hyperflexed) or hyperlordotic (hyperextended) reduces lateral hip mobility.
3. Motion should be maintained with rhythmic abdominal pelvic-hip exercise movements. These must be done properly. For example, with anterior and posterior pelvic rotations, the torso and head move predominantly upward and downward (vertically), respectively. Forward and backward movements are relatively slight.
4. For pelvic-spinal-hip complex (PSH-C) balance, lumbar lordosis and the pelvis should be neutral and the knees should rest below the level of the hips. If the knees are level with or above the hips while the pelvis and spine are in neutral, the result will be anterior hip compression, loss of hip mobility and low back tension. The end result is posterior pelvic rotation and spinal slump to reopen the hips and relieve the tension.

I. Standing

1. Weight should be distributed on the feet in such a manner so that rising up on the toes can be instantaneous without first having to shift (i.e., unlock) the weight forward from the heels toward the toes.
2. Standing incorrectly often results from sitting leaned back, habitually (see J-2).

J. Walking

1. Physiologic lateral hip movements are necessary to avoid compensatory (excessive) irritating lumbar movements.
2. Walking incorrectly, i.e., habitually leaned backward and downward and hyperextended and compressed at the thoracolumbar junction, often results from habitually sitting leaned back. The leaned-back habit is transferred from sitting to standing and walking.
3. Walking heel/toe rather than toe/heel provides a fulcrum for pelvic-spinal motion and generates biomechanically correct surface reactions from the floor for stability. It eliminates the need for undesirable stabilization, from the top down, by way of cervical and lumbar hyperlordosis.

Table 2-3. Classification of Sitting*

Type I Sitting upward and slightly forward as when working at a desk or computer.

Type II Sitting upright (vertical) as some people do when driving a car and at the dinner table. Another example is sitting up to talk, eye level to eye level.

Type III Sitting leaned backward up to 20° behind the vertical as when resting during work and as some people sit while driving.

Type IV Sitting leaned back more than 20° behind the vertical, relaxed.

The pelvis is rotated forward about 34°, 20° and 7° in Types I, II and III. A neutral lumbar lordosis should be maintained in Types I-IV. Active pelvic rotational movements should be carried out in Types I and II, especially in the sagittal plane, to prevent pressure and discomfort at the hip joints due to hyperflexion. Posterior rotation extends the hip joints.

*See Figs. 2-6, 2-7, 2-8.

When sitting at a desk or computer, Type I sitting is needed. Type II is also often appropriate. When sitting slumped, to reach Type I or II, the pelvis must initiate by rotating forward, and then the torso, head and neck move upward above it into on balance alignment. The occipital condyles rotate backward and upward and the neutral spinal curves are reestablished. (The pelvis is a torque converter. As it moves forward, the body moves upward. As it moves backward, the body moves downward.) When sitting at a desk or a computer, the upper body should not move forward and downward. Downward motion occurs if the pelvis first rotates posteriorly or if the upper body first moves forward and downward. In either case, the result is the familiar slump characterized by posterior rotation of the pelvis, a long convex thoracolumbar "C" curve in the sagittal plane, and often hyperextension of the craniovertebral joints with downward compression of the head on the spine. The skeletal axis "locks" in nonneutral, causing motion in all directions to be markedly restricted or absent. This is bad body use. In slumped sitting at a desk the body is actually, incorrectly, trying to be forward and backward at the same time, i.e., the lower half of the torso and pelvis are rotated and projected backward while the upper half of the torso (above the thoracic apex) and the head and the neck are forward.

The reader might wish to take a moment to sit on a chair and roll the pelvis posteriorly and anteriorly while keeping the chin horizontal to the ground. He will notice that the movement of the body is mostly vertically upward and slightly forward as the pelvis rolls anteriorly and the movement of the body is mostly vertically downward as the pelvis rolls posteriorly.

Working at a desk requires the upper half of the body to be positioned over the desk, but this should not eliminate the neutral alignment of the head, neck and spine. Neutral alignment allows mobility for turning the head and neck, for reaching with the upper extremities, for lateral shifts of the trunk and for maintaining the correct natural base of support which is the undersurface of the pelvis and the proximal thighs. In contrast, the sacrum is the unnatural base of support in a slumped body attitude (thoracolumbar and lumbar kyphosis) and the midposterior thighs provide the support when the body leans too far forward with hyper lumbar lordosis. In hyper lumbar lordosis, the upper weight centers are aligned fairly well over the pelvis, but the skeletal axis locks out of neutral, losing flexibility and mobility. To reiterate, with anterior pelvic rotation (neutral) at 20-34° below horizontal, the spine, neck and head can follow and are more easily maintained in neutral alignment.

When body movement is initiated at the pelvis, the abdominal muscles and gravity have important helping roles, which is not the case with either forward leaning or slumping. *The most neutral alignment is identified by the patient testing for availability and ease of instant active movement in three planes without first having to unlock joints or to shift body weight in order to move.* This simple test makes expensive testing equipment unnecessary. Furthermore, the patient can feel the ease of movement, can learn and reproduce it.

Table 2-4. Four types of sitting.

Types	I	II	III	IV
Examples of Locations	Desk; computer	Driver; dinner table	Driver; at rest "during" desk work	Relaxed
Body Postion	Upward and slightly forward	Upward "vertically"	Leaned back up to 20°	Leaned back more than 20°
Alignment in 3 Planes	Neutral balance	Neutral balance	Neutral balance	Neutral balance
Vertical Alignment	"On balance"	"On balance"	"Off balance" (weight supported by chair)	"Off balance" (weight supported by chair)
Sacral Angle	Forward tilt approximately 20°-34°	Forward tilt approximately 20°	0° to forward tilt approximately 10°	Backward tilt
Hip Flexion* (0° = full extension)	Approximately 75°-85°	Approximately 75°-85°	Approximately 70°	Less than 70°
Lumbar Lordosis**	Yes	Yes	Yes	Yes
Use Back Support	Rare	Frequent	Yes	Yes
Special Pelvic Support Device (on top of chair seat)	Yes	Yes	Yes	Not functional support; provides cushioning only

* Some patients require hip flexion of 90° or more.
** Some patients require lumbar flexion, i.e., flattening or even some kyphosis.

Rather than a static sedentary activity (which is the traditional way of thinking about sitting), it would be far better to consider sitting to be a noncompetitive athletic event. Performing active, rhythmic and organized abdominal-pelvic-spinal-hip movements into all planes and vertically is important for healthy sitting. A good chair is not a brace. In fact, it is wrong to be "held" or supported in one alignment.

The techniques used for rising from a chair and returning to sitting are also very important. The pelvic-spinal-hip complex (PSH-C) includes the lumbar portion of the spine, the lumbosacral joints, sacroiliac and hip joints, and all related soft tissues. In sitting and in most other activities, the PSH-C must act (initiate), not react, to help maintain the health and function of the entire somatic system.

A FUNCTIONAL APPROACH TO EVALUATING POSTURE

Most people define posture with phrases such as: "How you sit and how you stand," or "How you hold your body." The word "how" is used in the anatomical sense, mean-

Table 2-5. Pelvis — Body Center

1. The structural and functional support of the spine.
2. The pelvis is the center of the Pelvic-Spinal-Hip Complex (PSH-C)
3. Pelvic alignment determines spinal alignment because the spine follows the pelvis. The pelvis is a torque converter. The pelvis rotates at the hip joints.
4. The hip joint is the major joint of the pelvis and is vitally important for clinical movement of the spine and lower extremities in all planes, i.e., in all activities.
5. The anterior/posterior depth of the pelvis increases the moment for action of the hip extensor muscles.
6. The forward inclination of the femoral necks adds to #5.
7. The lower rectus abdominis muscles fine tune pelvic rotation and thus the degree of spinal curvatures in the sagittal plane.
8. The pelvis is the location of the body's net center of gravity. Its proximity to the ischial tuberosities (the fulcra for pelvic rotation) assists pelvic rotation.
9. The pelvis provides the natural base of support for the upper weight centers.
10. The pelvis provides the anatomical and biomechanical base for stability and mobility for the spine and extremities.
11. The pelvis connects the upper and lower portions of the body anatomically and kinesthetically, e.g., "the heel/coccyx connection" so important for normal stability and mobility in walking.
12. Movement into the three-dimensional space around the body is often initiated at the pelvis.
13. Effortless balance and ease of movement are maintained by initiating shifts of body weight at the pelvis.

ing static alignment, appearance, shape or contour, not in the physiological (functional) sense or in the sense of biomechanics, which refers to forces acting on the body, including gravity, muscles and surface reactions. (See Table 2-6 for a partial list of biomechanical forces.) But "how" should describe function, method or technique rather than appearance. Biomechanics has an important influence on body function.

In 1947, the Posture Committee of the American Academy of Orthopedic Surgeons reported that "posture is usually defined as the relative arrangement of the parts of the body."[4] In the author's opinion, a better definition would have been "anatomical, functional and biomechanical relationships of the parts of the body." Kendall et al.[4] stated that "posture is basically a matter of alignment" and emphasized muscle balancing through stretching and strengthening exercises to achieve better alignment. Kraus-Weber[3] emphasized the importance of alignment as well as flexibility when evaluating and treating posture. Either because of or in spite of these views,[3,4] most people think of posture only in terms of alignment.

Kendall et al.[4] recognized that "plumb-line tests" do not tell all there is about alignment. Those authors also referred to "segmental alignment faults," i.e., points not located along plumb lines. The "faults" included exaggerated spinal curves, faulty head alignment (e.g., head forward or tilted upward or downward), protruding abdomen, hyperextended or hyperflexed knees, and so on.

But sometimes a fault involves more than one specific joint. Plumb lines also do not take into account many of the joints, including the temporomandibulars and those of the feet. Further, there is disagreement as to where the plumb line should pass in relation to the

CHAPTER 2 Posture: The Process of Body Use; Principles and Determinants 25

Table 2-6. Balance of Forces (partial list).

		Direction	Force
1. **Alignment**			
a.	Neutral balanced alignment in 3 planes	↓	Body weight (gravity and body mass)
	and	↑	Surface reaction from seat surfaces and ground
b.	"On balance" alignment vertically*	↑	Lower abdominal muscles
		↑	Calf muscles
		↑↓	Other muscles
	Body Weight is over base of support and is counterbalanced by surface reactions.	↓	Tissue pressure, e.g., intervertebral discs
		↓↑	Connective tissue (fascia)
2. **Alignment**			
a.	Nonneutral alignment	↓	Body weight
	and	↓	Posterior spinal muscles and ligaments pull down (they hold the forward flexed trunk "up" as they pull down)
b.	"Off balance" alignment	↑	Tissue pressure, e.g., intervertebral discs
	Body weight is not over base of support and is not congruous with surface reactions	↑	Tight ligaments and muscles cause added tissue compression
		↑	Surface reaction but not as effective as in 1

* Includes Type I and II sitting

lumbar portion of the spine. Authors have placed this imaginary line anterior, posterior or through the lumbar vertebrae.

Other clinical methods use physical examination to evaluate regional structural alignment. One example is to observe how well the malar bones of the face are lined up vertically with the anterior edge of the sternum. Other examples are measuring the depths of the cervical and lumbar curves and the depths of the cervicothoracic and lumbosacral junctions.[3] By drawing a long vertical line that extends above and below the thoracic apex, one may determine the horizontal distance between that line to the depth of the midcervical curve. That distance should not be greater than 6 centimeters,[36] and the horizontal distances to both the cervicothoracic and lumbosacral junctions should not be greater than 1 inch.[3] With curves that are too deep, the alignments at these measured points are nonneutral. Although this interferes with movement, none of the above mentioned techniques test movement. Nonneutral alignment is also present when curves are too shallow. In other cases, as mentioned earlier, alignment is correct but there is hypomobility because of inflexibility.

Clinically, the process of body use can be evaluated objectively by examining alignments, flexibility, functional strength and especially *by noting the ease and quality of movement*. For example, weight is back too far onto the heels if the patient must first shift forward when instantly rising onto the toes. This tests the alignment at the start of the movement. As the patient's heels return to the ground and the weight is back too far, the examiner can feel excessive pressure on a finger placed at the patient's midthoracic spine. We can evaluate head and neck alignment by observing individually both lateral rotation of the neck and head flexion. With so-called "forward head alignment," (incorrectly referred to as "forward head posture") or if the head and neck are back too far in the sagittal plane, both head flexion and lateral rotation of the neck are restricted. Both are nonneutral alignments. To carry out these movements more completely and easily, neutral balanced and on balance alignments of the head and neck must be established. This also requires neutral alignment of the pelvis.

The patient learns to see and feel both restricted and free movements and uses these sensory inputs to recognize progressive changes in alignment. This is a simple and practical way to monitor the results of oral instructions and hands-on treatments. With training, patients learn quickly that joints in a more neutral alignment move better (greater range and ease) than joints in nonneutral. Thus, during static and dynamic activities, aligning the body according to ease of movement is far better than trying to be "straight." For example, while rising from a chair the patient can easily feel major differences between getting up by first moving his upper body upward and forward (correctly) maintaining neutral spinal alignment rather than first moving it downward and forward (incorrectly). In the former, he rises with greater ease by releasing the craniovertebral joints, stabilizing the pelvis, utilizing the quadriceps and hip extensors for power and by pushing off at the feet. In the latter instance, the craniovertebral joints are locked and compressed, the spine is first hyperflexed, then extended and the torso is lifted in a large arc, against gravity. When sitting in Types I or II at a desk or computer, neutral alignment and mobility of the craniovertebral joints, spine and hips are maintained. Although emphasis is on movement, it is also helpful to record structural relationships between body parts to evaluate changes with training. Also, a more neutral alignment is a predictor of better movement so long as the tissues are also flexible.

Objectively, another way to judge posture, as body use, is to analyze the mechanisms of injuries. Subjectively, the patient can evaluate his posture by noting pain, fatigue, comfort and discomfort, both at rest and during movement. Body attitudes and alignments such as slumping, a sunken chest, forward and rounded shoulders, all examples of bad body use, also all look unappealing. Thus, the lay person's assessment of bad posture, based usually on appearance, is often correct even though he has not tested movement. If movement were tested, it would be found to be greatly diminished or absent. Those alignments of "bad posture" lack vitality. They look tired and compressed. Standing in nonneutral alignment is tiring, partly because excessive and unnecessary muscle and ligament activity are needed to hold the body up. Nonneutral sitting is tiring, partly because correct breathing mechanics (using the diaphragm anteriorly, bilaterally and posteriorly) are interfered with and there is a loss of joint and soft tissue movement. Active movement is also a stimulus for breathing.

THE FIVE TYPES OF ALIGNMENT

Alignment is probably the single most important determinant of posture. An appreciation of alignment is vital for the evaluation of posture and for patient training. As previously indicated, alignment refers to the angular relationships between body parts either segmentally or regionally in the three cardinal planes and vertically. The frontal plane alignment is also described in relation to the midline. Table 2-7 lists five types of alignment. Three types are usually considered to be consistent with "good" posture. These are: 1) "neutral balanced alignment"; 2) "dynamically stabilized alignment" which is also referred to in the literature as "neutral spine"; and 3) "on balance alignment". Two

Table 2-7. Types of Alignment

a. Neutral Balanced
b. Dynamically Stabilized
c. On Balance
d. Nonneutral
e. Off Balance

types of alignment are usually considered to be consistent with "bad" posture. These are "nonneutral" and "off balance" alignments. In certain instances, both of these can be part of an overall good body use. In the same vein, in certain instances, both 1 and 3 can be part of an overall bad body use.

The five types of alignment will now be discussed in more detail.

Neutral Balanced Alignment (NBA)

This refers to functioning throughout the neutral range. This range encompasses the region from and including the physiologic barrier on one side to the opposite physiologic barrier in each of the three cardinal planes. These normal physiologic barriers defining the ends of neutral alignment are the result of normal muscle, tendon and fascial tensions. They represent the first resistance that develops during active movement of a joint. During normal postural sway, movements onto and off these physiologic barriers provide kinesthetic input for body awareness. There is some muscular activity during neutral alignment, enabling it to be flexible, mobile, stable and controlled.

Both static and dynamic activities occur in neutral alignment. The normal physiologic barriers define the end of neutral alignment and the end of the active range of motion. They also define the start of nonneutral alignment. Passive range of motion occurs in the space between the physiologic barrier and the anatomic barrier. The anatomic barrier is at the end of nonneutral alignment and is at the end of the passive range of motion. The anatomic barrier is due to the normal resistance of ligaments and bony elements of joints. Beyond it the joint subluxes. Accessory joint movements occur in the paraphysiologic space which is just before the anatomic barrier. Joint manipulation techniques of the thrust variety are performed through the paraphysiologic space[43] up to the anatomic barrier.

Neutral alignment can be defined in terms of:

1. Articulator anatomy which, in the spine, is midway in the normal range of motion.

2. Equal or balanced soft tissue tensions in three planes.

The second definition is more clinically relevant. The two definitions coincide in the normal spine, but in the extremity joints, they do not.[2] However, alignment may be midway or somewhere else within the normal range of motion between the physiologic barriers.

Dynamically Stabilized Alignment ("Neutral Spine")

This also is in the neutral range. Its hallmark is specific limitation of joint motion. The limitation is intentional, due to increased voluntary muscle activity. Dynamic stabilization decreases the arc of movement within the neutral range. The limited protected range of movement is closer to one of the two physiologic barriers. This can be so in each plane of motion. The purpose is to protect against pain, hypermobility and/or irritation of damaged or abnormal joints. The protected range is ideally pain-free. Aside from the limited motion, it is physiologically sound, occurring within the neutral range. Once the protected alignment for the segment(s) or region(s) is established, the person functions there. However, the precise protected alignment can change with different activities.

On Balance Alignment

"On balance" refers to aligning each body part vertically over its correct natural base of support (refer to Fig. 2-1). In Types I and II sitting, the upper weight centers (head and rib cage) are aligned in neutral in the sagittal and frontal planes over the pelvis, the natural base of support. The pelvis is also aligned in neutral and the hip joints are noncompressed and free to move. These characteristics are typical of Types I and II sitting. Devices that compress or limit hip joint movement are deleterious to the process of body use. Examples are kneeling seats and straps that encircle the knees and pelvis. "On balance" alignment applies to each individual spinal segment in relation to the one just below it as well as to the upper body weight centers (i.e., the head and rib cage) being aligned "on balance" over the pelvis in sitting and over the pelvis and feet in standing. It is important to realize that "on balance" (vertical) alignment and NBA usually occur together. (An exception is "on balance" but in the presence of decreased flexibility due to tightness from elastic resistance or stiffness from rigid resistance. Functioning throughout the neutral range is lost.)

The pelvis as body center is vital. One might think of "on balance" alignment as straight because there is vertical alignment of the weight centers. However, the patient is aware of being in "on balance" alignment not by structural landmarks but kinesthetically and functionally by noting the availability of easy, instant voluntary movement into all planes, and vertically.

When one sits "on balance" and moves from Type II to Type I, the head, neck and torso move upward and slightly forward. The actual movements are initiated at the pelvis as it rotates about the hip joints. The spine follows the pelvis. The movements are controlled by the abdominal, lumbar and iliacus muscles and are fine tuned by the lower abdominal muscles for distance, speed, acceleration and deceleration. The movements can be stopped at any point in the arc. Carrying out rhythmic, organized, controlled abdominal-pelvic-spinal-hip exercises teaches the importance of the pelvis in establishing correct alignment, movement and direction of movement. Such exercises also strengthen the muscles functionally, making it easier to sit in Types I and II. The "feel" of "on balance" alignment and the vertical movements of the upper body over the pelvis are even more dramatic as one moves in either direction between a controlled slump to Types I or II sitting. During those movements, the upper body should remain "free" and the head (Frankfort plane) remains level or flexed just 2-3°.

Nonneutral Alignment

This refers to functioning up against the anatomic barriers of joints, i.e., ligaments, joint capsules and bones (Fig. 2-3). Hyperflexion (kyphosis) and hyperextension (hyperlordosis) are examples of nonneutral alignment. Active motion is greatly diminished or lost, for the individual must first "unlock" to move in

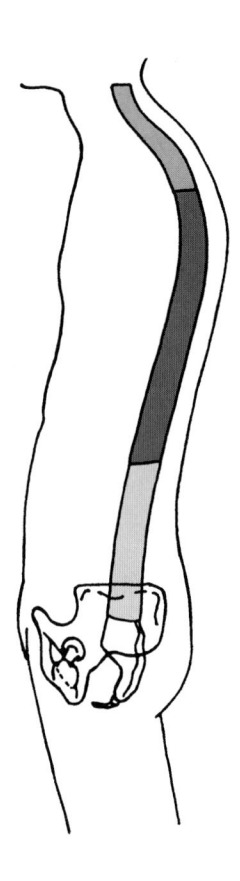

Fig. 2-3. Nonneutral Alignment. Standing with upper trunk leaned backward and downward. Spine and hips are locked in nonneutral alignment in the sagittal plane. The head is forward as a counterbalance. The sternum and upper ribs are restricted. The pelvis, hips and upper thighs sway forward. Hips are hyperextended and the pelvis is tilted backward.

the same plane. Furthermore, as per Freyette's third law of spinal motion, when movement occurs into one plane, movement into the other planes is diminished or lost.[17] When we sit or stand slumped and "locked down" in nonneutral and "off balance" alignments, we lose dynamic body movement, postural sway and the anterior, posterior and lateral lower chest breathing movements which result from normal diaphragmatic excursion.

Off Balance Alignment

This is a vertical alignment in which the upper weight centers are not aligned over their bases of support (Fig 2-4). "Off balance" and "nonneutral" alignments usually occur together. Static slumped sitting is an example. Instead of the natural base of support for

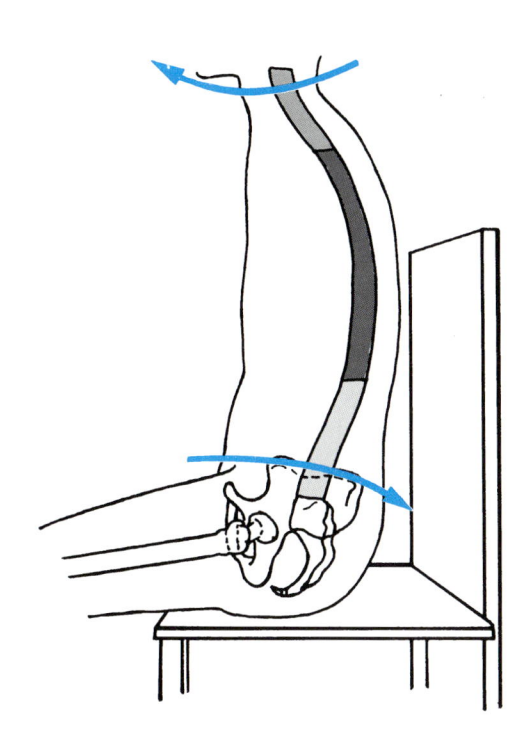

Fig. 2-4. Off Balance Alignment. Slumped sitting, not leaned back. Pelvis is rotated posteriorly; spine, which follows the pelvis, is kyphotic; craniovertebral joints are compressed. Alignments are nonneutral and "off balance." Stability depends upon ligamentous locking, anterior vertebral apposition, craniovertebral joint compression and fixation of the sacrum against the seat. Two reasons for slumping: 1) to provide pelvic stability (there is no support under the anterior pelvis to stabilize it in neutral); 2) to open the hip joints anteriorly ("extension") to relieve pressure and discomfort.[48]

body weight (the undersurface of the pelvis from ischial tuberosity to proximal thighs), there is an unnatural base of support for body weight, i.e., the posterior and inferior aspects of the sacrum. Associated with this are a long spinal "C" curve and the craniovertebral joints locked into extension. The body's weight rests directly on the sacrum. The joints throughout the pelvis and spine are in nonneutral alignment in the sagittal plane. Movement is lost.

ALIGNMENT AND POSTURE

Neutral balanced and on balance alignment are usually consistent with good posture. However, that is not always the case. Despite a tall, upright "on balance" appearance, a person may be inflexible because of tight fascia, tight muscles and/or joint capsules. In effect, that person is being held up "on balance" by these tight structures. When he is asked to bend forward or to sit in a "natural pelvic/lumbar slump," he cannot. Inflexibility due to tight tissues is a criterion of bad body use. Indeed, "on balance" alignment can be present despite overall bad body use. For that reason *movement is the ultimate clinical test of posture or body use.*

Clearly, alignment is only one of many determinants of posture, although it is an extremely important one. It should be noted that with dynamically stabilized alignment, the stabilized segments are functionally "not moved" or moved very little, but they should certainly retain the capability to move.

Nonneutral and off balance alignments are typically considered to be consistent with "bad" or "poor" posture. However, in certain instances, both can be part of an overall good body use. In certain activities, for short durations, these alignments provide the passive or active stability (*and local inflexibility, due to "locked" joints*) necessary for movements of another body part(s) or another body region(s) (Tables 2-1 and 2-2). Two examples are: 1) throwing a baseball and 2) bending forward by sequentially flexing the head on the neck, then the neck on the chest and so forth (see below). However, full body nonneutral and full body off balance alignments are never good use.

A person with scoliosis should not automatically be considered to have bad posture. If flexibility for ease of motion is retained in the curve, then there is good posture (good body use). Good body use also includes the controlled repetitive movements from neutral to nonneutral to neutral alignments when sitting or standing. These movements are initiated with active anterior/posterior pelvic tilt exercises, diagonal movements, figure eights and lateral pelvic shifts. The movements are controlled by abdominal, pelvic girdle and lumbar muscles.

It is difficult to sit upright continuously, statically, in anatomically correct neutral pelvic and spinal alignment (sacral angle 20-34° with neutral spinal curves above it) on a flat horizontal seat. It is difficult partly because of pressure in the anterior hip regions (Fig. 2-5). The hip joints out of neutral alignment.

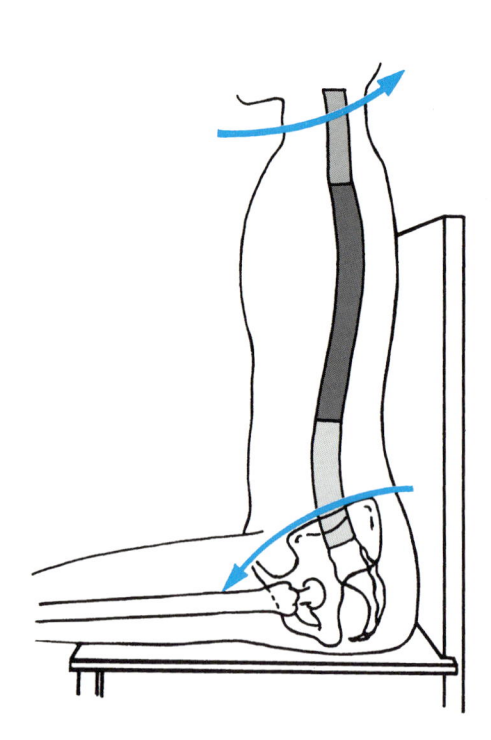

Fig. 2-5. Sitting upright to show NBA and "on balance" alignment on the way to standing (i.e., in transition). Sitting continuously upright on a flat surface with sacral angle and pelvis at upper range of neutral. Thighs are level, causing hyperflexion of hips, anterior hip pressure, and discomfort. The person would eventually slump for hip relief and to relieve the muscles.[48]

They are flexed (90°) and compressed for too long. In order to relieve anterior hip discomfort, unfortunately we often incorrectly rotate the pelvis posteriorly. This also causes spinal slumping (Fig. 2-4). Slumping extends the hip.[22] While sitting and carrying out the organized active functional movements already described, the hips are rhythmically moved in and out of neutral/nonneutral alignments. These exercises maintain hip mobility and comfort. They increase kinesthetic awareness at the hips and total body awareness because the movements occur at the pelvis, i.e., between the upper and lower portions of the body. Muscle fatigue is also a problem while sitting upright in neutral pelvic and spinal alignment. The organized functional movements prevent muscle fatigue by eliminating stagnation of tissue fluids, by increasing muscle blood flow and by increasing functional strength. Individual muscles rest between their contractions.

There are a number of important elements in sitting, especially nonsedentary sitting: neutral pelvis and spine; rhythmic controlled movements; on balance alignment; and freedom for the hip joints. One caveat is that a neutral pelvis without the knees resting lower than the hips will still cause compression at the anterior hips. Also, just lowering the knees below the level of the hips does not assure that the pelvis will be anteriorly rotated into neutral alignment. While lowering the knees does promote lumbar lordosis, it is, nevertheless, very common to see someone sitting with the knees lower than the hips, but with the pelvis rotated posteriorly and the spine slumped. Thus, neutral pelvic alignment must be maintained and controlled by balancing the forces from body weight, upward seat surface reaction, and muscle activity. As the pelvis and spine move through their ranges, direction, speed and distance must be controlled by the musculature. Otherwise we will use our internal locking mechanisms (ligament tension and bony compression) to hold ourselves up against the downward force of body weight. Every joint of the body should be able to function safely throughout its natural range of motion.

People like to move their bodies because movement feels good. Teaching the patient to move rhythmically is important to prevent slumping and stagnation in the tissues. Movement occurs most easily from a neutral alignment and it is important to train the patient properly. Movement is the benchmark of good posture, or body use.

Obviously, posture applies to ongoing or everyday activities as well as to more isolated single or repetitive events. For example, baseball pitchers have temporary, intermittent postural (body use) requirements for pitching that are not present in ordinary life. Good posture is body use which is based on correct anatomical relationships, physiology and biomechanics. These prevent somatic injury and allow pain-free activities in all body positions.

Good posture is also task related, it may occur in nonneutral alignment. e.g., bending forward or throwing a ball (Table 2-1). This appears to "break the rules" but one must keep in mind that good posture includes nonneutral alignment for short periods and/or with limited frequency of repetition for certain tasks and occupations. The same activities, in nonneutral, would be damaging (bad posture) if they were to continue for too long or if done too frequently. A dancer's turnout should not be continued during ordinary walking and certainly not in ordinary street shoes. If it were, the medial aspects of the feet and legs would be "sheared." Thus, duration and frequency are determinants of posture.

Even sitting in one place in neutral balanced and on balance alignments for too long without carrying out movement exercise means bad posture, as circulation of fluids in and out of muscles becomes relatively stagnant and muscles tire. Trigger points, weakness and spasm can occur along with muscle tension.[35] Eventually, alignment suffers when the tired muscles can no longer help support it. The individual slumps into generalized nonneutral alignment, which allows the overused muscles to stop contracting. However, in a short time, back muscles begin to ache because of the mechanical stretch tension and/or ischemia. It is important to realize that, when the body literally hangs on its ligaments, the ligaments are working even though they are passive structures. When the body is aligned in neutral, the ligaments are not working since the alignment is not at the end range.

In neutral the muscles must work intermittently to support the body. The muscles rest by contracting intermittently. The pumping action prevents them from tiring and otherwise becoming dysfunctional and painful. It is also important to keep the brain informed as to the length/tension[40] relationships of muscles and the kinesthetics of muscles and joints. This helps prevent injury by providing better proprioceptive control over movements, i.e., both planned voluntary active movements and at times of sudden unexpected movements, as occur with falls.

THE DETERMINANTS OF POSTURE

There are six basic *determinants* of posture: 1) mind factors, 2) physical factors, 3) duration and frequency, 4) comfort and relaxation, 5) adaptation and compensation, and 6) treatment (Appendix 2). Each determinant can be further characterized as either primarily intrinsic or extrinsic to the patient.

Note that what we refer to as the *principles* of posture are more prescriptive, oriented more toward treatment, than the determinants. For example, principle 17 states: "On balance alignment requires a mobile, stable pelvis... movement and body balance should initiate there." The sixty-seven principles we list in Appendix I can each be classified as falling under one or more of the determinants, and in fact are derived from them. Then we present the six determinants which comprise the basis for the more prescriptive principles. The 67 principles are not presented as an all-inclusive list.

Mind Factors (intrinsics)

Mind factors include body awareness, sensory memory, organization and sequence of motion,[9,10] motivation (too little or too much), and emotions. For example, when doing a posterior pelvic tilt the movement should be initiated by contracting the lower abdominal muscles and not by trying to press the back into the table or by squeezing the buttocks together. Mind factors are probably the most important aspect of posture, the main one in preventing bad body use, the "glue that binds." Without body awareness and correct organization of movement, all the other preventive measures and techniques are likely to have only temporary benefits because somatic function is less controlled and, therefore, less predictable. For example, hands-on mobilization techniques fall short over time unless the person is kinesthetically habilitated and/or rehabilitated.

Body awareness permits us to be aware of and to monitor movement while it is happening. Organization of movement includes preemptive anticipatory actions[13] as well as body leads (the body part that initiates movement) and the sequence in which parts move. Integrating body awareness with organization of movement is crucial. For example, only through training can most patients begin to use their abdominal muscles functionally during activities of daily living. We want the patient to develop kinesthetic awareness of the lower abdominal muscles, necessary for fine tuning pelvic rotation and alignment, and spinal alignment. Functional control of alignment is the goal, not flattening the back or achieving force strength in the abdominal muscles. Functional control includes functional strength, coordination, body centering at the pelvis and balanced soft tissue tension. The latter does not require anatomical or structural symmetry. An analogy is a biker turning a corner for, although the bike leans to one side, the forces are balanced. Ultimately, it is important that the person feels where the movement is taking place and is able to control the movement.

Almost all patients that we see (including those who are health professionals) have little or no awareness or understanding of how the body should move. Frankly, most individuals' minds and bodies are divorced. This may have occurred early in life. Even a relatively simple and natural activity such as sitting and rotating the pelvis forward and backward to move the body upward and downward is extremely difficult for most people to do when first asked; they are not centered at the pelvis and are not in functional control of their movement sequence. In fact, these movements are avoided and suppressed. One wonders how many people have functional sexual difficulties because they move mostly from the upper body instead of the pelvis.

It is very common to hear a new patient, as he stands in his slump, say, "Wait, I'll straighten up." To accomplish that, he moves the torso upward and the shoulders backward and locks the thoracic spinal segments in nonneutral, at the end of their extension ranges. The upper body, therefore, becomes tense and locked. He has converted a nonneutral slump (flexion) to a nonneutral rigid extension. This can easily be overcome by teaching the patient to release the upper body, but that can only be done if he can transfer control to the pelvis and feet.

In general, people are aware of their bodies only when they hurt, i.e., when there is a conflict. At those times, they carry out deliberate protective movements, for they quickly become aware of which movements hurt and which do not. To be aware of his body seems strange to the patient, for he has never thought about how to use his body and, more importantly, he has never been taught. It seems odd that it is so common to tell back pain patients to bend down "from their knees" without also explaining why; without training them in body centering, i.e., functional control of the pelvis for mobility and stability; and without training them to be able to monitor the alignment and freedom of motion of the upper weight centers in relation to the pelvis.

It has been said that humans do not have natural organization of movement. Different activities have different inhibitions. Also, humans must contend with rapidly changing environments, i.e., shoes, chairs, sofas, autos, planes, to name a few, in contrast to animals which have a more stable physical environment. Good body use requires the development of good habits and we should function by using those good habits. However, in everyday life we must also be able to become consciously aware of what we are doing in order to make changes. (This is often not applicable to the brain-damaged population.) If we are relegated to functioning by habit alone, we cannot be aware and we can not consciously make changes when things are not going right. We must be able to adapt consciously. For example, we may teach someone how to arise from a chair of specific design and height, but he must also be able to consciously adapt the technique of body use to any chair.

Sensory awareness also involves training in being able to monitor the intermediate functional and biomechanical aspects of body use: body centering; ease of movement into all planes; and balanced lengthening (releasing) of tissues. The latter provides light tissue tensions/countertensions which gives us awareness of the connectedness between body parts. Suffice to say that sensory awareness integrates the anatomy and function of the somatic system all the way from the individual muscles and joints to the total body alignments needed for correct physical body attitude during relaxation and in relatively static and dynamic activities.

We have already mentioned the problems that arise when patients overcorrect and strain in an effort to sit or stand up "straight." This interferes with movement; we want them to feel "ease." In our Posture 'n Motion* diagnostic and therapeutic technique, patients actively test their motions, regionally and segmentally, from a series of alignments to determine their awareness of movement, to increase that awareness and to locate the most ideal alignment by determining the alignment that allows the most freedom of movement. We have already stated that sometimes a purposeful local or regional nonneutral alignment is necessary to stabilize another moving part. Also, a dynamically stabilized alignment may be necessary to protect a painful, irritated or hypermobile segment or region. As a general rule, however, a stable and mobile alignment in NBA and on balance is best.

In the sagittal plane, "straight" should be described only in terms of an anatomical-functional link; the upper weight centers are aligned over the pelvis and each spinal segment is aligned over the one below it, within the spinal curve, allowing the most effortless balance and voluntary physiologic pain-free motion instantly in any direction with ease.

Clinically, there has been a failure to educate patients in how to achieve balanced alignment, how to be aware of it, and how to maintain it during activities. It is impossible for a person to consciously monitor posture from moment to moment by trying to concentrate on individual joint and muscle functions. We are dealing with a complex neuromusculoskeletal system with very rapid multimuscular function. To improve body use, we can train individual muscle functions, but these must be incorporated into the total motor activity. To achieve the goal of consistent better body use, the focus must be on the determinants and the techniques rather than on the end result.

Asking someone to stand or to sit anatomically straight for better posture (even if those terms were acceptable) would be analogous to asking someone to simply run faster in order to win a race. Running faster can be achieved with bad body use. This results in injuries because the body is not under control. It is important to emphasize that, to achieve consistent better body use, the focus

must be on techniques and not on the end result. Stated another way, we must focus on the intermediate steps: organization of movement; centering; awareness of the connectedness of body parts by momentary light physiologic tissue tensions involved in body use. "Sitting straight" and running faster are end results.

Reflexes, Habits, and Skills as Mind Factors

A habit is a nonsupervised automatic behavior which entails acting repeatedly in a certain way. We have already given the example of a person who rises from a chair with a certain fundamental body use regardless of his changing external or internal environment. The movement is performed essentially the same way every time because the habit allows for little if any physiologic or biomechanic adaptation. However, by being aware, we can adapt.

Patients with back pain are frequently taken aback when they realize that they have to *think* about how they use their bodies in getting out of a chair, in breathing, in the use of the pelvis, and so forth. At least bending the knees to initiate lifting, as practiced by many people with back pain, has generally made it into people's awareness.

Another good example of consciousness applied to movement is the tennis player whose game is not going well having to stop and consider the fundamentals, i.e., "Am I bending my knees?" or "Am I bringing the racquet back?" He must become aware. The automatic skills he has developed are now, temporarily, "supervised" activities which require the ability to adapt, train, and be aware.

Just as the tennis player can easily monitor his body use from moment to moment by his shot performance (the end result), we can monitor our body use in everyday activities by being aware of pain and stiffness. But we can be aware of the intermediate steps: freedom and direction of our movements into the three-dimensional space or kinesphere[9] around us (outer space); of any movements, including breathing movements, that are restricted to one plane; of the sensations associated with lengthening and light-

---

*A registered service mark of Lionel A. Walpin, M.D..

ness versus compression and heaviness; of the light, thread-like balanced tissue tensions and countertensions which provide the sense of dynamic connectedness between body parts, for example, head and shoulders and heel and coccyx; of alignment, flexibility, and of body centering which is so important.

Many health professionals already utilize the concept of organized movement to some extent. Patients with low back pain are routinely taught to initiate rising from a bed by first turning to the side, then lowering the lower extremities toward the floor and pushing the body up to the sitting position with the upper extremities. However, even this is too gross. The components of the movement sequence need to be further broken down or delineated and controlled. When turning to the side, how does one control the knee drop? Is the motion controlled properly by using abdominal and pelvic hip rotator muscles or does the weight of the extremities cause them to drop freely to the floor under the unopposed influence of gravity? This puts strain on the pelvis and back. Proper technique can control the location, speed and distance of spinal rotation and bending and will prevent and/or limit excessive lumbar hyperflexion and hyperextension.

CONTROLLED, RHYTHMIC SITTING EXERCISES

In neutral alignment, sitting, rhythmic exercises are very helpful for training patients to initiate body movement at the pelvis, reinforcing the pelvis' role as functional and structural body center. These abdominal pelvic lumbar exercises increase functional muscle strength, endurance and kinesthetics. The patient learns to control the direction, distance and speed of pelvic rotations and spinal movements. With control, the patient no longer "whiplashes" the pelvic, spinal or craniovertebral joints when doing anterior and posterior pelvic tilts. Ease of movement from neutral alignment makes doing these exercises possible.

The sitting exercises, initiated at the umbilicus by the abdominal muscles, include lateral shifts (with the least amount of lower extremity movement possible), anterior/posterior pelvic tilts, abdominal "clocks" (similar to Feldenkrais), and the inscription of figure-8's "drawn" both perpendicular and parallel to the floor. The pelvic movements mobilize the hip joints in the sagittal plane and also restore lateral hip movements which are so important for the normal function of the lumbar spine in walking. The posterior rotation phase of pelvic movement intermittently opens the anterior part of the hip joints, relieving discomfort. Furthermore, the posterior/anterior rotations "massage" the hip joints. Freedom of the hip joints and of the upper body is achieved, and diaphragmatic breathing becomes easier and fuller. Freedom of the hip joints is lost when we kneel on a forward-tilted seat and when straps surrounding the knees are anchored to the low back or posterior pelvis. In both situations the hip joints are compressed non-physiologically.

While seated, the feet should remain in contact with the floor. This is important for functional training of body use. Because each foot has 40 joints, feet provide balance, support and major proprioceptive input. Participation of the feet is lost when kneeling on a forward-tilted seat.

Clearly, discussion and demonstration of the fundamentals of posture, the process, has been sorely lacking. Patients get frustrated and end up going for neverending hands-on passive therapies, i.e., mobilization, manipulation, heat, massage, and so forth, without ever improving the mind factor determinants of body use. They seek the repeated "passive quick fix."

Further, exercise programs without proper body use are inadequate. Neutral balanced alignments, dynamic stabilization, organization and sequence of body movement and body centering are mentioned by few health professionals to their patients. People involved with the kinesthetics and the kinesiology of dance, however, are very familiar with the process of correct body use. Observe a dancer rising from the floor: movement is initiated and accomplished from a stable center which lifts and helps release the body. Dancers know that it is incorrect to pull the lower body up by compressing the head and neck downward for stability and raising the shoulders. The individual's body must be lifted up from below, and not pulled up from above.

Similarly, when a patient tries to stand straight, i.e., on balance, he should do so by first aligning the pelvis and releasing the upper body, maintaining mobility, not by trying to pull the upper body into some so-called "straight" (stiff) alignment. The latter restricts motion while the former permits it. After all, if someone tries to be structurally straight, how does he know if he is correctly straight, i.e., not too little or too much? If a person tries to become straight and overdoes it, he assumes a nonneutral restricted alignment. Furthermore, with activities requiring bending, twisting or walking, the mode of sitting or standing structurally straight cannot apply. For patients to understand and feel *the process of body use*, the emphasis of posture must be on function, i.e., movement, both at relative rest and dynamically.

In the opening sentence of the introduction to their outstanding textbook, Kendall et al.[4] state: "Good posture is a good habit." More recently, Bland,[19] an outstanding authority on musculoskeletal disorders, has stated in his textbook, "Bad posture is a bad habit," and "Good posture is a good habit that, once established, requires little voluntary effort to maintain."[19] The present author asks: How are those "good habits" to be established? Are more than just cookbook instructions given? Are they really good habits? Can the patient *feel* his/her body use? Really good habits are probably not being developed if it is cookbook.

When people function by habit only, bad habits easily creep in, remain and interfere with the process of good body use. We emphasize functional movement rather than static anatomical alignment, in contradistinction with past texts, we also emphasize the importance of awareness and finer control of movement, rather than only habitual activity.

Functional posture including functional movement is important in daily activities. Active exercise should be performed *correctly* to improve all the determinants of posture. For example, the supine patient may perform "knee drops" for rotational stretching of the lumbar spine and pelvis, but the technique used to drop the knees and then to reverse the movement may not be correct. Typically and incorrectly, the direction, speed and distance of the drop are due to the unopposed weight of the thighs and the return movement is typically started by extending the lumbar spine. It is far better for the patient to be kinesthetically aware, controlling the drop and return through the functional strength of the pelvic and abdominal muscles. The spine's alignment and the cephalad extent of the spine's rotation can be actively, consciously monitored and controlled. The movement is then predictable and safe and can be applied to daily activities such as rising from supine to sitting position in bed.

Functional strength must be distinguished from muscle strength for force (force strength). Crunch abdominal exercises utilize the upper abdominal muscles and cause compressed standing with attendant decreased mobility. Crunch exercises teach the patient little if anything about functional body use. It is worth noting that functional posture can also be improved by using gentle passive manual medicine techniques that mobilize and balance soft tissues and joints, increase flexibility, and improve proprioception and kinesthetics for better control of both muscle length and joint alignment. They improve the quality of reflexive and voluntary movements. All this helps to prevent injuries that result from unexpected, sudden movements and impacts.

Functional posture can also be improved through developments in the field of ergonomics. Environmental factors which physically contact the body and improve support, body awareness, and function are important. Chairs and special seat inserts, shoes and foot orthotics, bed pillows and mattresses are just a few.

The general public is under the misconception that ergonomic chairs will automatically improve "posture" and thus relieve back pain, neck pain and fatigue. But these chairs should not be thought of as braces for holding the body in a certain correct static alignment. Some so-called ergonomic chairs and other support devices actually interfere with function. Practically speaking, ergonomic chairs can only work well when the user knows how to and wants to use the body correctly.

PAIN AS A MIND FACTOR

Pain is another important mind factor that can contribute to poor posture. This happens in several ways. First, with acute pain one often adopts mechanically incorrect protective nonneutral alignment to avoid pain. With chronic pain, the psychologic response can lead to total nonneutral body alignment because of the accompanying depression. In the author's view, both situations can also cause further primary pain from nonneutral alignments and interference with movement. Recently, some authors have stated that bad posture is not painful. It depends upon how one defines posture and upon the envelope within which movement takes place. Painful movement can cause reflex weakness. Fear of painful movement can also cause functional neuromuscular weakness as a protective mechanism. An important approach in treating patients with chronic pain (i.e., prolonged pain with no ongoing organic basis demonstrable) is to utilize active movement. This helps to give the patient the confidence that movement is not harmful. Movement feels good and people like to move. Overcoming fear of movement by teaching body awareness and control of movement helps greatly. Thus, people can move in a controlled, predictable manner with more confidence. This is a far better approach than asking patients to "learn to live with" the chronic pain. Exercise properly carried out with good body is obviously important.

Physical Factors (intrinsic and extrinsic)

The soma (and its peripheral brain, the proprioceptors in muscles and joints), should not be divorced from the mind. That divorce may occur very early in life and/or throughout it, causing the development of unhealthy holding patterns of muscle. This may be aggravated by injuries, disease, pain, emotions and by the physical environment. For example, chairs designed poorly and giving poor support.

INTRINSIC PHYSICAL FACTORS

This category includes:

Body mass; weight (the effect of gravity on body mass results in body weight); all the specific structural components of the somatic system (including bone, shapes, lengths of muscles, fascias and other soft tissues); the important functional elements: alignment endurance, functional muscle strength, joint and soft tissue flexibility, release of excessive muscle contraction; inherent physical forces affecting alignment and overall body use, including muscle contraction, functional muscle strength, ligament tension, fascial drag, tissue pressure, synovial fluid pressure and joint surface tension (see Table 2-6, Balance of Forces, for a partial list of physical forces influencing the body).

Muscle

Since active movement is so essential to body use, a few comments will be made here about muscle. Functional muscle strength, i.e., strength due to neural factors, is more important than force strength. The central nervous system has an important role in integrating muscle with skeletal and arthrodial elements. Factors in the activation of muscle include the physiologic balance between synergists and antagonists, firing rate, the size of motor units. Preemptive anticipatory activity[13] and electromechanical delay[14] will be discussed further.

With training, muscle generates more force due to better activation, recruitment and coordination. Rapid coordination and alternation between concentric and eccentric contraction is important to prevent injury. Examples of muscles whose functional strength is especially important in body use are the lower abdominals and the diaphragm.

Relieving pain allows better recruitment, and also helps movement to occur. Movement per se then helps relieve pain further by enhancing availability of endogenous neurochemical pain suppressors. Even reflexes are altered by pain. The "H" reflex can disappear with pain and return with the administration of local anesthesia.

Muscle performance also depends on factors intrinsic to the muscle itself. Naturally or inherently longer muscles can undergo more shortening, while naturally shorter muscles often demonstrate more strength. Muscle fiber type, active and passive length/tension relationships,[40] and the metabolic capacity of the cardiovascular system are all important. With conditioning, the number of mitrochondria in muscles increases.

Negative physical factors include the mechanisms of muscle pain,[35] i.e., muscle tension, muscle spasm, muscle deficiency (weakness) and muscle trigger points. Another important consideration is loss of muscle flexibility. This can be loss of both physiologic elasticity (the ability of a muscle to let go of contraction) and mechanical elasticity (the ability of a muscle to yield to passive stretch). One can also consider relative flexibility.

Deconditioning syndromes affecting the somatic system are due to chronic disuse and are often more important than the original disorder or injury. These include joint stiffness with loss of normal arthrokinematics, ligament inelasticity, muscle inhibition, loss of cardiovascular and neurosensory endurance, and neuromuscular coordination deficiency due to loss of power and speed.

THE PELVIS AS BODY CENTER

A goal of good posture is to achieve the most effortless body balance. The upper weight centers (head and rib cage) should be aligned directly over the pelvis "on balance" anatomically and functionally. The pelvis is the functional and structural body center because: 1) it connects the upper and lower portions of the body anatomically, biomechanically and kinesthetically—an important example is the "heel-coccyx" connection; 2) it is the location of the body's net center of gravity; 3) it determines both spinal alignment and movement because the spine follows the pelvis; 4) it is the center of the pelvic-spinal-hip complex (PSH-C); 5) the pelvis provides the anatomical and biomechanical base for stability and mobility of the spine, allowing a fuller range of limb motion because of better limb placement; 6) it supports upper body weight centers; 7) movement into space (kinesphere) is often initiated at the pelvis and the most effortless balance and ease of movement are maintained by initiating shifts of body weight at the pelvis; 8) the structure of the pelvis is important because: a) the A-P diameter of the pelvis increases the moment arm through which the important hip extensor muscles function (these are the most important muscles for standing and walking); b) the anterior angulation of the femoral necks further increases the moment arm for the hip extensor muscles. Table 2-5 has a more complete listing.

Abdominal Muscles

The abdominal muscles have several functions: 1) they shorten from above against gravity, but the lower abdominals rotate and stabilize the pelvis, preventing hyper lumbar lordosis during sit-ups; 2) they stabilize and support the pelvis and spine; 3) as antigravity muscles, they lift the anterior pelvis; 4) they accelerate and decelerate pelvic rotation; 5) they have important roles in controlling and fine tuning pelvic and spinal alignment in the frontal and sagittal planes; and 6) they control and fine tune mobility at the lumbosacral joints and at the hip joints. By virtue of their force strength, the abdominal muscles do have an important role in supporting the lumbar spine. This is because of their continuity with the thoracolumbar fascia, posteriorly.[30] Inappropriate emphasis has often been placed on strengthening abdominals (upper) for force (to do sit-ups) and on achieving a "flat" muscular abdomen for appearance. The abdominal muscles have a vital role in the functional control of the alignment and mobility of the PSH-C that is far less known and/or utilized than it should be. The overwhelming majority of people, including health professionals themselves, do not have functional control of the pelvis. Training for function also increases strength, but training only for strength can interfere with functional control of the pelvis and spine. For example, doing crunch exercises to strengthen abdominal muscles as an end goal is often functionally counterproductive. Crunching can lead to the bad habit of compressed standing unless the person actively releases the trunk muscles and craniovertebral muscles. Later in this chapter, we shall discuss lengthening (releasing the torso and neck away from the stable pelvic platform).

A further point is that the active deceleration function of the rectus abdominis muscles (as they eccentrically contract) controls and fine tunes the amount of anterior pelvic rotation. As these muscles concentrically contract, the resulting upward lift on the pubic symphysis helps to rotate the pelvis posteriorly to decrease lumbar lordosis. The abdominal muscles are widely thought of as being productive of posterior pelvic tilt (rotation) and thus many people assume that contractions of these muscles produce lumbar kyphosis or at least lumbar "flattening." While that can occur in extreme situations, the fact is that the abdominal muscles are used effectively to fine tune neutral lumbar lordosis in order to produce neutral balanced alignment (NBA) and on balance alignment of the spine, rib cage, neck and head over the pelvis and feet. It is well to recall once again that the normal spinal curves are an essential feature of neutral alignment. It is not possible to correct a forward head alignment (so-called "forward head posture") unless pelvic rotation is corrected first. The pelvis must be brought into neutral alignment under the lumbar spine and under the head and neck. This is not to be accomplished by squeezing the buttocks together but rather by fine tuning pelvic rotation, backward and forward, with the lower abdominal, iliacus and back extensor muscles. This lifts the entire torso, neck and head. In contrast, the upper attachments of the rectus abdominis muscles pull downward on the sternum, decreasing lumbar lordosis, increasing thoracic kyphosis compressing the upper body. The pelvis rotates posteriorly toward nonneutral alignment.

The author refers to the rectus abdominis muscles as the "whoa" muscles for they must function (albeit actively) like reins for a horse (the pelvis). To control (limit) anterior pelvic rotation (forward motion) they must counter gravity. It would be very abusive to the pelvic-spinal-hip complex, and all the way up to the cranio-vertebral joints, if the pelvis were allowed to drop abruptly into full anterior rotation and/or full posterior rotation, because in those situations, the pelvic and spinal joints are jolted suddenly against their anatomic barriers and the soft tissues are suddenly stretched. The effect is just like whiplashing the neck and pelvis. Unfortunately, this is typical of patients. Thus, concentric contraction lifts the anterior pelvis and rotates it posteriorly around the hip joints and decreases lordosis. Eccentric contraction lowers the anterior pelvis and increases lordosis. The direction, distance and speed are controlled by the abdominal muscles. In the seated position, one carries out small forward and backward movements of the body's net center of gravity (located in the pelvis), by virtue of pelvic rotation about the axis of the hip joints. Ideally, the femoral heads should be stabilized by supporting the greater trochanters. The ischial tuberosities serve as the fulcra or pivot points for pelvic rotation. All this occurs under active control of the abdominal muscles, resulting in controlled functional rotation of the pelvis. Contrary to popular belief, the ischial tuberosities should not be considered to be the "sits" bones. In fact, one reason for slumping is to relieve the ischial tuberosities. Furthermore, controlled rhythmic organized abdominal pelvic-spinal-hip exercises should be carried out continually in Types I and II sitting. The ability of the pelvis to be both body center and the natural base of support while sitting is possible because of: the hip joints; the location of the net center of gravity in the pelvis at S2, just above the ischial tuberosities, and the action of the lower abdominal muscles which attach nearby to the pubic symphysis.

In sharp contrast, the upper body weight centers (head and rib cage) are located far above the pelvic fulcra. Thus, initiating movement at the upper weight centers causes large forward and backward arcs of motion of the torso in the sagittal plane (off balance with the pelvis) and large arcs of side bending in the frontal plane (off balance with the pelvis). Since the upper weight centers are then aligned off balance with regard to the natural base of support, excessive muscle activity is needed to support the body, i.e., to keep it from falling.

In sitting, with motion initiated at the pelvis (hips) by abdominal, pelvic and lumbar muscles, the pelvis rolls anteriorly and posteriorly, while the spine and head should respond by moving mostly upward and downward (vertical movement), NOT forward and backward. This explains the preservation of stability, flexibility and mobility throughout the pelvic-spinal-hip complex and the craniovertebral joints, the latter for easy head and neck movements and avoidance of downward compression of the skeletal axial. This preferred neutral alignment allows easier shoulder placement during upper extremity reaches both sideways and forward. It allows lateral shifts at the hip joints which helps maintain the alignment of the upper weight centers over the pelvis. In turn, this enables the upper extremities to release for easier and better reaching. In contrast, when movement is initiated with the upper body, the pelvis may be either dragged forward passively, along with the upper body (this also compresses the anterior hips) or the pelvis rotates posteriorly, causing slumping. Without pelvic control of body use, the result is somatic overuse, misuse, abuse and repetitive microtrauma with soft tissue injury and pain. This takes place throughout the entire body.

Finally, to reiterate an important point: when sitting in Types I or II, and when changing between Types I, II and III, moving the torso, neck and head upward and forward correctly, in neutral alignment, by fine tuning pelvic rotation, is a far different and much preferred body movement (and alignment) than is moving the torso, neck and head downward and forward as the primary or initiating event. Consider how much easier it is to sit and put on a pair of socks by bringing the hand forward by first rotating the pelvis forward. Contrast this hand position with that position resulting from backward pelvic rotation. Functionally correct abdominal-pelvic-spinal-hip movements strengthen the muscles. People who say they cannot sit in Types I and II find it easier and more enjoyable: as the muscles get stronger; when the hip joints are not compressed anteriorly; and as they learn to move.

Craniovertebral Joints (Occiput-C1-C2-C3)

The craniovertebral joints comprise a universal joint, allowing them to be the final adaptive mechanism for balancing the head. Thus, for best function, they should have natural freedom of movement in all directions. The patient makes fine adjustments in the alignment and actively inhibits (releases)[16] unnecessary suboccipital and superficial posterior and lateral neck muscle activities that would otherwise draw the head down into the neck. The release is subtle, giving a sense of lightness throughout the somatic system. In particular, the back of the head and upper neck feel as if they were moving upward and slightly forward due, in part, to the head not dropping as much as it would under the force of gravity alone. Simultaneously, the shoulder girdles should release and widen. By lengthening the neck, and widening the shoulders, there is light tension/countertension in the tissues, preventing strain in either direction.

The occipitoatlantal joint is normally aligned in slight kyphosis, causing the line of vision to be slightly below the horizontal (Frankfort plane). In actuality, there are five structural/functional curves in the spinal skeletal axis: the kyphotic curves are the occipitoatlantal, thoracic and sacrococcygeal, while the lordotic curves are the cervical and lumbar. It is helpful to point out the slight natural kyphosis at the occipitoatlantal region when training patients to release the occipitoatlantal joints and soft tissues.

The occipitoatlantal junction has many proprioceptors. There is no C1 dermatomal skin representation. This fact probably signifies the importance of kinesthetics from muscles and joints (myotomes and sclerotomes) at the C1 level. With occipitoatlantal release, proprioceptive control and alignment are improved throughout the body, as is the position and alignment of the head for better function of the brain's neural integrative sensory mechanism. Proper use of body center (the pelvis) supports and helps maintain the occipitoatlantal release because this provides a stable, mobile platform from which to release. In the author's experience, the Alexander Technique, which of course, is based on primary release of the craniovertebral joints, does not address the importance of pelvic control as do other body therapies based on techniques such as Feldenkrais, Bartenieff Fundamentals, and Pilates Exercise.

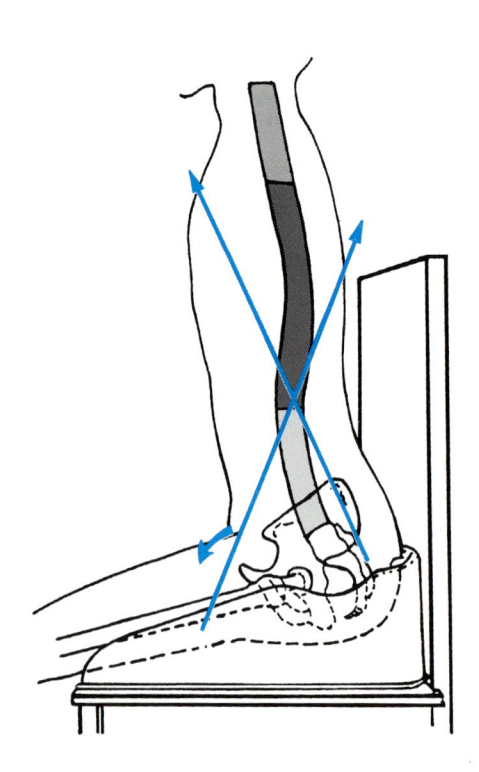

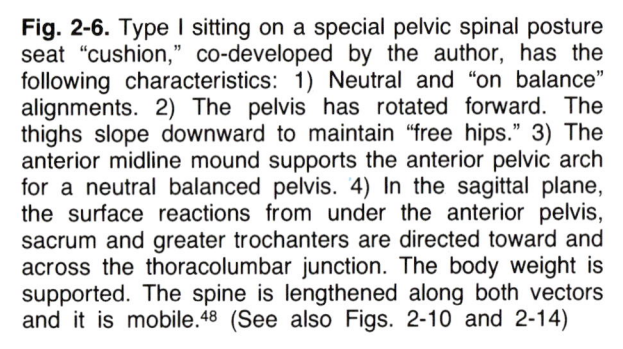

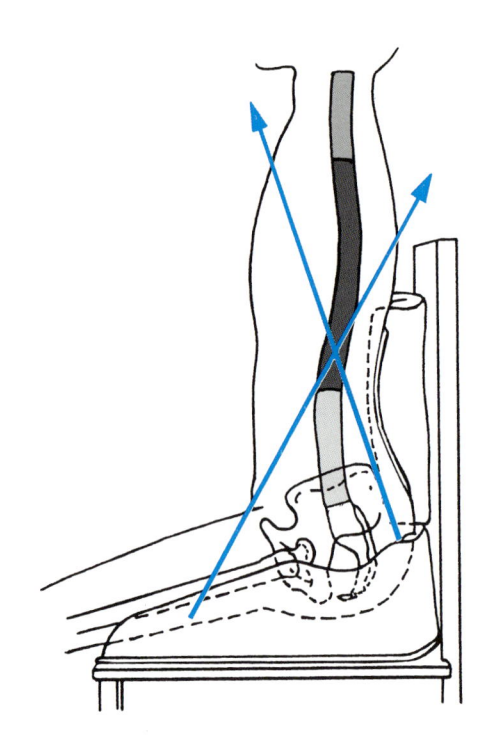

Fig. 2-6. Type I sitting on a special pelvic spinal posture seat "cushion," co-developed by the author, has the following characteristics: 1) Neutral and "on balance" alignments. 2) The pelvis has rotated forward. The thighs slope downward to maintain "free hips." 3) The anterior midline mound supports the anterior pelvic arch for a neutral balanced pelvis. 4) In the sagittal plane, the surface reactions from under the anterior pelvis, sacrum and greater trochanters are directed toward and across the thoracolumbar junction. The body weight is supported. The spine is lengthened along both vectors and it is mobile.[48] (See also Figs. 2-10 and 2-14)

Fig. 2-7. Type II sitting (See Table 2-3) on the special "cushion" in neutral balance and "on balance" alignments, with non-compressed hips (Compare Fig. 2-5). Thigh slopes reduce tissue tension at the posterior thighs and coccyx and aid lumbar lordosis. The special behind-the-back support (Fig. 2-17) contacts the back. (In Type II there is often no contact and in Type I there is none). The seat's surface reactions are directed to the spine in the sagittal plane. Lengthening (releasing) along both vectors simultaneously allows balanced tissue tension/countertension, increasing body awareness, correct alignment and freer movement.[48]

Feet

Each foot is a major source of proprioception and plays a major role in adaptation. The subtalar joint is a universal joint, as will be described in the section on walking and foot orthoses. During heel/toe walking, the foot transmits the floor's surface reactions "upward" to stabilize the knee, pelvis and lumbar spine. Heel strike also provides a fulcrum for normal movement of the pelvis and for the lumbar and upper portion of the spine. The surface reactions provide stability for those movements. Thus, walking heel/toe provides stability from below. In contrast, walking toe/heel requires stabilization from above downward.

The result of the latter is undesirable cervical and lumbar hyperkyphosis with "joint locking." This is bad body use, causing loss of motion, dysfunction, and pain. The author has seen patients after they have taken up ballet later in life and have begun to walk in the toe/heel fashion during ordinary activities. They developed nonneutral (hyperextension) of the cervical and lumbar regions with joint compression, loss of movement and pain. Signs and symptoms were relieved by reestablishing heel/toe gait, thereby reestablishing neutral alignment of the spinal curves.

Extrinsic Physical Factors (External or Environmental)

Forces in nature

Gravity, surface reactions from the ground, water and atmospheric pressures and wind resistance all affect the body's active mus-

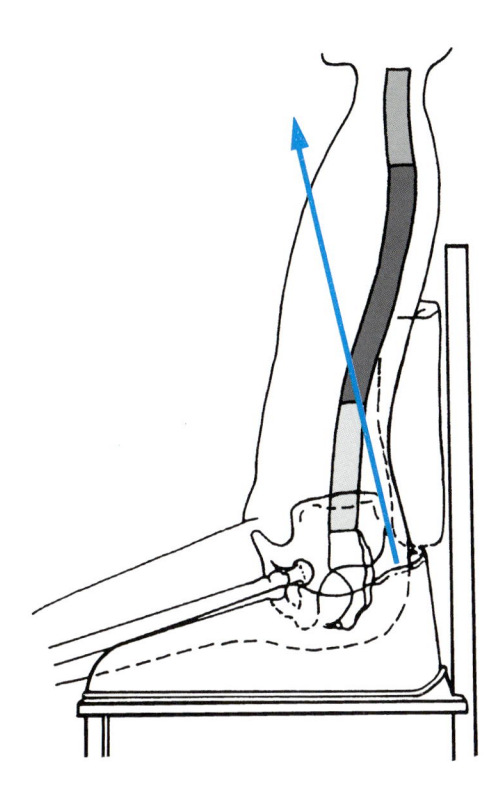

CHAPTER 2 Posture: The Process of Body Use; Principles and Determinants 41

Fig. 2-8. Type III sitting with much greater area of support for the back region up to the thoracic apex with a special back support codeveloped by the author. Compare this to Fig. 2-16. Avoids "draping over" of the thoracolumbar region, in fact, the upper torso lengthens. The pelvis is supported in neutral by the lower portion of the back support, which can be used without the special pelvic spinal support cushion, but with the cushion, the pelvis is further supported in neutral and the thighs slope downward, keeping the hips free.

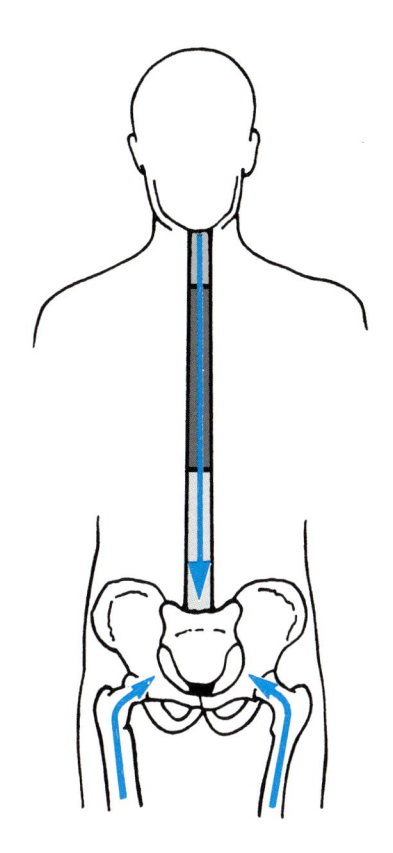

Fig. 2-9. Standing. The floor's surface reaction is directed back up to the pelvis and spine, to counter body weight.

cle requirements. All of these influence the amount of muscle activity that is needed to maintain the alignments required for good body use.

Devices that contact the body

These can be classified as orthotics if they are therapeutically designed to:

a. Relieve pain.
b. Improve or eliminate the mechanical factor(s) causing pain.
c. Prevent microtrauma by encouraging better anatomical, biomechanical and physiological relationships, i.e., good static and dynamic postures.
d. Provide immediate comfort at rest.
e. Provide comfort during movement.
f. Improve the underlying condition causing pain and dysfunction. "Progressive comfort" is therapeutic only if the underlying condition is improved.
g. Encourage correct movement, for movement feels good, relieves pain, provides kinesthetic input from skin, muscles, joints and fascia, promotes healing, and prevents disuse.
h. Provide sensory input for body awareness.
i. Provide anatomical support locally and to improve the function of the natural bases of support including the pelvis (body center) and the feet.
j. Provide surface reactions from the ground, seat and bed with enough magnitude and with proper direction to counterbalance the downward force of body weight.[7,8] (see Figs. 2-6, 2-7, 2-8, 2-9, 2-10) This provides stability externally.
k. Encourage the patient to lengthen (release) the body.
l. Help reduce pain of inflammatory origin.
m. Improve tissue structure and body function.

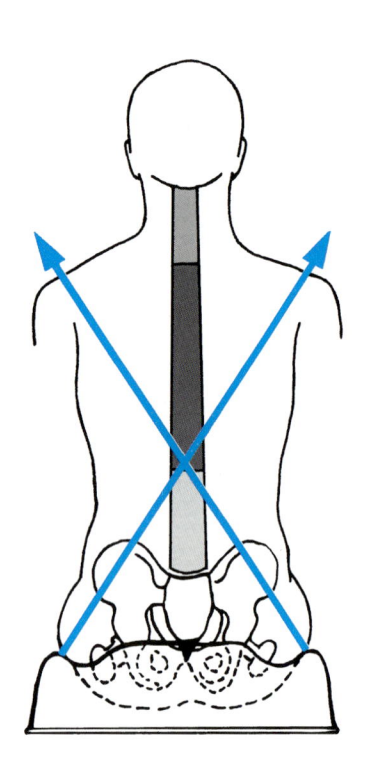

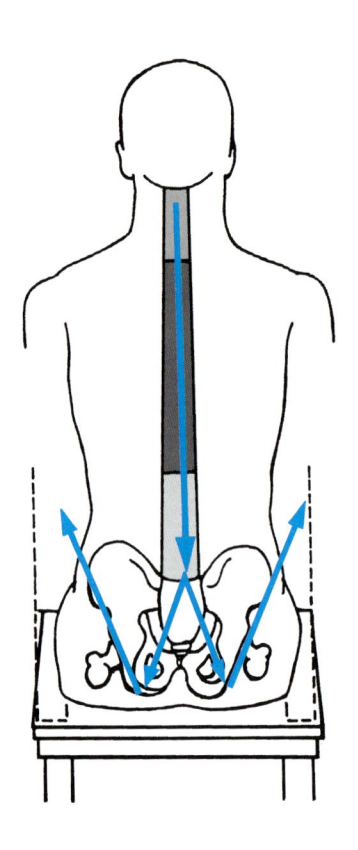

42 New Concepts in Craniomandibular and Chronic Pain Management

Fig. 2-10. Sitting on special pelvic spinal posture seat cushion. The surface reaction is directed from the trochanteric supports toward the contralateral shoulders in the frontal plane.[48]

Fig. 2-11. Sitting on a flat, firm seat. Surface reaction forces which are supposed to counter body weight are poorly directed, upward and outward, away from the body. For pelvic-spinal stability, slumped sitting results.[48]

Not every therapeutic device will do it all. However, the three most important criteria are: comfort at rest and with movement; improved body function from neutral alignment; and relief or improvement of the underlying physical problem.[8]

The nervous system has to know the location of body parts in order to help maintain good alignment. For example, when we sit too long in traditional seats and in the traditional sedentary, stagnant manner, we lose neutral alignment and mobility. Then, we fidget, trying to keep the nervous system informed of the location of body parts and to relieve pressure and discomfort. We also slump to help relieve pressure from the anterior hip joints and from the ischial tuberosities. Unfortunately, slumping causes other problems (See Fig. 2-4).

While seated, one needs body awareness and ease of movement and, of extreme importance, the balance of the upward and downward (body weight) force vectors. If external support from the chair is inadequate to help maintain a stable neutral alignment, then the body will rely on its ligament tension and excessive muscle use. A chair provides upward support: the amount depending on whether the seat is firm or soft (Figs. 2-11 and 2-12). In either case, chairs with traditional seat surfaces provide only general upward support to counterbalance body weight. If the chair is pulled away, the general upward support is removed and the user falls to the ground. Clearly, in order to provide true external stability for the body, the direction of the chair's upward surface reactions must be congruent with the downward forces of body weight to balance those forces. In other words, the upward forces must be "harnessed" and directed back to the body for support of the body. If the upward and downward forces are not congruent, there is torque and instability (Figs. 2-11 and 2-12) and the body locks down from above for stability (See Fig. 2-4).

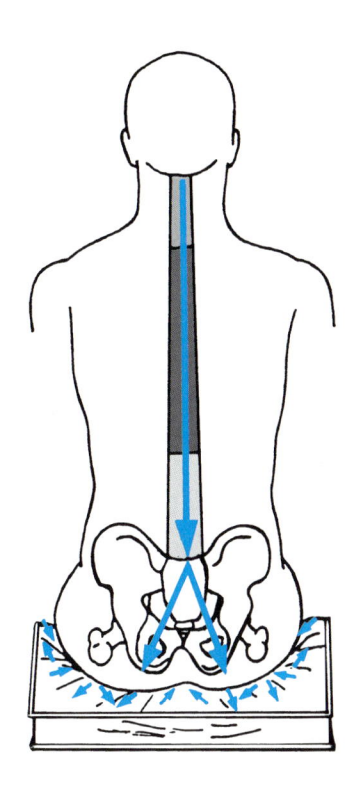

Fig. 2-12. Sitting on a soft seat. The surface reaction is weak and haphazard. For pelvic-spinal stability, slumped sitting results.[48]

The body needs to be stable. It is the basic requirement. The stability needs to be selective and physiologic so that mobility can continue in other parts of the body. Any moving part needs a stabilizing point from which to move: when the hip joints rotate they need a stable pelvis and when the arm is raised at the glenohumeral joint we need to selectively stabilize the shoulder girdle with the muscles that stabilize the scapula. If not, we lose selective stability and we resort to other sources of stability by locking up the entire upper quarter starting with the craniovertebral joints. Thus the body will sacrifice general mobility for stability if it cannot stabilize selectively. To accomplish this, it locks internally, nonphysiologically using excessive muscle activity; craniovertebral joint compression; hanging on pelvic-spinal ligaments; locking down into pelvic-spinal joints; anterior vertebral body compression. Another is sitting on the sacrum (an unnatural base of support). Clinically, the person is stable but sits in a stagnant sedentary slump (Fig. 2-4) because the stability is nonselective. It is general. Movement is lost. Sitting with the body's naturally rounded buttocks either on a flat, firm seat or on a soft seat is inherently unstable. The former is like placing an orange on a flat table. The latter is like falling on mud. Neither provides properly directed external surface reactions for support. The spine is compressed and locked, producing internal support. Sitting on a three-dimensional multicontoured surface that distributes body weight and directs surface reactions in directions that counter body weight is ideal. The seat surface should be moderately firm for support yet resilient to give proprioceptive cues. The multicontoured surface also provides proprioception. While an egg sitting in a smooth-surfaced egg cup is far more stable than an orange sitting on a flat table, sitting on a three-dimensional, multicontoured, seat surface that is firm, yet resilient, is best (See Fig. 2-14).

Newton's third law of gravity states that "every action has an equal and opposite reaction." When the action and reaction are congruent, there is stability and, when they are incongruent, there is instability. The body must achieve stability, and it does so however it can, even at the cost of overuse, misuse and abuse. In general, the direction of surface reaction forces is the most frequently overlooked and neglected determinant of posture. It is hardly ever mentioned in the literature. In the past few years, because of the increased interest in running and in gait laboratories, ground reaction forces have been mentioned with greater frequency. However, seat surface reactions have been referred to only once in the literature to the author's knowledge.[8]

The traditional flat and the soft seat surfaces of ordinary chairs, and many so-called "ergonomic chairs" and so-called posture corrective seating devices that have two-dimensional flat seat surfaces all fail to properly counteract (counterbalance) body weight (body mass and gravity). The less that surface reactions coincide with the downward force of gravity, the less that gravity can help us to maintain neutral alignment. A prevalent notion is that gravity is our enemy. But the fact is that, if we use it correctly, gravity is definitely our friend.

As for other supports, knee braces are designed to protect ligaments and to provide sensory awareness. They should have the least possible number of skin contacts consistent with the necessary amount of support. This prevents sensory distractions that would interfere with the nervous system's job of coordinating movement. Excessive brace contact points can also focus the athlete's attention to the knee and may also cause conscious overprotection.

Soft neck collars provide gentle support and proprioceptive cues. They keep us apprised of the position and relative alignment of the head and neck. They are not firm enough to prevent forceful movements. Yet they serve a useful function, for we can monitor our movement to the "early on" (i.e., first) contact between the collar, mandible or occiput. This helps us to limit ranges of motion and relieve muscles and joints from excessive activity.[8]

Duration and Frequency (Intrinsic)

Here we are talking about the duration and frequency of an activity or movement as a determinant of posture. As mentioned previously, when a region of nonneutral alignment provides stability for a flexible moving part, the nonneutral region is consistent with good body use: it is an adaptation. However, when the nonneutral alignment continues for too long, it is bad body use.

Every joint should be able to assume every alignment allowable by normal anatomy, biomechanics and physiology. However, some alignments should be assumed only intermittently and maintained for only brief periods, usually in the course of certain occupations. For example, most magazines show models in all sorts of poses that traditionally would be labeled as bad posture. When a baseball player leaps high in the air to catch a ball, he hyperextends the spine to provide stability for it and for the outstretched upper extremity. This is good body use despite the nonneutral alignment. With regard to the traditional limited way of defining good posture as standing straight or sitting straight, leaping in the air would not even fit into those limited parameters. Obviously, the traditional approach is neither practical nor accurate.

Thus, for any alignment to be evaluated in terms of its role in producing good or bad posture, one must consider all the circumstances including, but not limited to, the organization and sequence of movement used in getting into and out of the alignment, the effect of the alignment on the function of the remainder of the somatic system, and the duration for which the alignment is maintained.

Comfort and Relaxation

We have already referred to the importance of psychological factors in body use. Obviously, they are also important here, but this section concerns only the physical aspects of comfort and relaxation.

Comfort and relaxation are based on sound principles, physiologically and biomechanically, and require excellent external support. Knowing how to get into and out of the comfortable and relaxed alignments and positions is also essential. To physically relax, one should not habitually collapse. But all alignments that are possible due to natural, normal soft tissue flexibility, joint anatomy and arthrokinematics can be assumed intermittently and for relatively short durations. That would be "letting it all hang out," i.e., collapse. If habitual or for too long, it would be bad body use.

Comfort

In the author's experience, the issue of comfort is confusing to laymen and even to health professionals. This is certainly partly the result of Madison Avenue's emphasis on comfort. Comfort is important and necessary, but to consider only immediate comfort and comfort at rest is a mistake. With mechanical disorders of the moving parts and with the mechanical pain syndromes (to be described) immediate comfort or immediate discomfort can be deceiving.[8] Also, comfort and relaxation for one type of structure may mean overwork and physical stress and strain on others. For example, in slouched standing (Fig. 2-3) or slumped sitting (Fig. 2-4), many muscles relax (stop contracting), but the ligaments, joint capsules and bony elements of joints work passively to hold the body up. Then, when the alignment changes from nonneutral to "neutral balanced" and "on balance," the individual muscles can cyclically contract and rest, intermittently. The muscles support the body while the ligaments, joint capsules and bony elements rest. Thus, these structures and tissues have a reciprocal relationship. Relief of pain with movement can mean the passive (non-contractile) tissues (e.g., ligaments) are relieved of stress and strain but it can also mean that stagnant ischemic muscles are now able to contract and then rest, intermittently, improving their circulation.

Mechanical Pain Syndromes

Mechanical pain has been described[8,11] in detail. It is pain related to changes in alignment or movement. There are four types:

1. Pure alignment-related pain (traditionally called pure postural pain).
2. Pain of dysfunction.
3. Pain of contracture.
4. Pain of derangement.

Mechanical pain syndromes could also be called postural pain syndromes (body use syndromes). Posture is the common link for somatic health and fitness and in the diagnosis, treatment and rehabilitation of somatic disorders resulting from repetitive microtrauma, macrotrauma or specific diseases. Microtraumas can result from: bad habits; poorly designed or improperly used environmental factors, e.g., chairs and pillows; mental depression; nutritional deficiencies.

With pure alignment-related pain and with derangement pain, comfort is the goal. With the former, pain relief usually means there is a better alignment; with the latter, it usually means injured tissues, e.g., nerve roots, are relieved from further irritation or damage.[8]

With alignment and derangement pain, pain relief and comfort (at rest and in motion) are gauges of therapeutic benefit. With derangement pain, elimination of nerve root pain by protecting the nerve, regardless of alignment or position, is paramount.

In both dysfunction and contracture, complete or continuous comfort during treatment usually means there has been accommodation to the pain by the tissues. In those cases, the tissue abnormalities get worse over time. As one keeps accommodating the pain, the pain-free range of motion keeps shrinking.[8] For example, if it hurts sitting in neutral alignment, we slump progressively into nonneutral to avoid pain. Then, if and when pain reappears, we slump even more, trying to get comfortable again. Clearly, this increases bad body use. Voluntary active movement, diaphragmatic breathing and postural sway are greatly interfered with. Eventually, discomforts in other body areas appear. So we stand up, we bend or we stretch for temporary relief of the new discomforts and pains.

We must also consider the effect of time. When dealing with mechanical disorders and mechanical pain syndromes, it is common to find that almost any change in alignment may bring some comfort because abnormal tissues are temporarily relieved. Thus, immediate comfort may be deceiving. It may be due to the relative flexibility of tissues initially relieving stress from a less flexible area.[46] But over time, this could stress the normal area. Similarly, immediate discomfort may be deceiving. For example, patients may experience discomfort, early on, on a new mattress, pillow or chair but find that, after a few nights or days, the body has adapted and/or the device has "broken in" under the influence of body weight, shape and pattern of use.

It is not uncommon for someone to sit or lie down for three or four seconds and immediately declare that the chair or bed is uncomfortable. We must also be careful about judging comfort without considering the effect of movement. An individual may be comfortable while in a forward slump, but lateral movement in the frontal plane is restricted and uncomfortable. An alignment must be comfortable at rest and with motion to be consistent with good body use.

Physicians and other health professionals seem to have difficulty with this matter of comfort. Health professionals, especially physicians, clearly understand the fact that, although a patient with a knee effusion feels more comfortable lying supine at rest with the knee flexed on a pillow, that alignment should be avoided. It causes knee flexion contracture, and during standing and walking results in nonphysiologic intra-articular pressure and weight-bearing and loss of motion. Damage to the bony, cartilaginous and soft tissue elements of the joints occurs. Despite our appreciation of this, in other circumstances the negative aspects of comfort are often not even considered and comfort is generally accepted, incorrectly, as always being beneficial.

Clearly, when considering comfort we must consider the effect on all the tissues, over time, as well as the purpose of the comfort, i.e., is it merely accommodating a painful disorder regardless of physiologic and biomechanical principles (and overall clinical consequences), or is it relieving pain and allowing relaxation without neglecting or compromising those principles?

Posture and Pain

Recently, some clinicians have stated that bad posture does not cause pain. Of course, that would depend on how one defines posture. Although pain may not always be present with faulty posture, as the present author defines it (bad body use), such posture leads to, at least, a predisposition to pain. Such an individual is at greater risk to suffer joint, myofascial, ligamentous, nerve root and peripheral nerve injury from repetitive micro or macrotrauma.

Two common areas of dysfunction are T12-L1 and C2-C3. Pain may be absent because alignments and movements affecting those areas are purposefully avoided or the individual is too inflexible to incorporate the dysfunctional tissues into the movement. Another example is a derangement at C5-C6. Active extension movement would be painful. But pain is avoided by assuming a forward head/neck alignment that prevents extension at C5-C6. This can be voluntary or involuntary. (Relative flexibility[46] and compensatory poor posture result from decreased flexibility.) If acute, it is an adaptive compensation and, if chronic, it is nonadaptive (see below). The latter produces its own problems. Sometimes pain is prevented by structural changes (e.g., osteophytes) that block movements. Another reason for lack of pain with chronic bad postural alignment may be adaptation of the peripheral nociceptors and/or adaptation of the central nervous system.

With or without pain, people with bad posture often complain of other very important symptoms such as body fatigue, heaviness of a region, and generalized stiffness. The author has seen a number of victims of automobile accidents, months after the injury, who were referred because of pain, but, on careful questioning, admitted to having no pain. Instead, they felt miserable because of the other symptoms. They were surprised to learn that pain is only one symptom of a significant somatic disorder and that it is not always present. It follows that relief of pain is not always synonymous with recovery.

One author[11] defines bad or poor posture as "those which reduce or accentuate the normal curves enough to place the ligamentous structures under full stretch and to eventually be productive of pain." That definition is limited, for it does not incorporate the movement or the dynamic aspects of body use.

Relaxation

This term is related to comfort at rest, not during motion. Relaxation must not cause disuse, misuse or abuse. Chronic disuse is an important cause of the deconditioning syndrome. When resting in bed and when sitting leaned back in proper alignment (Type III sitting), the muscles can relax. In contrast, when sitting slumped, the muscles relax, i.e., are not contracting, but it is an unhealthy "relaxation" because the muscles are stagnant and ischemic, and they also do not provide normal kinesthetic input. The individual length/tension[40] relationships are disturbed because the joints are in nonneutral alignment. The muscles are unbalanced, i.e., some are too short, some are too long. Rhythmic organized controlled abdominal pelvic-spinal-hip exercises would allow the muscles to: relax intermittently; improve their circulation; improve the balance of their functional strengths and their lengths; and improve the sensory information from muscle.

ADAPTATION AND COMPENSATION (INTRINSIC)

Adaptation is defined as a change in structure, function or form that produces better adjustment of an animal or plant to its environment.[34] The key words are "better adjustment." *Compensation* is defined as the counterbalancing of a defect in the structure or function of a part by greater activity or development of another or other parts.[34]

The author views adaptive compensatory posture as good posture if it serves a useful purpose for the body as a whole. It follows that nonadaptive compensatory posture is bad body use. An example of the latter may be found in the patient who stabilizes the body from the top down with the craniovertebral joints, cervical spine and dental occlusion because of inadequate stability provided by the feet and pelvis. When that patient walks or stands statically on one foot, it seems that even greater excess muscle activity and joint compression are present at the head, face, neck and shoulders.

Anatomically and functionally, spinal curves can counter balance and compensate for each other. If one or more curves either increase or decrease, another can do the same in the opposite direction. Thus, the total body remains in weight balance (the person does not fall), but regionally and segmentally the tissues are out of balance. Again, scoliosis does not necessarily produce bad posture in the functional sense of body use. As stated previously, if the flexibility and mobility of the soft tissues and joints are maintained within the curves, the increased curvatures can still be consistent with good body use.

It is important for the pelvis to remain capable of compensating for curves higher in the spine. Lumbar curves are more difficult to compensate for than are thoracic and cervical curves. When the spine and pelvis compensate, the surface landmarks and/or weight centers may appear to be reasonably aligned one over the other "nearly on balance" but, in reality, the spinal segments may be either hyperflexed or hyperextended (nonneutral alignments), with increased curvatures. Alternatively, the spine's individual curves may be too straight (decreased) which is also nonneutral alignment of spinal segments. In either case, loss of motion, excessive abnormal soft tissue tension, and compressive forces occur due to imbalances.

TREATMENT
Rationale

Correct treatment for improving body use starts with correct diagnosis. Most often, this is arrived at solely by correlating anatomy, biomechanics and neuromuscular-articular function with the patient's presenting complaints, physical examination, and a detailed related history. The physical examination is a sequential analysis of static and dynamic structure and function of the total body as an integrated and interrelated unit of body regions and individual muscles, joints and connective tissues. Laboratory data is almost always of secondary importance except with a specific disorder such as a metabolic or inflammatory disease, a fracture or a herniated disc with active radiculopathy.

Sometimes a bad postural alignment results from one or more injuries from a single trauma or from repetitive microtraumas. Besides the initial injuries, adaptive and nonadaptive compensations can cause pain and stiffness. When the neck is thrown backward and forward, for example, symptoms can develop from several causes. When thrown backward from resting length without warning, the neck's anterior soft tissues suddenly activate the peripheral and central neuromuscular systems. There is immediate activation of muscle spindles in the overstretched anterior muscles, causing a spinal cord level reflex contraction of the (extrafusal) skeletal muscle fibers. The purpose is to restore the resting length of the muscle. This is the same as the knee-jerk mechanism (improperly referred to as a deep tendon reflex). The muscle is in direct continuity with the fascia, which is also traumatized. When the head and neck are thrown backward, the posterior soft tissues shorten and slacken. Then, as the head flies forward rapidly, the spindles in the posterior muscles are suddenly stretched and activated from the prior overshortened state, magnifying the effect of the change. Both the longer posterior skeletal muscles, which cover multiple segments, and often the shorter posterior segmental muscles, contract reflexively. The short rotatory muscles are also often affected.

In response to tissue injury, compensations develop to reduce pain, to balance the head correctly and to maintain neurosensory input. Pain often persists even after the acute and subacute inflammation subsides and even after adequate time for tissue healing has passed. The pain may be due to hypermobility of joints which results from inadequate ligament/bone attachment and ligament laxity. There may be pain due to hypomobility which results from shortened muscles, fascia, joint capsules and ligaments. Both can have associated osseofibrous and/or myofascial trigger points.[18,6] Movement is painful. Sudden stretching of the fascial/muscle unit causes reflex protective shortening. The sudden lengthening of these tissues during active or passive movements causes activation of muscle spindles resulting in muscle contraction, fascial strains, and resistance to movement, which are often painful.

Malalignments develop because of compensations and adaptations due to: muscle weakness; fascial drag resulting in excessive non-physiologic internal forces and abnormal kinesthetics; the sense of heaviness of body parts; fatigue; loss of arthrokinematics; painful movements; the desire for comfort at rest causing nonneutral alignments; joint and soft tissue imbalances; inflexibility of soft tissues (tight or resistant) or worse, stiffness (rigid), both with motion barriers; hyper or hypomobility of muscles and joints causing distortion of peripheral proprioceptors resulting in diminished, excessive and/or delayed signals to the spinal cord and brain. All dispose to further injuries.

Techniques

Treatment techniques must restore kinesthetics and movement; physiologic soft tissue lengths; muscle length/tension[40] relations; neuromuscular reflex responses; coordination between synergistic and antagonistic muscles; muscle and joint flexibility and mobility; functional strength; and endurance and physiologic alignments. Some treatment techniques are primarily directed at pain reduction, e.g., acupuncture and strain-counterstrain.[20] Others are primarily directed at tissue balance and function, e.g., muscle energy and myofascial release. Manual soft tissue techniques, including but not limited to myofascial release, craniosacral,[12] strain and counterstrain[20] and trigger point therapy[18,6] are others important for restoration of postural alignment.

In today's world, various injection techniques are also often helpful diagnostically and therapeutically, in addition to being cost effective. These include therapeutic injection for myofascial and osseofibrous trigger points and occasionally for tendinitis, bursitis, and arthritis; diagnostic trigger points, nerve blocks and epidural steroids.

Used in conjunction with other appropriate treatment methods, injections often shorten treatment significantly by improving accuracy of diagnosis, by relieving pain and increasing passive and active motions. Alignment improves, for the body no longer needs to follow the path of least pain. This is important today, in view of financial restraints imposed on patients and providers by today's insurance/economic climate. Also, since patients and health professionals travel more often than in the past, both are less available for protracted treatment programs. For example, when there is time for only one visit before a trip, a well-placed injection improves the likelihood that pain will be reduced. Also patients today are also often active in exercise and sports and want to resume them sooner. In acute and in some subacute cases, injections can play the major role. In chronic cases, they can be complementary.

Various active exercise techniques restore motion, flexibility, tissue length, functional strength and sometimes force strength. We often use active slow paced, short range of motion pain-free exercise, then faster paced short range exercise progressing to greater ranges of motion with slow and fast paced movement. Exercises to train rapid pain-free concentric and especially eccentric active muscle contractions are important because most sports injuries occur during eccentric deceleration movements. Cardiovascular type (non-impact) aerobic exercises are also important, particularly for treating fibromyalgia.

In the past, physical treatment was mostly physical modalities. Although relief was possible, it was usually short term. Physical modalities still have a role. Cold applications are valuable in acute injuries to relieve pain, to modulate inflammatory response, to prevent excessive swelling, and to relieve pain from tendinitis and bursitis. Moist heat is of particular value for muscle relaxation and for treating subacute and often chronic pains from muscle, fascia and ligaments and to relieve stiffness from rheumatoid and osteoarthritis. It is helpful in fibromyalgia. Some people also respond well to cold for muscle, fascial and ligamentous disorders. The choice of cold versus heat should depend on allowing sufficient blood flow for tissue nutrition, maintaining sufficient inflammatory response for the healing process to proceed yet avoiding excessive swelling and tissue pressure, muscle inhibition and atrophy and, of course, pain. Today, therapy should go far beyond modalities. We know that function and structure need to be restored through tissue remodeling. This occurs in response to manual therapy, body awareness training, movement therapy, physiologic physical stress from exercise and external supports. Certain specific body therapies, including Alexander Training, Feldenkrais, Bartenieff Fundamentals, Pilates exercise and others, can be important in helping to establish functional strength, tissue balance, body awareness and organization of movement. The latter, along with the control of surface reactions from both ground and seat surfaces for balancing downward and upward biomechanical forces, are the most overlooked elements of treatment even by otherwise well-trained and skilled doctors and therapists.

A few specific examples of observation and evaluation of body use will be described in the second part of this chapter.

The choice of individual treatment techniques and their sequence, duration and frequency should vary from patient to patient. In acute situations, relief of pain and prevention of tissue dysfunction s are paramount. Many times only a short treatment course is needed. However, if practical, even these patients would benefit from at least familiarity with body awareness and body movement. With therapy, even small improvements of tightness and/or contracture can cause one to feel much freer in movement and lighter, even if the examiner can barely detect increases in ranges of motion, and the patient's tissue resilience hardly feels palpably different. Nevertheless, the patient feels better because of decreased pain and because of subtle improvement in proprioception, sense of movements and better fine neuromuscular balance of his joints, muscles and connective tissues.

The extent of treatment often depends on the patient's ability to learn better body use. Detailed discussion of individual techniques for pain relief and soft tissue mobilization and stabilization is beyond the scope of this chapter. But a few points are well worth mentioning: 1) Any activity causing pain to radiate farther down an extremity should be stopped or modified. 2) Generally, treatment should be as pain free as possible especially for derangement, (mechanical pain category 4) and/or alignment (category 1) related pains. Pain related to tissue dysfunction (category 2) and/or contracture (category 3) may cause temporary pain. We simply wish to stress the importance of educating the patient about the meaning of posture, the importance of movement, and, of course, about the various principles and determinants of posture, including the proper role of comfort and relaxation.

Movement is important for healing of all somatic tissues and for natural pain control. Patients should learn to move and will want to because it feels good. Treatment should provide the patient with movement that can be incorporated into daily activities at work, in exercise, or in both sports and artistic athletics (e.g., dance).

When correcting dysfunctions, pain may temporarily increase during the first few repetitions of a movement. This is acceptable, and a recognized phenomenon, but movement that continues to cause the same or more pain should be discontinued.[11] Pain that radiates farther down to the lower extremity should be stopped. Any activity that causes pain to shift from the extremity to the low back is good (centralization of pain).[11] Other techniques used in treating dysfunctions avoid pain.[20] This is also true when treating contractures, but temporary increases of pain and soreness may also occur. Then, as new ranges of motion are achieved, pain may temporarily increase again. With dysfunction and with contracture, the addition of an anti-inflammatory medication is often helpful early on in the course of treatment. Pain relief is obviously important for sheer comfort, but it also allows the patient to concentrate on the essentials of the physical treatment program and to apply them to daily functions.

Stable neutral alignment, of course, is a major determinant of body use, perhaps the single most important, greatly affecting movement. To assist the treatment process, it is often helpful to ask oneself the following questions about alignment:

1. What type(s) of alignment does the patient manifest and want to achieve?
2. Where are the alignments present?
3. How do these alignments relate to the presence of symptoms, alleviation of symptoms and/or to specific functional losses?
4. Which ones of the following are providing the mobility and/or stability: muscle activity, ligament tension, joint locking or seat surface reaction?
5. How can we improve or correct the alignment? Which determinants need therapeutic intervention?

Societal and environmental demands have contributed to bad postural habits, including slumped sitting. Also, evidence exists that anteriorly the body has more muscle spindles than it has in the posterior muscles. This would tend to foster slumping because slacking the muscles avoids reflex muscle contraction and relieves pain from those muscles. Unfortunately, the slump provides comfort at rest but interferes with movement. Movement is restricted and can be painful. The slump worsens over time by adapting and compensating. It is estimated that about 50% of back and neck pains arise from anterior tissues, i.e., those that are relaxed by slumping forward. Clearly, the relief of pain by slumping is not synonymous with recovery. The relief of pain is just accommodating the dysfunction. Pain relief is temporary and the slump is progressive.

The importance of the pelvis, the body center, in developing balanced neutral alignment and ease of movement is crucial. Over the longer term, training and education help us learn to subjugate harmful reflexes and harmful habits to those alignments and movements which are "intelligent" and which provide comfort over time, along with safety and ease of movement. We can develop good functional habits and utilize helpful reflexes. Yet we should always be able to consciously monitor our proprioception and movements to make adaptations possible.

In fact, sometimes patients move best after they have been injured, for finally they are paying attention and maintaining self imposed, stabilized neutral balance. (This is true only for the spine–certainly not for the extremities.)

Elderly people often have difficulty rising from chairs and may fall backward frequently. For many, those problems would decrease if they had some familiarity with organization and sequence of movement and awareness of the pelvis' role for the initiation of body movement. Training in organization and sequence of movement and becoming aware of individual movements is analogous to someone at the piano playing several successive (sequential) chords on the piano rather than playing all the notes at once. If the pelvis were first rotated forward, beneath the upper weight centers and the knees moved anterior to the ankles, large "swings" of the upper body's center of gravity and the overuse of trunk and hip flexor muscles and back extensor muscles would be eliminated. Frequency of falling would decrease.

Exercise, important in the rehabilitative treatment process, has also become an activity of daily living. Health professionals must be involved in the choice of exercise, the equipment used for exercise and for pain relief and functional support and the technique of body use if we are to diminish the growing epidemic of somatic injuries. Based on a practice experience of over 20 years, for many or most patients whom we have seen for the first time, a major source of bad body use and a major place where bad body use is practiced and reinforced has been exercise. Exercise was most often performed only for a single, circumscribed goal: body appearance, general recreation, cardiopulmonary fitness and/or for force strength of a specific muscle(s). Principles and determinants ("Ps and Ds") that would have improved body (somatic) awareness, body centering, organization of movement and functional strength, had rarely already been learned. These, along with the other "Ps and Ds," are applicable to all exercise and should be taught by health professionals having practical knowledge of anatomy, biomechanics, physiology and somatic functions and dysfunctions. To help avoid patient exercise injuries, health professionals should have a greater role in preparing the body for exercise and in educating and training patients in body use.

Exercise has several beneficial aspects: 1) flexibility gained by warm-ups and stretching; 2) functional muscle strengthening by developing coordination between agonists and antagonists. (The latter is especially important for faster movements because joints are protected when initial active inhibition of the antagonist muscle switches to rapid facilitation and contraction of the antagonist to slow down the movement toward the end of the range.);[15] 3) balancing of the force strength of muscles through weight-lifting and other resistive exercises; 4) endurance training through aerobic exercise; 5) anaerobic fitness, and, of course, 6) internalization of good technique through education and training. Breathing exercises and technique are essential to all somatic treatment. They improve body awareness and movement into three planes as the inner space of the body expands into the outer space (kinesphere)[9] surrounding the body.

Overall, regarding pain relief and restoring tissue function and structure, treatment should be as specific as possible. Self body imaging and cues from oral instructions and/or hands-on physical contact are often enough in the presence of normal tissues (pure alignment pain) because alignment, body attitude and movement can improve rapidly.

In cases with dysfunctions and/or contractures with hypermobility or hypomobility, muscle weakness or muscle spasm, instructions and cueing are not enough. Hands-on mobilization treatment techniques are necessary. With hypermobility, special selective stabilization exercises and sclerotherapy (prolotherapy) injections[18] are available. External (environmental) supports, (e.g., seats or pillows) for added comfort, support and stabilization in neutral are also important.

With tissue dysfunction and tissue contracture, the midpoint of anatomical and functional neutral range shifts (see Figs. 2-1, 2-2). A spinal joint, pathomechanically restricted so as to be unable to flex, has had a shift in the neutral range and the midpoint of the neutral range ("neutral point") toward extension. Flexion is incomplete. Then, if the patient injures the "normal" anterior soft tissues, extension becomes acutely painful. Yet, as long as the kinetic chain remains open, he can still be comfortable flexed, in bed, in the fetal position because the kinetic chain remains open. The chronically short posterior tissues are not loaded, and the freshly injured anterior tissues are relaxed. However, standing and flexing the head and neck to the chest can cause back pain because the chronically shortened posterior tissues are now part of a closed kinetic chain and are under load in that kinetic chain. This can be a perplexing situation. When treating such a patient, after acute pain from the inciting episode is controlled, passive treatment of muscles to relieve spasm and eliminate protective reflexes should begin. Then, start local active exercise in the pain-free range. It helps if such a patient lies on his side with his fingers on the involved segment(s)—thus increasing his localization and awareness of movement—while slowly carrying out active, short-arc movements throughout the pain-free range. Then, advance the patient by having him carry out those movements while sitting and standing. Next, the exercise pace and the arcs of movement are increased (but always in the pain-free range). This approach helps to progressively increase pain-free physiologic motion, and to achieve a more balanced "neutral point," structurally and functionally, correcting the underlying problem.

With proper treatment of pain, management of pain and patient education and training, the causes of bad posture can be helped or eliminated in many cases. Goals vary. In chronic cases, this takes time, because tissue remodelling takes time. During that process, pain-free movements increase, but pain often continues when movement reaches the end of the movement range until abnormal tissue motion barriers no longer exist. At that time, normal ranges of motion have been reestablished and the quality and resilience of the tissues at the end ranges have become normal. During this gradual process, the pain fades. Sometimes pain decreases despite the presence of abnormal motion. Reasons vary. Probably peripheral nociceptors adapt.

EVALUATION–AN OVERVIEW

1. The somatic system is designed for motion. The ultimate goal of treatment is to improve motion, at least to some degree, qualitatively and quantitatively. This applies to individual joints, muscles and to the entire body. Interestingly, changes in joint and soft tissue mobility that are just perceptible to the examiner's fingers seem to be magnified by the patient's nervous system, for the patient feels significant changes in mobility even under these circumstances. For that reason, even one who is very stiff should be encouraged to increase motion, even slightly.
2. A complete hands-on examination evaluates all the joints, muscles and connective tissue (fascia, ligaments, tendons and joint capsules) for voluntary and involuntary[12] active movements, ordinary passive movements, and accessory joint play movements. A complete history and sophisticated physical examination of the somatic system correlated with anatomy, biomechanics and the patient's habits of body use are also essential.

When asking a patient about back pain and sitting, for example, it is important to ask at least how the patient sits, what type of seat is used, what and how movements are performed and how the patient gets into and out of a chair. All too often patients are merely asked, "Do you have pain sitting and is it worse than standing?"

Further, one learns a great deal about a patient's body awareness, tissue resiliency and mobility by visually observing how he or she moves and by palpating function of tissue, both at rest and during active voluntary movement. An example is to observe the patient's movement on a treadmill. Here, mobility of the scapula, trunk rotation, head/neck alignment and the heel/toe gait pattern can be evaluated. The examiner can even become quite adept at diagnosing segmental spinal restrictions and specific areas of joint dysfunction by correlating such observations with the history. Another important and basic procedure is to lightly rest the hand on the patient to evaluate inherent tissue motion.

Until recently, in injury evaluation, the functional concept of musculoskeletal disability rating was considered to be nonmedical. Medical evaluation was based on structure, i.e., loss of a part and losses of active and passive ranges of motion of an injured part (but not in the context of function). There are dramatic changes going on now. Functional testing is very much in vogue, as applied to motion analysis, pressure distribution, force plate studies of floor reactions in gait, joint angle measurements, aerobic and anaerobic cardiovascular fitness, endurance, pulmonary function, dynamic assessment of strength, lifting evaluation and job or sports-specific functional ability. The practical problems with functional testing are interpreting the individual tests, and then integrating their results. Furthermore, it is necessary to establish the validity of the instrumentation for all these tests.

Clinicians should not rely entirely on test data when assessing function. The importance of the sophisticated physical examination, to include specific structure and observation and palpation of function, cannot be overemphasized. Judges at athletic events such as Olympic gymnastics evaluate quality of technique and form. The author believes that health professionals should take a similar approach, adding the functional information to the history and to the remainder of the detailed physical examination in order to guide the patient to better body use. For example, dysfunctional body use while walking on a treadmill can be observed and ultimately corrected.

OBSERVATION AND PALPATION
Observation of Breathing

Observing a patient's breathing is a remarkable way of determining his awareness of the body's interrelated structure and function, including three-dimensional movement. Further, breathing exercise is an excellent way of developing a patient's skills in those areas.

To evaluate for correct, active diaphragmatic breathing, observe and palpate the lower rib cage anteriorly, laterally and posteriorly. With good body use, the spine is in neutral alignment, allowing the chest cavity to expand three-dimensionally into the "outer space" immediately around the body.[9] Expansion of the lower rib cage posteriorly is especially helpful for many patients with low back pain, because expanding it causes the thoracolumbar region to lengthen and widen, stretches the paralumbar muscles and fascia all the way down to the pelvis, and relieves thoracolumbar compression. As opposed to diaphragmatic breathing, breathing with accessory muscles of respiration strains the neck and the temporomandibular apparatus. Those muscles simply are not strong enough to repetitively lift the torso in breathing, and the practice also causes downward compression of the head on the neck. Breathing affects the entire body, and correct breathing promotes balanced alignments for good body use.

Observation of Rising from a Chair

Another important activity readily evaluated for body awareness and organization of movement is rising from a chair. External movement should be initiated at the body's center, the pelvis. In preparation for rising, preemptive anticipatory activity[13] and electromechanical delay[14] occur in appropriate muscles. The former creates so-called "dynamic stiffness" to improve muscle function, and the latter is the brief isometric contraction which stretches the series elastic component in muscle just prior to the external movement. Movement is then initiated at the pelvis by first rotating it forward until a sacral angle of about 34° is reached. This is approximately the upper end of its normal range of neutral alignment, i.e., 20-34°. Since the spine follows the pelvis, as the pelvis rotates forward, normal neutral spinal curves appear (assuming the spine is flexible). When anterior pelvic rotation nears the end of its range, the normal lumbar spine will also be near its full extension.

Initiating movement with the pelvis is far better than initiating it with the spine, especially when the latter is already in hyperkyphosis or hyperlordosis. It is easier for the pelvis to lift the spine (as the pelvis rotates forward) physiologically than it is for the spine to pull the pelvis along with it. One major reason for this is the fact that the body's net center of gravity is in the pelvis at the S2 level, just above the ischial tuberosities which are its pivot points for rotation. The pelvis actually rotates around the femoral heads which are close to: the ischial tuberosities, the lumbosacral joints and the lumbar portion of the spine. Thus, when the pelvis rotates even a small amount, it has a greater effect on the movements of the spine and torso above it. In contrast, if the spine and torso move first they must make very large movements in order to effect small movements in the pelvis. This results in large swings of the torso which cause off-balance and nonneutral alignments. When the spine is in nonneutral alignment, movement is limited. It is akin to the term "functional ankylosis."[15] Only when the pelvis is rotated forward can the upper body weight centers, the head and rib cage, be aligned over it. As the spine follows the pelvis, they are, in turn, automatically lifted predominantly upward and slightly forward. The body becomes taller. It is dynamically connected functionally and structurally. It is aligned for easier movement or for physiologic rest, without unnecessary exertion or physical stress.

As the pelvis rotates forward (iliacus muscle), the knees move forward, to or past the ankles. Then, to rise, muscle function is important: 1) Lower rectus abdominis muscles continue to support and stabilize the pelvis. They allow fine-tuned control of neutral pelvic alignment in two ways: a) by pulling up on the anterior pelvic arch and b) by releasing that pull. The lower rectus abdominus muscles decelerate anterior pelvic rotation. A patient can learn to place the pelvis in any degree of rotation he wishes, at any time; 2) The low back, buttock and thigh muscles push and lift the body off the ground by voluntary contractions and stretch reflexes;[16] 3) Some observers believe there is a natural reflex response from the feet that affords release and lengthening at the craniovertebral joints; and 4) Unnecessary and/or excessive contractions of thoracic and neck muscles, attached to the head, are actively inhibited (released), allowing the craniovertebral joints to remain free, noncompressed. This release is an "active undoing" rather than an "active doing." Inhibition has also been given another meaning, i.e., to increase the time interval between stimulus and response long enough to give us a choice of physical behavior. Loss of movement and proprioception at the O/A and at C1-C2-C3 joints cause and contribute to distorted proprioception and to restricted movement throughout the body.

Alexander referred to the use of the head and neck as the "primary control"[16] but, obviously, the craniovertebral joints are not the whole story. The head needs a mobile, stable base from which to release and lengthen. The pelvis, the body's center, and the feet provide this. As a result of stabilizing and releasing, the body can lengthen both above and below the pelvis. The released upper spine "floats" upward, perhaps aided by eccentric contractions of the deep short intervertebral muscles. During the process of lengthening, the muscles and connective tissues are more balanced on all sides of each of the joints. The posterior pelvis moves slightly caudally because the lower rectus abdominis muscle's lifting function rotates the pelvis posteriorly, normal hamstring tension rotates it posteriorly and the inherent weight of the posterior pelvis carries the pelvis caudally. An awareness of light, easy tension/countertension develops between the upper and lower portions of the body, primarily through the fascia and muscles, which are continuous. One might liken these connections to a fine thread of glass being stretched lightly at both ends. If it stretches too much, it breaks. If the two ends are brought together, it slackens. This balanced, light tension/countertension connection between body parts is mechanical, neuroreflexive and kinesthetic. In the body, the light tension/countertension provides awareness in both initiating and then sequencing body movement. As the connective tissue tugs on adjacent muscle, the muscle spindles are loaded, which initiates subclinical muscle stretch reflexes, eventually causing further tightness and imbalances in the muscle.

Often, people starting out in Alexander training painfully strain their necks as they try to lengthen. It occurs because they incorrectly try to lengthen the neck by actively moving the head/neck upward rather than correctly releasing (inhibiting) the muscles to let the neck "float" up, i.e., "undo rather than do." One of the Alexander Technique instructions is to *lengthen* the neck and *widen* the shoulders. The shape of the upper trapezius muscles and fascia is triangular. It attaches from shoulder to shoulder laterally, to the midline of the neck and along the base of the skull. With some concentration, the patient can feel light tension/countertension, a sense of connectedness horizontally from shoulder to shoulder and vertically from the back of the head, along the neck and thoracic portions of the spine. Simultaneous balanced lengthening and widening prevent undue attempts at overlengthening and overwidening. To balance the soft tissues and joints in the two planes, we must release in both directions simultaneously, for that is the only way we can lengthen the neck and widen the shoulders at the same time. Otherwise, as the neck would lengthen, the shoulders would narrow. Similarly, as the shoulders would widen, the neck would shorten and compress. To reiterate, we must elongate (release or inhibit) in both directions, simultaneously.

So, as we rise from a chair correctly, the upper body continuously moves upward and slightly forward, being physically lifted and supported by the pelvis and lower extremities. The torso, upper extremities, head and neck remain free. This is good body use. The emphasis is on body centering, soft tissue balance, body mobility, stability and functional strength—not on force strength.

In contrast, the typical "bad habit" method of rising from a chair is to initiate by moving the head and torso forward and downward, past the pelvis and knees, and then, extend the head on the neck. The body moves downward before it moves upward. This is bad body use. As the movements occur, there are: a large forward and downward excursion of the upper body weight's center of gravity, requiring lots of muscle work to bring it back up again; nonneutral alignment of the entire spine in the sagittal plane and head extension with compression downward into the neck. In essence, when the body is not centered, the pelvis cannot lead. When the head, neck and upper torso "lock" in nonneutral, they pull the lower torso and pelvis along with them, forward and downward. Overall, pelvic-spinal mobility is greatly diminshed because joints in nonneutral in one plane have mechanical limitation or loss of movement into other planes.[17] Also, muscle stretch reflexes and muscle length/tension relations are not physiologic.

Observation of Sitting Down

To sit down correctly, movement of the torso is initiated at the pelvis. The downward pull of the abdominal muscles at their attachments to the sternum and ribs contribute to the downward movement. The entire spine lengthens. While the lower torso moves downward, toward the chair, the upper torso and neck lengthen (float upward) as the muscles release. The craniovertebral joints remain free. The muscles and fascia are dynamically connected and light, balanced tension/countertension provides kinesthetic awareness. Lengthening of the entire spine, while moving from standing to sitting down, requires release (subtle movement) at both ends, in opposite directions. Neutral alignment helps this. In essence, the upper body releases, allowing it to remain lengthened (giving a sense of it moving upward) as we sit downward.

In contrast, when sitting down is performed incorrectly, the movement is initiated by the head extending on the neck and compressing it. The head literally pushes the neck and the remainder of the body downward into the chair. The entire spine is compressed, restricted and heavy; body awareness is severely compromised; and spinal joints are locked in nonneutral, prohibiting motion.

Observation of Other Activities

We also observe the following: sequence of movements while bending forward; head and neck movements while swallowing; weight distribution at the feet before, during and after rising on the toes; walking; and during all other activities. It is important to have an appreciation of the principles and determinants involved in each activity in order to teach the patient to make changes.

THE ROLE OF NONNEUTRAL ALIGNMENT IN POSTURE

In some activities, it is actually good posture, good body use, for the upper body weight centers to be temporarily anatomically "off balance," i.e., not aligned over the pelvis. Two examples follow:

1. In posturally correct walking, the "free" released head and neck (already lengthened) actually move upward and slightly forward. Thus, first, the upper body weight center is brought slightly ahead of the pelvis, i.e., "off balance." As a result, light tension/countertension develops between the back of the head and neck, the low back and the heels. This dynamic connectedness signals the brain to reestablish alignment and balance to prevent the body from falling forward and downward. Thus, the pelvic weight center is then shifted forward for realignment and rebalancing underneath the upper body, causing a forward step to be taken.

    Contrast this with the frequently seen posturally incorrect standing and walking habit characterized by the lower extremities and pelvis moving forward while the upper body torso continuously leans downward and backward (Fig. 2-3). Movement is confined to the sagittal plane. Walking in this matter is functionally inefficient and structurally damaging, causing, for example, hyperextension with compression at the thoracolumbar junction.

2. Bending forward while standing is the second example of good body use while in temporary "off balance" alignment. The spine's normal flexible curves allow independent movement of the three weight centers, i.e., the head, rib cage and pelvis. Thus, in normal (or customary) forward bending, the head, cervical, thoracic and lumbar portions of the spine flex in that

sequence. (Forward bending can also be performed by dynamically, selectively stabilizing the lumbar spine while bending forward at the hips.) As the head and torso move forward and downward out of neutral alignment, a distinct light stretch-tension develops in the posterior soft tissues throughout the length of the spine, and a subtle counter-tension develops in the posterior soft tissues connecting the pelvis to the heels. The tension/countertension provides proprioceptive cues for sensory awareness. Monitoring speed and distance according to sensory memory allows safer movement.

During forward bending, correctly performed, the upper body weight centers first move forward of the body's net center of gravity, located at the pelvis. When the lumbar flexion component is completed (normally 45°), the pelvis begins to rotate forward, then stops when forward bending is completed. Thus, there is progressive development of a distinct tension/countertension first above and then below the pelvis. This is a nonneutral stabilizing force helping us to keep the body from falling forward. It is good body use.

CLINICAL CASES AND TREATMENT

The total program used in our clinic is called Posture 'n Motion® and includes diagnosis and treatment. The individual patient is first analyzed from the perspective of the principles and determinants. Following that, a carefully selected progression of passive and active corrections to improve function and structure are introduced. We use a variety of methods, including modifications and combinations of prior works for body awareness, movement and pain relief (Table 2-8). We develop hands-on approaches for tissue mobilization and stabilization; visual, oral and hands-on cues and instructions for patients to use in achieving better body use through sensory awareness and functional exercise. We use specifically designed physical supports, e.g., neck pillows and pelvic and spinal posture supports (including supports to sit on as well as behind the back) to improve support, function and comfort. The use of automatic moist heat to help relieve pain and stiffness is often beneficial. Elastic bands provide sensory feedback.

Case 1

A young man presented with neck pain and forward head alignment. The craniovertebral joints (O-C1-C2-C3) were locked and compressed in extension. During swallowing, the tongue could be seen protruding anteriorly between the upper and lower teeth.

Treatment of this patient's neck pain and alignment included training in correct tongue placement during swallowing (one of the normal functions of the tongue is to provide an internal strut, or support, to stabilize the head during swallowing, since the tongue arises in the neck and its free end forms a functional articulation with the hard palate).

Other training included Alexander-type alignment, release and lengthening techniques; active stretch exercises (e.g., turtle exercises) to free the craniovertebral joints from extension locking; and manual medicine hands-on techniques to passively and actively mobilize the soft tissues that influence the craniovertebral joints. Training in pelvic control for body centering was also necessary: unless the pelvis is located beneath the upper weight centers, forward head alignment cannot be corrected.

Case 2

A 35-year-old female stood in poor alignment with her head and neck extended, causing the occipital condyles to be compressed downward and forward into the lateral masses of the atlas. Because of the transmitted downward compression, the posterior lower rib cage did not move during breathing. Poor abdominal muscle function resulted in excessive anterior tilting of the pelvis (the posterior pelvis was too cephalad and the anterior pelvis was too caudad). Lumbar hyperlordosis and tightness of the posterior paralumbar soft tissues were also present, as expected.

Correction of those problems first required stretching of the lumbar soft tissues and then improved abdominal muscle function to sup-

Table 2-8. Treatment

Manual Mobilization
    Myofascial release
    Craniosacral
    Articulation
    Stretch and spray
    Muscle energy (activation)
    Thrust

Stabilization
    Exercise for functional muscle strength
    Sclerotherapy/prolotherapy
    Surface support reactions

Body Awareness and Centering
    Alexander modifications
    Swiss Ball exercise
    Bartenieff modifications
    Exercise: pelvic-spinal-hip movements, sitting.
    Laban modifications
    Diaphragmatic breathing
    TherEx Rolls™ *

Exercise for Functional Strengthening and Movement
    Aerobic
    Diaphragmatic breathing (anteriorly, laterally, posteriorly)
    Stretch flexibility
    Isometric, isotonic, isokinetic
    Elastic bands, pulleys
    Pilates modifications
    Bartenieff modifications
    Body centering

Pain Relief
  Manual
    Strain/counter
    Strain stretch and spray
    Acupressure
  Injections
    Myofascial trigger points
    Osseofibrous trigger points (sclerotherapy)
    Epidural
    Acupuncture
  Modalities
    Electroacupuncture
    TENS
    Heat, cold

Supports for Function and Pain Relief
    Neck pillow
    Back support
    Pelvic spinal posture seat
    Orthotics - feet

* Trademark of Lionel A. Walpin, M.D.

---

port and "lift" the anterior pelvis. (Concomitantly with lower abdominal muscle strengthening, the paralumbar muscles are reciprocally inhibited and, as they relax, the pelvis' own weight causes it to move caudally.) The patient also required training in diaphragmatic breathing, with special emphasis on filling the posterior lower rib cage. As her lumbar muscles lengthened, the patient developed an awareness of light soft tissue tension (not hypertension) developing from the pelvis to the back of the head. Then, as she learned to release (actively inhibit) the posterior neck and shoulder girdle muscles attached to the head, her neck lengthened and the back of the head (occiput) moved lightly in an upward and slightly forward direction. This decompressed the craniovertebral joints.

The result was a balanced connection, without hypertension, between the upper and lower body soft tissues. This provided awareness of alignment during static sitting and standing, and during dynamic activities. Spinal alignment improved, for the spine became progressively more neutral, affording more freedom of movement throughout the body. This gradual process of change required patient training and soft tissue mobilization techniques.

SITTING

Sitting is a major source of body misuse and abuse. Although doctors and therapists often advise people with back pain about how to bend and lift, they rarely, if ever, instruct patients about sitting, other than to advise a "behind-the-back support." Typically, no instructions are given in terms of the different types of sitting, pelvic alignment, body centering and body movement. Furthermore, the behind-the-back supports mentioned can serve only a limited role. They make contact with the back when the user is leaning back in the chair (Type III sitting) and only sometimes in Type II sitting. When the patient is forward Type I (say at a desk or at a computer), the back does not contact the support, rendering it useless in those positions.

Sitting is a general term. Body weight is transferred mostly to the seat; some weight is transferred to the floor through the feet, and some weight is transferred to the backrest and armrests when the body contacts them. Sitting is traditionally considered to be a sedentary activity, but this is mistaken. In the author's opinion, sitting is a functional term that refers to body use in the seated position. The latter differs from other body positions because body weight is transferred mostly to the seat. Further, there are different types of sitting; it is not a single, generic activity. As already mentioned, we classify sitting according to the four categories below (See also Table 2-3).

Type I involves sitting upward and slightly forward when working at a desk or computer (Fig. 2-6).

Type II involves sitting upright (vertically), as some people do while driving. Other examples are sitting and talking at eye level, as when interviewing (Fig. 2-7). In this case, the Frankfort plane (drawn from the inferior orbit to the top of the external auditory meatus) is horizontal to the ground, or approximately 2° to 3° below that.

Type III involves sitting leaned backward up to 20° behind the vertical, as when resting during work, and as many people sit while driving (Fig. 2-8).

Type IV involves sitting leaned back more than 20° behind the vertical, relaxed, as in lounging.

In Types I, II and III, a neutral lumbar lordosis should be present. Even in Type IV, which involves general relaxation, neutral lumbar lordosis ideally should be maintained. In Types I and II, the knees are below the level of the hips with the pelvic-spinal-hip complex balanced in neutral. In Type III, the knees are below, at or above the level of the hips. In Types I, II and III, the trunk/thigh (hip) angle (less than 90°) should be more open than the thigh/leg (knee) angle. This prevents flexion/compression at the anterior hips (which is not only uncomfortable but also limits movement at the hips) and reduces the tension in the hamstrings. In Types I and II, upper weight centers are aligned on balance over the pelvis and are supported by the pelvis. The pelvis is in neutral alignment, rotated forward to approximately 34° and 20° below horizontal. In Types I and II active, organized, dynamic, rhythmic, controlled abdominal/pelvic/hip exercises are performed continually. In addition, postural sway continues in Types I and II. In Types III and IV, the back of the torso contacts the back of the chair. Types III and IV are basically sedentary and the body is at physiologic rest.

Types I and II sitting require forward pelvic rotation. In response to the forward rotation, the torso, neck and head move upward and a little forward because the pelvis is a torque converter. The head should remain level, or a few degrees flexed. It should not extend on the neck.

These alignments, movements and the sequence of movements are quite different from slumped sitting, a universal habit characterized by the pelvis rolling backward either before or after the head, neck and upper half of the torso (above the thoracic apex) have moved forward and downward. One must realize that it is impossible to sit at a desk correctly, when slumped, for the body is both forward (upper torso) and backward (lower torso) at the same time. Thus, when slumped, the head is projected forward and the pelvis is rotated backward. In Types I and II sitting, the body must be upward and forward; the upper weight centers should be balanced over the pelvis (head back, pelvis rotated forward), the body's natural base of support; the surface reactions from the chair's

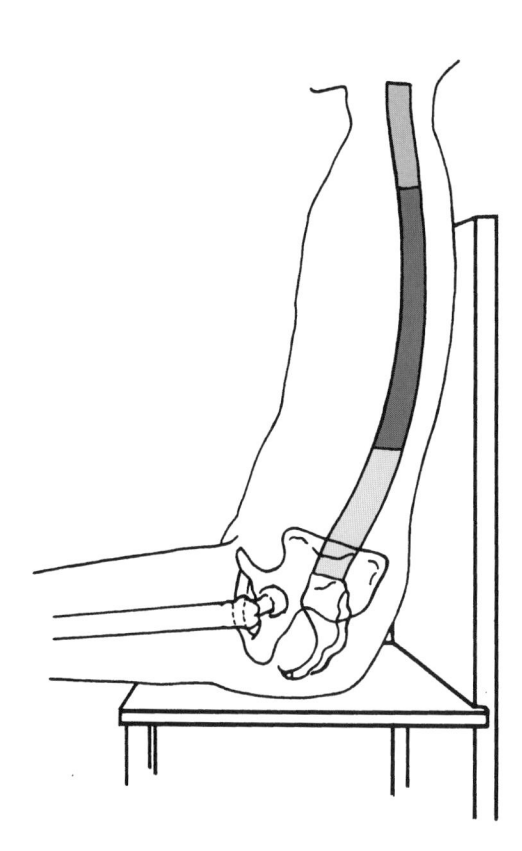

Fig. 2-13. Incorrect, slumped "Type III" (leaned back) sitting. Thoracolumbar compression and restriction of the lower chest and diaphragm are greatest, posteriorly.

seat should be coincident with the downward forces of gravity to counterbalance and to support those forces (which stabilize the body), and the pelvis, hips and spine should be in neutral alignment, allowing them freedom for continual active movement.

It is important to maintain healthy, anatomical, biomechanical and functional relationships within the pelvic-spinal-hip complex in all types of sitting. Clinically, there are five commonly observed "negatives" regarding sitting, all of which can be improved upon.

1. Traditionally, sitting is not comfortable for more than 5 minutes. By 15 minutes, there is lots of fidgeting and by 30 minutes, remaining seated is a distinct chore.
2. Slumped sitting is common, whether leaned back or not (Figs. 2-4 and 2-13).
3. Controlled, purposeful, rhythmic movements are rarely performed while sitting. Fidgeting or disorganized shifts of body weight and alignment are common. The latter includes the need to get up and move about, emphasizing the point that there is a basic need to move.
4. Leaned-back sitting (Type III), with or without a lumbar lordosis (Figs. 2-8, 2-13, 2-16), often carries over into leaned-back standing, with compressed nonneutral alignment, typically found at the thoracolumbar junction (Fig. 2-3).
5. Sitting upright with the pelvis in proper anterior rotation looks good, but if the knees are level with the hips (Fig. 2-5), the latter are too flexed and are compressed anteriorly. Additionally, tension exists in the posterior soft tissues of the thighs and pelvis. There are opposing forces in the soft tissues of the low back because the neutral pelvic-spinal alignment "causes" lumbar lordosis, while the posterior soft tissue tensions pull in the opposite direction, "causing" lumbar kyphosis. Those opposing forces are uncomfortable, causing fidgeting and slumping. Compare Fig. 2-5 with Fig. 2-7. In the latter, the knees are lower than the hips.

At least six elements must be considered when evaluating seating:

1. The chair
2. The location, height and tilt of the desk, table, steering wheel or windshield
3. The task, i.e., typing, eating, driving, resting or relaxing
4. Body alignment
5. Body mobility
6. Balancing of upward and downward forces

Slumped sitting is stagnant sitting. It is bad body use (Figs. 2-4). The pelvis and spine are locked in nonneutral alignment. Easy, active voluntary motion and postural sway are lost, and because of mechanical disadvantages, abdominal muscle function and diaphragmatic breathing are poor. The length/tension relationships[40] of the abdominal muscles and diaphragm are nonphysiologic. Also, diaphragmatic movement is mechanically blocked. In slumped sitting, the upper body weight centers are aligned off balance and the sacrum supports body weight. This is unhealthy, compressing the entire back and interfering with inherent myofascial and craniosacral rhythms. Slumping leads to fidgeting and the need to stand and stretch.

In correct natural sitting, the undersurface of the pelvis, from the ischial tuberosity to the proximal thighs, provides a natural base of support. In slumped sitting, the pelvis and the body gain their support and stability by locking down from above and by locking up from below. The head, C1 and C2 are extended and compressed. Below the C2-C3 facet joints, the spine is locked flexed all the way down through the pelvis. Diaphragmatic breathing and abdominal muscle function are dysfunctional; and back muscles, stretched over the spine's long kyphotic "C" curve, have little or no EMG activity. Pain is common and has several possible sources: muscles ache probably from ischemia and probably from increased intramuscular tissue fluids and elevated tissue pressure; myofascial and osseofibrous trigger points; hypomobility, often with painful, restricted motion, and hypermobility with clinical laxity or clinical instability causing painful movements.

While slumped, the body appears to be at rest but, in actuality, some individual muscles are at work stabilizing and supporting the body against the force of its weight. While slumped, most muscles are at physiologic rest (not contracting). The ligaments and other connective tissue attachments are at work, supporting the body at end range of motion. This overuse is a source of osseofibrous trigger points. In contrast, in neutral alignment, the joints are not aligned at the end range of motion. Thus, the ligament and joint capsules are at physiologic rest and muscles should contract voluntarily and rhythmically. Further, in neutral, the muscles and upward forces from the chair counterbalance downward forces. The more specific the direction of the upward forces, the more supportive they are so that less muscle activity is needed to support the body in neutral alignment. Performing rhythmic, controlled, purposeful movements allows the muscles to rest intermittently and prevents ischemia; prevents stagnation of fluids; improves blood flow and tissue nutrition; and improves physiologic and structural health of muscles, flexibility, endurance and functional strength. Pain from ischemia (due to stagnant sitting and compressed blood vessels) is typically relieved by movement. Pains from osseofibrous trigger points are relieved by movement that does not stress the dysfunctional irritated connective tissue to bone attachment. With rhythmic controlled movements, the ligaments and joint capsules can rest, pain lessens and stretched ligaments and compressed joints no longer are needed to stabilize the body.

As functional muscle strength and endurance improve, the muscles can relieve the ligaments and joint capsules more effectively. With tight connective tissues, movement can cause increased pain early on. Later, pain is typically relieved with movement, especially through the neutral range muscles.

Numerous causes of slumping have been mentioned in the literature. A few of the typical ones are: arm rests too-low; a seat too-deep (front to back), causing pressure at the backs of the knees; and a desk top too-low. Looking at the body, not the chair, one sees that the causes of slumping are: 1) lack of support under the anterior pelvic arch (pubic area); 2) compression and discomfort at the anterior aspect of the hip joints; 3) abdominal-pelvic-lumbar muscle fatigue; 4) relief of buttocks pressure; 5) the need to follow the path of least resistance to movement.

To expand on the five causes listed above, note that, first and foremost, 1) slumping results from the pelvis' need for support and stability. Thus, it rolls posteriorly to gain support from sacral weight-bearing and from posterior ligamentous locking of the pelvis and spine. There is natural instability when a round object is placed on a flat surface, e.g., an orange on a flat table. Similarly, because the pelvis and buttocks have rounded contours, there is instability on a flat seat. The body will then gain stability however it can: thus, it slumps onto the sacrum. Slumping also results from 2) a need to reopen the hip joints. The slump causes extension of the hips which decompresses the hips and helps relieve their discomfort.[22] Comparison of hip flexion angles in slumped and upright sitting has been described. The knees are lower than the hips with upright sitting; the hip angles can be the same as in slumping.²² Whether sitting or standing, neutral range pelvic and neutral spinal alignments should both continue. However, one can readily see that the anterior hip joints would be compressed while sitting with a neutral pelvis and spine with the knees aligned at or above the level of the hips. But, by rotating the pelvis posteriorly, the hip joints open, i.e., extend, for relief. Even if a flat seat surface is tilted forward, the pelvis will still rotate backward if there is lack of support under the anterior pelvis. Thus, four elements are necessary for correct sitting: Some forward tilt of the seat; support for the anterior pelvis; some hip extension and rhythmic pelvic-hip exercises that include anterior and posterior rotations of the pelvis. Slumping also results 3) from muscle fatigue when the abdominal, pelvic and low back muscles have not been functionally trained for supporting the body and for moving the body in the seated position. Those muscles are simply too weak. With slumping, the muscles stop contracting. Then, for support, the body hangs on its ligaments and compresses its bony elements or leans back on the chair. Excessive pressures on the under surface of the ischial tuberosities 4) results in posterior pelvic rotation to transfer the pressure to the posterior sacrum. The path of least resistance 5) relieves pain or discomfort resulting from relative inflexibility of tissues and from motion barriers.

Obviously, the chair is a critical element. But little attention has been paid to the actual seat surface despite the fact that most of the body weight is transferred to it. Four crucial factors regarding the chair's seat should be emphasized:

1. The chair exerts considerable general upward force on the body. But, to promote physiologic seating, these forces must be harnessed and directed back to the body.
2. The direction of the seat's surface reactions depends on its surface contours (surface geometry) and firmness.
3. The resiliency of the seat's surface contributes significantly to body awareness, sensory memory and to the performance of active voluntary body movement.

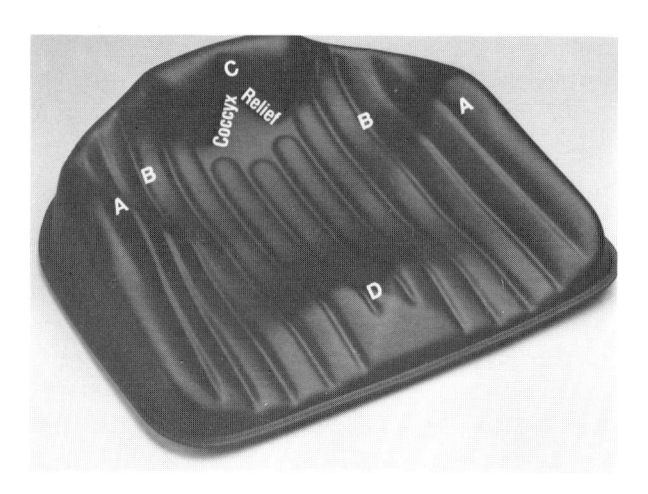

Fig. 2-14. Pelvic spinal posture seat, co-developed by author, with six support zones that balance the pelvis (the body center) to support neutral and "on balance" flexible spinal alignments: **A**, Trochanteric; **B**, Ischial; **C**, Sacral; **D**, Pubic and Thigh. "D" provides support and cueing for the anterior pelvis, helping to maintain the 20°-34° sacral angle.

4. The seat's specific geometric surface contour and general shape are important determinants of body alignment and stability. Regarding shape, an egg in an egg cup is far more stable than an orange on a flat surface. But, the smooth inner surface of an egg cup is not enough. The seat's surface should have a surface geometry to it and it should have a surface contour in addition to its general shape. The device shown in Fig. 2-14 was codeveloped by the author (See Fig. 2-10).

One might expect that posterior pelvic rotation and slumping could be eliminated by merely tilting the seat's surface forward 5-15°. This may help but, unfortunately, the pelvis can and often does rotate posteriorly even on a forward-tilted seat. There are three reasons for this: First, forward-tilted seats typically have flat surfaces. Thus, there is no surface contour for support of the anterior pelvic arch. Second, because there are no thigh slopes which would allow the knees to be aligned lower than the hips, the hip joints do not extend. Third, patients also need to be instructed about how to sit centered at the pelvis in neutral pelvic alignment. These instructions are rarely given.

The pelvis, the structural and functional foundation of the spine, is situated between the lumbosacral joint and the hip joints. A recent report discussed the correlation between back pain and decreased hip and lumbar mobilities.[28] Correct movement is important for structure, function and pain relief. That is why we teach rhythmic, controlled sitting exercises.

In Types I and II sitting, the alignment of the pelvis and the spinal segments should be in the same ranges as in standing (Figs. 2-1, 2-6, and 2-7). Pelvic neutral balanced alignment is about 20-34° below horizontal. The spinal segments should be in neutral balanced alignment with neutral range lumbar and cervical lordotic curves and neutral thoracic and occipitoatlantal kyphotic curves.

Technically, the term "neutral" does not apply to the joints of the cervical spine nor to the occipitoatlantal joints. Nevertheless, there is a physiologic range of easy motion between the anatomic barriers of those joints. Thus the use of the term. The result is a mobile, stable pelvic-spinal-hip complex.

The factors necessary to retain a neutral balanced stable alignment while sitting are: correct support from the seat providing a balance of upward and downward forces for stability; body centering at the pelvis; freedom of movement of the hip joints; coordinated, *functionally* strong muscles that can support neutral balanced pelvic-spinal alignment and make possible continual (intermittent) rhythmic controlled organized abdominal-pelvic-spinal-hip movements, in both Types I and II sitting. These movements, functional muscle strengthening and muscle coordination, require training.

Upward forces include the surface reactions from the seat surfaces (reactions to body weight), internal resistance of the tissues (for example, the intervertebral discs), and the upward pull of the lower abdominal muscles on the anterior arch of the pelvis. Downward forces include body weight; the downward pull of muscles, e.g., the upper abdominals and anterior and posterior ligaments of the spine (Table 2-6). Regarding upward forces, on a flat, firm seat reactions to body weight are directed upward and outward (Fig. 2-11). On a soft cushion, surface reactions to body weight dissipate; they are haphazard, attenuated and poorly supportive. In fact, sitting on a soft cushion is like falling onto a muddy surface, i.e., the surface reactions "splatter" (Fig. 2-12). These types of seats cannot correctly counterbalance body weight. They do not give effective support. The result is torque and instability because the external support beneath the pelvis and spine is poor. Thus, the body relies on its internal locking mechanisms for support, i.e., tense ligaments and compressed joints. When possible, the body also leans backward on the upright of the chair for external support.

Ordinary seats and cushions and most so-called ergonomic chairs and therapeutic supports do not provide specific contoured support zones for the anterior arch of the pelvis, the trochanters and sacrum. Also, the materials with which they are made (often wood) have no resiliency and do not provide kinesthetic input for body awareness, or sensory memory (e.g., how far the pelvis has rotated anteriorly). These are major factors why the pelvis is rarely rotated forward into neutral alignment. This also interferes both with pelvic support and the fine-tuning of pelvic rotation by the lower rectus abdominis muscles. These muscles contract most easily at their resting lengths. That occurs when the pelvis is in neutral balanced alignment. In the absence of these intrinsic and extrinsic support mechanisms, above and below the anterior pelvic arch, the pelvis, seeking stability, rotates posteriorly causing pelvic-spinal slumping. Another cause of slumping is hip joint compression, anteriorly. The pelvis rotates posteriorly to extend the hips and relieve the anterior hip discomfort.

Some seating devices, which claim to correct posture by placing a strap behind the lumbar spine and anchoring it in front, around the knees or upper tibias, interfere with movements of the pelvic-spinal-hip complex and also cause hip joint compression.[44] In the author's opinion, this type of device can create bad body use and should only be used by people who are especially weak or in such pain that they could not otherwise carry out the activity. With that device, the body is biomechanically braced and passively suffers physiologically and structurally. When the device is removed, there is nothing holding the body up and it slumps. As stated, there is a role for this device but, in most situations, it is incorrect to support the body passively by compressing joints. The latter diminishes proprioceptive input, it greatly restricts movement and injures joints.

Needed simultaneously are: neutral pelvic alignment (20-34° below horizontal); knees lowered to below hip level and rhythmic controlled exercise movements. These avoid hip flexion, anterior hip compression, and slumping. Interestingly, the hip joint angle is the same when comparing posterior pelvic rotation (slumping) with leveled knees and hips versus anterior pelvic rotation (neutral alignment) with the knees lower than the hips.[22] Keegan recommended a trunk/thigh angle of 105° minimum.[23] (At that time, a fully extended hip was referred to as 180°; today it is referred to as 0°. Thus, today Keegan would say 75° or less.) In theory, 135°[23] (45° in today's terminology) is optimal. However, it is not practical, for the person would slide forward and downward out of the chair. Nevertheless, one can sit aligned at 100-105° (75-80° today) and intermittently can open the trunk/thigh angle more by performing controlled posterior pelvic rotational exercise movements. (The latter are part of the rhythmic sitting exercises described in this chapter.) Performing these exercises is much easier when sitting on a multicontoured seat surface that counters the downward force of body weight.

The pelvic-spinal-hip complex is a functional and anatomical unit. To maintain a neutral balanced pelvic-spinal alignment (Types I and II sitting), the upper body weight centers must be "on balance" over the pelvis. This is achieved by first rotating the pelvis anteriorly. The pelvis functions as a torque converter. The lower rectus abdominis muscles are decelerators of anterior pelvic rotation. Thus, the spine, which follows the pelvis, is literally lifted by the pelvis. The spine lengthens in neutral balanced alignment and the depths of the spinal curves are physiologically decreased. In Type III sitting (Fig. 2-8), the spine should also remain within neutral alignment. However, in Type III, because the body's upper weight centers are behind the base of support (the pelvis), additional support behind the back is required. An X-ray (Fig. 2-15 A)[7,8] taken with the subject sitting on a flat, firm surface, shows his "natural" slump. Note that the head and upper torso are anterior while the pelvis and lower torso are posterior. The two regions have moved in opposite directions away from each other. The upper body weight centers are aligned "off balance" in relation to the pelvis. Note that the L4-L5-S1 disc spaces and facet joints have narrowed posteriorly despite the lumbar and sacral kyphosis. The latter observation is contrary to the popularly held assumption that those lower disc spaces and joints always open with flexion. The author has published this finding previously.[8] In another study by the author, a subject was X-rayed while seated in a chair that was tilted 15° forward, then 15° backward and then at 0° of tilt. The same observations were made. This probably depends on the fact that, in sitting, there is a closed kinetic chain because the pelvis is "held" by body weight against the seat. In contrast, a person sidelying with the knees and head drawn together (as for a lumbar puncture) has an open chain at both ends. In sitting, as the lower lumbar vertebrae rotate into kyphosis, their posterior-inferior surfaces move caudally. This narrows the facet joints and the disc spaces posteriorly. Ultimately, the degree of posterior narrowing and compression seems to depend upon the relative motions between L4, L5 and the sacrum. This may also help explain why some patients do better clinically with flexion exercises and some do better with extension exercises. It may also depend on the relative movements of L5 and S1. The second X-ray (Fig. 2-15 B)[7,8] demonstrates neutral balanced alignment of the upper body and pelvis. Again, they have moved in opposite directions, but toward each other. The alignment is on balance.

When the seat surface reactions are supportive, and the downward and upward forces are congruous, there is stability. For several years, we have utilized the author's special pelvic-spinal posture seat for Types I, II and III sitting (Fig. 2-14). This device has several important features, including, but not limited to, multicontoured surface, six pelvic support zones, thigh supports which slope downward and forward 10°, and a specific recessed area for the coccyx. The device has been briefly described previously,[7,8] includ-

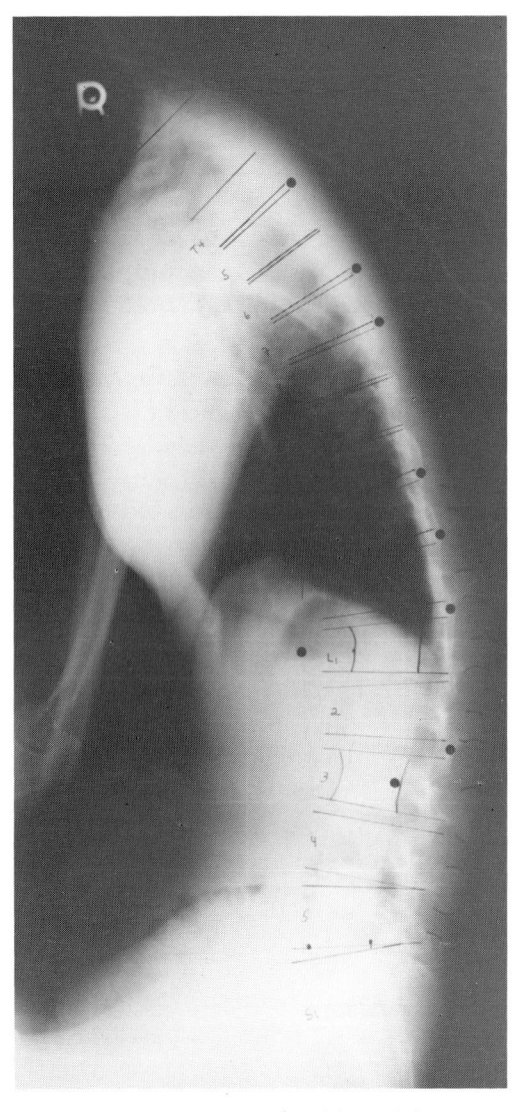

Fig. 2-15. A, Lateral view of subject sitting on a flat surface.[8]

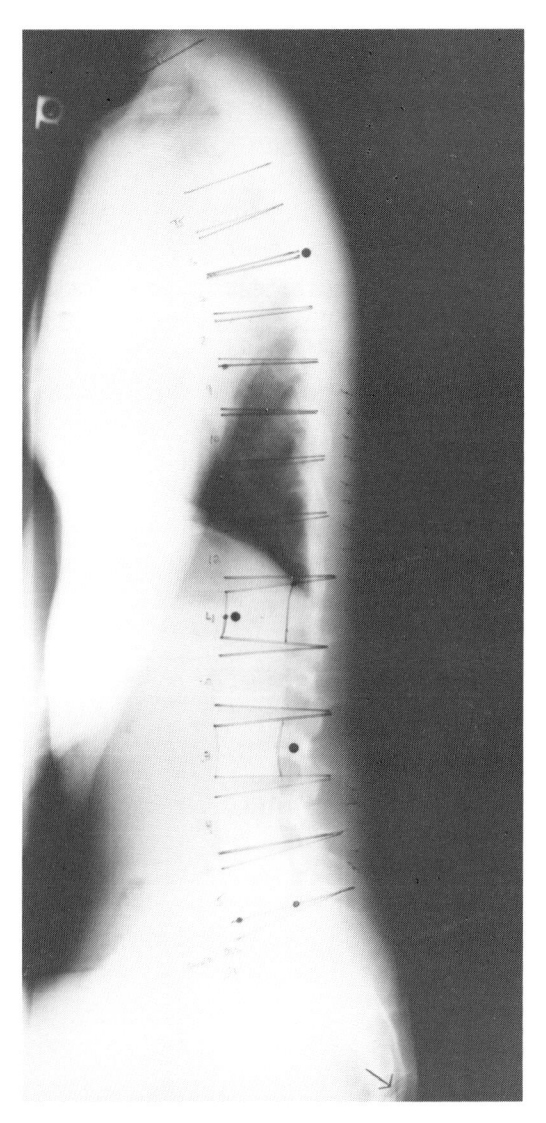

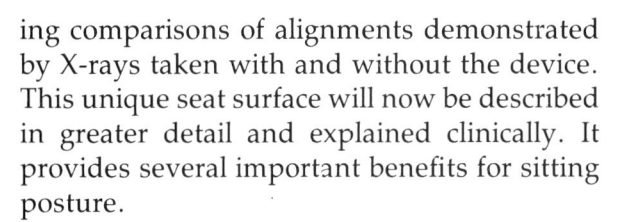

Fig. 2-15. B, Lateral view, same subject, now sitting on a pelvic spinal posture seat. (Subject knew the goal—"to sit comfortably taller, at ease, in an upward and slightly forward direction.")[8]

ing comparisons of alignments demonstrated by X-rays taken with and without the device. This unique seat surface will now be described in greater detail and explained clinically. It provides several important benefits for sitting posture.

1. Two trochanteric supports counter the downward forces of body weight and direct the chair's surface reactions upward, forward and medially toward the skeletal axis in the sagittal plane (Figs. 2-6 through 2-8) and toward their respective opposite shoulders in the frontal plane (Fig. 2-10). In sitting, femoral necks are nonfunctional in this regard (compare standing, Fig. 2-9). The trochaneric support zones also support the pelvis laterally to counter external rotation of the hips. (The anterior midline mound counters internal rotation of the hips.) The ischial supports direct the surface reactions upward and forward. The patient can then release and lengthen along the surface reaction vectors.

2. Pressures on the coccyx, sacroiliac joints and ischial tuberosities are lessened because considerable weight is borne above them by the trochanteric support zones. (Trochanteric pressure has been complained of by only 1 out of 400

patients. That was a very thin female with great sensitivity due to a low pain threshold. The problem was relieved by providing her with the next wider-sized seat.) The design also provides a specific coccyx relief zone, and the thigh slopes provide additional coccyx relief.

3. The sacral support mechanically blocks the pelvis from rolling posteriorly and also "reminds" the user not to allow posterior rotation.

4. The six support zones provide sensory reference points. This improves body awareness, which helps the patient correct pelvic alignment, pelvic-spinal-hip balance, and movement in all directions.

5. Pelvic, spinal and abdominal exercises can effectively be performed using the seat.

6. Because of the materials' resilience and "memory," they provide proprioceptive input and assist body movement.

7. There is no wood or metal. Vibrations are absorbed, not augmented.

8. The device can also be used for movements similar to those which occur in a rocking chair. These are different from the rhythmic, organized specific pelvic-spinal-hip exercises we use.

9. The pelvis can easily be actively (and even passively) maintained in neutral alignment in both Type I and in Type II. This provides a natural base of support for the spine. The body's net center of gravity is at the level of S2, which is just above the fulcra for pelvic rotation, the ischial tuberosities, and just above the axis for pelvic rotation, the hip joints. Thus, gravity can assist in the achievement of neutral pelvic alignment because, when the body weight is concentrated in front of the ischial tuberosities, the pelvis rotates forward under the influence of gravity. However, to prevent too much anterior pelvic rotation and lumbar hyperlordosis, the pelvis must be stabilized, supported, and fine-tuned by the abdominal muscles and surface reactions. This is greatly helped by this device. The mechanism has already been refered to. The pelvis can also be maintained in mild forward tilt in Type III.

10. The lumbar spine follows the pelvis. The entire spine and head can more easily be aligned on balance over the pelvis, and each spinal segment can be more easily balanced in neutral alignment over the natural base of support, immediately below it. Even if we should react reflexly from stimulation of peripheral proprioceptors, we will be safer and perform better if the pelvis is already controlled.

11. With the pelvis rotated anteriorly in Types I and II sitting, the anterior midline mound supports the anterior pelvic arch above it. The anterior arch rests near or on the mound when the thighs are well apart. Usually, the thighs are closer together and the mound's support is transmitted through the thighs to the anterior pelvis. The abdominal muscles (rectus abdominii), which insert at the top of the pubic symphysis, can contract gently, for they are at resting length and their points of insertion at the pelvis are supported from below. Thigh adductor muscles are better stabilized because of the mound. These muscles also stabilize the arch from below.

12. With this seat, in all types of sitting, the thighs can be supported in about 10° of downward forward slope. This prevents hyperflexion of the hip joints even with simultaneous neutral pelvic alignment. The forward downward slope is greater with the model used for desk sitting than with the model used for car sitting because the former has 3° more forward pitch. (It is important to recognize, however, that the knees are typically higher than the hips when one sits on a low seat or when the person has long legs.) With long legs, the chair must at least be higher to prevent this.

Freedom of the hip joints is very important, for that allows active rhythmic controlled movements of the PSH-C and helps prevent compression and discomfort at the anterior hip joints. It also relieves tension and strain in the posterior soft tissues at the thighs, hips and lower back. If one "sits up" in neutral spinal alignment but with the knees at or above the level of the hips, there is a conflict: the lumbar lordosis is countered by the pos-

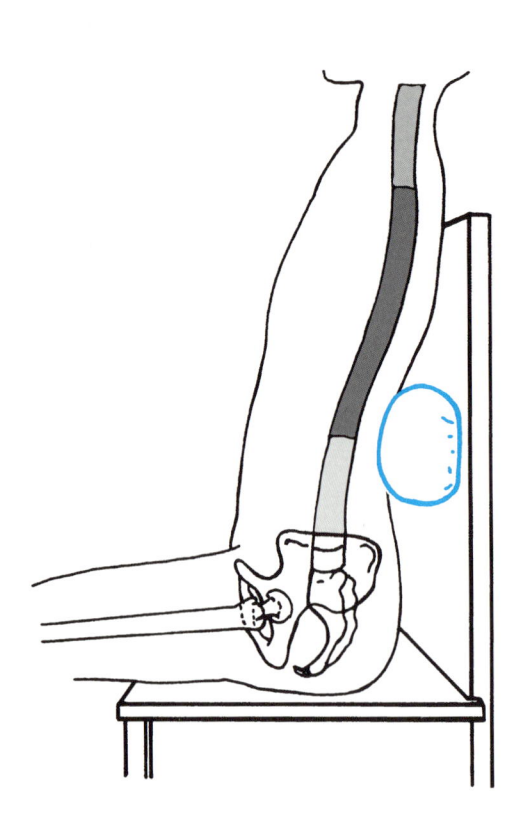

66 New Concepts in Craniomandibular and Chronic Pain Management

Fig. 2-16. Type III sitting with focal forward pressure exerted on lumbar spine using a tubular-shaped pillow (lumbar roll). The spine is focally in nonneutral (extended position) and above the pillow the thoracolumbar region "drapes" backward, over it, increasing thoracolumbar restriction. Thighs are level. If the person were sitting upright, it would casue anterior hip pressure and the person would need to slump or stand up.

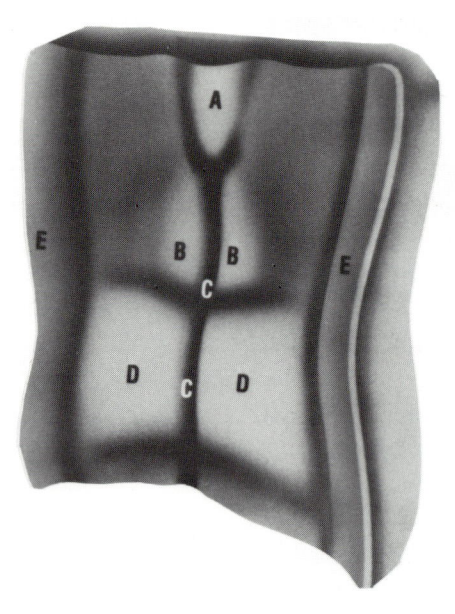

Fig. 2-17. Back support with Multiplane Surface contour (codeveloped by the author): **A**, Thoracic Support Mound; **B**, Paraspinal Muscle Support; **C**, Spinal Relief Valley; **D**, Lumbar Supports; **E**, Contoured Side Huggers.[8]

terior soft tissues of the thighs and pelvis which pull the pelvis toward posterior rotation and the lumbar lordosis toward kyphosis. This is uncomfortable physical stress at the low back and hips. The forward slope helps relieve the tension in the posterior soft tissues which reduces strain at the coccyx. As previously pointed out, it is often inadequate, inappropriate and sometimes harmful to use lumbar rolls or some other type of behind the back supports only, while neglecting the other elements of the PSH-C. It is one functional/structural unit and, ideally, it should be addressed in its totality. The models used for sitting at a desk provide the additional 3° of forward tilt which is very helpful for Type I sitting. Qualitatively, this provides a similar forward tilt as do forward tilted chairs. However, the latter do not have a multicontoured surface. Their flat seat surfaces do not pro-

vide the type of physical support or the body awareness that helps promote anterior pelvic rotation in neutral. As previously stated, the seat's surface, under the pelvis (shape, surface geometry, thigh slopes and resiliency) is extremely important in Type I and Type II sitting. Additionally, in Type III (and sometimes in Type II) a support placed behind the back is very important. In the author's opinion, the surface geometry of a behind-the-back support (Fig. 2-17) should include a forward (convex) midline mound for support at and just below the apex of the thoracic portion of the spine. Sitting upright (vertically) with or without a behind-the-back support, e.g., a lumbar roll, can result in anterior hip compression and discomfort if the thigh/trunk angle is 90°; the roll pushes the lumbar spine forward into lordosis and the anterior hip joints will be compressed. The way to prevent this is to provide the proper seat surface under the pelvis (Figs. 2-5 and 2-7).

WALKING AND FOOT ORTHOSES

Events at the foot-shoe-ground interfaces are important determinants of body balance and walking. Each foot has 26 bones and 40 joints. There are three major joints or functional regions: the hindfoot, containing the subtalar joint, which allows the foot to be a mobile adapter; the midfoot, containing the midtarsal joints, which allow the foot to be a rigid lever; and the forefoot, containing the metatarsophalangeal joint of the large toe. Hyperextension of the latter produces the windlass effect and the return of the medial longitudinal arch just before toe-off.

The subtalar joint provides adaptation to the ground, absorbs shock, is a control for the midtarsal joints, and serves as a torque converter. In other words, as the foot rotates on the "Z" axis for pronation/supination, the leg rotates on the "Y" axis for internal/external rotation. This hindfoot torque conversion accounts for the significant biomechanical influence of the foot on the leg, hip and spine. The mobile adaptor function occurs from just after heel strike through the first 25% of stance phase. From 26% to toe-off, the midtarsal joints convert the foot to a progressively increasing rigid lever for forward propulsion and push off.

Clearly, the foot is complex, biomechanically, neurophysiologically and anatomically, and has important relationships with posture throughout the body. For example, if instead of first heel striking the individual touches the forefoot to the ground first, the ground surface reaction will be inadequate, causing the knee, spine and pelvis to be unstable. The compensation is to stabilize from above downward by hyperextending the cervical and lumbar portions of the spine. The foot is a major source of proprioception and its many joints and functions allow it to adapt and to compensate for ground irregularities and for changes in postural alignment and movement elsewhere in the body.

Foot orthoses are corrective devices that assist posture in standing, walking and running by providing comfort, support of structure, and support and control of biomechanics. To be an orthotic, the device must "maintain the foot in neutral position."[24] Not all orthoses are the same. There is a great array of devices, falling into four general categories.

Accommodative devices

These are intended to provide comfort and some structural support for the foot, but generally offer little to no biomechanical support or biomechanical control of the foot. Examples are:

a. Heel and sole lift(s) to equalize lower extremity length. This does have biomechanical effects on the pelvis and spine. It eliminates the need for adaptive spinal curves that would result from a short leg.

b. Individual pads placed in the shoe. Examples are the navicular pad for support of the medial longitudinal arch and the metatarsal pad which is placed behind the metatarsal head to relieve pressure.

c. One-piece soft (flexible) devices for comfort and some supports made of leather and rubber laminates or other soft materials. These contain several accommodative pads, placed between the upper and lower coverings. These so-called "orthotics," made in both metatarsal length and full length, are only props for various parts of the foot and do not help the support or control of biomechanics. Specifically, the subtalar joint is not controlled because these devices are not designed to control the three-plane motion of the foot. They really do not begin to work until midstance, i.e., after heel strike and the transition to normal pronation. Therefore, as a biomechanical orthotic, they are antiquated, at best being accommodative.

These devices are "fitted" by having the standing patient imprint his/her foot in a foam box, without the benefit of placing the subtalar joint in neutral alignment. In other words, the functional and structural relationships of the leg to the subtalar joint are not taken into account. This is outmoded and explains the fitting problems and the biomechanical deficiencies that patients experience. The imprinted foam is sent to a factory where accommodative pads are inserted inside the one-piece devices. A number of doctors have commented on the greatly similar appearance of these devices made for their various patients. This probably attests to the "general" nature of these accommodative corrections.

d. One-piece, soft (flexible) full-length, shock-absorbing inserts are available to health professionals. An array of accomodative modules, also made of shock-absorbing material, are applied for in-office use. These modules are placed underneath the full-length shoe insert. The latter can be cut to proper length.

The accommodative devices in b, c, and d (above) can provide comfort and support for sore, stiff feet. They are flexible and provide for some proprioceptive input. However, the hindfoot is not properly supported or controlled. In fact, normal pronation may be interfered with, particularly when a medial wedge is placed under the heel. This is because the hindfoot may slide forward and laterally. The medial heel wedge is a common "correction" provided in those devices (group c, above) supplied from the factory. The wedge is supposed to prop up the subtalar joints, i.e., to prevent excessive pronation, but it does not guide the triplane motion of the subtalar joint into normal pronation. These devices frequently utilize corrective pads, the location of which should be precise, to avoid increased symptoms of pain and pressure. It is apparent that adjustments in the location of the corrections can be made more readily with the modular in-office system (d), than with the completed device provided by the factory.

Preformed triplane functional devices

Preformed triplane functional devices that support the biomechanics of the foot are semi-rigid (semiflexible) orthotics that guide the hindfoot in the manner of a true orthotic. This is often a good way to provide orthotics. It provides biomechanical structural support as well as comfort and proprioceptive input. Furthermore, the devices are available immediately. Orthotic adjustments can be made. The preforms are available in a variety of firmnesses, although at the soft end of the spectrum, little or no biomechanical support or control is provided.

Functional orthotics made from a plaster impression cast

Functional orthotics made from a plaster impression cast afford a more precisely controlled method benefitting two very different populations. The cast is obtained from the nonweight-bearing foot with the subtalar joint held passively in neutral alignment. Feet with normal flexibility utilize the biomechanical support and control provided by these orthotics which guide the feet through normal pronation and resupination. These are effective for walking and at slower jogging speeds, i.e., 5-6 minutes/kilometer. Above that speed, the runner has decreasing heel contact.[25] Specific postings can be added to the orthotics. Diseased feet, even though not flexible, also benefit because specific dysfunctions and lesions require precise support and control. However, diabetics usually do not use these rigid orthotics.

Functional orthotics and semifunctional/semiaccommodative orthotics.

Both of these are made from a foam impression taken, supine or sitting, with the subtalar joint in neutral alignment. The author has found these to be excellent.

SLEEPING

The average person spends about one-third of each 24-hour period in bed, sleep being the longest continuous daily activity. During sleep, we are at particular risk of aggravating preexistent disorders or suddenly developing acute pain and dysfunction of the neck, temporomandibular joints, upper extremities, or the low back. The reasons include: poor support from pillows and mattresses; awkward, prolonged static alignments causing gradual onset of pain; or poorly controlled, rapid body movements causing sudden onset of pain. The altered state of awareness during sleep is an important contributing factor.

Prone sleeping should be discouraged for the following reasons: it causes twisting rotation of the head/neck complex; lateral pressure on the jaw and lumbar hyperextension. With the head/neck rotated, the craniovertebral joints are compressed and irritated; lateral pressure on the jaw irritates the temporomandibular joint (TMJ) and associated muscles. The joint is also placed a little out

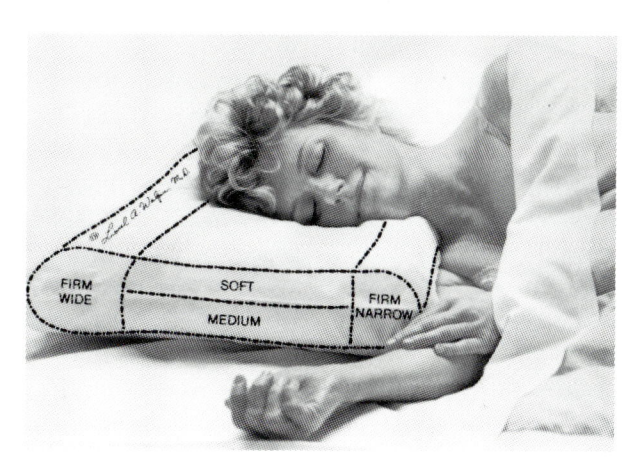

Fig. 2-18. Neck pillow. Four combinations of head and neck support in sidelying and backlying body positions.[8]

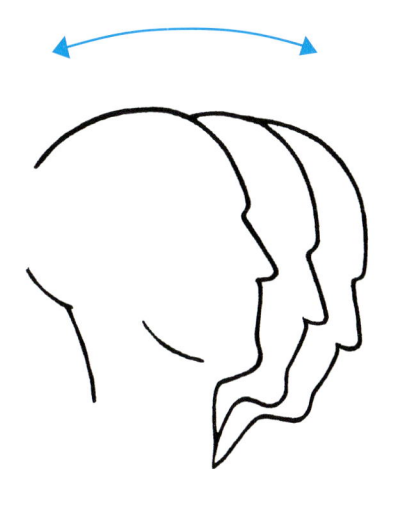

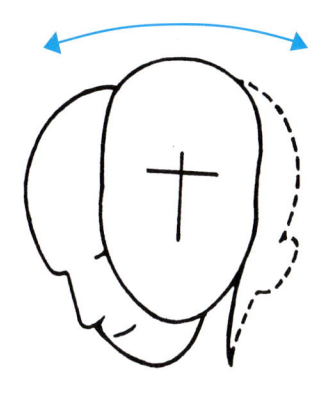

Fig. 2-19. Diagrammatic representation of head and neck positions and alignments achievable with special neck pillow. During backlying, the head and neck can be neutral (normal lordosis), forward flexed or extended. During sidelying, the head and neck can be neutral or laterally flexed, upward or downward, with or without rotation.[8]

of alignment. If the person grinds the joint, irritation and the potential for damage to the joint are further increased. Prolonged lumbar hyperextension compresses the facet joint.

Other problems are associated with sleeping because of pressure on the hand or arm while resting on them. The former aggravates or precipitates the carpal tunnel syndrome. Patients with this condition commonly awaken during the night complaining of numbness and tingling affecting the thumb, index, middle and radial one-half of the ring fingers. The patient typically shakes the hand for relief. It is very important to ask the patient where the hand was when he/she awakened. Often, it has been under the pillow, compressed by the head. Ulnar neuropathy with numbness and tingling of the little and ulnar one-half of the ring fingers commonly results from sleeping with the elbow bent to 90° while the upper extremity is under the pillow. The main reason people sleep that way is to support the head and neck, for many pillows do not give adequate support, nor do they stay in place.

In our work, we utilize a special versatile head and neck pillow design codeveloped by the author. It is four pillows in one (Fig. 2-18). The important principle of this pillow relates to the fact that "the four sides of the neck are not equally painful or equally restricted, thus it is advantageous to be able to place the head and neck in different alignments and attitudes while in sidelying and backlying body positions (Fig. 2-19)." By simply turning the pillow around and/or over, the user can select from four combinations of head and neck support for sheer comfort and/or for specific therapeutic benefits. This pillow has already been described in great detail.[8] In addition to all the benefits mentioned, this pillow protects the ulnar nerve.

CONCLUSION

In 1947, the report of the Posture Committee of the American Academy of Orthopaedic Surgeons stated: "Posture is usually defined as the relative arrangement of the parts of the body. Good posture is that state of muscular and skeletal balance which protects the supporting structures of the body against injury or progressive deformity irrespective of the attitude (erect, lying, squatting, stooping) in which these structures are working or resting. Under such conditions, the muscles will function most efficiently and the optimum positions are afforded for the thoracic and abdominal organs. Poor posture is a faulty relationship of the various parts of the body which produces increased strain on supporting structures and in which there is less efficient balance of the body over its base of support."[4]

Obviously, the author agrees with the overall message set forth in that early report. However, if one examines it more carefully, one sees that posture is defined as "anatomical alignment" and the terms "attitude" and "position" (i.e., erect, lying and so forth) are used interchangeably. This probably led to vagaries and miscommunication between doctors, therapists and patients. Also, the report made no mention of surface reaction forces nor of quality or quantity of movement. One may ask why, forty-one years later, many health professionals and most lay people are unclear about the concept of posture and ways to improve it. Why is the word "posture" still used nonspecifically as a buzz word for relationships of body parts and appearance? The reasons appear to be multiple.

There had been a general lack of interest and motivation. A notable exception was Hans Kraus, M.D., in 1947[3] and Billig, in 1949.[47]

As an outgrowth of the medical profession's remarkable achievements in World War II, the attention of surgeons, internists and general practitioners continued to be directed to the phenomenal growth of the technical aspects of diagnosis and treatment rather than to "hands-on" medicine. Although allopathic medicine has continued to make remarkable contributions to everyone's health care, it is ironic that more recently it has been criticized for not being more holistic and "hands-on." This is unfortunate, for were it not for the acute pressures of World War II, the medical profession would undoubtedly have been able to gradually cultivate the seeds of holism and "hands-on" medicine that were already planted.

Nevertheless, because of the work and teachings of its "handful of giants" in the fields of musculoskeletal and manual medicine, the medical profession (especially some physiatrists and some rheumatologists) is becoming increasingly proficient in specific somatic clinical diagnoses based on palpation and observation of patients at rest and in motion and in the manual medicine treatment of somatic disorders of dysfunctional (nondisease) origin.

The public was also enraptured by the technical advances. Physicians found that emphasizing and correlating with history, physical examination and lifestyle of a patient was almost never enough. They turned to more and more tests to assure the public they were not old-fashioned and out-of-date.

Medical specialists in Physical Medicine and Rehabilitation (physiatrists), physical therapists and occupational therapists were very busy managing patients with spinal cord injuries, amputations and other major impairments. Unfortunately, some of the principles used in the management of that patient population are exactly opposite to those needed for the "walking wounded" population. Paraplegics, for example, are taught to stand "hanging" downward and backward on the "Y" ligaments at the hips.[8] Today, physiatrists and therapists in increasing numbers are applying their knowledge of the neuromuscoloskeletal system to the diagnosis and treatment of mechanical pain and somatic dysfunction. This includes the use of manual medicine techniques and whole body therapies.

In the past, dentists were almost universally involved with teeth, not the stomatognathic system. Today, that is changing primarily because of dentists' interest in temporomandibular disorders.

Chiropractors were "adjusting" (passively manipulating) individual joints. Today, increasing numbers of chiropractors recognize the importance of treating the somatic system effectively with nonthrust, mobilization-type techniques, and some recognize the importance of active movement and exercise for success of treatment.

Osteopaths, traditionally trained holistically, were becoming less interested in manipulative techniques and functional management of the somatic system and more interested in the allopathic approach. Today, osteopathy is also returning to its heritage, i.e., to the philosophies of its founders.

Another major problem area was that the ideas set forth in the 1947 report could not be practically implemented into patient care. Methods or techniques to achieve good posture and to correct poor posture were known to relatively few health professionals because of the emphasis on disease and local dysfunction rather than on integrated total body use. The art of gentle manual techniques for the correction of soft tissue and joint dysfunctions was hardly utilized by most health professionals. Interest in exercise was low, and exercise techniques had not been developed because knowledge of cardiovascular and musculoskeletal physiology had not matured. Ergonomics, including knowledge of the importance of surface reactions, was in its infancy.

Today, as indicated, this is all changing. The work of health professionals in multiple disciplines, including medical doctors, doctors of dentistry, osteopathy and chiropractic, physical and occupational therapists, movement analysts, exercise physiologists and ergonomic engineers is focusing on disorders of the somatic system. It is the hope of the present author that, by presenting posture functionally as body use, by organizing principles and determinants of posture, and by emphasizing the importance of body awareness and organization of movement, ideas such as those set forth in the 1947 report can be clarified, expanded and used more widely with increased effectiveness of clinical diagnosis and treatment of the somatic system. One cannot begin to imagine diagnosis and/or management of the cardiac or pulmonary systems without relying on dynamics. A static approach to posture also makes it impossible to analyze and manage the somatic system. Movement is the benchmark of good body use and correct movement is the hallmark.

APPENDIX 1

Principles of Posture

1. Posture is functional; it is the process of body (somatic) use and is determined by many factors (Appendix 2).

2. Posture should not be confused with position, alignment, shape, contour, form or pose.

3. The emphasis is on tissue balance, body mobility, stability and functional muscle strength, NOT simply on maximal muscle strength or force strength. Correct tissue balance means there are ideal vector quantities of the force couples acting about a joint(s) to prevent microtrauma; further, tissue lengths about a joint(s) are balanced, i.e., not too long or too short.

4. The body's center of gravity is the exact center of weight or the point about which the body would rotate freely if it were free to do so. It is where the weight is exactly equal on all sides.

5. Balance is the state of equilibrium where the center of gravity is over the base of support.

6. The body's center of gravity should remain over the correct, natural base of support with the individual body segments in neutral balance and "on balance" alignment. When sitting, the base of support is the pelvis, which is rotated anteriorly and below horizontal, approximately 34° in Type I and approximately 20° in Type II sitting.

7. Clinically, posture is best evaluated by the presence of easy instant physiologic pain-free neutral range movement into three planes from a neutral balanced stable alignment and upward and downward movement in "on balance" alignment. All physiologic motions should be available.

8. If motion is easier, then alignment and body use are better (the exception is dynamic stabilization, for motion is limited to the protected range).

9. Breathing is an excellent way to evaluate and improve motion and kinesthetics.

10. Posture is not "how we sit or stand or hold our bodies."

11. The body is a series of curves and triangles. Thus, trying to feel "straight" results in increased strain and unhealthy holding patterns.

12. Trying to be "straight," as in a straight line, results in increased stiffness, fatigue and strain because of unhealthy holding patterns. There is confusion between mind and body. It is difficult, even impossible, to concentrate on the goal of movement while being "tied up" trying to be straight. The brain receives few, if any, signals from straight structures.

13. Plumb line assessments are inadequate. They do not reflect dynamics or static faults or regional alignment.

14. Good posture is not synonymous with straight and erect. Alignment has been called "straight," but in the sagittal plane this can only refer to the relationships of body regions to each other, e.g., the head to the pelvis. In the frontal plane, "straight" refers to those same regional relationships and also to orientation about the midline.

15. "Straight" is difficult or impossible to relate to anatomically. The exception is the combination of "on balance" and "neutral balanced" alignments wherein the upper weight centers are aligned straight over the pelvis in the frontal and sagittal planes and the normal neutral flexible sagittal curves are maintained.

16. The pelvis is the body's center, structurally and functionally. It is the foundation of the spine. Pelvic (hip) movements and moments (torque at the hip joints) are clinically more important than the small sacroiliac movements.

17. "On balance" alignment requires a mobile, stable pelvis. Movement and body balance should initiate there. The pelvis is a torque converter for, as it rotates forward, the spine and torso move upward and a little forward. As the pelvis rotates backward, the spine and torso move downward and a little backward.

18. Very short duration "off balance" alignment can be good posture.

19. "Off balance" and nonneutral alignments can be good posture only if they provide stability for the movement of another body part or region.

20. The soma should not be divorced from the mind.

21. We should not function by good habits alone. We must also be able to consciously adapt and correct.

22. Awareness helps prevent bad habits.

23. Sensory awareness is monitoring the intermediate functional and biomechanical aspects of body use, e.g., ease of movement, dynamic connectedness or light tension/countertension in the connective tissues between body parts.

24. The body is an integrated, interrelated, anatomical, biomechanical and functional unit.

25. The craniovertebral joints must be free and the feet must be biomechanically balanced and functionally supported. These areas are major sites for kinesthetic input, kinesiologic control and adaptive responses. The C1 sensory root has no skin representation. It is all deep sensation, indicating the importance of kinesthetics from C1-level innervated muscles and joints.

26. Postural sway, part of neutral balanced alignment, in standing and sitting (Types I and II) entails movement on and off physiologic barriers to provide kinesthetic input.

27. Nonneutral alignment results in loss of movement and body awareness.

28. Joints in nonneutral in one plane lose motion in other planes.

29. Orthopedic-type devices provide sensory input and structural and functional support to improve posture.

30. Surface reactions from the ground and seat must counterbalance body weight properly to maintain "neutral balance" and "on balance" alignments. Surface reactions are the most neglected determinant of posture.

31. To be therapeutic, a support should be more than a "prop" for comfort. It should help improve the underlying problem.

32. Comfort can be a trap and progressive comfort may actually mean progressive bad posture. Comfort during movement is a more important guide to good body use than comfort at rest (see 65, 66).

33. Pelvic-spinal alignment should be in the same functional range in Types I and II sitting as they are in standing. In Types III and IV, they are different than in standing.

34. The entire pelvic-spinal-hip complex (PSH-C) must be controlled and balanced in sitting. In Types I and II the pelvis is rotated forward and the knees are lower than the hips. The pelvis is rotated forward 20-34°.

35. In Types I and II sitting, the hip angles should be flexed about 75-85° with normal neutral spinal curves. The pelvis must be supported anteriorly, laterally and posteriorly and the hips must be free to move.

36. Sitting on a flat seat surface in neutral pelvic-spinal alignment with or without a lumbar lordosis support behind the back, in Types I and II sitting, is inadequate. This often progresses to slumping in order to free the hips from compression and discomfort, anteriorly.

37. Types III and IV sitting are relaxing but can lead to the bad habit of leaned back, compressed nonneutral standing and walking and

loss of postural sway. Training and education can prevent this.

38. The four sides of the neck are not equally painful or equally restricted. Thus it is advantageous to be able to place the head and neck into different alignments and attitudes in backlying and sidelying sleeping positions.

39. Flexed elbow alignment during sleep can cause or aggravate an ulnar neuropathy at the elbow.

40. Sleeping with the hand under the pillow and head can precipitate symptoms of carpal tunnel syndrome.

41. Sleeping with the hand or arm under the pillow is usually due to insufficient support of the neck by the pillow.

42. Bruxing while the jaw is deflected to one side by the hand or arm under the pillow, during sleep, aggravates the temporomandibular joint.

43. "Ergonomic" chairs fail to help us if we do not also use our bodies correctly when sitting in them. The goals of relaxation and comfort can be inappropriate and can lead to disuse, misuse and abuse. Furthermore, comfort must include comfort during motion.

44. The design of the chair's seat surface is vital for posture of the pelvic-spinal-hip complex.

45. The design of back supports is important, but simply placing a support behind the back may be inadequate.

46. A pelvic support is more important in Types I and II sitting and a back support is most important in Types III and IV.

47. A foot support is an orthotic only if it controls neutral balanced alignment of the subtalar joint.

48. Neutral is a point located 2/3 of the distance from full pronation and 1/3 of the distance from full supination in the normal foot.

49. Pronation is normal in the first 25% of the stance phase.

50. Heel contact pronation should not exceed 5-8° on a flat surface.

51. Heel/toe gait is important, for the heel provides a fulcrum for pelvic-spinal movement, the floor reaction affords stability, and the heel eliminates the need for cervical and lumbar hyperlordosis to stabilize from above, downward.

52. The rear foot is a mobile adaptor. The midfoot develops stability and contributes to the rigid lever for toe off and forward propulsion. The forefoot provides the windlass effect for development of medial longitudinal arch.

53. The talus is a torque converter between the foot and leg, i.e., pronation of foot/internal rotation leg; supination of foot/external rotation leg.

54. A foot orthotic controls the biomechanics of the foot more at slower running speeds because there is more heel and midfoot contact at slower speeds.

55. A person running a kilometer in three minutes has very little heel contact. A rigid posted orthotic would be nonfunctional.

56. There are ideal vector quantities of the force couples acting about the joints.

57. Clincal stabilization requires: body centering at the pelvis; selective stabilization of one side of a moving joint(s); functional muscle strength; mobility of spinal and extremity joints; counterbalancing of body weight and surface reactions with the body in neutral alignment.

58. Accommodative orthotics such as the "stand-in-the-box to measure" type do not control biomechanics. They are nonfunctional and serve as props under the foot.

59. Every joint of the body should be capable of mobility (flexibility) by functioning in neutral alignment.

60. Every joint of the body should be capable of functioning in neutral alignment, stabilized by normal muscle activity. Movement requires a selectively stabilized point or region from which to move. For example, the glenohumeral joint requires a stabilized scapula. The pelvis, body center, is another vital area that must be selectively stabilized.

61. Every joint, with the possible exception of the temporomandibular joint, should be capable of providing stability for another joint or joints by functioning in nonneutral alignment.

62. To normalize joint movement, active exercise is not enough. It requires passive mobilization or manipulation. To accomplish this, one side of the joint is stabilized and the other is mobilized.

63. Acute compensations are adaptive (useful) when they relieve pain.

64. Chronic compensations are adaptive if they serve a useful purpose for the entire organism. With relative inflexibility, compensations in alignment take place at areas of relative flexibility. With a motion barrier, movement

takes place at the next available joint in the movement sequence.

65. To move more easily in comfort requires neutral alignment (see 32).

66. Chronically slumping away from pain to gain comfort is not adequate because then movement from the slumped, nonneutral alignment is restricted (see 32).

67. Fatigue can result from lack of a stable base of support because excessive muscle activity is needed to hold the body against gravity.

APPENDIX 2

Determinants of Posture

I. Mind Factors
  A. Body Awareness and Sensory Memory
    1. Proprioception/kinesthesia and ease of movement
    2. Conscious supervision of movement
    3. Body lengthening and simultaneously balanced widening
    4. Dynamic connectedness
    5. Physiologic barriers
    6. Postural sway
    7. Tension/countertension
    8. Breathing
    9. Inhibition of inappropriate and excessive muscle activity
  B. Other
    1. Skills
    2. Preemptive anticipatory actions
    3. Organization and sequence of movement
    4. Pain
    5. Psychologic
II. Physical Factors
  A. Inherent
    1. Somatic Tissues (see text)
    2. Neurosensory and neuromotor
    3. Tissue Structure and Function
      a. Soft tissue length, alignment, flexibility
      b. Functional muscle strength, endurance
      c. Joint surface shape, smooth- ness, arthrokinematics
      d. Joint flexibility and stretch
      e. Adaptability
      f. Sensation-nociception, proprioception
      g. Nutrition
    4. Joint Alignment
      a. Neutral balance in 3 planes
      b. "On balance"
      c. Dynamic stabilization in neutral range (protected range)— "neutral spine"
      d. Nonneutral
      e. Motion barriers
      f. Flexibility
      g. Stability
    5. Body Center—Pelvis
      a. Connects the upper and lower body
      b. Supports the upper weight centers
      c. Easy shifts of the center of gravity
      d. Balances the upper weight centers by shifting underneath them; "on balance" alignment versus "off balance"
      e. "Initiates" body movement (leads the body)
    6. Movement
      a. Active voluntary
      b. Active involuntary (craniosacral)
      c. Passive
      d. Passive accessory (joint play)
    7. Exercise
      a. Goals:
        1) Flexibility
        2) Functional muscle strengthening and balancing
        3) Endurance
        4) Training and education in body use, e.g., organization and sequence of movement; body centering; muscle function for fine-tuning alignment
        5) Power
        6) Coordination
        7) Speed/velocity
        8) Stability ih6pc
      b. Techniques of exercise
      c. Compatibility of tissues and exercise equipment
  B. Environmental Factors
    1. Natural

            a. Gravity
            b. Wind
        2. Ergonomic
            a. Provide support for body stability
            b. Provide surface contact for sensory input and body awareness
            c. Provide flexibility by allowing body flexibility, mobility and adaptability
            d. Provide surface reactions, for example, from seat surface and ground
            e. Control (harness) the direction of surface reactions from seat and ground
            f. Balance of upward and downward internal and external forces
        3. Surface Reactions
III. Duration and Frequency
IV. Comfort and Relaxation
    A. Comfort
        1. Not always best, alter the acute compensation (adaptation) to pain
        2. May be accommodating a dysfunction
        3. "Long term" comfort is most important—immediate comfort or immediate discomfort can be deceiving (the body may need to adapt)
        4. Comfort during movement is a more important gauge of body use than is comfort at rest
    B. Relaxation
        1. Relaxation occurs at rest
        2. It must not cause disuse, misuse or abuse
        3. Relaxing does not have to mean collapsing
V. Adaptation
    Three critical areas:
    A. Craniovertebral joints
    B. Feet
    C. Thoracolumbar
VI. Treatment Techniques
    A. Mobilization/manipulation
    B. Stabilization (selective)
    C. Integration of body awareness, organization and sequence
    D. Exercise
    E. Pain relief/control
    F. Supports, for example: seat surfaces
    G. Nutrition

REFERENCES

1. Ward RC (principal investigator). Glossary of Osteopathic Terminology. *JAOA*. 1981;80:119-134.
2. Kimberly P. Formulating a prescription for osteopathic manipulative treatment. *JAOA*. 1979;43-50.
3. Kraus H, Eisemanger-Weber S. Quantitative tabulation of posture evaluation based on structural and functional measurements (a report). *Physiother Rev*. 1946;76:235-242.
4. Kendall HO, Kendall FP, Boynton DA. *Posture and Pain*. New York, NY: Kreiger; 1977:1-7.
5. Levine HL, Finnegan EM. Overuse and vocal disorders: cause and effect. *Med Probl Perform Art*. 1986;1817-19.
6. Travell JG, Simon DG. Myofascial Pain and Dysfunction. In: *The Trigger Point Manual*. Baltimore, MD: Williams and Wilkens; 1983.
7. Walpin LA. Back pain: the important role of a unique pelvic spinal posture aid. Presented at American Academy of Physical Medicine and Rehabilitation, 1985.
8. Walpin LA. The role of orthotic devices for managing neck disorders. *Physical Medicine and Rehabilitation: State of the Art Reviews*. Redford J, ed. 1987; Vol. 1, No. 1, 25-43.
9. Bartenieff I, Lewis D. *Body Movement: Coping with the Environment*. New York, NY: Gordon and Breach; 1980.
10. Dowd I. *Taking Roots To Fly. Seven Articles on Functional Anatomy*, 1981.
11. McKenzie RA. *The Lumbar Spine: Mechanical Diagnosis and Therapy*. Spinal Publications, 1981.
12. Magoun HI. *Osteopathy In The Cranial Field*. 3rd Ed. Kirksville, MO: JL Printing Co; 1976.
13. Roberts TDM. *The Role of Vestibular and Neck Receptors In Locomotion*. Herman R, Grillner S, Stein P, Stuart D, eds. New York, NY: Plenum Press; 1976.
14. Norman RW, Komi PV. Electromechanical delay in skeletal muscle. *Acta Physiol Scan*. 1979;106:241-248.
15. Janda V. *Muscles, Central Nervous Motor Regulation and Back Problems*. New York, NY: Plenum Press; 1977.
16. Jones FP. *A Study of The Alexander Technique. Body Awareness in Action*. New York, NY: Schocken Press; 1979:46,143.
17. Fryette G. American Osteopathic Association Convention, 1918.
18. Hackett G. *Ligament and Tendon Relaxation Treated by Prolotherapy*. Springfield, Ill: Charles C. Thomas; 1958.
19. Bland JH. *Disorders of the Cervical Spine. Diagnosis and Medical Management*. Philadelphia, PA: WB Saunders; 1987:269-273.

20. Jones LH. *Strain and Counterstrain.* American Academy of Osteopathy, 1981.
21. Maigne R. *Orthopedic Medicine. A New Approach to Vertebral Manipulations.* Springfield, Ill: Charles C. Thomas; 1972.
22. Bendix T, Biering-Sorensen F. Posture of the trunk when sitting on forward inclining seats. *Scand J Rehab Med.* 1983;15:197-203.
23. Keegan JJ. Alterations of the lumbar curve related to posture and seating *JBJS.* 1953;35A:589-603.
24. McKenzie DC. The role of the shoe and orthotics. *Med Sports Sci.* 1987;23:30-38.
25. Pagliano J. Management of pronated and supinated feet. *Med Sports Sci.* 1987;23:155-160.
26. Walpin L. Bedroom posture: the critical role of a unique pillow in relieving upper spine and shoulder girdle pain. Presented at the American Congress of Physical Medicine and Rehabilitation, 1977.
27. Dishman R. *Dynamic Chiropractic.* 1988;6:(16) 32.
28. Mellin G. Correlations of hip mobility with degree of back pain and lumbar spinal mobility in chronic low back pain patients. *Spine.* 1988:668-670.
29. Hicks JE, Gerber LH. Rehabilitation of the patient with arthritis and connective tissue disease. In: DeLisa JA, ed. *Rehabilitation Medicine Principles and Practice.* Philadelphia, PA: Lippincott; 1988:765-794.
30. Bogduk N, Twomey LT. *Clinical Anatomy of the Lumbar Spine.* New York, NY: Churchill Livingstone; 1987:84-89.
31. Mohl ND. Introduction to occlusion. In: Mohl ND, Zarb GA, Carlsson GE, Rugh JD, eds. *A Textbook of Occlusion.* Chicago, Ill: Quintessence; 1988:15-23.
32. Farfan HF. Biomechanics of the lumbar spine. In: Kirkaldy-Willis WH, ed. *Managing Low Back Pain.* 2nd ed. New York, NY: Churchill Livingstone; 1988.
33. McKenzie RA. *Back Letter.* 1988.
34. *Webster's New World Dictionary of the American Language, Second College Edition.* Guralnik DB, ed. New York, NY: Simon & Schuster; 1986.
35. Kraus H. *Diagnosis and Treatment of Muscle Pain.* Chicago, Ill: Quintessence; 1988.
36. Rocabado M. Biomechanical relationship of the cranial, cervical and hyoid regions. *J Craniomandibular Pract.* 1983;7:61-66.
37. Kraus H, Eisemanger-Weber S. Fundamental Considerations of posture exercises. *Physiother Rev.* 1947;27:361-367.
38. Sahrmann SA. Adult Posturing. In: Kraus S, ed. *TMJ Disorders: Management of the Craniomandibular Complex.* New York, NY: Churchill Livingstone; 1988:295-309.
39. *The World Book Dictionary.* Barnhart CL, ed. Chicago, Ill: Doubleday and Co; 1970.
40. Stolov WC. Musculoskeletal problems. mobility problems of the muscle-joint unit. In: Basmajian JV, Kirby RL, eds. *Medical Rehabilitation.* Baltimore, MD: Williams and Wilkens; 1984:196-205.
41. Yunis MB. Diagnosis, etiology and management of fibromyalgia syndrome: an update. *Comprehensive Therapy.* 1988;14:8-20.
42. Yunis MB. Primary fibromyalgia syndrome: current concepts. *Comprehensive Therapy.* 1984;10:21-28.
43. Grice A. A biomechanical approach to cervical and dorsal adjusting. In: Haldeman S, ed. *Modern Developments in the Principles and Practice of Chiropractic.* New York, NY: Appleton-Century-Crofts; 1980:331-358.
44. *Orthopedic Product News.* Gralla Publications, January, 1989.
45. Upledger JE, Vredevoogd JD. *Craniosacral Therapy.* Chicago, Ill: Eastland Press; 1983:19.
46. Sahrmann S. Lecture at Rehab '89 – Abbey/Foster. Los Angeles, CA; 1989.
47. Billig HE, Loewendahl E. *Mobilization of the Human Body. Newer Concepts in Body Mechanics.* Stanford, CA: Stanford University Press; 1949.
48. Walpin LA. *Bottoms-Up® Pelvic Spinal Posture Seat: Principles and Functions.* 1988.

Chapter 3

Diagnosis and Treatment of Muscle Pain

Hans Kraus, MD

There are four types of muscle pain: muscle deficiency, tension, spasm, triggerpoint.

Muscle deficiency results from decreased strength, decreased flexibility, or a combination of both.[1] Typical examples are low back pain caused by weak abdominal muscles, frequently after pregnancy, or back pain caused by stiff back muscles.[2] Pain in the extremities after recuperation from injury is also often attributable to weak, stiff muscles.

After prolonged immobilization, it is necessary to increase therapeutic exercise gradually in order to avoid overtaxing the capacity of the injured limb. We frequently see patients after well-healed fractures walking too soon or overexerting their arms, possibly because their orthopedists encouraged them to do so. Overexertion will cause pain and disability even in the healthy, let alone the injured.[3]

Before an exercise program is introduced, muscles must be tested for strength and flexibility.[1] Muscle strength is assessed by observing the muscle's ability to contract, to overcome gravity and resistance, and to fully bear weight in comparison with the healthy extremity. Tightness and lack of flexibility are gauged by registering the range of joint movement on a goniometer.

In back patients, we gauge strength and flexibility of key posture muscles by means of the Kraus-Weber Test[2] (Fig. 3-1).

If the test indicates muscle deficiency, then a therapeutic exercise program following a well-designed pattern should be prescribed. Each exercise program should start with easy movements (assisted if necessary) and progress gradually to movements against gravity and resistance. Lack of flexibility, which restricts range of motion, is treated similarly; starting with a limbering motion and advancing to active, then passive stretches.

The program[1,2,3] consists of 1) relaxation, 2) gentle movements, 3) more strenuous movements and stretches, and 4) workout. The sequence is then reversed as a cool-off. Each exercise should be repeated three to four times only, followed by other movements involving different muscle groups. Multirepetition exercises should be avoided because they stiffen muscles (Fig. 3-2).

Two to three sessions a week are needed for satisfactory progress; they should continue until maximum attainable function is reached. The patient should learn the exercises step by step so that he or she can perform them at home between treatment sessions. The same exercise principles applies to the masticatory muscles.

The benefit of exercise has been demonstrated by the "Y's Way to a Healthy Back" program which is offered in a thousand YMCA's in this country. Over 300,000 patients have completed these six-week exercise sessions and many continue them at home. Of over 1000 people who were surveyed, 82% showed improvement.[4] According to a one-year follow-up, medical costs and job absenteeism were both reduced by 50%.

Tension pain occurs when a muscle contracts and stays contracted beyond functional need. *Tension* can occur in any muscle. Everybody is familiar with tension headache, but few people understand that back pain and other muscular pain may stem from the same cause.

Tension may result from emotional, situational, or positional stress. A typical example is pain in the neck and trapezius occurring

SIX BASIC MUSCLE TESTS

TEST 1. Lie on your back, hands behind your neck, legs straight. Keeping your legs straight, raise both feet 10 inches off the floor and hold for 10 seconds. This is a test of your hip-flexing muscles.

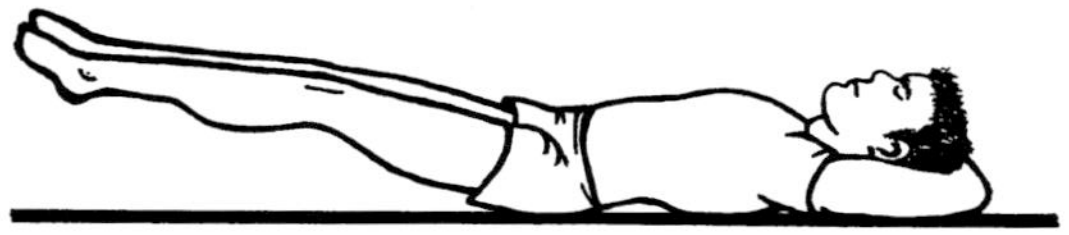

TEST 2. Lie on your back, hands behind your neck, feet under a heavy object which will not topple over. Try to "roll" up to a sitting position. This tests your hip-flexing and abdominal muscles.

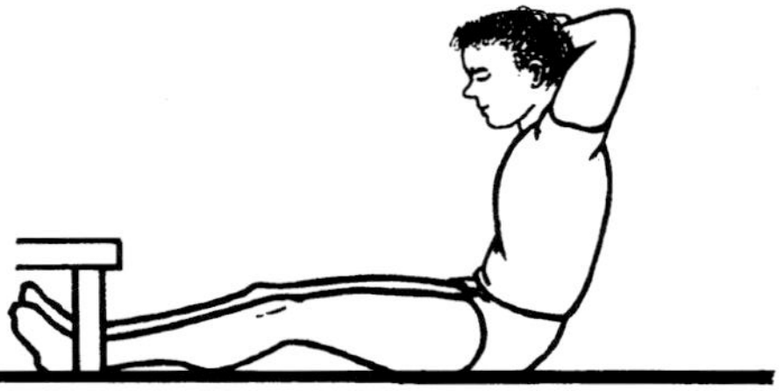

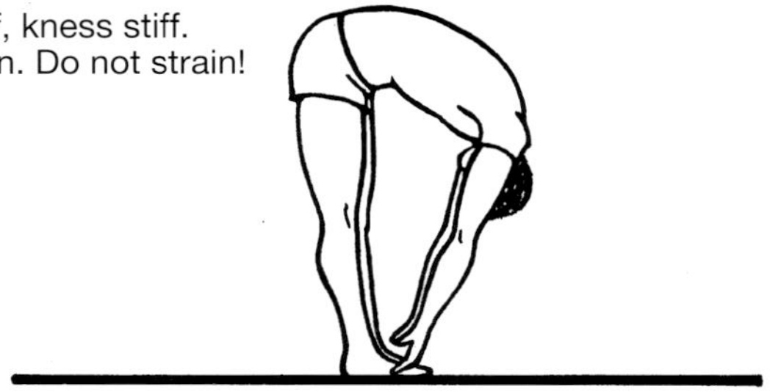

TEST 3. Lie on your back, hands behind your neck, knees flexed, feet under a heavy object which will not topple over. Again try to "roll" up to a sitting position. This is a test of your abdominal muscles.

TEST 4. Lie on your stomach with a pillow under your abdomen, hands behind your neck. With someone holding your feet and hips down, raise your trunk and hold for 10 seconds. This tests the upper back muscles.

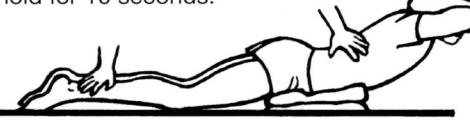

TEST 5. Taking the same position as that used for Test 4, but this time having someone holding your shoulders and hips down, try to raise your legs and hold for 10 seconds. This tests the muscles of the lower back.

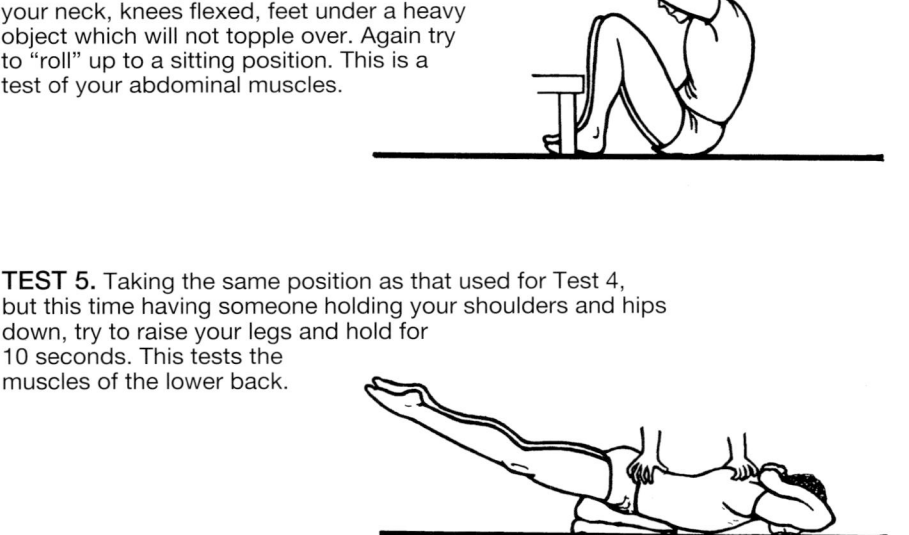

TEST 6. Stand erect with shoes off, knees stiff. Slowly reach down as far as you can. Do not strain!

Fig. 3-1. These six standardized tests of muscular function may help to "pinpoint" deficiencies of strength or flexibility (Test 6). They are done as slowly and smoothly as possible. Avoid jerky movements. Do not strain. Stop and rest briefly after each test.

Exercise 1
Take a deep breath, then exhale slowly. Now, shrug and breathe in. Exhale as you let ho of the shrug.

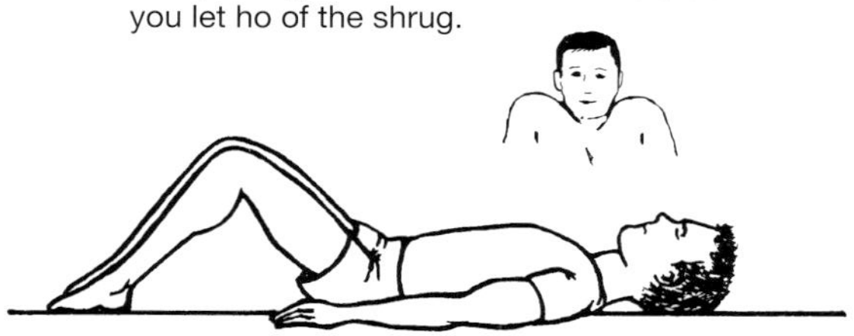

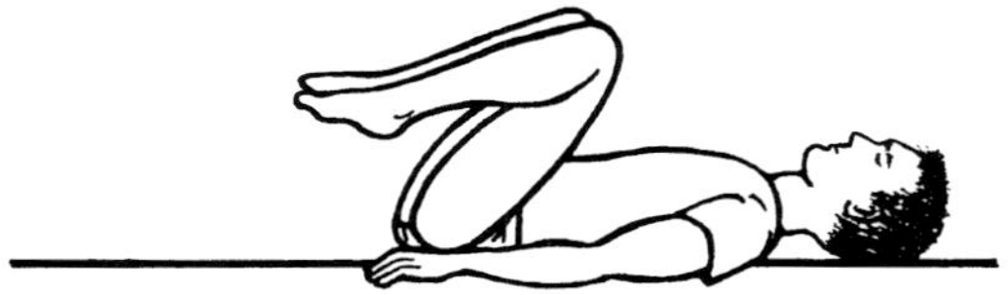

Exercise 2
Position yourself comfortably with your back on the floor and both knees bent. Close your eyes. Take a deep breath and exhale slowly. Slide your right leg forward and then slide it back. Slide the left leg forward and then back. Take another deep breath. Tighten both fists, then let go.

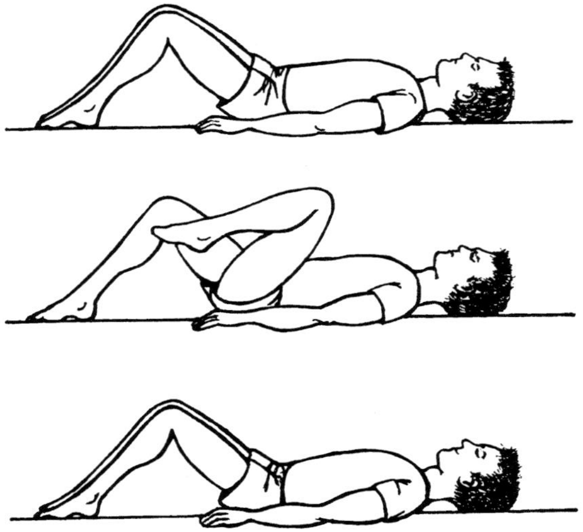

Exercise 3
Lie on your left side with your head resting comfortably on your arm. Keep both knees flexed and hips slightly flexed. Slide your right knee as close to your head as is comfortably possible, then slowly extend the leg until it is completely straight. The leg is dead weight; you do not lift your right leg, slide it on the left leg. Do the exercise three times, then turn to your right side and repeat the exercise with your left leg. Remember, *the top leg is dead weight.*

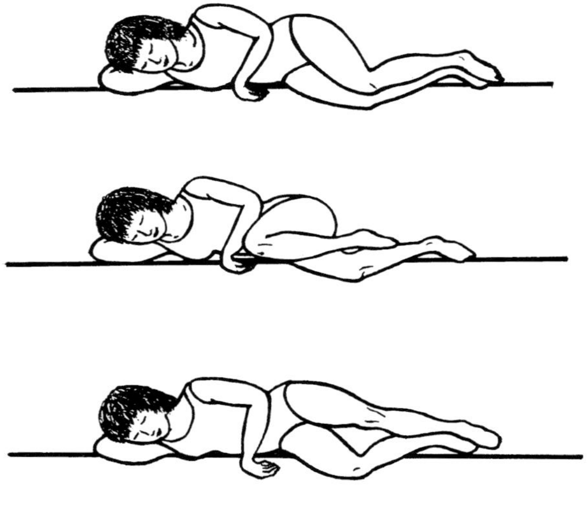

Exercise 4
Lie on your stomach. Let your head rest comfortably on your folded hands and point your toes inward. Now, tighten your seat muscles. Hold that position for two seconds, then let go.

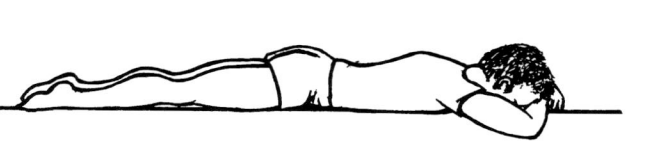

Exercise 5
Lie on your back and flex both knees. Pull both knees up to your chest. Then, lower your legs gradually to the floor in the flexed position. Do not raise your hips off the floor.

Exercise 6
Assume a kneeling position, resting on your hands and knees. Arch your back like a cat and drop your head at the same time. Now, reverse the arch by bringing up your head and forming a "U" with your spine.

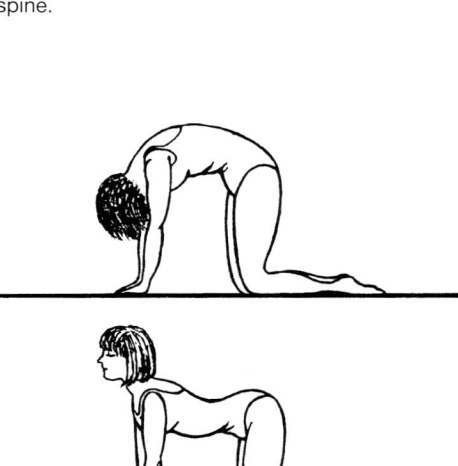

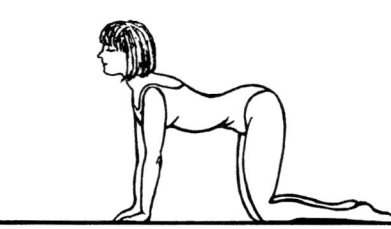

Fig. 3-2. Therapeutic exercise program.

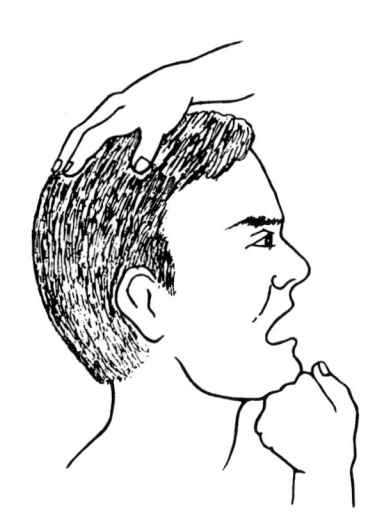

Fig. 3-3. Resistance relaxes antagonist of contracting muscle.

in people who frequently squeeze the telephone between their ear and shoulder while at work.

Treatment of tension must include changes in work habits and lifestyle. Tranquilizers or psychotherapy may be needed temporarily. Relaxation exercises should be the first step in any exercise program.[3] Further, hypnosis[6] can be very effective in producing deep relaxation: hypnotizable patients can enjoy several brief periods of self-hypnosis during a hectic day. Once patients have learned to relax, vigorous exercise can achieve a similar result, e.g., DeVries reports that jogging can be more relaxing than Meprobamate.

Tooth-grinding or the inability to open the mouth sufficiently is usually tension-related. Rehabilitation exercises and relaxation training are often helpful. Resistance applied under the chin while the patient opens his or her mouth and relaxes the occluding muscles (Fig. 3-3) is useful here.

Muscle spasm in acute cases is characterized by severe pain, limitation of motion resulting in manifest dysfunction, and an antalgic position. We prefer to treat this state of muscle pain with electrotherapy: tetanizing current for 10 minutes on trunk and neck muscles, followed by sinusoidal current for 10 minutes; for muscles spasm of the limbs, we use only sinusoidal current for 15 minutes.[1,2,3]

Electrotherapy is followed by gentle exercises made pain-free by ethyl chloride spray.[8]

We use limbering movement, movement within easy range; we never stretch muscles in the acute stage. We have found ethyl chloride or even ice massage[9] to be more effective than Fluori-Methane.[10] Relief of pain and increased range of motion indicate successful treatment. Treatment on seven to ten successive days is usually necessary to relieve acute spasm. This method does not succeed if major pathology is present. Immediate mobilization is especially important in acute back episodes; bed rest should be avoided.

Partial ligament tears — or muscle strains — also respond far better to immediate mobilization than to immobilization and rest.[3,11,12] Exercise, without any weight bearing, is recommended for the lower extremity, but crutches must be used until walking is painfree. The upper extremity should be treated similarly, with gentle exercise that is increased gradually. The patient should be given a sling, and instructions should be given to take it off and exercise at frequent intervals.

Muscle spasm of masticatory muscles responds well to ethyl chloride and gentle chewing motion. To prevent the patient's inhaling the ethyl chloride spray, protect nose and mouth and keep the face averted; have the patient exhale while spraying.

When the acute attack has been managed, muscle tests should be performed, and suspected triggerpoints palpated. Relief of pain is not the final aim. To achieve long-range results, proper rehabilitation must follow. This is especially true for occupational and athletic injuries. A worker who has to lift 100 pounds will experience recurring back pain if he returns to work when he is capable of lifting only 50 pounds. A skier with a knee injury will risk reinjury if he resumes his sport before his leg is fully reconditioned.[3]

Triggerpoints are tender nodules, usually localized close to the insertion and origin of a muscle or aponeurosis. Max Lange[13] first mentioned triggerpoints in 1932; Glogowski[14] and Wallraff described them as small areas of degenerated muscle tissue. Triggerpoints can be caused by prolonged muscle spasm, tension, or chronic muscle strain. Endocrine imbalance, menopause, hypothyroidism, and

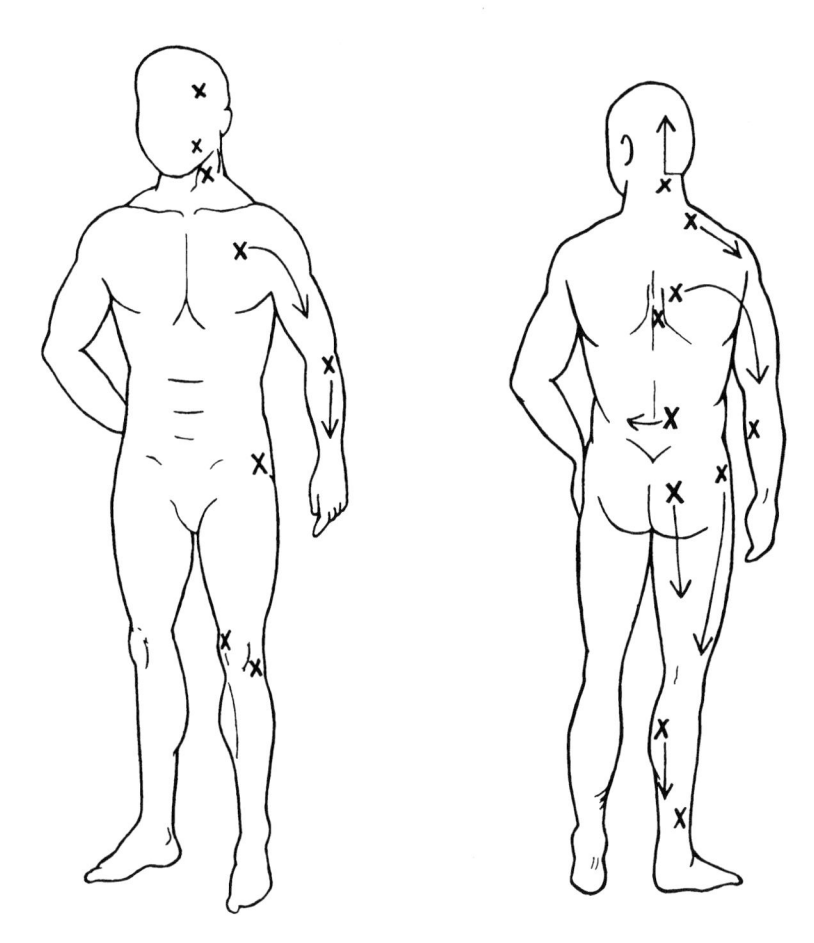

Fig. 3-4. Most frequently found triggerpoints and pain radiation.

so on frequently cause general muscle ache, tenderness, and triggerpoints.[15]

Diagnosis is made by palpation for localized tenderness. Muscle spasm may show generalized tenderness of the whole muscle, but tense muscles are not tender. Probing often produces avoidance movement and an expression of pain.[16] History reveals typical pain patterns,[2,3,17] as seen in Figure 3-4, and described below.

1. Suboccipital triggerpoint producing posterior headache.
2. Sternomastoid triggerpoint causing dizziness.
3. Posterior neck triggerpoint causing neck stiffness.
4. Trapezius triggerpoint radiating to neck and arm.
5. Scalenus triggerpoint resulting in peripheral entrapment of cervical plexors and simulating disc disease.

6. Triggerpoint in infraspinatus radiating to posterior aspect of arm and curtailing inward rotation; this condition is often misdiagnosed as bursitis.
7. Pectoral muscle triggerpoints, left and right, leading to arm pain and suggesting angina.
8. Triggerpoints near humeral condyles, mostly lateral and sometimes medial (tennis elbow), radiating to forearm and frequently combined with a triggerpoint in forearm muscle.
9. Interscapular triggerpoint causing upper back pain (round back).
10. Trigger point in sacrospinal muscles radiating toward upper back (same effect produced by triggerpoints in quadratus).
11. Triggerpoints in gluteus maximus radiating to posterior aspect of thigh.
12. Triggerpoint in gluteus medius tensor frequently radiating to lateral aspect of thigh

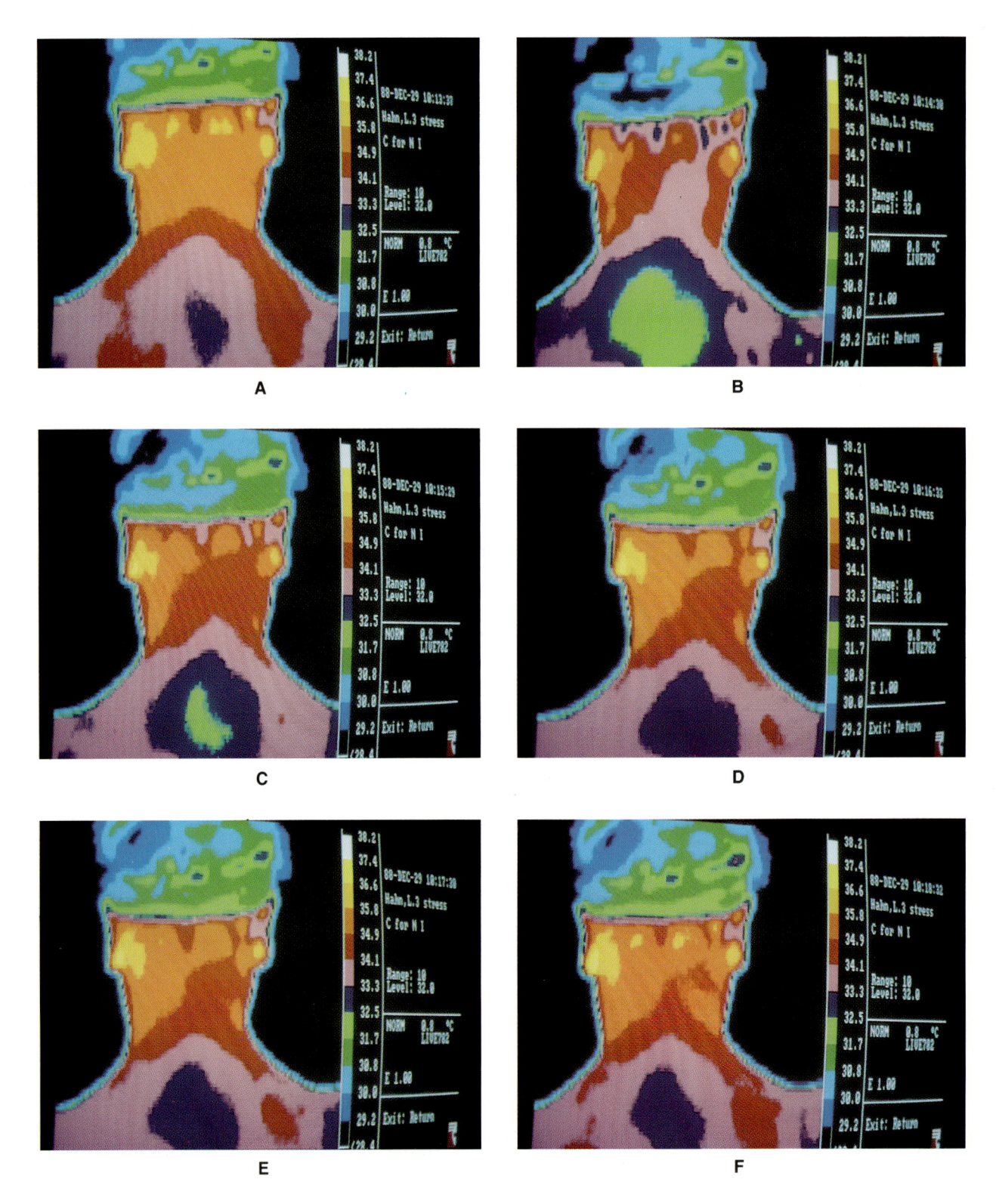

Fig. 3-5. Protocol for documentation: Suboccipital trigger points producing posterior headache. **A**, a pre-alcohol and baseline photograph; **B**, one minute post alcohol spray; **C**, two minutes post alcohol spray; **D**, three minutes post alcohol spray; **E**, four minutes post alcohol spray; **F**, five minutes post alcohol spray. It is noted that the trigger point areas turn cold following the alcohol spray. Cooling ends within three minutes and the area returns to what represents a true trigger point level at five minutes. Thermal artifacts, such as vascular shunts, are removed by this protocol. The yellow area indicates the increased heat emission of a suboccipital trigger point.

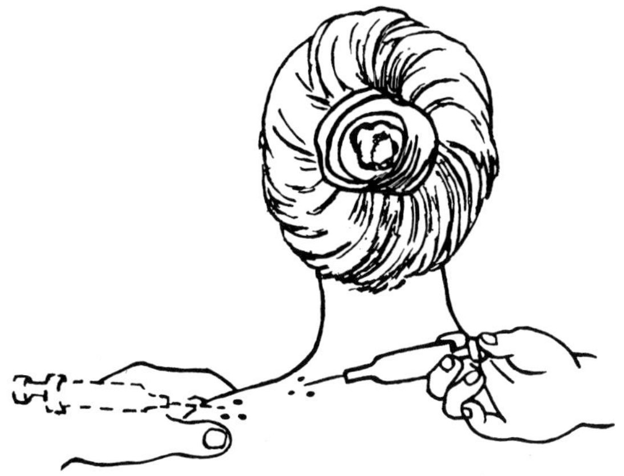

Fig. 3-6. Injection of triggerpoint in trapezius muscle.

and causing entrapment of lateral femoral cutaneous nerve.

13. Triggerpoint in origin of rectus femoris radiating to patella.
14. Triggerpoint in vastus intermedius radiating to patella and patella femoral ligament.
15. Triggerpoint in piriformis causing true sciatic nerve compression (peripheral nerve entrapment); frequently misdiagnosed as disc disease.
16. Triggerpoint in vastus lateralis and fascia lateralis causing knee pain.
17. Triggerpoint in head of triceps surae causing knee pain and radiating toward heel.
18. Triggerpoint in soleus radiating toward heel; often misdiagnosed as Achilles tendinitis.
19. Triggerpoint in interossel muscles; most often misdiagnosed as neuroma.
20. Triggerpoint in masticatoris muscle; frequently caused by temporomandibular joint problem.

Triggerpoints – as well as muscle spasm – may cause peripheral nerve entrapment, which is frequently mistaken for nerve root pressure. Semi-objective quantification is possible with Fischer's pressure gauge.[18] This instrument registers a decreased pain threshold as compared to the contralateral side.

Thermography can also be used to visualize triggerpoints (Fig. 3-5). Both pain threshold measurement and thermography demonstrate disappearance of triggerpoints after successful treatment (see Chapter 4 by Dr. Weinstein).

Triggerpoints should be treated after muscle spasm has been relieved, at which time they can be clearly identified. Mark the tender spots with a scratch on the skin, then needle the painful area. Explore the insertion and origin of the muscle with a needle and inject lidocaine or saline. (The needle causes pain in the triggerpoints, whereas normal muscle remains painfree.) Observe careful sterile technique (Fig. 3-6).

On three consecutive days after the injection, follow up by using tetanizing current for 10 minutes, sinusoidal current for 10 minutes, ethyl chloride, and gentle movement. During this time the patient must avoid prolonged sitting, standing, and walking.

Triggerpoints in masticatory muscles frequently cause tension and spasm in the neck and trapezius areas, which in turn generate new triggerpoints. Although triggerpoints may stem from true orthopedic problems (TMJ and bite problems), tension and spasm may be the only cause of pain. Conservative treatment can help the patient without bite plates or surgery.

Inasmuch as the skeletal muscle may be the only immediate cause of pain, it should be examined and treated before more aggressive measures are considered. Many patients diagnosed as having disc disease can recover completely with adequate treatment of their muscles.

Many acute and chronic injuries to muscle and ligament, as well as minor fractures, can be treated successfully by the methods described above, without the need for immobilization or surgery.

REFERENCES

1. Kraus H. *Therapeutic Exercise.* Springfield, Ill: Charles C Thomas; 1949: 33-34, 62-64.
2. Kraus H. *Clinical Treatment of Neck and Back Pain.* New York, NY: McGraw Hill; 1970.
3. Kraus H. Evaluation and treatment of muscle function in athletic injury. *Amer J Surg.* September 1959;98:353-362.
4. Kraus H, Nagler W, Melleby A. Evaluation of an exercise program for back pain. *Am Fam Physician.* September 1983:153,154.

5. Sainsbury P, Gibson TG. Symptoms in anxiety and tension and the accompanying physiological changes in the muscular system. *J Neurol Neurosurg Phychiat*. August 1954:17.
6. Spiegel H, Speigel D. *Trance and Treatment: Clinical Uses of Hypnosis*. New York, NY: Basic Books; 1978.
7. DeVries HA, Adams GM. Electromyographic comparison of single doses of exercises and meprobamate as to effects on muscular relaxation. *Am J Phys Med*. August 1954;51.
8. Kraus H. Use of surface anesthesia in the treatment of painful motion. *JAMA*. June 1941;116:2582-2583.
9. Waylonis GW. The Physiological effects of ice massage. *Arch Phys Med*. May 1952;33:291-298.
10. Travell J. Ethyl chloride spray for painful muscle spasm. *Arch Phys Med*. 1967;48:37-41.
11. Salter S, et al. The biological effect of continuous passive motion on the healing of full thickness defects in articular cartilage. *J Bone Joint Surg*. 1974.
12. Dorelle S, Hecter P, Killis. Early controlled mobilization following extensor tendon repair in zone V-VI of the hand: preliminary report. *Contemp Orthopedics*. October 1985;11.
13. Lange M. *Die Muskelharten (Myogelosen)*. Munich, Germany: JF Lehmann;1931.
14. Glogowski G, Wallraff J. Ein Beltrag zur Klinik und Histologie der Muskelharten (Myogelosen). *Ztschr Orthop*. 1951;80:237-268.
15. Sonkin L. Myofascial pain in metabolic disorder. *Med Times*. April 1983;43-51.
16. Gillette HF. Office management of musculoskeletal pain. *Texas J Med*. January 1966;62:47-53.
17. Travel J, Simons D. *Myofascial Pain and Dysfunction: The Triggerpoint Manual*. Baltimore, MD: Williams and Wilkins;1983.
18. Fischer A. Advances in documentation of pain and soft tissue pathology. *Med Times*. December 1983:24-31.

Chapter 4

Scoliosis Evaluation & Documentation With Computerized Infrared Thermography

S. Alan Weinstein, DO
Gay Weinstein, RTT

The widespread implementation of routine school screening examinations for the early detection of scoliosis, in the United States and elsewhere, has resulted in the referral of a large number of children for further evaluation. After reviewing cases of idiopathic adolescent scoliosis identified through regular or experimental screening programs,[1-3] many clinical researchers have advocated regular screening of school populations in certain age groups or grades.

The major objection to such screening is that it exposes a large number of children to periodically repeated radiography, the majority of whom have minor curvatures which do not currently, and may not ever, require treatment.[4,5] These critics argue that more economical and less hazardous diagnostic alternatives should be sought out.

In this chapter, after briefly considering the potential clinical significance of preliminary screening, discussing findings of scoliosis, and introducing the fundamental principles of thermographic evaluation, the application of this technology to the assessment of scoliotic disorders and postural analysis will be presented succinctly.

SCOLIOSIS: A BRIEF OVERVIEW

In the early seventeenth century, Thomas Adams argued that "he is a better physician that keeps diseases off of us, than he that cures them being on us."[6] Notwithstanding many recent clinical advances in the field, the contemporary physician still encounters difficulty in establishing the true prevalence of scoliosis and finds himself unable to identify a means for accurately determining which patients have a disorder that will progress significantly after it has been recognized clinically.

Prevalence studies based upon school screening programs would appear to suggest an incidence ranging from 0.3 to 15.3 percent.[1-4,6-8] Careful examination of this literature readily reveals that these substantial differences in possible prevalence reflect differing detection methods, different proportions of children evaluated radiographically, and differing definitions of scoliosis. When only larger curves (> 10%) are considered as positive findings, the prevalence rates narrow to approximately 1 to 3 percent, and most likely average 1.5 to 2 percent.[2,6,8,]

Since only the larger curves require treatment, a knowledge of the risks of curve progression is necessary to enable practitioners to devise proper follow-up programs for continued periodic evaluation of each patient, one which establishes an optimal, and therefore cost-effective, means for the continued evaluation of the patient. Available studies on the natural progression of idiopathic scoliosis during the patient's growth period are difficult to compare and interpret due to differences in measurement techniques, in the degree of curvature at the time of initial diagnosis, and in the duration of follow-up after the initial diagnosis has been established.

Studies that followed all spinal curves detected in school screening programs tended to produce low progression rates, in the range of 5 to 6 percent of the patients followed.[1,3] However, when one considers only initial curves of 10 percent or greater, progression is far more common—usually in the range of 20 to 60 percent of the patients, with the highest percentages observed among individuals with initial curvatures of 20 to 40 percent.[9-12] From this data, it would seen quite evident that the risk of progression, and therefore the need for adequate follow-up evaluations, is quite high among those patients who evidence substantial curvature at the time of initial clinical recognition of the problem.

Unfortunately, most contemporary patient follow-up programs in scoliosis place substantial reliance upon periodic radiography, with the result that many children may be excessively exposed to unnecessary radiation. Realistically, this exposure may not be justified except in the presence of a compelling clinical need for a sophisticated radiological workup when substantive treatment is required. However, recent advances in contemporary medical technology are now providing alternatives for simpler, less invasive procedures for the evaluation of the spine in children with scoliosis.

Magnetic resonance imaging, a procedure with no known biological risk, has been reported to be clinically useful for this purpose.[13] This procedure, while potentially quite accurate and sensitive in this application, remains an expensive procedure that may never prove to be cost-effective in routine use. Computerized infrared electronic thermography, however, has been previously reported to be useful for the routine evaluation of adolescents with scoliosis.[13]

THERMOGRAPHY: AN INTRODUCTION

Historically, the concept of thermography can be traced to Hippocrates, who is recognized as the first clinician to apply thin layers of moistened earth to various body regions for the purpose of demonstrating body surface temperature differences.[14]

During the past two decades, computerized infrared electronic thermography has become increasingly important for the assessment of one of medicine's oldest problems: pain. In this clinical application, thermography does not detect pain directly, but instead passively records the body surface temperature alterations that reflect cutaneous vascular response to pain, as well as that which may be associated with other irritating stimuli present in underlying musculoskeletal tissues.[15] Most importantly, it provides these imaging evaluations without reliance upon any radiation source.[10] The clinical use of thermal imaging for the evaluation of pain was first described in 1964.[16,17] Since that time, it has become widely recognized that infrared thermography provides a valuable clinical tool for the assessment of pain in a variety of disorders: stress fractures,[18] myofascial pain,[19] reflex sympathetic dystrophy,[20] nerve entrapment disorders,[21] thoracic outlet syndrome,[22] facet joint pain,[23] bone and joint inflammatory disorders,[24] and radicular syndromes of the cervical and lumbar spine.[25-35]

The techniques employed in computerized infrared electronic thermography, although somewhat complex, can be mastered and appropriately applied in most clinical settings. The procedures which we will initially describe were developed over 25 years of application to the evaluation of pain; thereafter, we will examine the specific procedure that has been found accurate and reliable for the evaluation of the postural deformities associated with scoliosis.

There are several reliable instruments available for use in clinical thermography. It is beyond the scope of this discussion to provide a comparative evaluation of the relative merits of these different units. The experience of this author has been primarily with two units: the AGA Thermovision Model 720 and the AGA Discon Model 782 electronic thermography units.

The standard procedure followed for the thermographic evaluation of patients with complaints of pain is as follows. Thermographic evaluations are conducted in a draft-free room where the temperature is maintained between 68 and 78°F. In advance of the procedure, patients are advised not to smoke, apply hot packs or topical medications to the area of suspicion, use TENS units or have physical therapy for 4 to 24 hours prior to the thermographic procedure. After disrobing as necessary to expose the body region involved, the patient is allowed to equilibrate in the surrounding thermal environment for 15 minutes, customarily in the view of the technician, who has already instructed the patient to remain relatively still and not touch the area involved in the pain complaint. Thereafter, standard thermographic photographs are obtained covering the patient's area of pain and all neuroanatomically-related areas of actual or potential pain radiation per protocol of ANMT. A 0.8-1.0° centigrade temperature difference affecting at least 25% of the surface area of a single dermatome when compared to its contralateral dermatome is the minimum criterion for recognition of a body surface temperature abnormality indicative of pain.

Infrared thermographic documentation of a suspected or previously recognized scoliosis is a somewhat less complex procedure than that required for the evaluation of a complaint of pain. Other than the thermographic unit itself, only five minor accessory tools are required:

Accessories for Postural Measurement
- HAMA – DSR System
- Vivitar Instant Slide Printer
- Polaroid 665 Film
- Protractor
- Colored Pen

The technique for thermographic postural analysis is carried out in the following manner. This procedure may be performed as a separate thermographic assessment seeking evidence of postural abnormalities, including pelvic tilt and/or scoliosis, or it may be performed as an adjunctive study accompanying a thoracic or lumbar thermographic evaluation being conducted for some other clinical indication.

The steps in the postural study are as follows:

1. A marker, consisting of either tape or X-ray marker, is placed on the patient's back, over the skin covering the first thoracic vertebra (T1).
2. An alcohol spray is applied to the skin surface of the back, directed to the area over the spine.
3. Next, a wait of at least three minutes is imposed to assure the complete evaporation of the residual alcohol.
4. The examining thermographic camera should be positioned appropriately for the intended procedure. The contralateral parts of the back should be parallel to each other to the extent achievable in each individual case, with adequate surface area available to permit proper assessment.
5. The photograph(s) is (are) then obtained of the entire back.
6. The 35 mm film is then developed and mounted in a standard slide.
7. The slide is placed into a Vivitar Slide Printer which contains Polaroid 665 film, and is printed.
8. The Polaroid 665 film image is then assessed in the manner described and illustrated in the following discussion.

The physical landmarks for the scoliosis evaluation are schematically depicted in Figure 4-1A: the first thoracic vertebra (T1) appropriately marked as previously described, the spinal stripe, the two posterior iliac spines (PSIS) and, finally, the gluteal cleft. A standard thermographic image of the same area, with the identical anatomical landmarks identified, is presented in Figure 4-1B.

Figure 4-2A demonstrates the initial assessment, determination of the horizontal pelvic alignment by means of a line drawn between the two posterior superior iliac spines. Figure 4-2B depicts the same line drawn on a standard thermographic image obtained using a normal volunteer.

In the next step, as shown schematically in Figure 4-3A, a second line is drawn from the midpoint of T1 to the midpoint of the line previously drawn between the two posterior superior iliac spines. The same procedure has been applied to a representative normal thermogram in Figure 4-3B. A finding that the

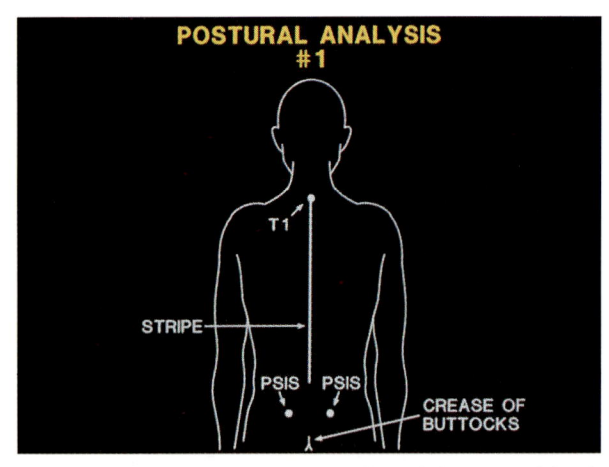

88 New Concepts in Craniomandibular and Chronic Pain Management

Fig. 4-1A. Schematic representation of the normal back and those landmarks which are necessary.

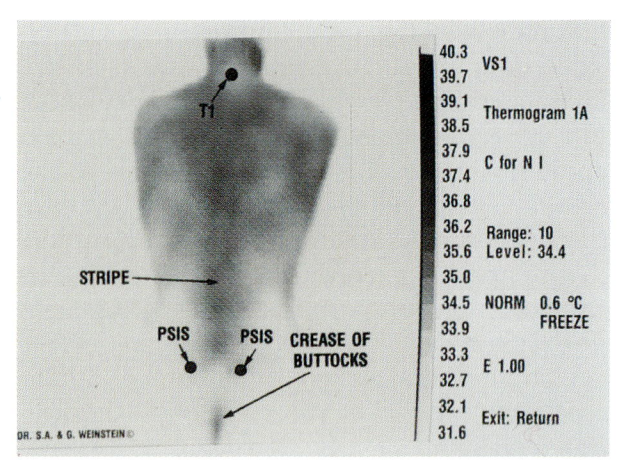

Fig. 4-1B. Demonstrates a thermogram of the same area labeled appropriately.

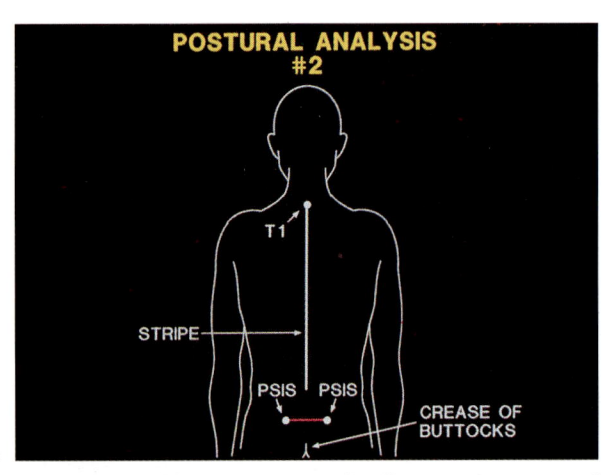

Fig. 4-2A. This demonstrates the first measurement of the pelvic tilt with a line being drawn between the two posterior superior iliac spines.

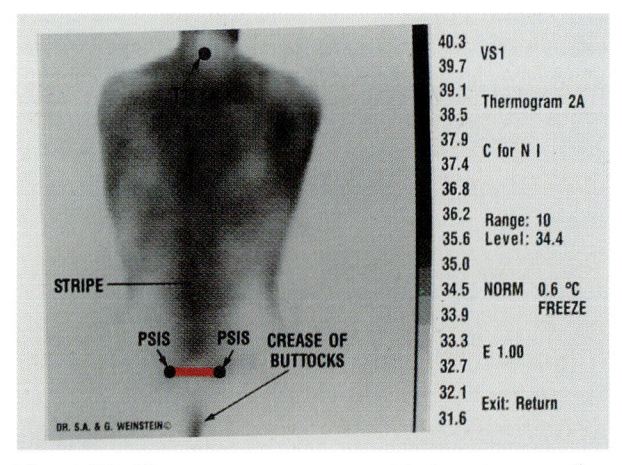

Fig. 4-2B. The same measurement being done on the thermogram.

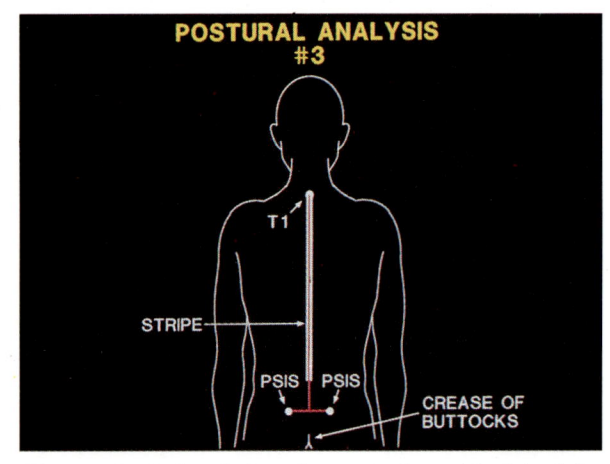

Fig. 4-3A. A line being drawn to the midpoint of the line between the two posterior superior iliac spines from the T1 midline.

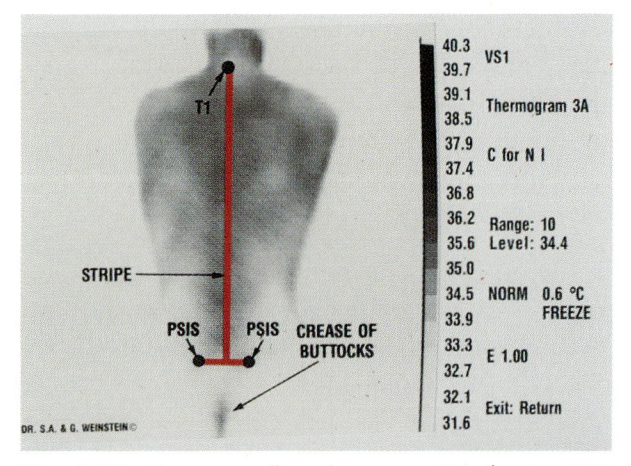

Fig. 4-3B. The same line drawn on the thermogram itself. If a 90° angle occurs, i.e., a perpendicular line, and if the thoracic and lumbar stripes are maintained in the midline, this represents a normal, as there is no curvature or pelvic tilt.

two lines intersect at a 90° angle and that the thoracic and lumbar stripes representing the spine appear clearly in the midline demonstrates that there is no curvature in the spinal column nor any pelvic tilt or misalignment. Thus, Figure 4-3B demonstrates a thermographic representation of the normal state.

In contrast, we will now examine the abnormal state. Figure 4-4A schematically portrays an abnormal back disorder with clear evidence of scoliosis and an obvious pelvic tilt. The associated Figure 4-4B presents the thermogram obtained in that clinical situation.

Repeating the process previously shown for a normal back, the alignment of the pelvis is found not to be horizontal (Figures 4-5A and B) when a line is drawn between the two posterior superior iliac spines. The addition of the standard perpendicular line, extending from T1 downward to its intersection with the line previously drawn between the PSIS (Figures 4-6A and B) presents the first evidence of the depicted abnormality. As can be seen in Figure 4-6B, the thermographic representation of the thoracic stripe is no longer in the normal perpendicular state. Moreover, when this perpendicular line intersects with the line drawn between the two PSIS points, two unequal angles are created rather than the two 90° angles found in the normal state.

Once these preliminary findings have been established, the clinician can now proceed to document the measurement of the primary thoracic curve (Figures 4-7A and B) with this measurement taken from the midline by means of a linear projection along the angle of the curve. The angle between this line and the perpendicular midline represents the primary curvature of the scoliotic spine. This measurement is then followed by the determination of the compensatory scoliotic curve (Figures 4-8A and B) on the same thermogram.

The above illustrations of the normal and the scoliotic back pattern, respectively, clearly demonstrate the utility of thermographic imaging for the initial documentation of scoliosis and for the continued periodic re-evaluation of the patient for the full duration of the individual's growth period or until continued progression of the scoliotic curvature renders extensive radiography and therapeutic intervention necessary.

There is clearly a contemporary need for a non-invasive, cost-effective means for the periodic evaluation of the spinal column in children with scoliosis. While it is quite evident that extensive neuroradiologic evaluations (myelography, computerized tomography, or MRI techniques) may be necessary in patients with demonstrated progressive neurologic or spinal abnormalities and in any patient requiring surgical correction,[36] the majority of patients are periodically re-evaluated by routine radiography for extended periods of time until the need for therapeutic intervention arises or the requirement for any such intervention is rendered moot by reason of age, modest degree of deformity, and/or absence or progression of minor deformity. One recent study found that almost 90% of all children referred to orthopedic surgeons for evaluation of the possible presence of scoliosis were subjected to at least one series of radiological evaluations.[37] Given the customary 5 to 7 percent of referral from routine school screening programs,[2-9] this would clearly indicate that approximately 5 percent of the entire pediatric population of the United States is currently being exposed to radiation once or several times, solely for the evaluation of possible scoliosis.

Magnetic resonance imaging (MRI) has been repeatedly proposed as an alternate means for the necessary periodic follow-up evaluations of individuals with scoliosis.[38-40] While MRI has as yet no known biological risk and may be accurate for purposes of recognition and evaluation of such lesions, such procedures are expensive and very likely not cost-effective for repeated periodic follow-up evaluations in the majority of patients with scoliosis.

Computerized infrared electronic thermography offers a viable alternative to either standard radiography (with its burden of radiation exposure) or MRI (with its burden of expense). In contrast, thermography does not involve exposure to radiation and offers a cost-effective alternative to MRI. In addition, thermographic evaluations are non-invasive, relatively easily performed in all patients with scoliosis, and accurate for the detection of this disorder, as demonstrated in the proce-

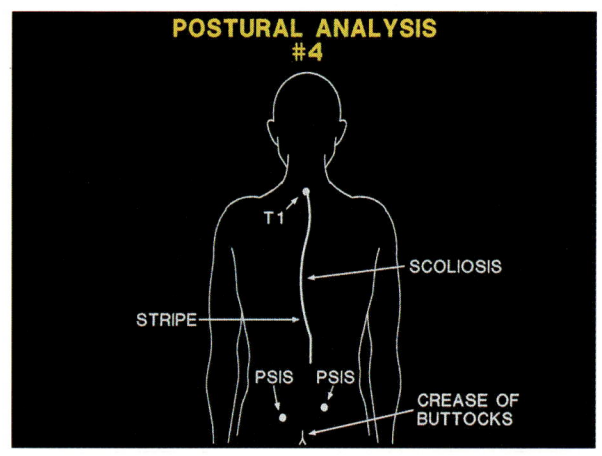

90 New Concepts in Craniomandibular and Chronic Pain Management

Fig. 4-4A. An abnormal back pattern with a scoliosis and obvious pelvic tilt being demonstrated.

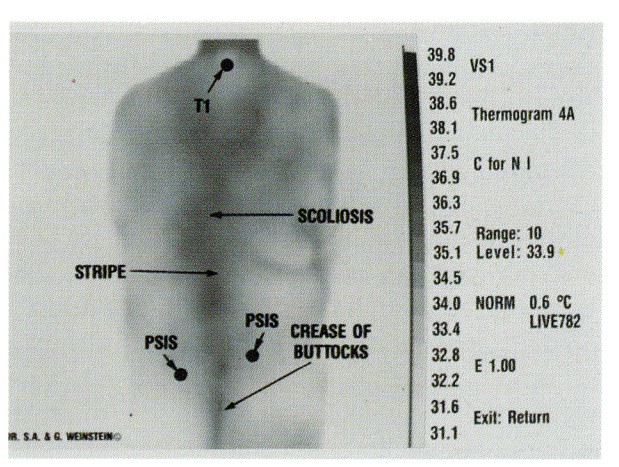

Fig. 4-4B. A thermogram with similar problems.

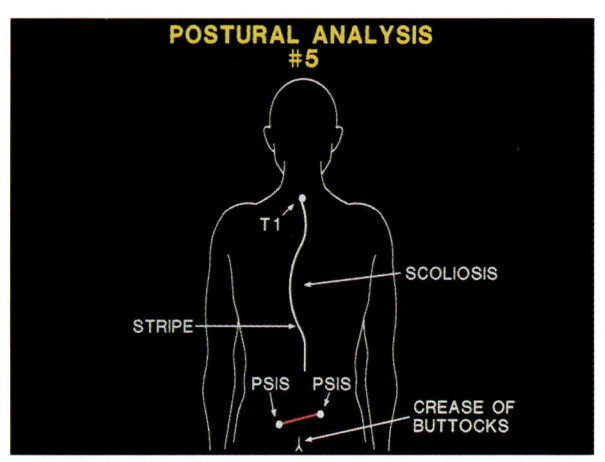

Fig. 4-5A. A measurement line being drawn between the two posterior superior iliac spines as had previously been done in Figure 4-2A.

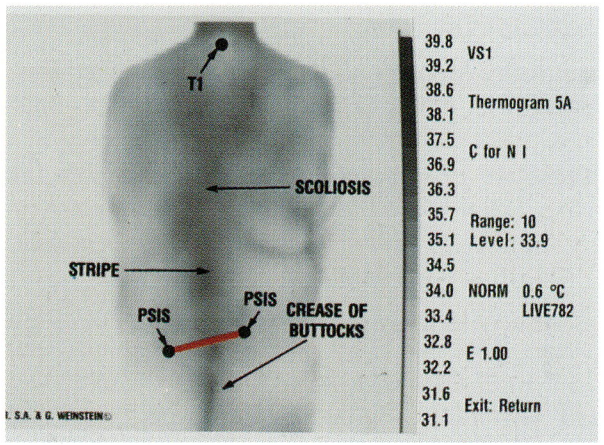

Fig. 4-5B. The same measurement being taken in a thermogram.

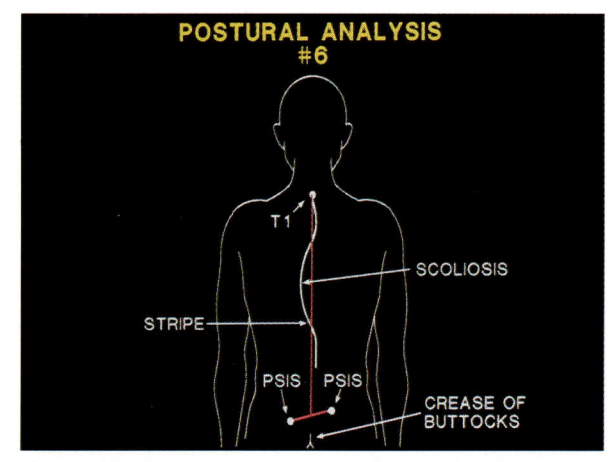

Fig. 4-6A. The second measurement line being drawn from the midpoint of the line between the two posterior superior iliac spines to T1.

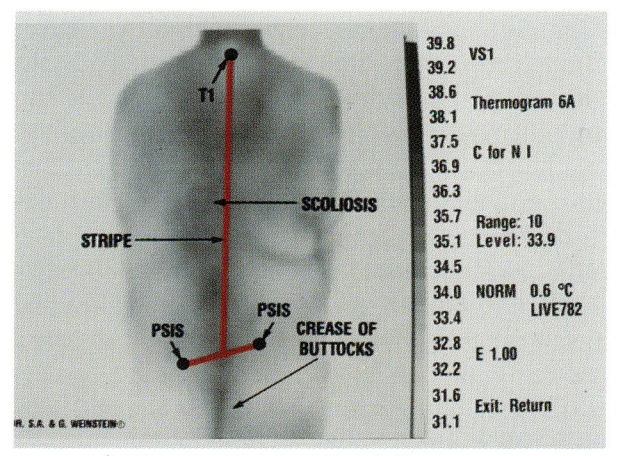

Fig. 4-6B. A thermogram with similar measurements. Now the stripe is no longer directly on the line. Also, there is an angle created between the two posterior iliac spines as had been mentioned. Since this is no longer a perpendicular, there is a pelvic tilt, with the angle being measured to show the angle of tilt.

CHAPTER 4 Scoliosis Evaluation & Documentation with Computerized Infrared Thermography 91

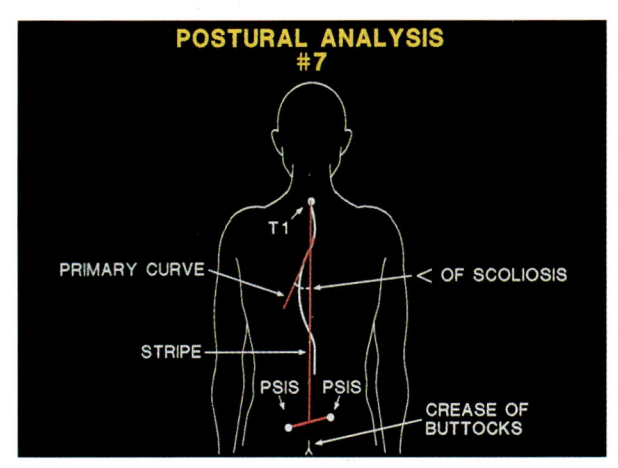

Fig. 4-7A. Measurement of the primary curve from the midline with a line moving along the angle of the curve. The angle between this line and the midline is the primary curvature of the scoliosis.

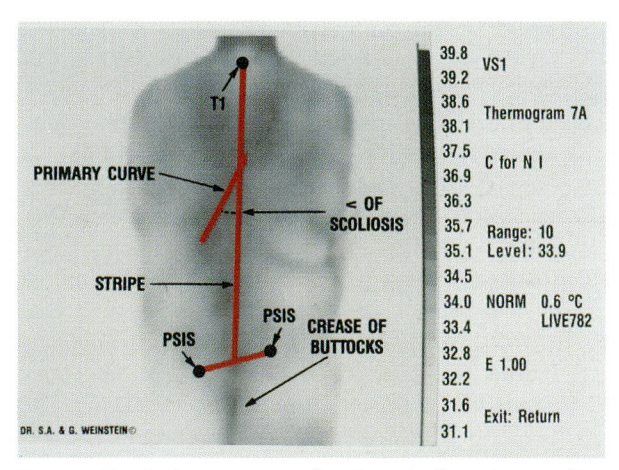

Fig. 4-7B. A thermogram showing similar abnormality.

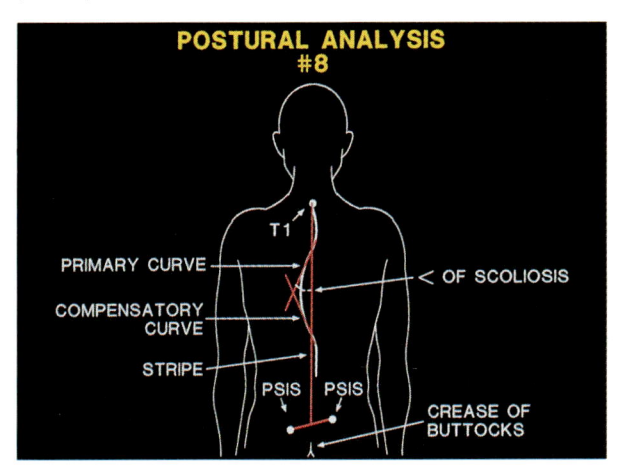

Fig. 4-8A. The measurement line for the compensatory curve in a scoliosis.

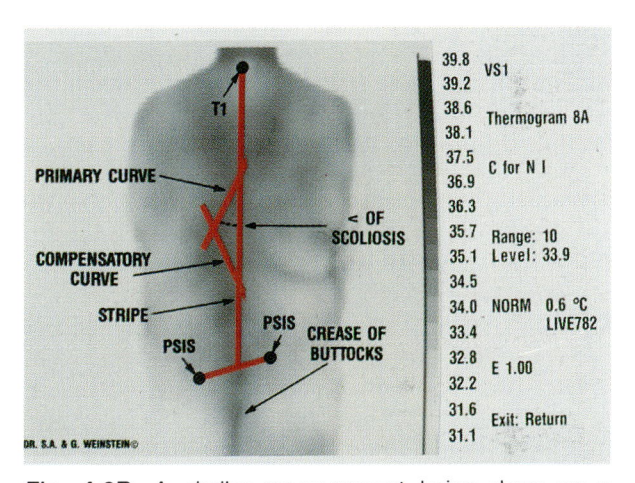

Fig. 4-8B. A similar measurement being done on a thermogram.

dures and illustrations provided herein. With no contraindication to this procedure, no risk involvement, and relative simplicity, it is obvious that thermographic postural analysis is a viable procedure of the 90's.

The illustrations above indicate that a normal back and/or a pelvic tilt or a scoliotic pattern may well be measured by appropriate thermographic evaluation. This renders great value to the physician, as in doing his primary thermogram a postural analysis may occur. This may be done in such a way as to remove the necessity for unnecessary x-ray evaluation. It would, therefore, appear that this may well represent a primary modality for the screening of school children without x-ray exposure and with considerably less cost.

REFERENCES

1. Brooks HL, Azen SP, Gerberg E, Brooks R, Chan L. Scoliosis: a prospective epidemiological study. *J Bone Joint Surg.* 1975;57(A):968-972.
2. Lonstein JE, Bjorlund S, Wanninger MH, Nelson RP. Voluntary school screening for scoliosis in Minnesota. *J Bone Joint Surg.* 1982;64(A):481-488.
3. Rogala EJ, Drummond DS, Gurr J. Scoliosis: incidence and natural history. *J Bone Joint Surg.* 1978;60(A):173-176.
4. Dickson RA, Stamper P, Sharp AM, Harker P. School screening for scoliosis: cohort study of clinical course. *Brit Med J.* 1980;281:65-67.
5. Warren M, Leaver J, Alvik A. School screening for scoliosis. *Lancet.* 1981;2:52.
6. Asher M, Greene P, Orrick J. A six year report: spinal deformity screening in Kansas school children. *J Kansas Med Soc.* 1980;81:968-971.
7. Leaver JM, Alvik A, Warren MD. Prescriptive

screening for adolescent idiopathic scoliosis: a review of the incidence. *Int J Epidemiol.* 1982;11:101-111.
8. Lonstein JE. Screening for spinal deformities in Minnesota schools. *Clin Orthoped.* 1972;126:33-42.
9. Bunnell WP. The natural history of idiopathic scoliosis before skeletal maturity. *Spine.* 1986;11:773-776.
10. Clarisse PH. *Prognostic Evolution of Idiopathic Scoliosis of At Least 10 to 29 Degrees during Follow-up.* Lyon, France: 1974. Thesis.
11. Picault C, et al. Natural History of idiopathic scoliosis in girls and boys. *Spine.* 1986;11:777-778.
12. Lonstein JE, Carlson MJ. The prediction of curve progression in untreated idiopathic scoliosis during growth. *J Bone Joint Surg.* 1984;64(A):1061-1071.
13. Cooke ED, Carter LM, Pilcher MF. Identifying scoliosis in the adolescent with thermography: a preliminary study. *Clin Orthoped.* 1980;148:172-176.
14. Bar-Sella A. Infrared thermography–a historical perspective. *Postgrad Med.* (Suppl) 1986;March:104-106.
15. Schnitzlein HN. The neuroanatomy and physiology related to thermography. In: *Clin Proc Acad Neuro-muscular Thermography.* June 1985; Dallas, TEX/New York, NY: McGraw Hill Book Company, Postgraduate Medicine, Custom Communications; 1986;21:5.
16. Heinz ER, Goldberg H, Taveras JM. Experiences with thermography in neurological patients. *Ann NY Acad Sci.* 1964;121:177-189.
17. Albert SM, Glickman H, Kallish. Thermography in orthopedics. *Ann NY Acad Sci.* 1964;121:157-170.
18. Devereaux MN, Parr GR, Lachmann SM, Page-Thomas P, Hazleman BL. The diagnosis of stress fractures in athletes. *JAMA.* 1984;252:531-533.
19. Fischer AA. Thermography in differential diagnosis and documentation of painful conditions. *Curr Ther Physiatry Phys Med Rehab.* 1984:131-45.
20. Uematsu S, Hendler N, Hungerford D, Long D, Ono N. Thermography and electromyography in the differential diagnosis of chronic pain syndromes and reflex sympathetic dystrophy. *Electromyogr Clin Neurophysiol.* 1981;21:165-182.
21. Nakano KK. Liquid crystal contact thermography in the evaluation of patients with upper limb entrapment neuropathies. *J Neurol Orthop Surg.* 1984;5:97-102.
22. Richardson RR, Torres H, Analitis S, Downie J. Traumatic thoracic outlet syndrome: a six case report. *J Neurol Orthop Surg.* 1983;4:327-337.
23. McFadden JW. Thermography used to diagnose the facet syndrome–case report. *J Neurol Orthop Surg.* 1983;4:353-357.
24. Ching C, Wexler CE. Peripheral thermographic manifestations of lumbar disc disease. *Appl Rad.* 1978;100:53-59.

25. Dagi TF, Abernathy M, Luessenhop AJ, Stotsky G. Electronic thermography in the diagnosis of lumbosacral radiculopathy. Paper presented at the 33rd Annual Meeting of the Congress of Neurological Surgeons; 1983.
26. Pochaczevsky R, Wexler CE, Meyers PH, Epstein JA, Marc JA. Liquid crystal thermography of the spine and extremities: its value in the diagnosis of spinal root syndromes. *J Neurosurg.* 1982;56:386-395.
27. Wexler CE. Thermographic of trauma (spine). *Acta Thermographica.* 1980;5:3-10.
28. Wexler CE. Cervical thoracic and lumbar thermography: a clinical evaluation. *J Neurol Orthop Surg.* 1981;2:183-185.
29. Pochaczevsky R. Assessment of back pain by contact thermography of extremity dermatomes. *Orthop Rev.* 1983;12:183-185.
30. Nakano K. Liquid crystal contact thermography (LCT) in the clinical evaluation of traumatic low back pain (LBP). *J Neurol Orthop Surg.* 1984;5:206-212.
31. Uematsu S, Hendler N, Hungerford D, Long D, Ono N. Thermography and electromyography in the differential diagnosis of chronic pain syndromes and reflex sympathetic dystrophy. *Electromyogr Clin Neurophysiol.* 1981;21:162-182.
32. Raskin MM; Viamonte M Jr, ed. *Clinical Thermography.* Chicago, Ill: American College of Radiology; 1971:51-55.
33. Tichauer ER. The objective corroboration of back pain through thermography. *J Occup Med.* 1977;19:727-731.
34. Wexler CE. Lumbar, thoracic and cervical thermography. *J Neur & Orthop Surg.* 1979;1(1):37-41.
35. Wexler CE. Cervical, thoracic and lumbar thermography. *J Neuro & Orthop Surg.* 1981;2:183-185.
36. AAOS Committee on Communications and Publications. A statement regarding school screening programs for the early detection of scoliosis. *American Academy of Orthopedic Surgeons Bulletin.* 1984;32(1):27.
37. Morais T, Bernier M, Turcotte F. Age- and Sex-specific prevalence of scoliosis and the value of school screening programs. *Amer J Public Health.* 1985;75:1377-1380.
38. Nokes SR, Murtagh FR, Jones JD III, et al. Childhood scoliosis: MR imaging. *Radiology.* 1987;64:791-797.
39. Han JS, Kaufman B, Yousef SFE, et al. NMR imaging of the spine. *Amer J Nucleomag Reson.* 1983;4:1151-1159.
40. Han JS, Benson JE, Kaufman B, et al. Demonstration of diastematomyelia and associated abnormalities with MR imaging. *Amer J Nucleomag Reson.* 1985;6:215-219.

Chapter 5

Prevention and Restoration of Abnormal Upper Quarter Posture

Jeffrey S. Mannheimer, MA, PT

INTRODUCTION

The prime factor that brings patients to a medical clinician is pain. It is pain that most often leads to dysfunction and a resultant inability to effectively maintain one's vocation and activities of daily living. Loss of function and its inherent consequences frequently leads to further pain, physical and emotional, compounding the nature of the patient's complaint.

Postural abnormalities are a major factor in the production of pain and dysfunction. Along with proper nutrition, postural assessment and education is one of the most important overlooked entities in the education and training of all physicians, dentists, and therapists.

Traumatic events such as automobile accidents frequently produce the acute onset of pain which subsequently leads to dysfunction if not properly addressed. In the eyes of an experienced and aware clinician, the soft tissue trauma resulting from severe flexion-extension injuries of the cervical spine, often called whiplash, understandably leads to postural abnormalities. It is, however, quite common for the experienced and aware clinician to be the last medical practitioner that a patient sees, and only in the later sub-acute or chronic stages of pain and dysfunction. The initial approach by the primary care physician frequently consists solely of symptomatic pain relief. But instruction of the patient in the maintenance of proper posture and body mechanics for the involved area is also needed to minimize stress, strain, and the compressive and irritative forces that result in functional loss.

Cumulative stress and strain without any specific traumatic event probably constitutes an even more common underlying cause of pain and the resultant dysfunction that we see in clinical practice. Since this type of pain and dysfunction does not have a well understood etiology, the possibility of chronic, cumulative stress and strain is not usually considered in a typical clinical evaluation. It then becomes extremely easy for the physician or dentist to practice medicine solely by consulting the Physicians' Desk Reference. It is just as easy for physical therapists, chiropractors, and other professionals to practice solely through the application of symptomatic modalities, with or without manual therapy. Again, neither approach is sufficiently comprehensive to successfully treat pain of musculoskeletal origin, unless instruction in proper body mechanics, and corrective postural techniques, and exercises are incorporated into the therapeutic paradigm.[1] A knowledge of ergonomics is also imperative when the work environment is a causative factor.

The overwhelming majority of patients rarely consider postural factors such as working, sitting, and sleeping positions as prime contributors to their complaints. Therefore, when the treating clinician fails to emphasize what is occurring at work or home, the pain and associated dysfunction is perpetuated.

Definitions of posture, as well as discussions of general body awareness and segmental movement, have already been covered in this text. It is the intent of this chapter to highlight the common postural changes induced by an individual's lifestyle or work habits pri-

Table 5-1. The Upper Quarter Musculoskeletal Relationships

Cranium + Cranial bone/suture articulations
Mandible + Hyoid
TMJ's
Dentition (occlusion)
Suboccipital spine
Mid-lower cervical spine
Cervicothoracic junction
Upper thoracic spine
Ribs 1 & 2
Sternum
Shoulder girdle + related articulations
Interrelated: fascia, ligaments, tendons, neural innervbation, circulation and lymphatic drainage

Table 5-2. Hyoid Bone Articulations

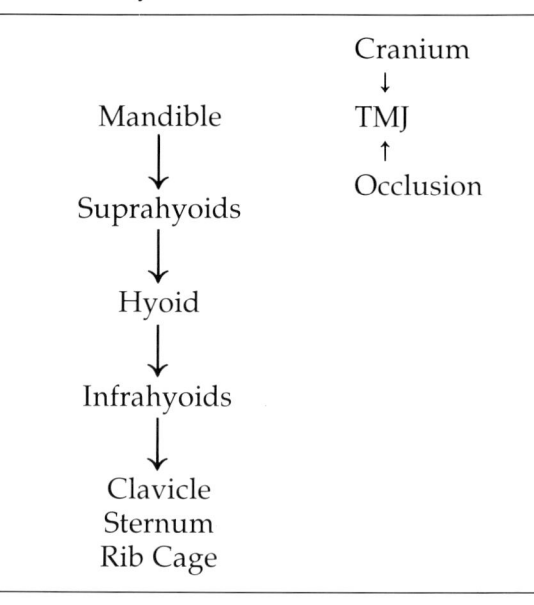

Mandible
↓
Suprahyoids
↓
Hyoid
↓
Infrahyoids
↓
Clavicle
Sternum
Rib Cage

Cranium
↓
TMJ
↑
Occlusion

marily as these relate to the craniomandibular and cervical-shoulder girdle complex commonly known as the upper quarter. I will refer to more distal regions such as the lumbosacral area as they relate to and affect the upper quarter.

BIOMECHANICAL RELATIONSHIPS OF THE UPPER QUARTER

The relationship between the head, neck, and shoulder girdle—as well as the surrounding joint and soft tissue structures—is a complex one. Traumatic and cumulative postural or occlusal abnormalities that affect one structure frequently contribute to pain or dysfunction in an adjacent region. The upper quarter therefore must be considered as a functional unit, since at any time the position of one structure can influence another. Because much material is covered elsewhere in this text, my focus at this point will be on the cervical spine.

The cervical spine is divided into two sections, the suboccipital and mid-to-lower cervical spine. The suboccipital spine consists of the articulations between occiput, atlas (C1) and axis (C2). The occiput has strong ligamentous and muscular connections to the atlas and axis. Any imbalance of this musculature can easily alter the normal position of the head on the neck.[2] The occiput can bend forward and backward (flexion and extension) upon the atlas as well as bend to the side and rotate. These motions can be performed independently of the rest of the cervical spine. It is important to understand that sidebending and rotation in the suboccipital area occur independently of one another, while in the mid-to-lower cervical spine they occur together.[3]

A recent study has shown that the greatest degree of flexion occurs at the atlas-axis and not at the occiput-atlas articulation. Extension, however, is greatest at the occiput-atlas, twice that which occurs at the atlas-axis, while sidebending occurs equally at both axes. The greatest degree of intervertebral motion in the spine is axial rotation at the atlas-axis.[4]

The connection between each upper quarter structure occurs by direct joint articulation and/or soft tissue attachments via ligaments, fascia and muscle. Neural innervation as well as circulatory and lymphatic vessels comprise the complete system (Table 5-1). The hyoid bone has no direct articulation with any other bone. As a result, its anatomical position is totally dependent upon the relative degree of muscular tension of the supra and infrahyoids.[5] The suprahyoid muscles provide the biomechanical relationship between the mandible, temporal bone, and hyoid bone. The infrahyoids in turn connect the hyoid bone to the clavicle, sternum, and rib cage (Table 5-2).

The mid-and-lower cervical spine, where the majority of cervical motion occurs, consists of the C3-C7 vertebrae. The last cervical vertebrae and the first two thoracic vertebrae comprise the region known as the cervicothoracic junction.

For several reasons, the first and second ribs must be included in any upper quarter postural analysis. The scalenii which originate from the cervical spine insert upon ribs 1 and 2. The costovertebral joints or articulations between the ribs and vertebrae can easily influence one another. Specifically, elevation of the first rib can result in a rotational fault of the first thoracic vertebrae, which may in turn produce compression at the brachial plexus. The ribs also articulate with the sternum, and the infrahyoids provide a soft tissue relationship between the hyoid bone and the manubrium of the sternum.

The shoulder girdle is comprised of the clavicle, scapula, acromion, sternum, upper thoracic and lower cervical spines and the glenohumeral, sternoclavicular, and acromioclavicular joints. The scapulothoracic area must also be included in our analysis. Postural alterations can easily affect shoulder and upper extremity functions. A prime area of concern at this region is the supraclavicular fossa and the neural, vascular, lymphatic, and musculotendinous attachments therein.

NORMAL (ORTHOSTATIC) POSTURE

A normal, or orthostatic, upper quarter posture requires proper orientation of the cranium on the suboccipital spine, normal rest position of the tongue, centric relation or loose-packed positioning of the TMJ's, a normal cervical lordosis, slight upper thoracic kyphosis, and scapular retraction.

Normal erect posture is present when a plumb line falls slightly behind the apex of the coronal suture, through the external auditory meatus and odontoid process and just posterior to the cervical vertebral bodies. It continues through the glenohumeral joint, lumbar vertebral bodies, and sacral promontory. In the lower extremity, it falls slightly posterior to the center of the hip joint, slightly anterior to the center of the knee joint, through the calcaneo-cuboid joint, and finally just anterior to the lateral malleolus.[3]

The center of gravity of the skull is located at the bisection of the vestibular apparatus (otic plane) of the inner ear.[6] In addition, there are three planes of reference which optimally should be parallel to one another. These are the pupilar, otic and occlusal planes established by lines drawn through the eyes, ears, and maxillary/mandibular teeth respectively. Alterations occur when observation shows one eye or ear to be higher or lower than its counterpart, possibly due to uneven cranial growth, congenital anomaly or trauma. Measurement of ramus height may reveal uneven growth or development of one side of the mandible. Finally, the head may be held or fixed in a sidebent position on the cervical spine, thus altering the planes of reference.[7]

Regarding the TMJ, a close-packed position is considered to occur at a maximally congruent point where further movement cannot be accomplished and the ligaments surrounding it are taut. The TMJ is thought to have two close-packed positions, one anterior and one posterior.[8]

The posterior close-packed position, according to Rocabado, exists when the mandible is at its most retruded point and the condyle cannot go further. An anterior close-packed position exists when the condyles are against the eminence of the temporal bone upon maximal opening when further movement is not possible. Any point away from the posterior or anterior close-packed positions in which the periarticular connective tissues maintain 70-80 percent of their normal visco-elastic nature is considered to represent a loose-packed joint.[8]

Hesse is of the opinion that the TMJ does not possess a close-packed position. It is, however, nearly close-packed when full occlusion of the dental arches occurs. He feels that this is questionable because the restraining capsule and ligaments are not maximally tightened during maximal intercuspation.[9]

Centric relation (CR) is defined as the most anterosuperior position of the mandibular condyles in the glenoid fossa with the menisci in proper location. This differs from what is termed centric occlusion (CO) which exists when tooth contact occurs in the CR position. This is not always considered to occur at maximal intercuspation due to malocclusion.[10]

There should exist a slight degree of flexion of the cranium on the sub-occipital spine. Greater specificity however is warranted since

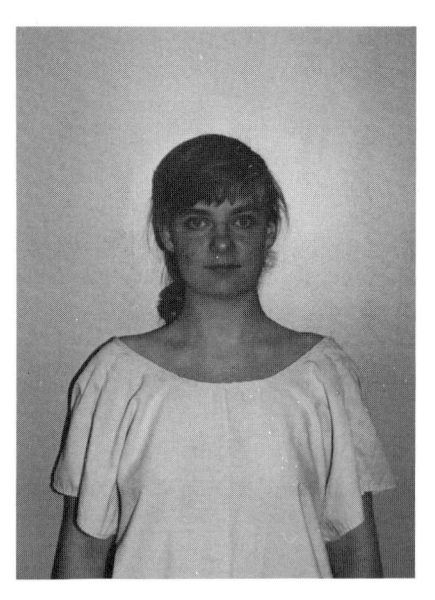

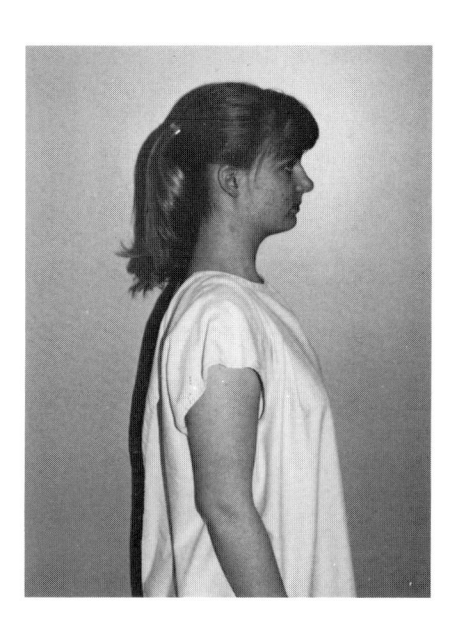

Fig. 5-1. A and B. Normal Upper Quarter Posture.

the cervical spine actually has two normal physiological curves. There is the lower cervical lordosis and a reversal or slight kyphosis of the upper cervical spine.[11] This allows for simultaneous flexion and extension of the upper cervical region independent of the lower cervical. Simultaneous extension of the upper cervical spine (lordosis) and flexion of the lower (kyphosis) occurs with bilateral contraction of the sternocleido-mastoid (SCM) muscles.

It should also be noted that for the purpose of postural analysis, in the presence of complete flexion, a slight lordosis of the upper and a kyphosis of the lower cervical spine are present. A complete lordosis occurs in the presence of full extension. A complete kyphosis, however, can also exist if the head (occiput) is forward bent to end range on the neck during full cervical flexion.[11]

Rocabado, a pioneer in the field of craniomandibular dysfunction, has delineated the radiographic relationships of this area. There is a nodding range of 15 degrees from the midline into the direction of flexion and extension of the head on the neck. This occurs in the suboccipital spine.[5]

The tongue is normally held against the palate by negative pressure. The tip of the tongue should lightly touch the posterior aspect of the maxillary incisors. The center of the tongue should be located about midway between the crowns of the maxillary molars and the palatal vault. It is also very important to understand that the tongue is a muscle which is suspended like a hammock between the styloid process of the temporal bone and the anterior portion of the mandible. Its resting position may thus be altered by either a change in the degree of flexion/extension of the cranium on the suboccipital spine, or a change in the resting position of the mandible.[5,7,8,10,12]

The cervical spine should have a 30-35° lordosis present. The lordotic curvature results in the passage of the line of gravity posterior to the vertebral bodies. The compressive force of gravity will thus be altered by a change in the lordotic curve.[3,11]

The hyoid bone should be situated just anterior and inferior to the vertebral body of C3 with the posterior horn level with the C2-3 intervertebral disc. There are fourteen muscles that attach to the hyoid bone. The supra- and infrahyoid length/tension relationship is again dependent on the status of the craniovertebral posture at any given time.

Mandibular resting position is governed by numerous factors, including the length/tension relationship of the masticatory and hyoid muscles, craniovertebral posture, disc-condyle association, and the occlusal entities covered in Chapter 12.

The shoulders should be slightly retracted from the line of gravity and the clavicles situated just posterior to the first rib. The clavicles should be horizontal, without promi-

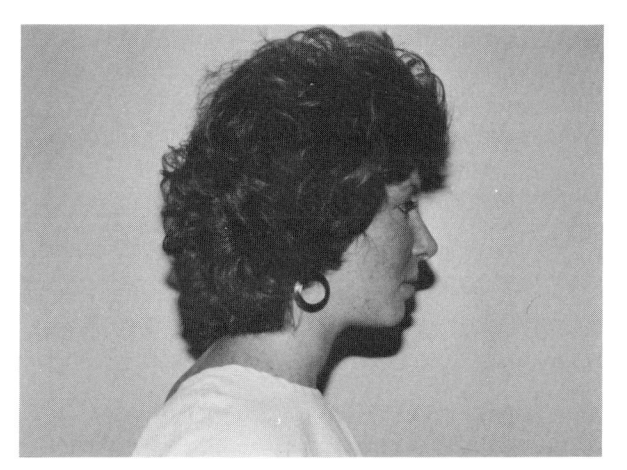

Fig. 5-2. Provocation Testing. **A**, Initial standing posture with minimal symptomatology.

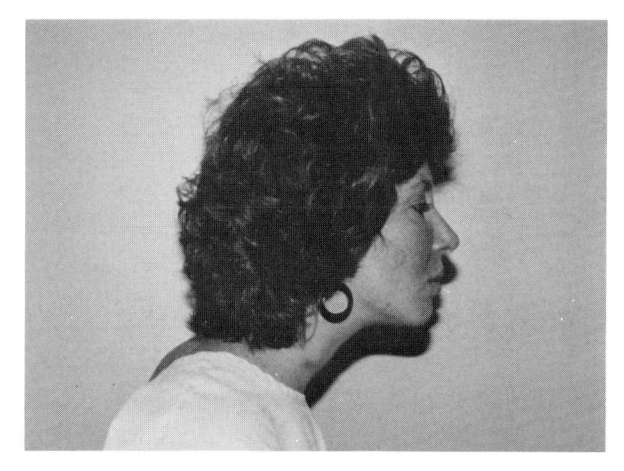

Fig. 5-2. B, Exaggeration of FHP with posterior cranial rotation quickly reproduced chief complaints of dizziness, blurred vision, facial pain and headaches in an individual employed as a hairdresser.

nence of the acromioclavicular or sternoclavicular joints. The angulation of the sternocleidomastoid muscles from origin to insertion normally is about 45-60°. The depth of the supraclavicular sulcus should be equal bilaterally. Posteriorly scapular spines should be horizontal without prominence of the vertebral borders. The spinous processes of the first and second thoracic vertebrae should be in line with those of C7 and T3.

The aforementioned anatomical relationships are required to maintain a normal or orthostatic posture.[7,8,13,14] Figure 5-1 illustrates normal standing posture.

ABNORMAL POSTURE

In general, postural abnormalities can be classified according to the three major curves of the spine. Abnormalities in the lumbar, thoracic, and cervical regions can all result in alteration of normal orthostatic head and neck posture. Since the focus of this chapter is the craniocervical relationship, it must be stated that this changes frequently with postural alterations that occur when sleeping, sitting, and working. The craniocervical region must have the ability to adapt to such alterations, but this ability is predetermined by the degree of soft tissue elasticity and joint mobility in each individual at a given time.

In the presence of normal joint and soft tissue function, an individual's physiologic adaptation range allows for short periods of stress and strain. This ability is, however, limited even in the presence of normal range of motion (ROM) if previous postural abnormalities—congenital, traumatically acquired, or from cumulative faulty habits—have promoted changes in posture.

The ability of the body to adapt is remarkable. This author has evaluated many individuals with abnormal posture but no significant pain or functional complaints. It is, nevertheless, my firm belief that such individuals are prone to problems if they are exposed to acute trauma or the cumulative stress and strain of poor postural habits over prolonged periods.[15]

Recent studies have shown that abnormal posture alone does not necessarily predispose an individual to subsequent back and neck pain or mandibular dysfunction.[16,17] These studies, however, did not consider prime factors such as occupation or sitting, sleeping and working postures. They thus overlooked any effects of cumulative stress and strain that may become significantly more pronounced than that observed during the postural assessment at the time of the study.

The objective part of an evaluation should include placing the craniocervical region into positions of extreme postural faults that may serve to rapidly reproduce the patient's subjective complaints. Accentuation of forward head posture (FHP) and quadrant positioning, with compression if necessary, constitutes such a provocation.[18-20] We have been

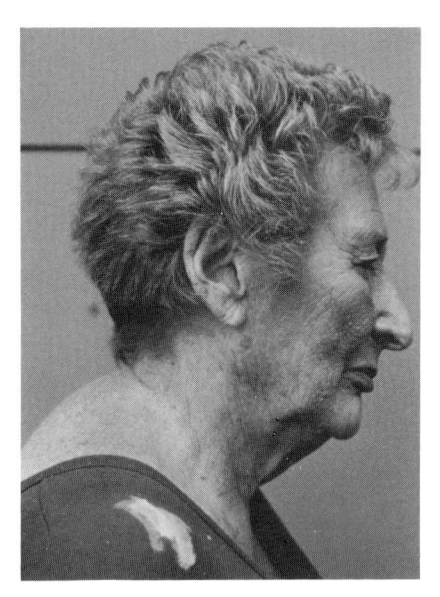

Fig. 5-3. Kyphosis of Cervicothoracic Junction. **A**, Note the approximation of the lower cervical and upper thoracic spinous processes.

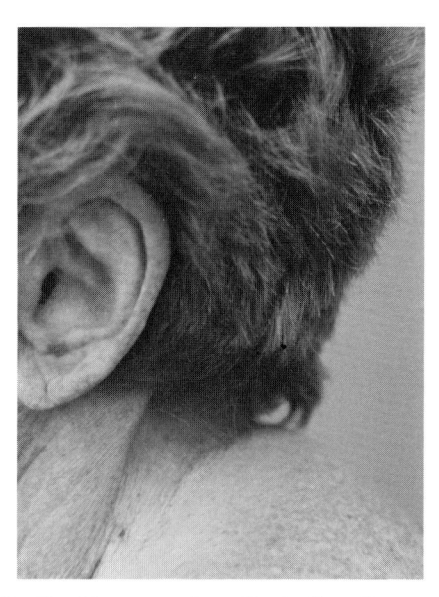

Fig. 5-3. B, Close-up view illustrating the associated posterior cranial rotation. History of craniofacial pain related to sub-occipital compression.

able to easily reproduce or exaggerate symptoms by using this approach, which at times has been as simple as placing the patient solely in their normal sleeping, sitting, or working posture, then exaggerating it if abnormal (Fig. 5-2, A and B).

When one analyzes posture, the patient should be observed from the anterior, posterior and lateral views. In addition, the analysis should begin from the feet and proceed to the cranium. Emphasis is placed upon the lumbar, thoracic, and cervical regions, in increasing importance. One should also observe the feet for asymmetry in the medial plantar arch or pronation/supination. The examiner should then analyze the knees and hips for deviations from the normal, as established by Kendall.[15] Any abnormality in the lower quarter may easily have an effect on leg length and hence pelvic symmetry, and consequently produce a change in the normal curvature of the spine. The body must therefore be looked at as a kinetic chain where a fault in one link may spread proximally and distally. The ability of this kinetic chain to adapt is in turn affected by the aging process, which may be associated with osteoporosis or spondylosis. The degree of spondylosis or degenerative arthritis is in fact enhanced by improper posture.

The effects of muscular stress and associated tension on bony attachments results in the laying down of increased calcium for enhanced structural support to counteract abnormal forces acting upon the spine. In the presence of abnormal posture, cumulative effects thus play a major role in spondylosis. The spondylosis in turn hinders or reduces joint mobility, resulting in further soft tissue restriction. The end result is a decreased physiologic adaptive range, producing more pain complaints (Fig. 5-3, A and B).

The Lumbar Spine and Its Influence on the Craniocervical Area

A loss of normal lumbar lordosis is frequently associated with FHP. In my years of clinical experience, patients with low back or sciatic pain often present with a decreased lumbar lordosis. The lumbar spine may in fact be totally flat, without any visible lordotic curvature. With loss of normal lumbar lordosis, the structural lines of force acting upon the intervertebral disc are altered.[3] Normally, when the lordosis is present, the nucleus pulposus of the disc is positioned anterior to the midline. With a decrease of the lordotic curve, an increasing reversal of forces creates posterior nuclear migration.[21] Dependent upon the degree and duration of the posterior compressive force, the nucleus exerts a strain on the outer annulus fibrosus,

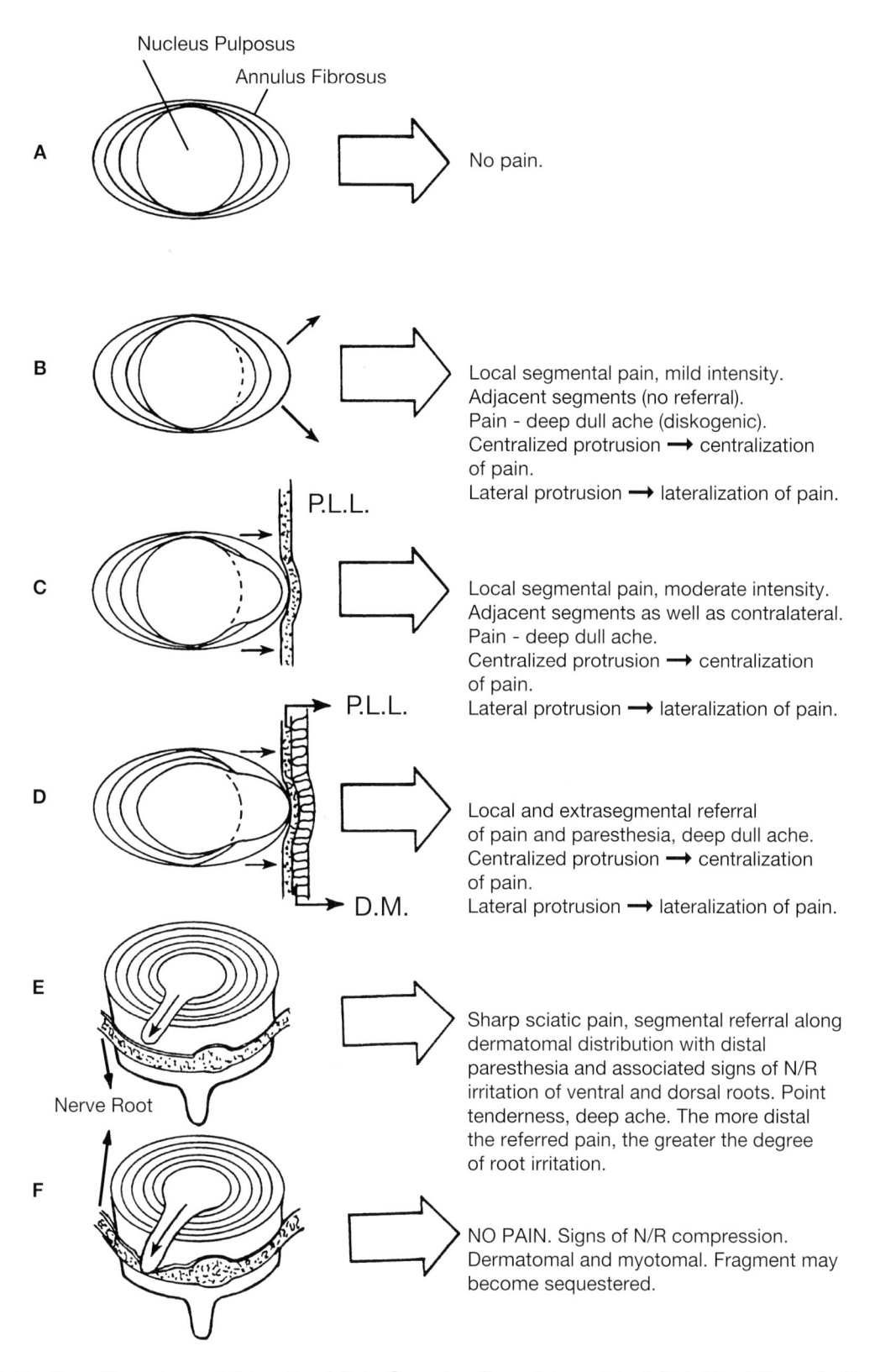

CHAPTER 5   Prevention and Restoration of Abnormal Upper Quarter Posture   99

A Nucleus Pulposus / Annulus Fibrosus → No pain.

B → Local segmental pain, mild intensity.
Adjacent segments (no referral).
Pain - deep dull ache (diskogenic).
Centralized protrusion → centralization of pain.
Lateral protrusion → lateralization of pain.

C P.L.L. → Local segmental pain, moderate intensity.
Adjacent segments as well as contralateral.
Pain - deep dull ache.
Centralized protrusion → centralization of pain.
Lateral protrusion → lateralization of pain.

D P.L.L. / D.M. → Local and extrasegmental referral of pain and paresthesia, deep dull ache.
Centralized protrusion → centralization of pain.
Lateral protrusion → lateralization of pain.

E Nerve Root → Sharp sciatic pain, segmental referral along dermatomal distribution with distal paresthesia and associated signs of N/R irritation of ventral and dorsal roots. Point tenderness, deep ache. The more distal the referred pain, the greater the degree of root irritation.

F → NO PAIN. Signs of N/R compression.ABC Dermatomal and myotomal. Fragment may become sequestered.

Fig. 5-4. Position, Character and Intensity of Pain Occurring From Intervertebral Disk Herniations. **A**, Norma disk. No bulging, fissures or tracts and therefore no pain. **B**, Herniation into annulus. Periphery of annulus remains intact. **C**, Annular bulge or herniation has irritated the posterior longitudinal ligament. The annulus remains intact, and pain is intensified. **D**, Annular bulge, giving rise to local and extrasegmental pain rreferral. **E**, Posterolateral protrusion resulting in nerve root irritation. Pain is sharp and referred in a dermatomal pattern. **F**, Complete root compression, which would result in sensory loss (no pain) and unilateral paralysis. from Mannheimer, JS and Lampe, GN.[52] *Clinical Transcutaneous Electrical Nerve Stimulation.* FA Davis, Philadelphia, PA. 1984.

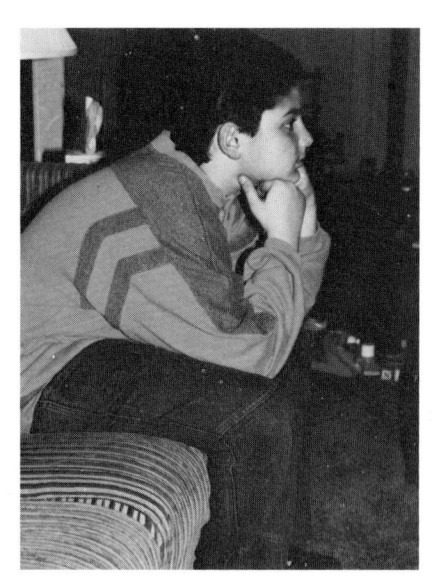

Fig. 5-5. Slumped Sitting Posture While Watching Television. **A**, The lumbar lordosis is lost and the position assumed promotes a FHP. Couches with low and thick back rests do not allow for craniocervical support.

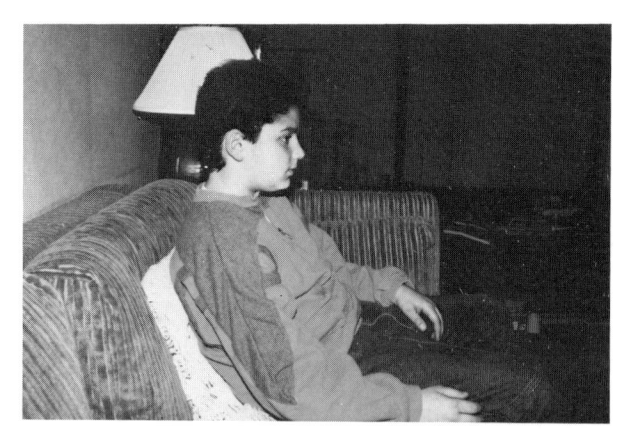

Fig. 5-5. B, When the head is supported by the hands in a slumped position, sub-occipital and TMJ compression is increased.

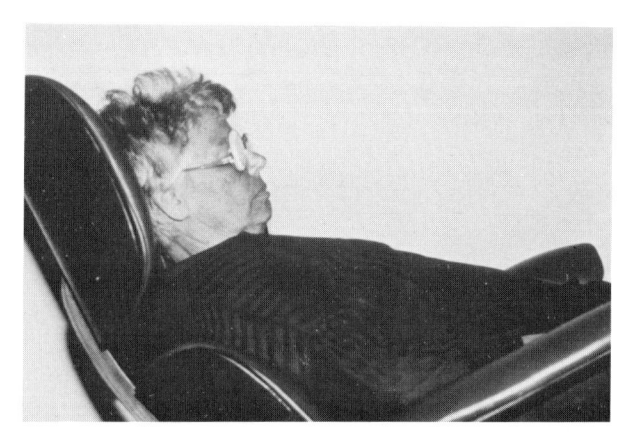

Fig. 5-6. Slumped Sitting Posture. Note that this may also occur from sliding down in the seat of a chair.

which has afferent innervation, and gives rise to low back pain. Continual improper posture may result in a progression of annular bulging and increasing pain intensity upon the posterior longitudinal ligament or anterior dura mater.[21,22] Each of these structures is innervated by the sinuvertebral nerve. Finally, posterolateral movement away from the thin posterior longitudinal ligament gives rise to unilateral low back pain with the possibility of referral into the lower extremity (Fig. 5-4).

Cumulative factors usually related to sitting and working postures lead to reduction in lumbar lordosis with increased spondylosis, decreased mobility, and the production of low back or lower extremity referral. Occupational factors have been studied extensively and show a high degree of correlation between the development of low back pain and working in a forward bent position.[23,24]

Prolonged sitting at work promotes shortening of the rectus-abdominis and iliopsoas muscles, resulting in a constant anterior torsion on the pelvis. The lumbar spine is thus forced to flex, causing a decrease in the lordotic curve. Perhaps even more significant is the effect upon the lumbar spine of sitting in a slouched position without use of a lumbar lordotic support.

The majority of seats in vehicles are not ergonomically designed. They do not contain a built-in lordotic support and/or do not consider the size of the driver. A seat that forces the driver to have his knees at or above waist level also serves to flatten the lumbar spine.

Individuals who work at computer terminals or at desks throughout the day are prone to the same cumulative effects on the low back. In fact, if these same individuals spend time driving home in a poor sitting posture or sit slouched on a soft chair at night, the cumulative effects are greatly magnified. Also in direct relationship is sitting up in bed while reading or watching television. Figures 5-5 and 5-6 depict improper posture while sitting on a couch and lounge chair, respectively.

Perhaps overlooked is the effect of a flat lumbar spine on craniocervical posture. As soon as one assumes a slouched sitting posture, the head immediately inclines forward. The greater the slouch, the greater the extent of the FHP. If the individual is watching television, driving or performing any other activity that requires the eyes to be horizontal, the head must also be extended or rotated posteriorly to an increased degree. Extension of the head or cranium on the upper cervical spine is synonomous with the term posterior rotation and may be used alternatively throughout this chapter. These two terms differ, however, from the movement known as axial extension, which is a backward gliding of the head on the neck without any posterior rotatory movement. Axial extension is demonstrated in the restorative section of this chapter and may also be called head retraction. The resultant effects give rise to a FHP with increased TMJ and suboccipital compression.

The causes of low back pain are many. A complete discussion of each is beyond the scope of this chapter. It has, however, been estimated that 50 to 90 percent of the diagnoses given for low back pain are relatively imprecise, including words such as muscle strain, ligamentous sprain, or lumbago.[25,26]

A simple muscle or ligamentous strain will commonly produce a dull achy pain in the low back. Wyke equates back strain with what is called primary fatigue backache.[27] Fatigue of a specific region causes localized pain and tenderness. This is frequently brought on by improper posture, activity, work, or recreational habits. Primary backache may occur during the last trimester of pregnancy, degenerative disk disease, rheumatoid arthritis, osteoarthritis, osteoporosis, visceral pathology, and even from constant wearing of high-heeled shoes or pronation of the foot.[28]

Most mechanical disorders of the lumbar spine occur from a forward bent position. The position of forward bending of the lumbar spine, especially when sitting, produces the greatest degree of intradiskal pressure and creates a force component that causes the nucleus to track backward against the annulus.[21,22,26]

An annular tear or fissure can occur from sudden, forceful movement or repeated (gradual-cumulative onset) stresses resulting in derangement. Objectively, one of the first signs of posterior displacement of the nucleus is a loss of the normal lordosis.[29] Forward bending causes the nucleus to move posteriorly toward the highly innervated tissues behind it, resulting in pain. The protruding nucleus causes an enlargement of the posterior intervertebral space, forcing the lumbar spine into a forward bent position and hence flattening the low back.

Another factor which may also affect orthostatic head and neck posture is pelvic asymmetry. This dysfunction can contribute to leg-length discrepancies, resulting in a sidebent or rotated head position.

The pelvis consists of the two ilia on either side of the sacrum. The articulations in between are called the sacroiliac joints. Probably the most common dysfunction of this joint is either an anterior or posterior rotation of one ilium on the sacrum. The acetabulum exists within the ilium, and its articulation with the head of the femur forms the hip joint. Any posterior or anterior movement of one ilium on the sacrum thus results in a leg length discrepancy.[30,31]

It is thought that at least 10 percent of the population have structural leg-length discrepancies of 1 cm or more.[32] Denslow and Korr have experimented with heel lifts to produce postural changes, resulting in segments receiving afferent input from paraspinal muscle tension.[33-37] Their early work led to the use of the term "Facilitated segment," which is related to the characteristics of an osteopathic lesion. An osteopathic lesion of an intervertebral joint and adjacent vertebrae exhibits hypomobility, positional faults, pain and tenderness, muscular tension, and reflex changes in skin and muscle as well as vasomotor and visceromotor changes.[34-38] Robinson has shown electromyographic changes of masticatory muscles from a leg length discrepancy contributing to a malocclusion.[39]

The Thoracic Spine and its Influence On the Cervical Area

Loss of lumbar lordosis contributes markedly to an increase in the kyphotic curvature of the thoracic spine, as does FHP. A combination of the two may result in flattening of the mid-thoracic area, due to the need to maintain an upright posture, and the development of an increased kyphotic curvature of the cervicothoracic junction, usually referred to as a dowager's hump.

One of the overlooked factors of increased thoracic kyphosis is approximation of the abdominal-visceral contents. This may result in the hindrance of normal diaphragmatic excursion. Since the diaphragm is active only upon inspiration, a decrease in its contractile range may reduce the amount of oxygen inspired, or make breathing more laborious.[40] The individual may very well have to recruit the accessory muscles of respiration, which primarily consist of those in the cervical area, specifically, the sternocleido mastoid muscles (SCM) and scalenes, with their insertion upon the clavicle, sternum, and first and second ribs. A concomitant side effect is exaggeration of FHP due to hyperactivity of the anterior cervical musculature, including the pectorals and intercostals.[41]

Perhaps even more deleterious effects occur when a combination of FHP and increased upper thoracic kyphosis produces dysfunction and pain of the shoulder girdle, supraclavicular fossa, and thoracic inlet. A separate section is needed to discuss those syndromes, frequently seen in association with TMJ dysfunction, but in fact precipitated by abnormal posture.

Common Pain Syndromes of the Upper Quarter

TMJ problems are not the cause of the many syndromes which are about to be mentioned. Postural stress in which compressive and irritative forces along with improper body mechanics combine to produce pain and dysfunction are the prime etiological factors. In fact, this can be a cumulative or continual process in which pain and dysfunction at one region leads to additional problems at another.

The shoulder girdle is unable to remain in its orthostatic position in the presence of prolonged FHP with associated upper thoracic kyphosis. Due to the soft tissue connections (origin and insertion) of muscles such as the trapezius, abnormal or increased tension is exerted upon the shoulder girdle. Shortening of the upper trapezius and levator scapulae occurs due to posterior rotation of the cranium and approximation of the occiput to the suboccipital spine, cervicothoracic junction, and shoulder girdle. The middle and lower trapezius, as well as the rhomboids, are placed on stretch as the increased thoracic kyphosis promotes abduction and protraction of the scapulae. This in turn creates a forward migration of the shoulder girdle due to shortening of the pectorals. The insertion of the pectoralis minor on the coracoid process of the scapula in turn contributes to a forward or round-shouldered posture. The omohyoid may also promote scapular migration due to its origin from the superior border of the scapula and insertion upon the hyoid bone.

Maintenance of a round shouldered posture causes approximation of the acromioclavicular and sternoclavicular joints. This will inhibit the normal elevation and posterior rotation of the clavicle that occurs with shoulder elevation. In addition, normal scapular rotation is altered, and the composite pattern gives rise to impingement and entrapment syndromes as well as to strain of the rotator cuff muscles of the shoulder.

An individual who engages in any repetitive activity with the upper extremities in the presence of a sustained forward-head, round-shouldered posture (FHRSP) is a prime candidate for shoulder pain and dysfunction. This will usually occur in the dominant arm. Such individuals frequently present with diagnoses of tendinitis, bursitis, rotator cuff tears, and associated aches and pains due to trigger point production.[42,22]

Pain in the posterolateral shoulder region may even be referred as a result of suprascapular nerve entrapment. The suprascapular nerve innervates the acromioclavicular and glenohumeral joints as well as the infraspinatus. Brachial plexus traction from the C5-6 roots to the suprascapular notch results from the tension placed on the nerve relative to the FHRSP.[8,41]

The dorsal scapular nerve may be entrapped by the middle scalene muscles through which it passes. FHRSP can lead to hyperactivity of this muscle, producing nerve irritation or compression. Pain is referred to the rhom-

Table 5-3. The Characteristics of Neurovascular Compression Syndrome

SYNDROME TYPES

Scalenus anticus
Scapulocostal
Thoracic outlet
Hyperabduction (pectoralis minor)
Costoclavicular

All involve compression of subclavian artery, vein and lower cord of brachial plexus.

LOCATION

Interscalene space
Costoclavicular space
Axilla, pectoralis minor tendon and coracoid process

SYMPTOMS

Neurologic	Vascular	Characteristics
Weakness (ulnar)	Ischemia	Intermittent or chronic;
Numbness	Decreased temperature	increased by: movement,
Heaviness	Discoloration (cyanosis)	inspiration, hypertrophy,
Paresthesia	Trophic changes	trauma, emphysema, or
	Edema	posture—round shoulders,
	Claudication	alar scapulae
	Decreased pulse	

boids and levator scapulae, which are innervated by the dorsal scapular nerve. Severe entrapment may even produce muscle atrophy and weakness if nerve impulse transmission is hindered by compression.[8,41,42]

Perhaps even more demonstrative is pain referral as a result of neurovascular compression at the thoracic inlet. This region is bordered by the first thoracic vertebra posteriorly, the superior border of the manubrium of the sternum anteriorly, and by the first rib laterally. Primary structures of importance include the subclavian artery and vein, plus the lower trunk of the brachial plexus.[41,42]

Pain and dysfunction syndromes commonly associated with this section of the upper quarter include the thoracic inlet, scalenus anticus, costoclavicular, hyperabduction (pectoralis minor) and scapulocostal (levator scapular) syndromes. The etiology may be congenital (from a cervical rib) or postural (from FHRSP, hyperactivity of the anterior scalene muscle, or compression resulting from soft tissue adhesions).

Neurovascular compression of the thoracic inlet can also occur from postural abnormalities produced by pendulous breasts, obesity, and occupational requirements. Work that necessitates repeated elevation of the arm, reaching, or a sustained elevated position in the presence of a preexisting FHRSP can easily lead to a neurovascular compression syndrome (NVCS). It is interesting to note that these syndromes occur frequently in females between the ages of 20-40,[41] a population similar to that of TMJ dysfunction.

Table 5-3 outlines signs and symptoms that commonly occur with neurovascular compression syndromes in the shoulder girdle region of the upper quarter. Neurologic signs can range from paresthesia (as a result of nerve irritation) to weakness, atrophy, and sensory deficit due to longstanding compression. Vascular compression may even lead to ischemia, discoloration, trophic changes, Raynaud's disease, and gangrene.[43]

Raynaud's is a vasoconstrictive disorder that frequently has an emotional etiology. It

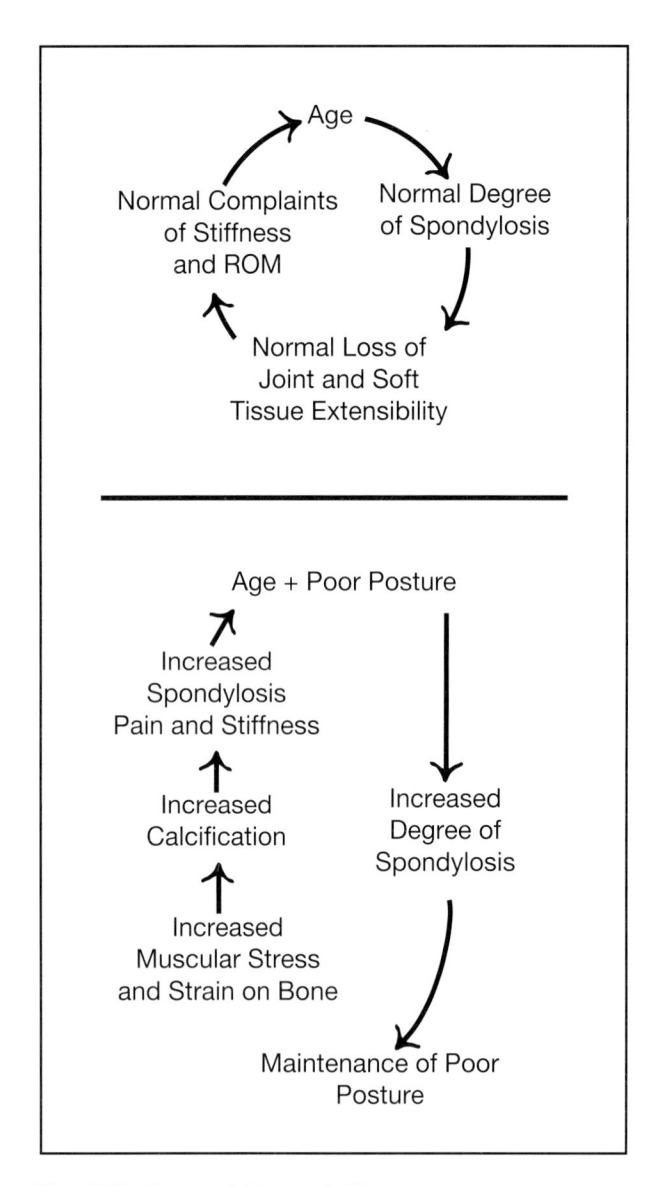

Fig. 5-7. Age and Postural Changes

is most common in young to middle-aged females and commonly associated with systemic conditions such as rheumatoid arthritis, scleroderma, polyarthritis nodosa, and systemic lupus erythematosis.[44-47] Raynaud's involves the upper extremity more than the lower extremity and may affect the edge of the ears and tip of the nose as well as the hands or feet. Symptoms may be similar to that of NVCS with paresthesia, and since it occurs in the same population group seen with postural and TMJ syndromes, it cannot be excluded. Postural factors are most evident when the patient is sitting or standing. Nocturnal paresthesia, however, may awaken the patient and is a common sign which occurs when the lower trunk of the brachial plexus is lifted off the first rib while supine. In this position, compression is decreased, and nociceptive impulses can travel proximal to the lesion to the somatosensory cortex where discomfort is perceived. In an upright position with improper posture, compression may predominate, hindering nociceptive transmission and the subsequent appreciation of pain. Note, however, that vascular signs may predominate during the day.

The aforementioned are the most common syndromes that occur at the shoulder girdle region from postural dysfunction. The etiology of pain in this region necessitates a comprehensive evaluation of the cervical and thoracic spine, shoulder girdle, and sites of entrapment. There is a close overlap of pain referral from all of these structures, and the quality plus location of pain may be very similar. The development of trigger points and their respective distribution of pain, as well as cervical spine dysfunctions with distal referral, must be delineated. This author frequently encounters patients that have a combination of factors, all of which may be traced back to an acute traumatic or cumulative postural etiology.

By distinct observation of posture, and by performing various provocation tests and movements, differentiation of etiology can be achieved. The clinician should thus become familiar with tests for shoulder girdle, thoracic inlet, and cervical spine involvement. Delineation of cervical spine involvement by compression/distraction movements, shoulder abduction, and brachial plexus tension tests are also helpful.[22,42,46-48] The existence of many tests frequently means that no individual test is sufficiently specific when it comes to distinct delineation of the causative structure in this complex area. The clinician's experience and the performance of a comprehensive evaluation thus play a major role.

The Cervical Spine and its Effect Upon Head Posture

The spinal section ultimately affected by distal structures, which thus may influence its proximal structure, is the cervical spine. A discussion of the numerous syndromes that can occur in the presence of cervical spine dysfunction is, again, beyond the scope of this chapter. However, excessive postural abnormalities frequently compound degenerative arthritic processes (spondylosis) that normally occur with age and may lead to discogenic changes that can result in nerve root and dural sheath irritation, compression, and stretch.[49] The net effect may be increased local and distal, lateral, or proximal pain referral (Fig. 5-7).

As previously mentioned, the cervical spine can be subdivided into the upper or suboccipital and mid-lower units. Generally, involvement of the C5-T2 nerve roots can produce distal referral into the upper extremity including the vertebral border of the scapula to the level of the inferior angle. The C4 roots will refer laterally to the acromion, and the C1-4 proximally to the cranium.

In order to fully understand the distribution of pain arising from the cervical spine, one must also review the respective dermatomal, myotomal, and scleratomal relationships. Generally, there is a fairly uniform segmental relationship among the three. However, only the myotome and sclerotome distinctly correspond. According to Hilton's law, the nerve supply of the myotome acting on a specific joint provides for the innervation of that joint as well as its overlying dermatome.[50] This correspondence, however, is not apparent at the head, pectoral region, scapula, intrathoracic structures, hand, buttock, and scrotum.[22,50]

For the purpose of this discussion, the scapula and intrathoracic areas are of prime importance. The dermatomal region extending from the spine of the scapula to its inferior angle is innervated by the T3-T7 nerve roots. In direct contrast, the musculature which acts upon the scapula is all cervical myotome. Cloward, in his research with cervical discography, showed that the innervation of the anterior myotome differed by two segments from that of the corresponding dermatome. The difference was more pronounced with the posterior myotome, sometimes approaching six segments.[51] Figure 5-8 illustrates the characteristics of discogenic pain. Cloward demonstrated that irritation of the C3-4 disk caused discogenic pain at the level of the C7 spinous process. This is the area covered by the upper trapezius (C3-4 myotome). Pain will be perceived at the midline from central herniation, and at the same level but alongside the vertebral border of the scapula with lateralization. Pain will be referred to the T3, T5, and T7 levels with pathology of the C4-5, C5-6, and C6-7 disks, respectively.[51]

It is important to note that pain from the above cervical disk derangements is felt in the thoracic dermatomes. This pain is not superficial: it is deep, dull, and achy, commonly producing myalgic or trigger points in the scapular musculature innervated by the cervical spine.[52] The location of the pain may mislead the clinician to suspect a thoracic pathology, but delineation of pain quality and correlation via manual compression/distraction tests of the cervical spine will frequently establish that the lesion is at the cervical level.

Analysis of FHP requires observation from anterior, posterior and lateral views while the individual is standing in their "normal" (relaxed) posture. However, if the patient's working posture is markedly different, it should also be reproduced and analyzed. Consideration must be given to the posture assumed when sitting (home or work), driving, and sleeping. In the standing position, posture should be viewed with the shoes both on and off. In the seated position, attention should be directed to the type of chair and work that is being performed.

Normal SCM angulation from mastoid to sternoclavicular joint should be 45-60°. As this angulation approaches 90°, FHP increases. The SCM angulation can be quickly and simply determined by placing a pen alongside the neck from the mastoid process to the sternoclavicular joint. Another quick method involves measuring the angle formed by a line connecting the tragus of the ear to the tip of the C7 spinous process in relation to a horizontal line from C7. Measuring the horizontal distance from a vertical plumb line posterior to the apex of the thoracic spine to the surface of the mid-cerivcal region has also been utilized. The normal distance should be 6-8 cm. More sophisticated techniques have been developed for research purposes and can yield very specific objective data.

106 New Concepts in Craniomandibular and Chronic Pain Management

CERVICAL DISKOGENIC

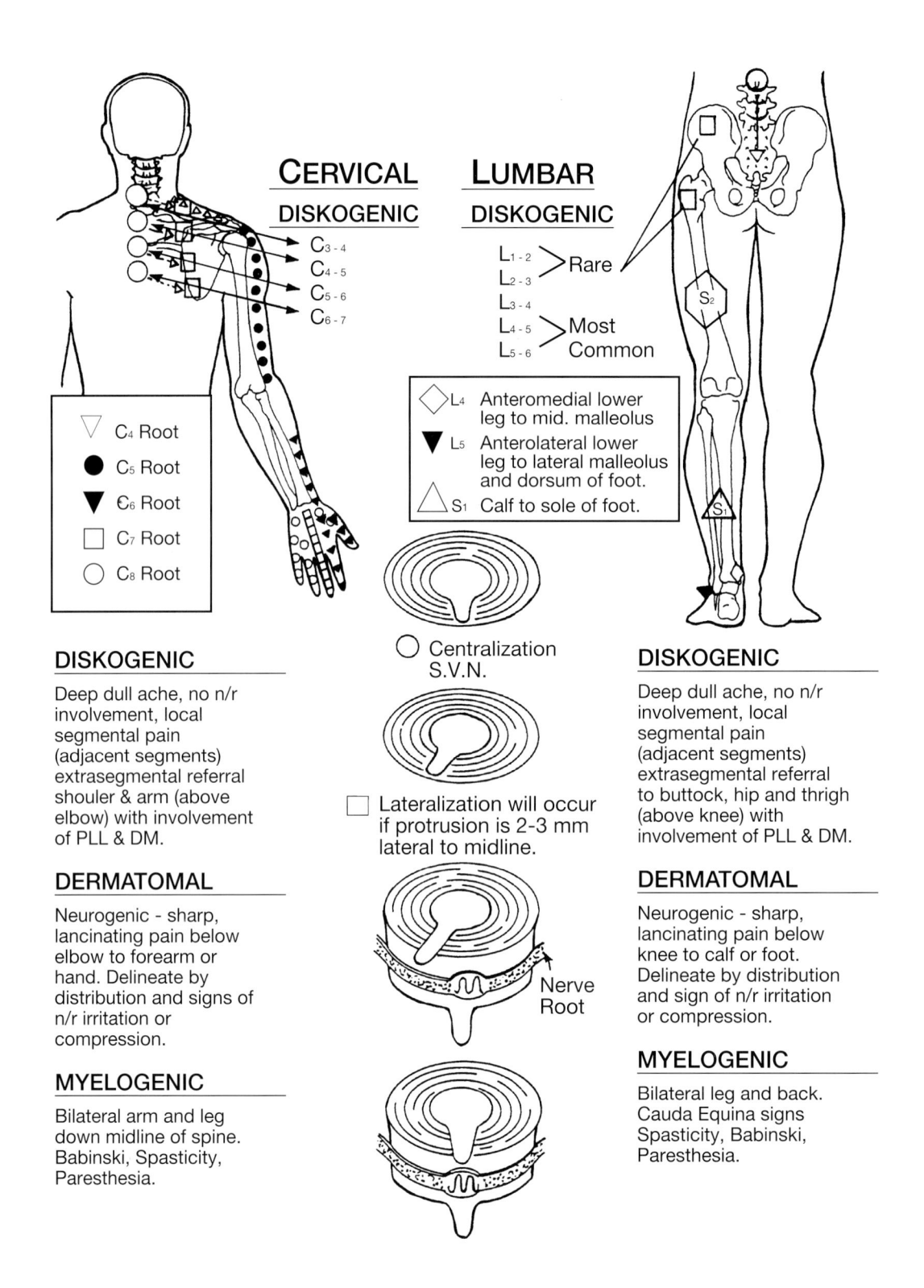

→ C_{3-4}
→ C_{4-5}
→ C_{5-6}
→ C_{6-7}

▽ C_4 Root
● C_5 Root
▼ C_6 Root
□ C_7 Root
○ C_8 Root

LUMBAR DISKOGENIC

L_{1-2}
L_{2-3} ⎬ Rare
L_{3-4}
L_{4-5}
L_{5-6} ⎬ Most Common

◇ L_4 Anteromedial lower leg to mid. malleolus
▼ L_5 Anterolateral lower leg to lateral malleolus and dorsum of foot.
△ S_1 Calf to sole of foot.

○ Centralization S.V.N.

□ Lateralization will occur if protrusion is 2-3 mm lateral to midline.

Nerve Root

DISKOGENIC

Deep dull ache, no n/r involvement, local segmental pain (adjacent segments) extrasegmental referral shouler & arm (above elbow) with involvement of PLL & DM.

DERMATOMAL

Neurogenic - sharp, lancinating pain below elbow to forearm or hand. Delineate by distribution and signs of n/r irritation or compression.

MYELOGENIC

Bilateral arm and leg down midline of spine. Babinski, Spasticity, Paresthesia.

DISKOGENIC

Deep dull ache, no n/r involvement, local segmental pain (adjacent segments) extrasegmental referral to buttock, hip and thrigh (above knee) with involvement of PLL & DM.

DERMATOMAL

Neurogenic - sharp, lancinating pain below knee to calf or foot. Delineate by distribution and sign of n/r irritation or compression.

MYELOGENIC

Bilateral leg and back. Cauda Equina signs Spasticity, Babinski, Paresthesia.

Fig. 5-8. The Pattern and Characteristics of Pain Resulting from Intervertebral Disk Pathology. from Mannheimer, JS and Lampe, GN.[52]

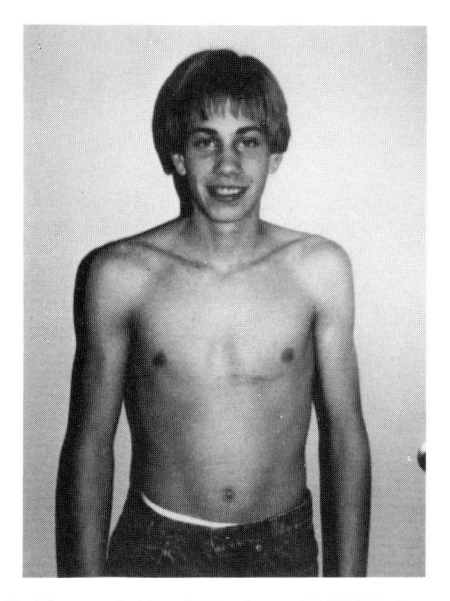

Fig. 5-9. Forward Head Posture. FHRSP in a young man without pain or dysfunction. He is, however, prone to develop craniomandibular and/or cervical spine pain due to cumulative stress and strain or as a result of acute trauma. **A**, Anterior view, note clavicular angulation and depth of the supraclavicular sulci.

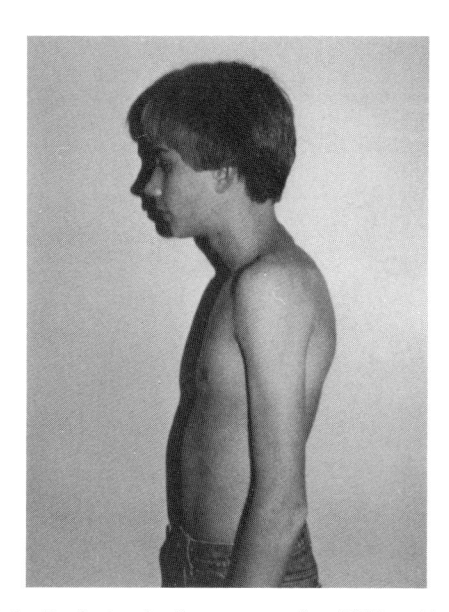

Fig. 5-9. B, Lateral view, note the FHP with round shoulders.

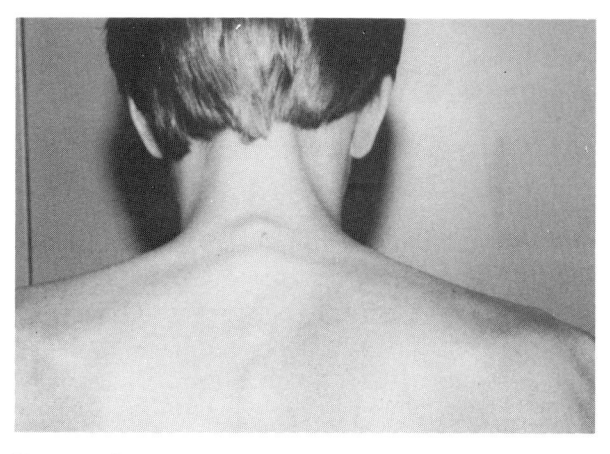

Fig. 5-9. C, Posterior view, Note prominence of spinous processes in the cervicothoracic junction.

In addition to FHP, clavicular angulation should be observed (Fig. 5-9). Elevation of the clavicle from hyperactivity of the clavicular head of the SCM can increase the depth of the supraclavicular sulcus. This may accompany shoulder girdle asymmetry and relate more to unilateral muscle guarding of the scalenes and of the levator scapulae. The presence of edema in the supraclavicular sulcus has also been observed, primarily in elderly individuals with longstanding FHP. This may signify lymphatic pooling resulting from neurovascular compression syndromes.

Forward Head Posture

All of the previously discussed postural faults will give rise to a FHP, of which there are two variations. One may occur after acute trauma, such as a hyperextension injury, producing reflex guarding or contraction of the longus colli, SCM's and scalenes. This results in a loss of normal cervical lordosis, producing FHP with a straight cervical spine.[54] This posture can progress to the point of causing normal cervical lordosis to become inverted (Fig. 5-10).

A cervical strain produced by concurrent hyperflexion and hyperextension will also cause reflex guarding of the posterior cervical musculature. Most commonly this involves the splenius and semispinalis capitus, upper trapezius, and levator scapulae. Extension of the occiput on the upper cervical spine occurs. In addition, hyperactivity of the SCMs increases the degree of posterior cranial rotation or extension due to their mastoid attachment. A significant degree of posterior cranial rotation and approximation to the upper cervical spine mechanically produces increased cervical lordosis. This may occur in conjunc-

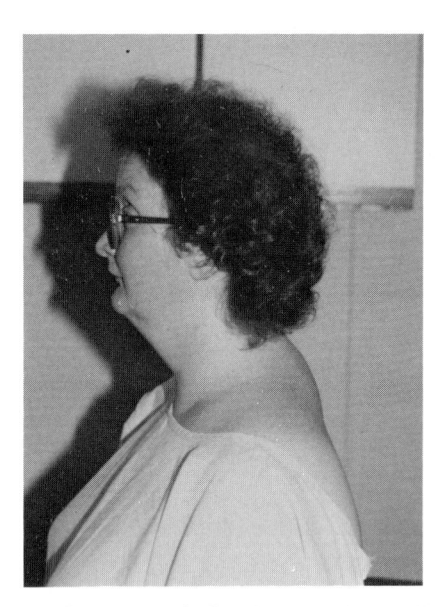

Fig. 5-10. Reversal of Cervical Lordosis. Note the presence of an inverted midlower cervical spine lordosis (kyphosis) and upper cervical lordosis. A developmental history of associated micro and retrognathia exists.

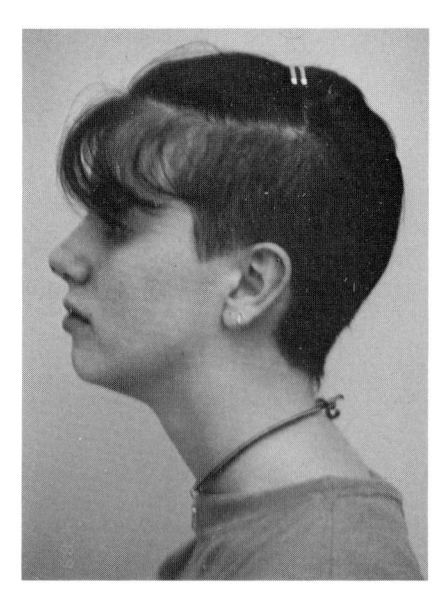

Fig. 5-11. Forward Head Posture with Posterior Cranial Rotation and Increased Cervical Lordosis. Eighteen-year-old female with bilateral TMJ internal derangements. No traumatic history, but cumulative etiology possibly related to abnormal posture.

tion with FHP, producing intensified discomfort in the craniofacial area, as will be discussed.

Gradual development of FHP in the absence of trauma usually culminates in a posture of associated posterior cranial rotation. A habitual slumped posture, causing the head to migrate forward, will also necessitate posterior cranial rotation to promote proper eye level. Figures 5-11 and 5-12 illustrate FHP with and without posterior cranial rotation, respectively.

Discogenic changes resulting in posterior nuclear migration can also culminate in FHP. The majority of cervical disc herniations occur at the mid to lower cervical region. In the presence of discogenic changes, posterior central nuclear migration can alter the normal resting position of the articular surfaces, producing a space-occupying lesion. McKenzie has termed this the derangement syndrome.[21] The posterior borders of adjacent vertebrae will separate and the anterior borders approximate one another, causing profound alteration of normal lordosis, with the patient assuming a FHP.

FHP without significant posterior cranial rotation may be an antalgic position. The need to avoid the discomfort which occurs when normal cervical posture results in the pinching of a posterior bulging disc is the likely scenario. Without proper therapeutic intervention, a prolonged FHP can serve to produce even greater posterior nuclear migration as the anterior loading maintains posterior positioning of the nucleus.

The sequelae of pain and dysfunction resulting from prolonged maintenance of a FHP can be profound. The majority of individuals develop associated posterior cranial rotation to some degree.

Another region subject to significant mechanical stress in the presence of FHP is the cervicothoracic junction. Many individuals complain of pain in the area lateral to the cervicothoracic junction, where the upper trapezius and levator scapulae cross each other. Due to the anatomical approximation of the occiput to the shoulder girdle, in the presence of a FHP with posterior cranial rotation, the levator scapulae and upper trapezius muscles shorten. There is, of course, associated sternocleidomastoid and pectoral tightness, all existing as part of the FHRSP. This leads to development of the proximal or crossed shoulder syndrome, further stressing the craniocervical and cervicothoracic regions.[55] Pain in this area will be much more intense on the

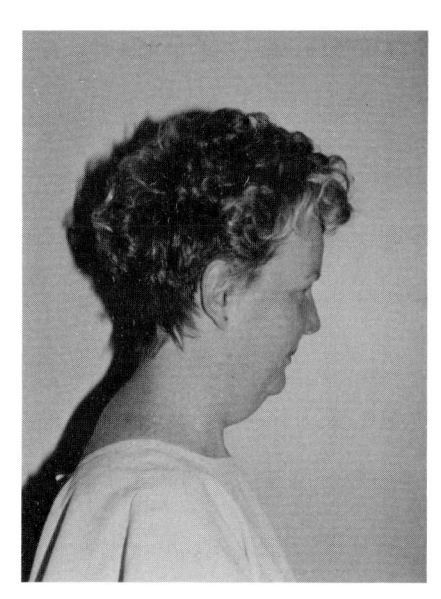

Fig. 5-12. Forward Head Posture without Posterior Cranial Rotation. Note accentuation of cervicothoracic junction.

side of the dominant arm; increased upper thoracic kyphosis or dowager's hump may develop.

Upper Thoracic Kyposis

Figures 5-3, 10, and 12 show exaggerated kyphosis of the upper thoracic spine and/or cervicothoracic junction, commonly referred to as dowager's hump. This is present most often in the elderly, the result of a long-standing slumped posture with an associated forward head. Cumulative mechanical stress results in a stretch of the interspinous ligaments and facet joint capsules with progressive accumulation of excess calcium to stabilize the region. Spinal stress and strain thus ultimately lead to spondylosis and a posture that becomes fixated.

In younger patients, the development of such a posture can be reduced or significantly eliminated by comprehensive therapeutic techniques combined with patient education. The postural deformation is more plastic in the young, making restructuring possible. Although younger patients with this postural abnormality usually present with only minimal restriction of cervical mobility, their mobility can gradually and consistently diminish without proper therapeutic intervention.

The Suboccipital Spine

The suboccipital spine (occiput, atlas, and axis) contains very important neural and circulatory components. Dense mechanoreceptor innervation exists in the ligaments, facet joints, and capsules of the atlas and axis, and to some degree of C 3.[2,19,55-57] Balance and equilibrium are highly dependent on normal input of non-nociceptive activity from this region. Note, however, that visual and vestibular signals combine with those of proprioception to stabilize gaze during most natural movements of the head.[56] The interaction among all three sources of afferent input occurs at the vestibular nucleus. Any disruption or imbalance of normal proprioceptive input, such as by degenerative changes or nerve root irritation, can result in nystagmus or vertigo.[56] It is important for the clinician to obtain a thorough evaluation of the eye, ear, nose, and throat, and of neurological status whenever these symptoms occur. A consult to a specialist is advised, as etiology may also be due to peripheral neuropathy, orthostatic hypotension, sensory deficits due to disease or a central nervous system disorder.

Temporal bone integrity is of prime importance in any analysis of nystagmus, vertigo, or dizziness, since the vestibular labyrinth is located within the temporal bone. Any fracture of the temporal bone can thus trigger the aforementioned problems and give rise to nausea and vomiting.[57]

Nystagmus, an involuntary repetitive movement of the eyes, is the most positive sign of a vestibular disorder. Dizziness refers to a sensation of altered spatial orientation. These differ from vertigo, which is described as a floating or swimming head or rotatory movement of a hallucinatory nature. In the presence of vertigo, sudden head movement can result in loss of balance.[56,57]

Hyperactivity of the sternocleidomastoid muscles and concomitant trigger point development can cause similiar complaints. Travell and Simons have delineated how the clavicular head can produce spatial disorientation, dizziness, and even vertigo. Nausea is commonly associated. A paroxysmal dry cough, sore throat, lacrimation, reddening or ptosis of the eye along with blurred vision are related

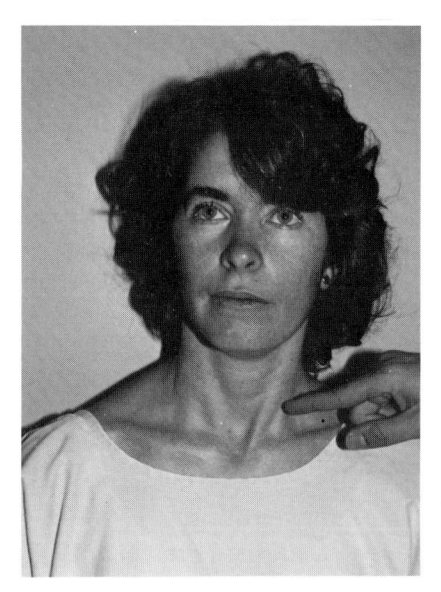

Fig. 5-13. Unilateral Hyperactivity of the SCM. **A**, Anterior view, note the prominence of the left SCM tendinous insertions and the position of the head in left sidebending and right rotation.

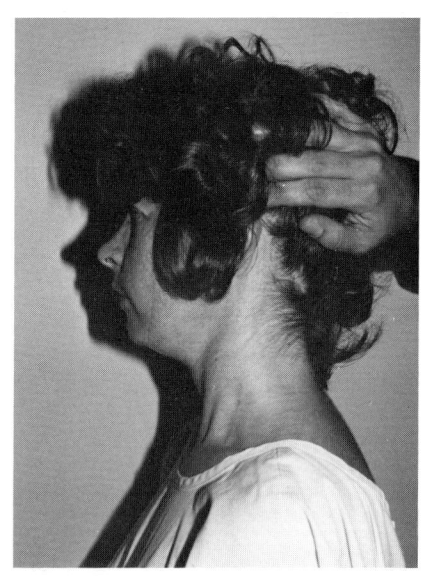

Fig. 5-13. B, Lateral view, note the prominence of the SCM tendons.

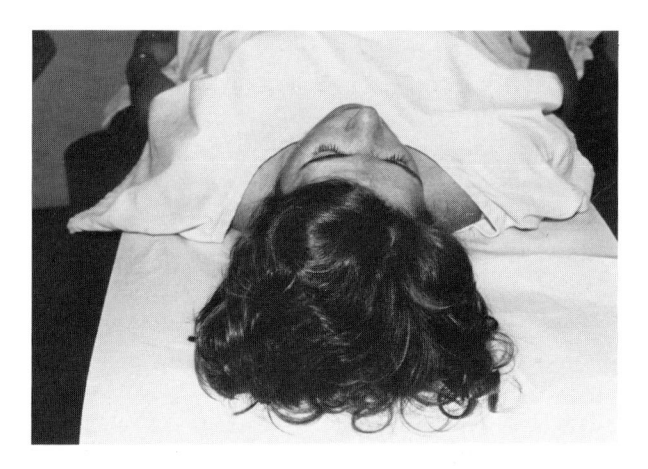

Fig. 5-13. C, Note the resting position of the head in slight left sidebending and right rotation.

to the sternal head. The sternocleidomastoid muscle is considered to be the prime muscular source of proprioceptive input relative to orientation of the head in space. The composite picture of local and referred pain includes the cheek, maxilla, supraorbital ridge, orbit of the eye, external auditory meatus, pharynx, skin, TMJ and forehead. Forehead pain can be ipsilateral, contralateral, or bilateral.[42]

The sternocleidomastoid muscles play a major role in cervical proprioception, and any disruption to its normal function and rest length can be quite profound. Figure 5-13 illustrates the position of the head in the presence of hyperactivity of the left sternocleidomastoid muscle.

Another highly significant anatomical relationship can now be presented. The temporal bone articulates with the sphenoid, parietal, mandible, zygomatic and occipital bones. The anatomy of the temporal bone, along with its articulations, muscular and ligamental attachments, in addition to the sense organs and cranial nerves that it houses or provides pathways for, is more extensive than any other cranial bone. Eight complete pages are devoted to it in Gray's Anatomy, and thus only a few succinct anatomical facts will be discussed here.[58]

The sternocleidomastoid, temporalis, posterior-digastric, longus capitus, splenius capitus, masseter, and stylohyoideus all attach to the temporal bone. If one is in agreement with the controversial tenets of cranial osteopathy, then slight movement of the cranial bones is thought to occur. Thus, hyperactivity of a muscle such as the sternocleidomastoid (which contributes to FHP and posterior rotation of the cranium) may also pull the mastoid process down and forward, resulting in what has been termed internal rotation of the temporal bones. However, this may only occur in the presence of sternocleidomastoid hyperactivity with a preexisting end range posterior cranial rotation. The splenius capitus, longus capitus, and posterior digastric can also contribute to this proposed movement. There are other movements of the temporal bones that are discussed in the literature, and the reader is directed here to some references for greater depth of knowledge.[59-63]

Dysfunction of the temporal bones has also been associated with malocclusion, lightheadedness, syncope, headache, retro-orbital eye pressure, nausea, dizziness, nystagmus, vertigo, and tinnitus.[60-63] The nerves that course through the temporal bone include the facial, glossopharyngeal, vagus, chorda tympani, acoustic, and trigeminal semilunar ganglion. Many blood vessels also pass through the temporal bones.[58]

Frequently, patients with temporomandibular joint dysfunction relate some of the aforementioned symptoms indicative of upper cervical dysfunction. The innervation of this region also encompasses the trigeminocervical complex, which—when irritated—can give rise to craniofacial pain along with pharyngeal, laryngeal, aural, or visual symptoms, with or without those of a vestibular nature.

The spinal tract of the trigeminal nerve descends into the upper cervical spinal cord to the level of C2-C4. There are thus synaptic connections between the trigeminal nerve and the upper cervical spine. Furthermore, the nucleus caudalis of the trigeminal nerve contains a substantia gelatinosa region which is similar in structure and function to, and continuous with, that of the dorsal horn of the spinal cord.[64-70]

The sternocleidomastoid muscles have dual innervation—cranial (accessory) and ventral rami of C2 and C3. The accessory nerve also innervates the upper trapezius via a plexus formed with C3 and C4 ventral rami and has a branch that joins the vagus nerve. Each sternocleidomastoid muscle acts synergistically with its homolateral upper trapezius during active sidebending.[54,55] As compound nerves have more than one nucleus of origin and termination, there are anastomoses between the accessory nerves and the hypoglossal, which joins the sensory nuclei of the trigeminal nerve. The proximal fibers of cranial nerves 5, 7, 9, and 10 are thus all associated with the sensory nucleus of the trigeminal nerve and have sympathetic connections with the upper cervical spine via the nucleus caudalis. A significant percentage of afferent fibers from the sensory nucleus of the trigeminal nerve cross the midline, while a smaller amount remain ipsilateral.[58,67,71-73]

Trigeminal nerve terminals and the upper three cervical nerves combine into a single column of grey matter and cannot be differentiated anatomically. It is thus considered to be a single nucleus (trigeminocervical), and the prime center involved in the mediation of nociception from the craniocervical region.[57,72]

HEADACHES

Here we will discuss only headaches of a musculoskeletal etiology—namely muscle contraction or tension headaches precipitated by postural and degenerative changes of the cervical spine. Involvement of the upper cervical facet joints C1-3 results in irritation of the occipital nerves that primarily originate from the C2-3 segments. The C1 root is not considered to have a cutaneous distribution, but it may provide some sensory innervation to the anterior half of the head since stimulation of C1 rootlets has produced orbital, frontal, and vertex pain.[22,65,71,74] Guarding of the splenius and semispinalis capitus produces suboccipital, occipital and vertex pain. The greater occipital nerve courses through the semispinalis capitus and occipital attachment of the upper trapezius muscles.[42,74]

The trigger point referral pattern is thus indicative of the distribution of the greater occipital nerve. Involvement of the upper trapezius commonly produces pain referral in an occipital-temporal and retro-orbital distribution. Associated dizziness or vertigo may be related to reflex activation of the sternocleidomastoid, levator scapulae, or infraspinatus.[42] I feel that persistence of pain in the temporalis muscles also can give rise to concomitant referral to the maxillary teeth as described by Travell.[42] Any prolonged guarding of the temporalis may also cause limitation of mandibular movement due to its elevation and retrusive force on the mandible. Upper trapezius strain is also seen in buxom women with associated FHRSP that utilize thin and tight bra straps. This serves to increase pressure on the upper trapezius. It is suggested that the bra straps be made wider and overlie the acromion instead of the upper trapezius.

The course of the vertebral artery brings it into close contact with the uncovertebral joints.[75] The vertebral artery also comes into play with postural dysfunction that compresses the suboccipital region. Any irritation or compression of the posterior cervical sympathetic network can result in intracranial vasoconstriction hindering circulation to the cranial nerves, producing widespread symptoms.

Nerves which arise from the cervical part of the sympathetic trunk and cervical roots anastomose with each other around the vertebral artery.[76] They thus may be irritated or compressed by degenerative changes at Luschka's joints and other vertebral structures as distal as C6. The most prominent area of involvement is at the C2-3 level.[77]

The upper three cervical nerves innervate the ligaments and joints of C1-3, the anterior and posterior musculature, the sternocleidomastoid and trapezius, as well as the posterior cranial dura mater and vertebral artery. The dura mater is considered to be very sensitive at the cranial base in that stimulation of the tentorium cerebelli and falx cerebri refers pain to the forehead.[75] Neural connections in this area become even more intimate since the ventral ramus of C2 has meningeal branches to the hypoglossal and vagus nerves innervating the lateral walls of the posterior cranial fossa.[72,75]

The trigeminocervical complex can be implicated as a source of pain in the mouth and throat. The glossopharyngeal nerve innervates the base of the tongue and soft palate.[67] A burning or stabbing pain of a paroxysmal nature not unlike that of trigeminal neuralgia can occur. This, however, is perceived at the posterior aspect of the tongue, throat, and the middle ear.[45,78]

Involvement of the vagus nerve may produce superior laryngeal neuralgia which has similar characteristics to those of glossopharyngeal neuralgia. Pain is perceived at the base of the tongue as well as the glottis, and may even be referred to the upper thoracic region.[45,67,78]

Pain in the tongue and cervical region has been termed the neck-tongue or cervicolingual syndrome, usually precipitated by a sudden rotational movement of the head that stretches the capsule of atlas-axis.[57,72,79] Ipsilateral numbness of the tongue occurs with a concomitant unilateral occipital headache and postauricular pain.

The Barre-Lieou syndrome is thought to occur as a result of irritation of the sympathetic fibers surrounding the vertebral artery or from an osteophyte arising from the uncovertebral joints. The symptom complex can include pain anywhere in the head or neck (vertebral artery courses to C6 vertebrae), impaired hearing, tinnitus, vestibular problems, blurred vision, hoarseness, nasal irritation, tearing of the eye, hot flushes, and sweating. Pain may be continuous but variable, and described as a throbbing, burning, stinging, pricking, or a creeping sensation.[80]

The dense neural interplay in the cervical spine also includes the sinuvertebral nerve of C3, which has an extensive distribution. All other sinuvertebral nerves, except that of C1 and C2, innervate the outer third of the annulus fibrosus of the disc at its level, as well as the one above. Other innervated structures include the posterior longitudinal ligament and anterior dura mater.[81] Intervertebral discs are absent at the occipito-atlantal and atlas-axis articulations.

The sinuvertebral nerve of C3, however, also innervates the ligaments of the atlanto-axial complex and the paramedian dura of the posterior cranial fossa. The sinuvertebral nerves of C1 and C2 join that of C3, and they collectively mediate pain from the cruciate ligaments, tentorial membrane, and dura mater of the posterior cranial fossa.[81]

Edmeads lists seven signs to delineate the origin of a headache from the cervical spine.[65]

1. Persistent suboccipital or occipital pain, usually intense and unilateral.
2. Cervical movements bring on or change the headache.
3. Abnormal head and neck posture such as a forward head.
4. Tenderness in the suboccipital or nuchal region, particularly if unilateral headache is produced by deep suboccipital pressure.
5. Significant and painful hypomobility.

Table 5-4. Prolonged Forward Head-Round Shoulder Posture. Effects upon the spine.

Cervical	Thoracic & Shoulder Girdle	Lumbar

INCREASED
  Suboccipital and TMJ compression. Accentuated cervical lordosis or straightening dependent upon the degree of thoracic kyphosis and posterior rotation of cranium.
 	
INCREASED
  Compression on trigeminal spinal tract and occipital nerves.
 	
INCREASED
  Cranio-facial pain.
 	
INCREASED
  Mandibular repositioning and occlusal alteration.
	INCREASED
	  CT kyphosis. Flat mid-thoracic spine. Supraclavicular compression.
	
	INCREASED
	  Shoulder impingement. Scapular abduction, protraction, and elevation. Internal rotation of the GH joint.
	
	DECREASED
	  Diaphragmatic excursion.
	
	INCREASED
	  Activity of accessory muscles of respiration.
		DECREASED
		  Lordosis.
		
		INCREASED
		  Pressure on intervetebral discs promoting strain on annular fibers.
		
		INCREASED
		  Spondylosis and posterior nuclear migration.

6. Craniocervical dysfunction.
7. Symptomatology indicative of the upper cervical spine and nerve roots.

FHP in association with posterior cranial rotation can therefore lead to widespread symptomatology in the head, face, mouth, and neck that is commonly misinterpreted as TMJ dysfunction. This may occur from acute trauma or cumulatively from upper cervical spondylosis.[82] Again, a comprehensive evaluation is required to adequately determine the etiology of the pain and dysfunction as originating from either the upper cervical spine or the TMJ. Quite often, as will be discussed, both the upper cervical and craniomandibular regions are involved, leading to an overlapping distribution and increased level of discomfort. Therapeutic intervention by both the dentist and physical therapist, who must work together, is then needed. Without such a clinical interplay, treatment of one region may negate or interfere with treatment of the other.

Postural factors thus play a prime role in the craniocervical area and represent a distinct etiological entity in the development of TMJ pain and dysfunction. Table 5-4 outlines the general effects of prolonged FHP on the spine.

CRANIOCERVICAL POSTURE AND TMJ DYSFUNCTION

Rocabado and Kraus have written extensively about the effects of craniocervical posture on TMJ function. Here, we will review their salient points and follow with supporting observations from a clinical perspective.

The function and resting position of the head has been shown to be directly dependent upon the posture of the cervical spine. Head posture, however, always dominates, and when dealing with the upper quarter, any dysfunction will lead to a compensatory change in head position. The head's center of gravity is located slightly anterior to the cervical spine.[6] Unless the posterior muscular antagonists exert a sufficient counterforce, the head will fall forward on the cervical spine. Since the anterior cervical musculature is primarily composed of small, thin muscles, the posterior cervical musculature has no problem maintaining balance.[5,7,8,12,13]

The need for maintenance of the horizontal line of vision is ultimately of prime importance. Alteration, however, can occur from any one or a combination of events previously mentioned. In the presence of normal craniocervical posture, the bipupilar, otic, and transverse occlusal planes should all be hori-

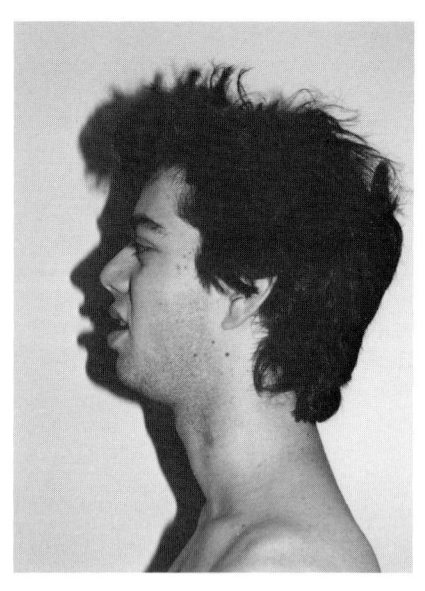

Fig. 5-14. Forward Head Posture with Posterior Cranial Rotation and Anterior Open Bite. **A**, Lateral view, note the presence of posterior cranial rotation and FHP.

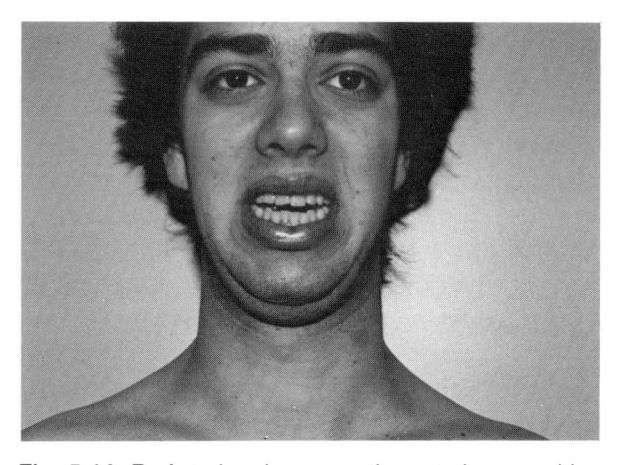

Fig. 5-14. B, Anterior view, note the anterior open bite.

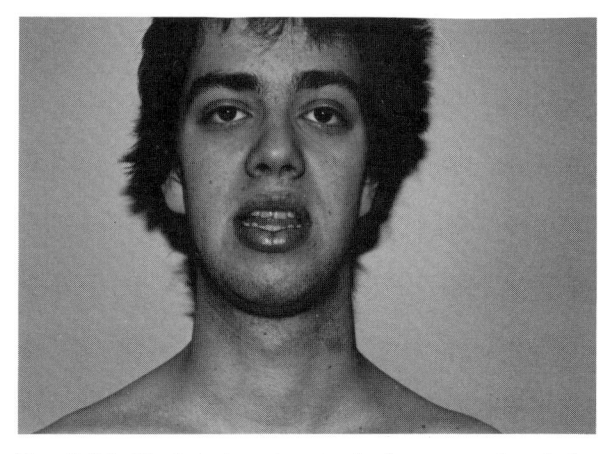

Fig. 5-14. C, Anterior view, note increase of anterior open bite when tongue is on the floor of the mouth.

zontal and parallel to one another.[7,8] As discussed in the previous section, maintenance of this relationship requires normal proprioceptive input from the dense mechanoreceptor network of the suboccipital spine.

The factors that account for the normal resting position of the mandible have long been debated. The author agrees with Kraus that a more appropriate term than resting position is upright postural position of the mandible.[13,83] This position is obviously strongly influenced by the craniocervical relationship, and by the adaptive posture, which is dependent upon muscle tone and tissue elasticity.

The resting position of the mandible in the presence of normal masticatory muscle function and posture should allow for a freeway space of about 2-4 mm. Individuals who present with a skeletal open bite have an increased freeway space.[14] This is usually associated with a narrow, oval-shaped face, narrow nasal apertures, a high narrow palate and a constricted pharyngeal space. Such a combination promotes mouth breathing.

Mouth breathing cannot, however, be effectively performed with the tongue in its normal rest position on the palate. The tongue thus drops down. In order to further increase the airway, the head is extended on the suboccipital spine.[13,83] The result may eventually irritate the trigeminocervical complex in the suboccipital region, and also promote adaptation into a FHP to maintain proper vision.[84-87]

Figure 5-14 shows an individual with an anterior open bite recorded at 3 mm without the mandibular appliance that he had been using, and 7 mm with the appliance in place. There was also a significant degree of posterior cranial rotation. His chief complaints at the time of the referral consisted of a constant achy pain at both TMJs, plus retroorbital and masseter discomfort. Pain also was present at the cervicothoracic junction, upper trapezius, levator scapulae, and suboccipital fossa bilaterally. Although he exhibited normal mandibular mobility, there was a reciprocal click at the right TMJ and tenderness to palpation of the right medial pterygoid, the anterior digastric, and infrahyoid region. The tongue was kept on the floor of the mouth. Progressive appliance revisions were suggested to decrease the anterior open bite as treatment for postural restoration was initiated.

Daly studied the effect on head posture of creating an anterior open bite.[88] An opening of 8mm was induced in a normal population without any craniocervical dysfunction. All subjects had a class 1 occlusion and a freeway space that did not exceed 5mm. Head extension occurred in 90 percent of the subjects after one hour of bite opening. The literature strongly supports the notion that head posture changes to maintain the ability to breathe, swallow and speak easily.[13,59,88] In further support, Vig and associates demonstrated experimentally induced extension of the head in the presence of nasal obstruction. The average amount of extension was recorded at 3.6°.[89]

Hellsing and associates studied 30 adult nasal breathers who had competent lips, complete detention, and no masticatory or spinal disorder.[90] They found that nasal airway obstruction caused an immediate extension of the head and reduced posterior cervical and anterior temporalis activity with mandibular depression in 28 of the 30 subjects. The range of extension varied between 2.4-3.0°. Activity of the suprahyoids increased to allow for mandibular depression (anterior digastric) and stabilization of the hyoid bone (geniohyoid) for an open airway.

Posterior cranial rotation or extension of the cranium on the upper cervical spine will also cause a change in the resting position of the mandible. An understanding of the biomechanics involved requires knowledge of the soft tissue changes that occur between the mandible, hyoid bone, and cervical spine.

A prolonged FHP leads to shortening of the posterior neck extensors and a stretch or elongation of the anterior neck flexors. This produces flexion of the mid-to-lower cervical spine and extension of the upper cervical spine, reducing normal cervical lordosis and promoting FHP.

The normal length-tension relationship of the hyoid bone becomes altered. The mandible is forced into a down-and-back (depressed and retruded) position as increased suprahyoid muscle tension occurs.[91] The maxillomandibular distance thus increases. It is important at this juncture to visualize the entire mandible. The mandibular condyles are forced up and forward as the body of the mandible is pulled down and back. The range of mandibular movement or repositioning is directly proportional to the degree of posterior cranial rotation. In turn, the greater the amount of posterior cranial rotation, the greater the increase in freeway space and suboccipital compression.

In the presence of acute trauma, such as from a cervical strain, the amount of condylar translation increases with the degree of hyperextension of the head on the upper cervical spine. Such a sudden movement may well result in a stretch or tear of the retrodiscal tissue, increasing the likelihood of internal derangement.[53]

Flexion of the head on the cervical spine produces the opposite scenario of up and forward mandibular movement and a decrease in freeway space. The position of the head in relation to the cervical spine also affects the activity of the masticatory muscles. Generally, when the head is extended upon the cervical spine, masticatory muscle activity causes elevation and retrusion of the mandible. With the head flexed upon the cervical spine, there is a small degree of tension, causing depression and retrusion of the mandible.[88]

Initial studies (on animals and man) show some divergence from a more recent study. Funakoshi's studies revealed a major increase in temporalis, moderate increase in masseter, and no increase in digastric muscle activity with head extension.[92,93] In man, Boyd found that activity increased in the anterior temporalis, but decreased in the masseter and anterior digastric during extension. Flexion of the head produced a decrease in anterior temporalis and an increase in masseter and anterior digastric activity.[94]

When the effects of both hyoid muscle tension and masticatory activity are considered jointly, the composite pattern of head-on-neck extension is associated with mandibular elevation and retrusion.[88] This position most commonly occurs with FHP.[13] If such a posture is acquired early in development, the degree of mandibular elevation and retrusion, along with suboccipital compression, can lead to major pain and dysfunction syndromes later in life.[95] This will be most apparent as high school, college, and work days require increased sitting.

Classic early studies and more recent experimentation using electromyography confirm the aforementioned postural effects on the mandible and freeway space.[92,93,95-99] Forsberg and associates, in a study of 30 adults, recorded the EMG activity of the cervical and masticatory muscles in positions of 5, 10, and 20 degrees of extension and flexion with the mandible at rest.[100] As extension of the head increased, they found that posterior cervical muscle activity decreased progressively. This was attributed to a change in the center of gravity of the head, which required less muscular activity to maintain balance. Sternocleidomastoid activity only increased significantly at 20 degrees of extension, with no change occurring in flexion. A forward shift in the center of gravity upon flexion results in increased posterior cervical muscle activity.

Increased EMG activity was recorded in both the infra and suprahyoid muscles with head extension. This was attributed to the passive stretch of the suprahyoids resulting in upward displacement of the hyoid bone and corresponding contraction of the infrahyoids to maintain stability.[100] The supra and infrahyoids also responded with increased activity at 20 degrees of head flexion, attributed to the need to maintain normal hyoid position and airway patency or to avoid occlusal contact (as reported during the experiment). Masseter activity increased in rotation at 10 and 20 degrees of head extension.

Contrary to other studies, Forsberg and associates did not observe definitive evidence of increased activity in the anterior temporalis during flexion or extension of the head.[88-100] This again is most likely related to the short duration and static requirements of their study.

Postural development, facial morphology and adaptation, as has previously been mentioned, begins early in life and can ultimately influence the position of the craniocervical complex.[15,84,95] It has generally been concluded that retrognathism occurs more frequently with increased extension of the head on the neck, and prognathism with flexion.[84] Excessive adenoid development in the nasopharynx may be another contributory entity in that it promotes a forward and downward position of the tongue and concomitant extension of the head, both of which serve to increase the airway in the presence of nasal obstruction.[101]

Hellsing and associates recently reexamined this relationship among 8, 11, and 15-year-old children. They concluded that lumbar, thoracic, and cervical curvatures were sex and age dependent among the 125 healthy children studied. A decrease in cervical lordosis and increase in thoracic kyphosis and lumbar lordosis occurred with increasing age in both males and females. They did not find a correlation between thoracic kyphosis and cervical lordosis as is seen in elderly individuals. A decrease or straightening of the cervical lordosis correlated with extension of the head, cervical mandibular angulation, and anterior facial height. Hellsing and associates measured the cervical lordosis from C2-C6, and thus differentiated upper cervical spine posture from that of the mid-lower region.[102,103] Alteration of the hyoid bone was also demonstrated with repositioning of the mandible.[95,104]

Tallgren and Solow studied 191 adults with relatively normal dentition, occlusion, and similar cervical spine curvature to determine the relationship between the hyoid bone, head posture, and facial morphology.[105] They found a positive correlation among the 20-29, 30-49 and 50-81-year-old age groups, in which an increased hyomandibular distance occurred with a large inclination of the mandible. Head position in relation to the vertical reference line was significantly more extended in the two older groups than in the youngest group. This indicated that marked extension of the head on the cervical spine with forward inclination of the cervical column was associated with a large hyocervical distance.[105]

The position of the hyoid bone also directly influences the resting position of the tongue and consequently, deglutition. What effect then does FHP have upon the tongue and what problems can ensue? The tip of the tongue should normally be positioned against the posterior aspect of the maxillary incisors. It should not push against them, just make slight contact.[106] In addition, the anterior half of the tongue should lie against the palate, a position which is enhanced by negative pressure, since it is suspended from the styloid process of the inferior surface of the temporal bone to the anterior region of the mandible.

In the presence of FHP, posterior cranial rotation (extension of occiput on the suboccipital spine) results in anterior movement of the styloid process, bringing it in closer contact to the mentonium symphysis and decreasing the sling-like tension. In addition, elevation of the hyoid bone slackens the inferior extrinsic muscular attachment. The end result is that the tongue drops down from the palate to the floor of the mouth where it may press on the posterior surface of the mandibular incisors.[106] If the tongue is held on the floor of the mouth for a prolonged period of time, the altered proprioceptive activity will favor mouth breathing and also contribute to development of an anterior open bite.[7,8]

Protrusion of the tongue is performed by the genioglossus. Posterior cranial rotation has been shown to cause increased activity of the genioglossus. The combination of postural changes and increased genioglossus activity are prime factors in the development of a tongue thrust swallow.[106,107] In the presence of associated increased mandibular elevation and retrusion possibly contributing to anterior disc dislocation, the tongue in its position on the floor of the mouth may also be used as a decompressive appliance by the patient.

Figure 5-15 illustrates a scalloped tongue due to a FHP and cumulatively developed internal derangements. The patient has kept the tongue between the teeth for a prolonged period of time to decompress the TMJs, resulting in a scalloped appearance around the periphery.

The initial contact of the maxillary and mandibular teeth depends in part upon the dentition as well as the craniomandibular posture. When active cervical mobility is within normal limits and craniocervical posture is good, there should be no significant tooth contact when swallowing. FHP, however, promotes intercuspation when swallowing, as the tongue is thrust forward against the incisors, allowing increased posterior tooth contact. This decreases the effectiveness of the middle and posterior parts of the tongue during

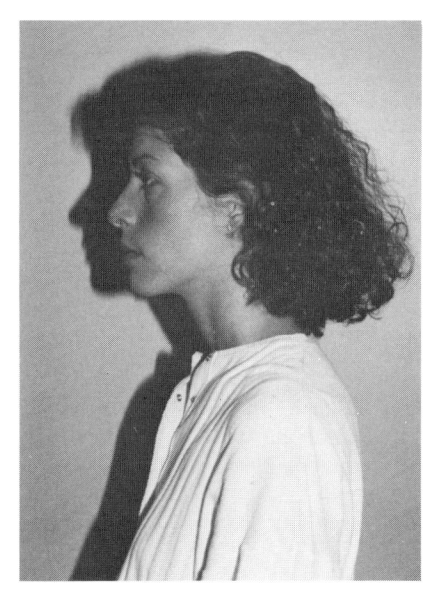

Fig. 5-15. Scalloped Tongue. **A**, Lateral view of FHP.

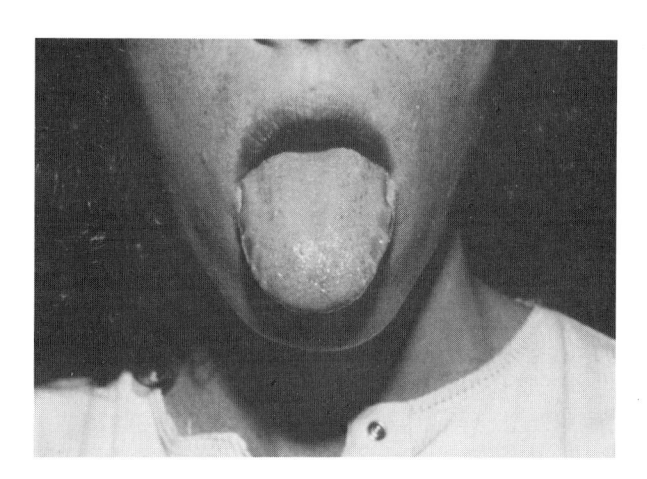

Fig. 5-15. B, Forward head posture promoting loss of the normal suspension system of the tongue. The tongue sits on the floor of the mouth and may be placed between the teeth as a decompressive appliance resulting in a scalloped appearance about the periphery.

the oral stage of swallowing in which it must press up on the palate and assist in movement of the bolus of food or water.[13,83,107] Increased activity of the anterior cervical musculature (longus cervicis and colli) serves to compound the tension in the hyoid region. Tightness in the throat and a globus sensation may occur, thus making swallowing more difficult.

Further, increased tooth contact promotes hyperactivity of the muscles of mastication with associated soreness and achy pain. Trigger points may develop and lead to pain referral within the craniomandibular complex

Table 5-5. Prolonged Forward Head Posture: effects upon the mandible and associated soft tissues

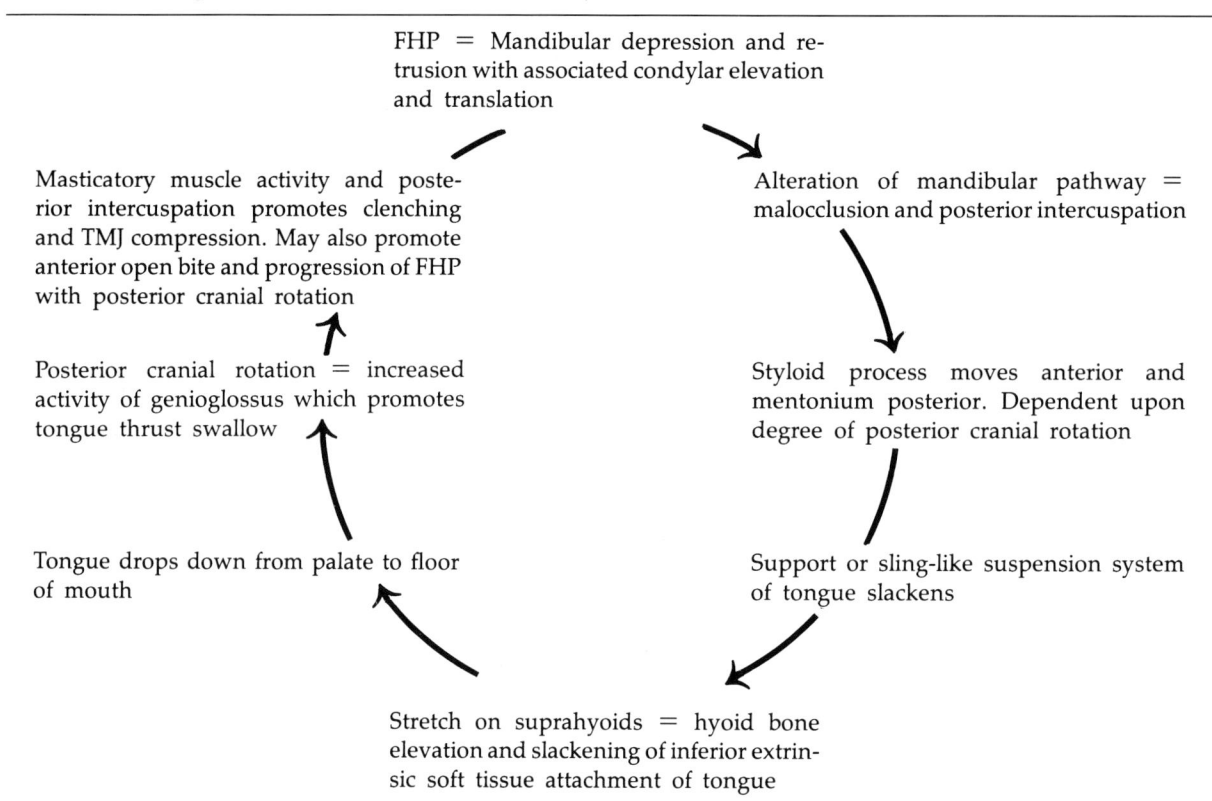

FHP = Mandibular depression and retrusion with associated condylar elevation and translation

Masticatory muscle activity and posterior intercuspation promotes clenching and TMJ compression. May also promote anterior open bite and progression of FHP with posterior cranial rotation

Alteration of mandibular pathway = malocclusion and posterior intercuspation

Posterior cranial rotation = increased activity of genioglossus which promotes tongue thrust swallow

Styloid process moves anterior and mentonium posterior. Dependent upon degree of posterior cranial rotation

Tongue drops down from palate to floor of mouth

Support or sling-like suspension system of tongue slackens

Stretch on suprahyoids = hyoid bone elevation and slackening of inferior extrinsic soft tissue attachment of tongue

---

and anterior cervical area, and a fullness in the floor of the mouth. When the FHP is maintained, the elevation and retrusive force upon the mandible also changes the normal pathways of TMJ function and can lead to premature tooth contact and malocclusion. The net result may be increased masticatory activity, bruxism, and TMJ symptomatology.

FHP with posterior cranial rotation promotes an initial occlusal contact that is more posterior than normal. This increased molar contact may serve to increase TMJ compression.[13,83,107] Occlusal interference has been shown to induce excitation of periodontal ligament mechanoreceptors, facilitating motoneurons in the trigeminal motor nucleus, thus promoting clenching. Specific excitation of the masseter has been induced by stimulation of periodontal and gingival receptors in man.[92,93]

It is easy to perceive mandibular repositioning and more posterior intercuspation by just lightly tapping the teeth together while in a normal seated posture in comparison to a marked FHP. The difference in contact is easily discernable. Another method is to lightly keep the maxillary and mandibular teeth in contact while in normal posture and feel the repositioning of the mandible as the FHP is slowly assumed.

When FHP exists concomitantly with a sidebent or rotated position of the head, an additional change is proposed. Rocabado states that the mandible will deviate contralateral to the sidebent or rotated position of the head. Occlusal contact will thus be more pronounced on the buccal cusps in the premolar and molar region contralateral to the position of the head. If the head is rotated and sidebent to the same side, rotation dominates mandibular position, and occlusal contact occurs on the side of rotation.[7,8] Funakoshi and associates have demonstrated increased EMG activity of the left temporalis and masseter in comparison to the right with the head positioned in left rotation.[93] This factor has also been researched by Wheaton (Chapter 6), who found the mandible to be positioned opposite to the side of head tilt and towards the side of increased temporalis activity.

The incidence of FHP in patients with TMJ pain or dysfunction is profound. Clinically, we see this in no less than two-thirds of our craniomandibular patients. Before discussing the implication of FHP in the management of craniomandibular dysfunction, however, the causes of improper posture will be analyzed. This is of prime importance: if the development of abnormal posture is prevented, the incidence of craniomandibular-cervical pain and dysfunction will diminish significantly. Table 5-5 outlines the effects of a prolonged FHP on the mandible and masticatory apparatus.

CUMULATIVE FACTORS IN THE DEVELOPMENT OF ABNORMAL HEAD AND NECK POSTURE

Cumulative factors play a leading role in the development of FHP and its associated problems. Basic activities of daily living and the postures or positions assumed during them are most significant. Everyone must sit, stand, or lie down for varying periods every day. These are the three basic positions that everyone assumes. But body posture in each of these positions can differ markedly from person to person. Many individuals have developed FHP simply from the way they sit.

Sitting

Sitting has become the most frequent position that man assumes. Postural adaptation begins early in life, as soon as a child starts to sit unaided. Simply the time spent watching television while sitting slumped in a soft chair, couch, beanbag, or on the floor may trigger a habitual slumped posture. Figure 5-5 illustrates an improper sitting postion while watching television. Once the child is old enough to begin school, the type of chair, bench, or desk in which they sit also frequently promotes a slumped posture. Zacharkow has completed an excellent and thorough review of the postures that school children have assumed in various types of desks and chairs.[109] Many of these positions encourage a FHRSP, and if that posture is also assumed at home, it becomes a cumulative factor in the development of pain and

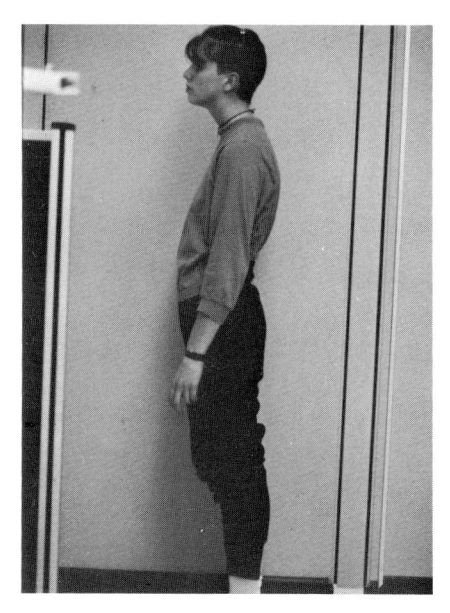

Fig. 5-16. Postural Dysfunction. Eighteen-year-old female with genu recurvatum, increased lumbar lordosis, thoracic kyphosis, round shoulders, forward head and posterior cranial rotation.

dysfunction which may not become evident until the teenage years.[109]

Prolonged sitting with the head and neck in a forward flexed position results in extreme flexion of the lower cervical and upper thoracic spine. A recent study has shown that normal, healthy subjects who assumed this posture developed low cervical and upper thoracic pain in fifteen minutes. Pain disappeared fifteen minutes after the provocation ceased, but nine of the subjects experienced a return of pain during the same evening or next morning. Pain persisted for up to four days in some of the subjects. Pain referral to the arms and head was a concomitant complaint, and some subjects developed nausea, tiredness, and dizziness as well.[110]

A prolonged FHP, especially at school, requires posterior cranial rotation and subsequent extension of the occiput on the upper cervical spine in order for the student to observe the blackboard or pay attention in class.[108-111] The composite effects of the above postural abnormalities have previously been shown to cause abnormal compressive forces upon the upper cervical spine and temporomandibular joints. Figures 5-11 and 5-16 illustrate an eighteen-year-old female art major with these marked postural abnormalities. The major contributory factor in her case was prolonged sitting on a backless stool while leaning forward to paint and draw. Without any history of trauma, this patient developed craniofacial pain and bilateral anterior displaced TMJ menisci. It is quite possible that the retrusive force exerted upon the mandible by the FHP with associated posterior cranial rotation was a significant factor in the development of TMJ dysfunction. If such postural factors begin early, even a retrognathic mandible may occur.

Prolonged thoracic spine loading from a kyphotic posture has also been implicated in the development of Scheuermann's disease, producing anterior vertebral wedging and increased ossification of the thoracic vertebrae. Also known as vertebral epiphysitis, the condition produces associated fatigue and pain in the back and limbs. It is most commonly seen between ages of 10-25.[112,113]

Hamstring and pectoral shortening may also occur from a prolonged slumped posture. The shortened hamstrings may then promote posterior pelvic rotation when the upright standing position is assumed. This serves to produce a further decrease in lumbar lordosis (already decreased when in the slumped posture). Furthermore, a relaxed abdominal wall may occur due to approximation of the sternum to the pelvis, creating a downward and forward force upon the viscera that can lead to depression of the diaphragm.

Not only does the slumped sitting posture promote a FHRSP, but it is also the position that produces the greatest intradiscal pressure in the lumbar spine. Unsupported sitting increases intradiscal pressure in the lumbar spine by 40 percent in comparison to an upright standing position. Reclining reduces the pressure by 50-80 percent.[114]

Figure 5-17 illustrates an individual with a flat lumbar spine, increased thoracic kyphosis, forward head round shouldered posture and posterior cranial rotation. This degree of postural deformity has developed through years of neglect and lack of education as to corrective postural techniques. Unsupported sitting causes the pelvis to rotate posteriorly, thus decreasing lumbar lordosis and promoting a flexed or kyphotic posture. The facet joints of the lumbar spine do not absorb the load when in a kyphotic sitting posture. The

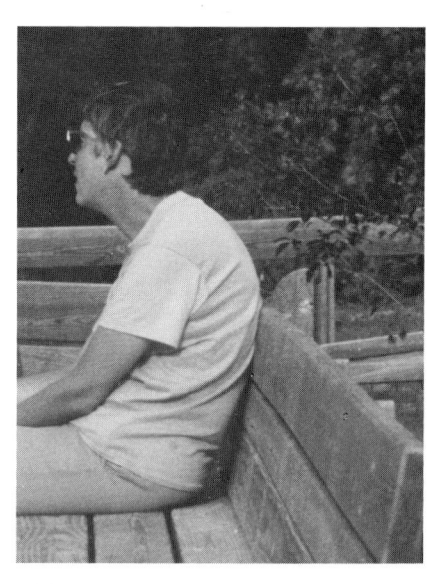

Fig. 5-17. Postural Neglect. Note the slumped posture producing loss of the lumbar lordosis, increased thoracic kyphosis, FHP and increased posterior cranial rotation.

compressive force is thus transmitted to the intervertebral discs, contributing to degeneration and strain of the posterior annular wall, which if maintained can cause irreparable damage. Maintenance of a flexed spinal posture has been shown to weaken or tear the annulus fibrosus, decrease the fluid contact of the nucleus pulposus and thus promote a herniation or derangement.[115-118]

Driving while in a slumped posture can also have significant cumulative effects. Research has shown that men who spend at least one-half of their work day driving are three times as likely to develop a lumbar herniated nucleus pulposus. Truck driving compounds the likelihood of a herniated nucleus pulposus fivefold due to associated vibrational forces. The factor of vibration is also apparent on motorcycles, buses, tractors, and bicycles, all of which may involve unsupported sitting. The mechanical properties of lumbar intervertebral discs begin to show significant changes after only one hour of static (office) or vibration (driving) sitting.[117,118]

Cumulative factors thus weigh heavily in industrial situations where low back pain and concomitant injury plus lost work time have become expensive. Static work postures not only involving sitting, but also bending, twisting, lifting, vibration, and driving have also been implicated. Any task that involves crouching or stooping due to inadequate head clearance or cramped work areas also contributes to increased lumbar stress. Welders, plumbers, and mechanics are prime examples, with dentists not far behind.

Jobs that require reaching forward also necessitate leaning forward if sitting in a chair. If the task is repetitive or involves a reach of more than 15″ in front of the body, a loss of lumbar lordosis will occur. The type of chair may not even make a difference when repetitive forward reaching is required. A recent study comparing preferences during reaching while seated in a fixed backward reclining, forward-reclining, or tiltable seat did not reveal any significant difference.[119,120]

The shape of the seat, however, may contribute to increased low back pain. When the seat has a scoop shape, the femurs tend to internally rotate and the trochanters move superiorly. This can compress the sciatic nerve just lateral to the ischial tuberosity and give rise to pain referral into the lower extremities.[108]

In a normal lordotic sitting posture, the line of gravity passes anterior to the cervical spine, necessitating slight-to-moderate activity of the posterior neck musculature to maintain proper head position. Chairs with backrests that push the shoulders forward also result in increased upper trapezius activity and promote an associated FHP. This is primarily true in narrow chairs with rounded or semicircular backs, as well as chairs with large and thick back pillows. Related is the need to forward bend the trunk in order to stand up from a very soft chair, thus also promoting a FHP.[121,122]

Cumulative factors also play a prime role when proper arm support is not available during prolonged sitting in a slumped posture. The greater the degree of the slump and associated FHP the greater the increase in upper trapezius and other posterior muscle activity. Any workstation (desk or worksurface with or without a chair) that requires the worker to assume a FHP contributes markedly to neck and shoulder pain. This is frequently encountered in keypunch operators, typists, draftsmen, bank tellers, computer programmers and other similar occupations that involve the performance of highly repetitive manual skills in a relatively fixed position.[123-128]

The upper trapezius is the muscle most likely to develop trigger points. A complete discussion of anatomical and physiological factors relative to trigger points can be found in Chapter 3 by Kraus, as well as in the work of Travell and Simons.[42] The upper trapezius must be continuously active when the head and neck need to be maintained in a vertical position to keep the eyes level.

Other etiological factors that serve to increase stress on the cervical musculature include desks that are too low or horizontal, as well as too great a distance between the desk and chair. If the distance to the desk or work station is sufficient to necessitate elevation of the arms to 30 degrees or more without support, the trunk will need to adapt by forward flexion. This will promote a FHRSP, especially when the elevation reaches 45 degrees.[129-131] Prolonged sitting at horizontal desks promotes a FHRSP. Posterior cranial rotation and associated suboccipital compression may also occur, depending upon how often the individual must view material with the head upright.

VIDEO DISPLAY TERMINALS

The increased use of computers in the workplace as well as at home has also contributed to the incidence of FHP. The relative position of the head, neck, and trunk is dependent upon the specific location of the video display terminal (VDT) as well as that of any documents being read. Improper positioning of the VDT—too low or too far—will lead to the development of a FHP. A keyboard that is not detachable will negate the ability of the operator to adjust sitting position. Figure 5-18 illustrates improper VDT and source document positioning. Source documents that are positioned flat on the desk or work surface require increased cervical spine flexion. When this is associated with a FHP, the strain on the posterior cervical musculature increases markedly. Furthermore, there is a corresponding increase in compressive force upon the cervical spine that can lead to intervertebral disc degeneration.[108,110,111,122,130,132]

Bifocals tend to further compound abnormal postural faults associated with display

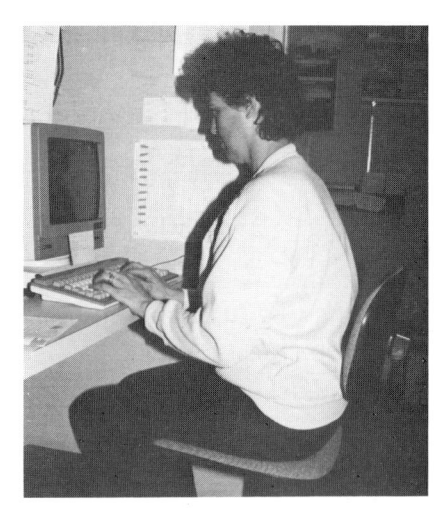

Fig. 5-18. Improper VDT Placement. Note that the monitor is placed too low requiring forward inclination of the head. The worker is also not utilizing the backrest.

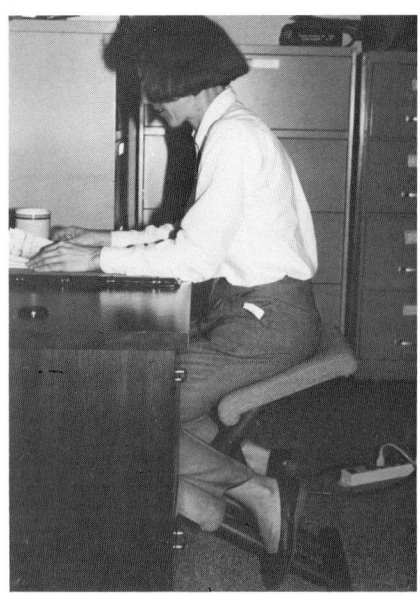

Fig. 5-19. Balans Chair. Provides for maintenance of proper lumbar and trunk posture but promotes forward inclination of the head and neck when used with a horizontal work surface.

terminals. The operator with bifocals needs to extend and posteriorly rotate the head to properly view the screen, thus leading to increased suboccipital compression. Improperly fitted glasses may also drop to one side or slide forward, necessitating head adjustment into a position of strain. Nearsightedness must be corrected, as this also promotes the development of a FHP.[108]

The position of the feet and legs must also be considered. If the legs cannot be placed directly underneath the work surface a sitting position on the anterior aspect of the chair will occur. This is seen frequently in punch press operators and certain types of assembly work.[133] Whenever there is inadequate room to position the feet under the workplace the worker will look for alternate placement. This usually takes the form of foot placement upon stools, braces or supports for the desk or workstation. If the elevation of the foot support is sufficient to raise the knees above waist level a decrease in the lumbar lordosis occurs with a tendency towards forward inclination of the head.

In an attempt to minimize lumbar intradiscal pressure and resultant low back pain from prolonged sitting, the Balans chair was developed in Norway. The Balans chair does not have back support, but its design necessitates knee and hip flexion, foot placement under the seat, and a downward slope of the thighs. The angle of hip flexion is around 60 degrees (as compared to 90 degrees in a standard chair) with the knees supported to counteract any forward slant of the body off the seat. This position promotes maintenance of lumbar lordosis to decrease lumbar strain, as well as an upright position of the trunk and head which tends to negate a FHP.[134,135] However, when used with a horizontal desk or work surface that is too far from the chair, a forward and downward inclination of the head and neck occurs, thus increasing posterior cervical activity (Fig. 5-19).

Individuals in the Balans chair demonstrated lower initial paraspinal EMG activity in both the lumbar and cervical areas than when in a standard sitting position in a conventional chair. EMG activity, however, gradually increased in both areas when the position was maintained beyond 30 minutes. Final EMG recordings were higher in the kneeling position on the Balans in comparison to a conventional chair.[135]

SLEEPING

Prior to sleep, many people spend a significant period of time reading or watching television in bed. The position assumed in this instance most often involves leaning or sitting up against the headboard or wall with one or more pillows placed behind the upper back and head, as illustrated in figures 5-20 A, B, C. The legs may be positioned either with full knee extension on the bed or in a degree of flexion with a pillow under the knees. This position again produces forward flexion of the trunk, loss of lumbar lordosis, and a concomitant FHP. The height and location of the television monitor may serve to increase the FHP or posterior cranial rotation, as previously discussed in the section on video display terminals.

Sleeping in the supine position on one thick pillow or more than one pillow raises the head into a forward inclined posture (Fig. 5-21), also placing considerable strain upon the cervicothoracic junction. A burning pain or ache commonly develops due to stretch of the interspinous ligaments. The sternocleidomastoids are shortened, and this, if prolonged, not only leads to a FHP, but also to the development of trigger points. Many individuals assume a similar position when lying supine on a couch with the head supported on an armrest, headboard, thick seat, or back cushion (Fig. 5-20 C). Maintenance of this anterior head posture for prolonged periods day after day produces adaptive structural changes in the anterior and posterior cervical region that eventually may become permanent.

Sleeping in the prone position with or without a pillow may promote mandibular deviation, and will definitely lead to strain of the cervical joints or soft tissue due to prolonged end range rotation (Fig. 5-22). This is most apparent in the upper cervical region on the side to which the head is rotated and is a common cause of suboccipital irritation or compression with pain referral to the cranium. Sleeping in a supine position without a pillow promotes posterior cranial rotation (Fig. 5-23).

Prolonged standing over a low workstation can also lead to loss of the lumbar lordosis, an increased thoracic kyphosis and associated FHRSP. This is commonly seen in cafeteria and assembly line workers as well as pharmacists or anyone performing work at a counter. Figure 5-24 illustrates the FHP and figure 5-25 the standing work position of a pharmaceutical assistant. Closely associated with counter work are activities performed at home such as cooking, washing dishes and ironing.

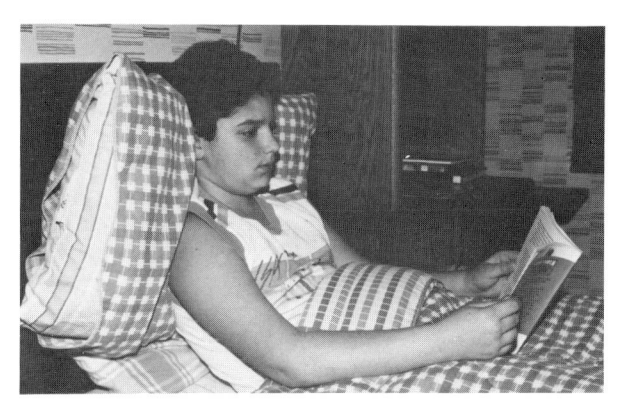

Fig. 5-20. A and **B**, Reading or Watching TV in Bed. The lumbar lordosis is lost and pillows push the head forward.

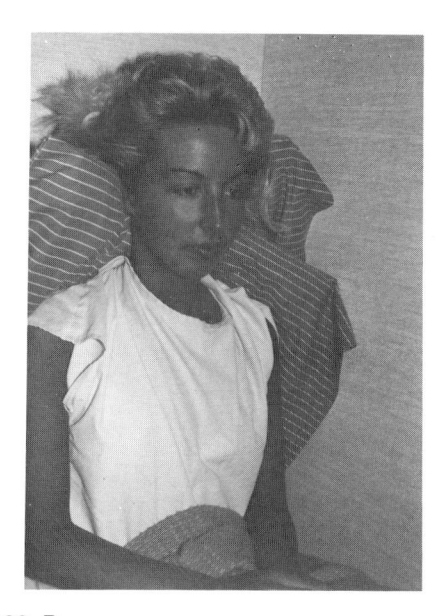

Fig. 5-20 B.

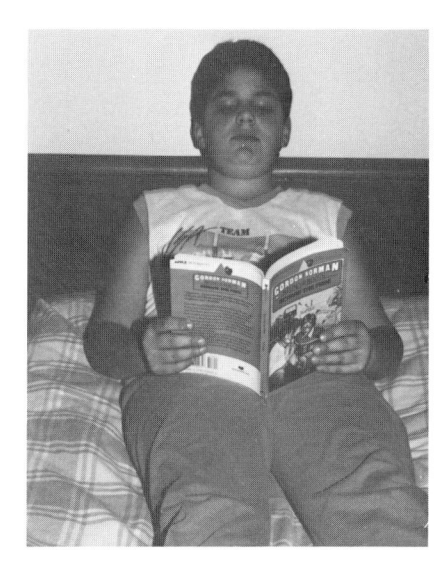

Fig. 5-20. C, Reading with head supported on headboard provides the greatest degree of forward inclination of the head.

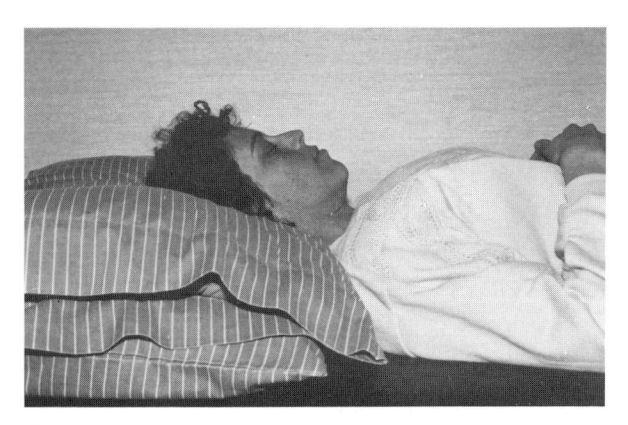

Fig. 5-21. Improper Sleeping Position. Sleeping supine on two pillows. The head is inclined forward for a prolonged period of time, contributing to the development of a FHP.

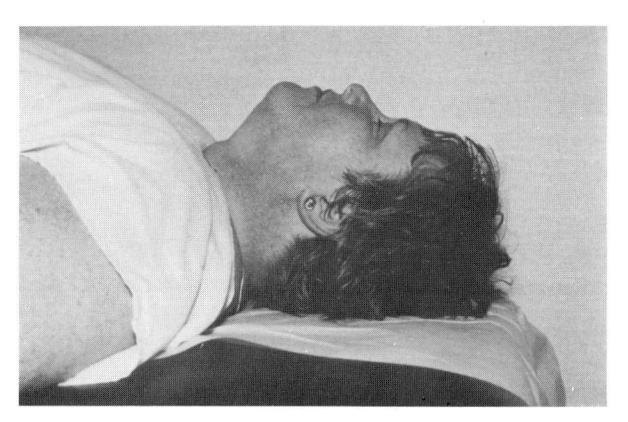

Fig. 5-23. Improper Sleeping Posture. Note the degree of posterior cranial rotation when lying supine without proper head and neck support in the presence of a FHP. Headaches, dizziness, blurred vision and facial pain may become evident during the night or upon assuming an upright position.

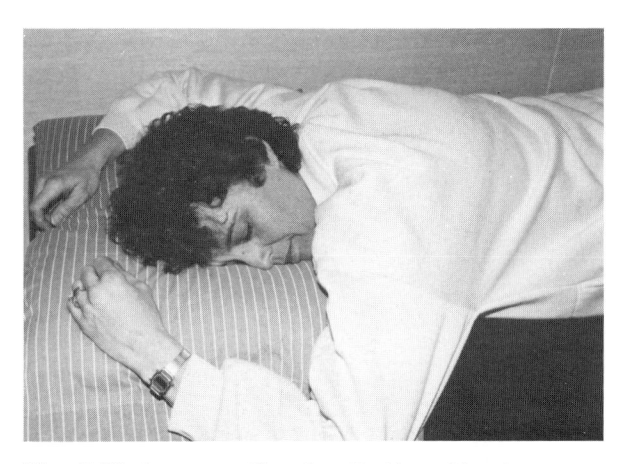

Fig. 5-22. Improper Sleeping Position. Sleeping prone with head in full rotation. This position may initially feel very comfortable but it produces compression forces upon the upper cervical spine. Elevation of the arms overhead may contribute to neurovascular compression of the supraclavicular region.

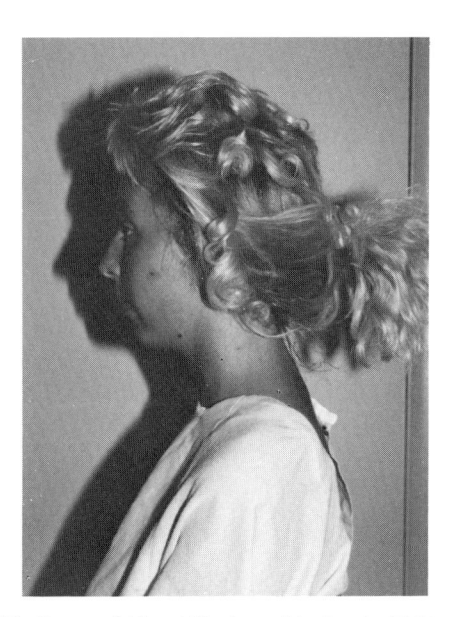

Fig. 5-24. Forward Head Posture. Moderate FHP seen in a pharmaceutical assistant. Note that there is a minimal degree of posterior cranial rotation. The work position as illustrated in Fig. 5-25 requires forward inclination of the head.

Other jobs may require the worker to function in the standing position under a workstation that does not allow adequate headroom. This is commonly encountered by the plumber, auto mechanic or coal miner who may have to either crouch forward and/or look overhead. Prolonged work in this position leads to sub-occipital compression and an associated FHP dependent upon the extent of the upright position. A job that requires any repetitive or prolonged overhead work with tools or merely reading displays or monitor dials can result in similar discomfort. Figure 5-26 illustrates the repetitive work of a painter and subsequent sub-occipital compression and increased lumbar strain.

ACUTE TRAUMA

Individuals with a preexisting FHP are sitting ducks for the development of severe whiplash injuries to both the cervical and craniomandibular areas. A previous publication by this author has outlined the mech-

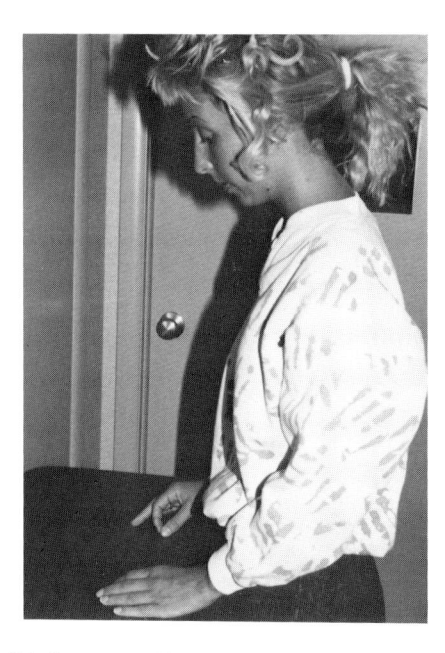

Fig. 5-25. Improper Working Posture. Typical working posture of a pharmaceutical assistant which promotes a forward inclination of the head. Ergonomic modifications and periodic interruption by postural corrective exercise (head retraction) is needed.

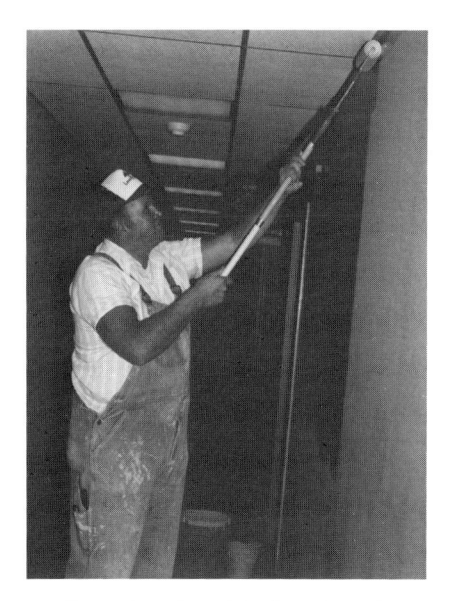

Fig. 5-26. Posterior Cranial Rotation During Work. **A**, Painter exhibiting posterior cranial rotation during painting.

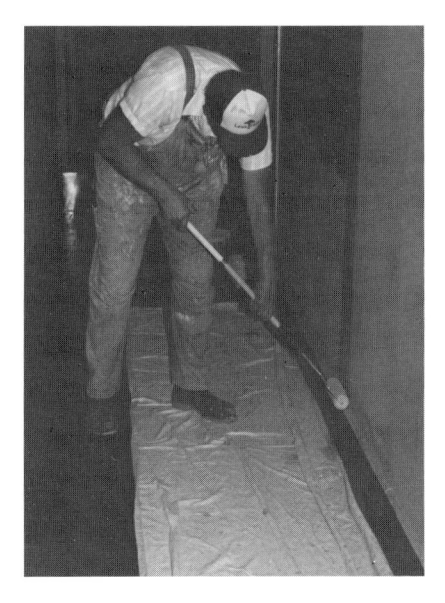

Fig. 5-26. B, Forward bending of lumbar spine when painting.

anism of injury resulting from flexion/extension and lateral flexion injuries of the cervical spine.[53] Mandibular whiplash is a concomitant injury. Separate from an acute mandibular whiplash is the rapid development of a FHP as a result of acute trauma and its subsequent effect upon the mandible.

When the auto accident does not produce initial trauma to the TMJs, maintenance of the FHP can lead to prolonged compressive forces and minor to moderate dysfunction that may eventually make the craniofacial pain more severe than the cervical discomfort. Insufficient awareness of the mechanism of injury, late referral for definitive therapeutic intervention and failure on the part of many clinicians to recognize the interrelationship of upper quarter structures may significantly contribute to long rehabilitation courses.[53]

A whiplash injury produces forces which act upon the cervical spine as well as the craniomandibular region. In a typical hyperflexion injury of the cervical spine, a strain or stretch of the posterior cervical musculature occurs. This most commonly involves the short suboccipital extensors, the upper trapezius, and levator scapulae. Secondary muscle spasm produces posterior cranial rotation and extension of the occiput upon the upper cervical spine. The signs and symptoms resulting from suboccipital compression have previously been discussed.

Sudden cervical hyperextension stretches, strains, or tears structures in the anterior compartment, most commonly the longus colli, sternocleidomastoids, and scalenes. Secondary muscle spasm of the longus colli decreases cervical lordosis, and shortening of the sternocleidomastoids contributes to further posterior cranial rotation and upper cer-

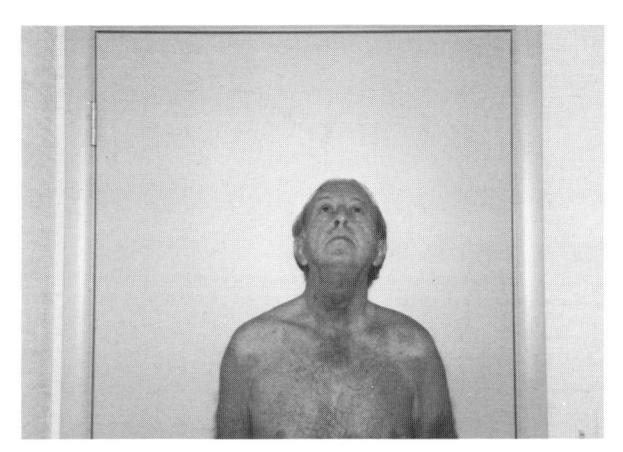

Fig. 5-27. Cervical Hyperextension Injury. Note the ecchymosis extending from the suprahyoid region to mid-sternum.

Table 5-6. Whiplash: effect on cervical spine.

Direction of Injury

A Hyperflexion = reflex guarding of posterior cervical musculature = ↑ suboccipital compression

PLUS

B Hyperextension = reflex guarding of anterior cervical musculature = ↓ cervical lordosis

EQUALS

C Combination = FHP with posterior cranial rotation = pain and dysfunction of craniomandibular and cervical structures.

FHP with posterior cranial rotation, furthermore, promotes mandibular depression and retrusion with associated condylar elevation and translation.

vical compression. Figure 5-27 illustrates the anterior ecchymosis which developed due to a soft tissue stretch or tear from an acute hyperextension injury. A preexisting FHP and improper positioning of the head rest may have contributed to the extent of the injury. Guarding of the scalenes increases the degree of forward head movement as well as thoracic inlet compression due to elevation of the first two ribs. SCM guarding may compound the neurovascular compression of the thoracic inlet by elevating the sternum and clavicles as well.

The whole scenario ends in the development of a FHRSP, with its inherent effects upon the mandible. Table 5-6 outlines the sequence of events which culminate in a FHP as a result of a cervical whiplash injury. Dependent upon the degree of flexion-extension, other structures such as the cranium, larynx, esophagus, intervertebral discs, vertebral bodies, and possibly the spinal cord can also sustain damage.

Cervical collars of either hard or soft material are frequently prescribed for use after whiplash injuries, as well as in the presence of spondylosis or disc herniation. But prolonged continuous use (beyond 2-3 weeks) without initiation of a weaning program and concomitant manual therapy plus active ROM exercise promotes muscle shortening, atrophy, and weakness. Perhaps even more important is how the collar is worn.

A cervical collar that is higher anteriorly than posteriorly exerts an upward force upon the chin and pushes the head into posterior rotation on the upper cervical spine. Compression of the trigeminocervical network intensifies and may promote increased craniofacial pain, dizziness, nausea, and other symptoms. Maintenance of the eyes in a horizontal plane results in forward inclination of the head, and again the composite FHP occurs.[136]

Hard cervical collars and orthoses, such as the Philadelphia Collar, are at times needed to provide immobilization of the cervical spine in the presence of irritation that may damage the spinal cord, nerve roots, or vertebral arteries. Prolonged use of cervical collars, as well as mechanical mandibular traction, are additional factors contributing to TMJ pain and dysfunction. If a cervical collar is needed, it should provide proper cervical support in both the upright and supine positions without causing mandibular or suboccipital compression. Figure 5-28 illustrates a new cervical collar that meets these requirements and also is adjustable.

Acute injury to the TMJs is also possible. Insufficient time for the supra and infrahyoids to relax and assume normal rest length may contribute to anchoring of the mandible. As the head posteriorly rotates in the presence of an anchored mandible, excessive mouth opening will occur. The net result is that the mandible is pulled back and down while the condyles excessively translate anteriorly.

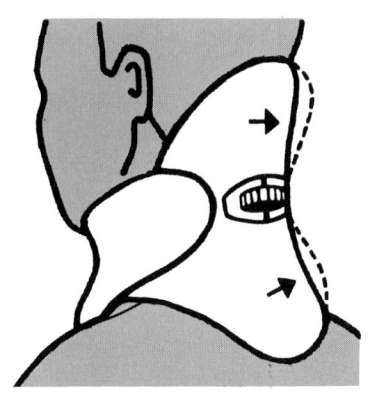

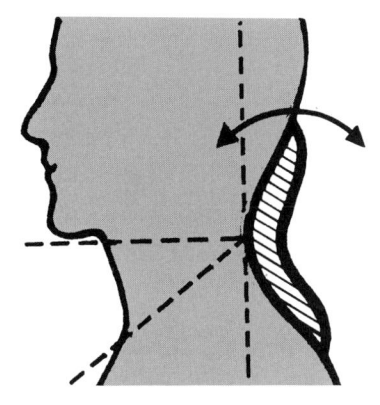

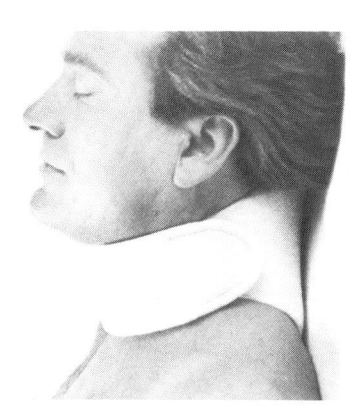

Fig. 5-28. Cerviflex. An adjustable posterior support allows for correction of the cervical lordosis and does not promote mandibular elevation or forward inclination of the head. Reproduced with permission of Bauerfiend, 5570-M Tulane Drive, Atlanta, Georgia 30336.

This may lead to a stretch of the retrodiscal tissue.[53]

The possibilty of an acute internal derangement increases with the degree of hyperextension of the cranium. A retrodiscal tear may cause a laxity in the elastic superior zone, which in the presence of guarding of the superior belly of the lateral pterygoid may combine to produce anteromedial TMJ disc displacement. A preexisting FHP may have already produced mandibular hypomobility, resulting in increased damage such as condylar head fractures against the eminence of the temporal bone.

PREVENTION AND RESTORATION BODY MECHANICS AND ERGONOMICS

Prevention of abnormal head and neck posture must begin at home where the majority of time is spent. Good sleeping posture necessitates a firm mattress and use of proper cervical and head support. Sleeping supine without a pillow or use of a very thin pillow is not recommended. Posterior cranial rotation and upper cervical compression occurs when sleeping supine without a proper pillow, as illustrated in Figure 5-23. The prone position should also be avoided. Supine or sidelying positions are recommended with the use of a cervical pillow or cervical roll placed within the pillow case to maintain proper posture. Figures 5-29 and 5-30 illustrate sleeping positions.

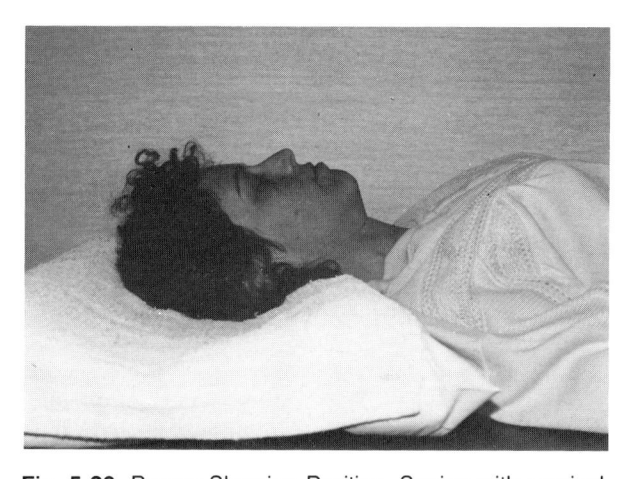

Fig. 5-29. Proper Sleeping Position. Supine with cervical pillow. Note contour of pillow maintaining the cervical lordosis without forward inclination of the head.

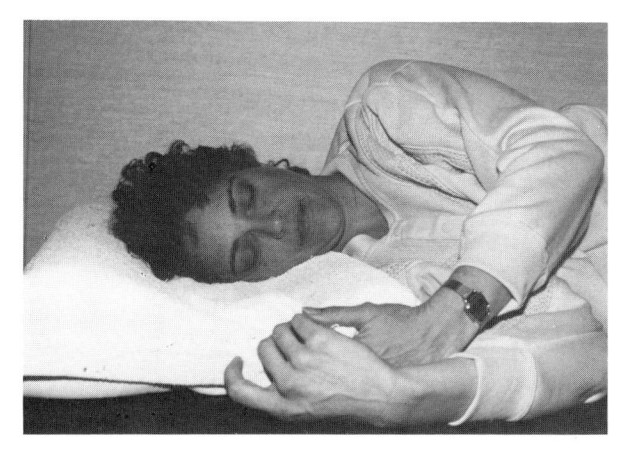

Fig. 5-30. Proper Sleeping Position. Sidelying with cervical pillow. Note contour which maintains the head in neutral position minimizing any upper cervical compression.

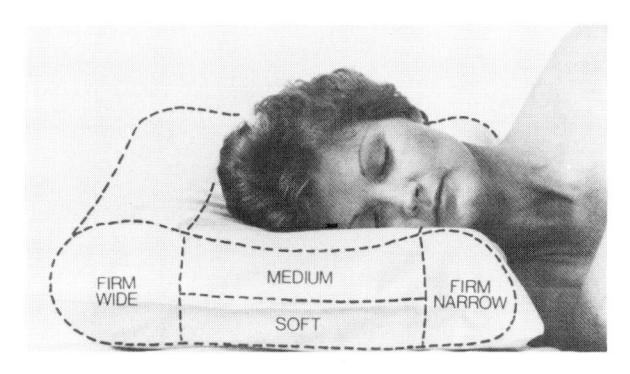

Fig. 5-31. Wal-Pil-O. Proper support and alignment of the head and neck by use of the Wal-Pil-O. Note the choice of supports available when sidelying or supine. Reproduced with permission of Pleasing Patients Unlimited.

Specially designed pillows that provide proper support in both supine and sidelying positions are becoming increasingly available. One of the first was designed by Dr. Lionel Walpin and is known as the Wal-Pil-O. This pillow, illustrated in figure 5-31, can be adjusted to provide four different combinations of head and neck support in either the supine or sidelying position and is available in different sizes and heights.

In the supine position, restoration of the normal cervical lordosis is promoted and a neutral midline posture can be maintained when sidelying. When a FHP already exists, with shortened upper trapezius and suboccipitals, supine lying with the Wal-Pil-O in the medium center, side border position can provide a stretch.

The Mckenzie cervical roll is a foam rubber insert that can be placed in front of the pillow within the pillow case to maintain the cervical lordosis. This of course may contribute to an increased FHP with or without posterior cranial rotation if used with a pillow that is too thick. Pillows must be adapted to an individual's posture and body type. It is not uncommon to spend the night at a hotel sleeping with a pillow that is as hard and thick as a tree trunk only to awaken with significant discomfort.

Due to the many different body types and upper quarter postures, it is recommended that a few different pillows be available in any practitioner's clinic for patients to evaluate. The use of a proper pillow can easily be negated by sleeping on a mattress that does not provide firm support. A mattress that sags in the middle pushes the trunk into forward flexion when supine or sidebending, thus promoting either a FHP or unilateral suboccipital compression. If reading or watching television in bed is a necessity, use of an adjustable wedge can provide adequate trunk and head support in an inclined position. This is also helpful for the individual with a hiatus hernia who cannot lie supine. The wedge should provide support from the waist to the occiput, and the addition of a cervical roll may serve to enhance head and neck support.

ERGONOMICS

The science that deals with the problem of job design to minimize injury and enhance efficiency is known as ergonomics. Ergonomic principles are now playing an increasing role in the design of chairs, work stations, tools, desks, and other objects used on the job.

Many different types of chairs are now being designed with emphasis on maintenance of lumbar lordosis. When a lumbar support is provided to promote an anterior pelvic tilt and posterior movement of the trunk, a lordotic posture is promoted, and forward inclination of the head is minimized. This results in a considerable decrease in lumbar intradiscal pressure, hinders the development of low back pain, and promotes proper craniocervical posture.[137]

Chairs that are not designed with backrests which promote lumbar lordosis can be modified by simply adding a lumbar roll or pillow. Figure 5-32 illustrates the use of a lumbar support pillow when reading. If a recliner that does not have a thick head rest is available, it is recommended for reading when a lumbar pillow is added. In the absence of a recliner, we suggest that a hard chair be placed against a wall, and a cervical roll and lumbar support added so that the head maintains light contact with the wall. This relaxes the posterior cervical musculature and maintains cervical lordosis. The placement of one or two pillows under the upper arms, as

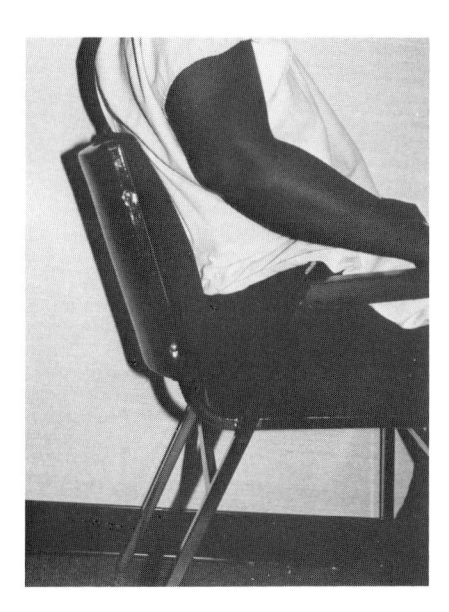

Fig. 5-32. Lumbar Lordotic Support Pillow. Maintenance of the lumbar lordosis is easily performed when utilizing a lumbar pillow and sitting upright in a hard chair.

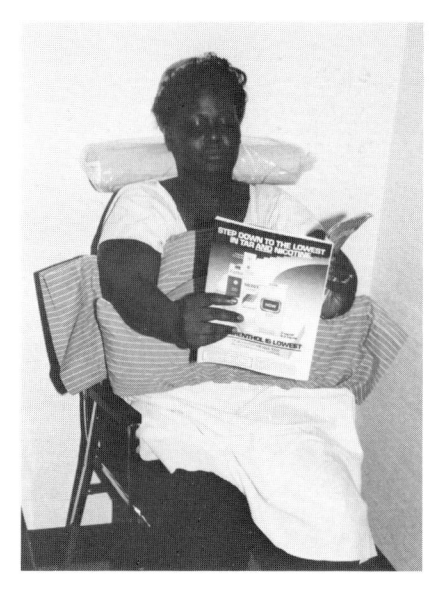

Fig. 5-33. Adaptive Sitting. Note that the head is easily maintained in an upright position by the use of a lumbar pillow and cervical roll which allows for the occiput to rest gently upon the posterior wall. The pillows provide arm support for reading material to reduce strain on the shoulder girdle area.

illustrated, minimizes stress on the shoulder girdle muscles (Fig. 5-33).

Chair height and angle of inclination must be adjustable, especially when working with a video display terminal or a keyboard that is not separate from the monitor. Studies with video display terminal operators show a preference for a backward inclination of the trunk with full and high back support that requires a downward gaze angulation of only 5-20 degrees to the center of the screen and source documents. The recommended eye-to-screen distance is 16-24 inches.[108,119,138-141]

Forearm and wrist supports significantly decrease trapezius muscle and lumbar disc loading. It is also recommended that forearm angle match that of the keyboard inclination. The keyboard is best positioned at elbow level, with a slope of about 30 degrees, but should optimally be adjustable.[140-145]

The feet must be able to be placed flat on the floor directly under the work station. This necessitates an adjustable seat height, and a seat back that can be inclined. Seat height should be adjusted to 3-5 cm above the popliteal crease, and the desk or work surface 3-5 cm above elbow level. The seat should be wide enough to support both buttocks, and the front edge should be rounded to allow for easy changes of leg position. The thighs are best kept parallel to the floor, and the knees should not be above hip level or lordosis will be reduced. These measurements should be performed with the worker in an upright sitting position with relaxed shoulders.[119,120,133]

A desk or work station with a surface that can be adjusted from horizontal to 45 degrees of inclination also serves to decrease static load upon the musculature of the head, neck and shoulders. The best example of this is the artist's adjustable desk. Research has demonstrated that as the incline of a desk increases, the cervical and lumbar spine assume a more extended position and the trunk becomes more upright. In addition, the worker should be instructed to alternate between standing, sitting, and supported sitting postures.[129,133] An adjunctive pelvic spinal posture seat can provide stability as well as allow for safe pelvic mobility. This can be placed on top of the seat of a standard chair (Fig. 5-34).

In the presence of a fixed flat work surface, an adjunctive device (Fig. 5-35) may be helpful. This allows for an inclination that can minimize forward movement of the head and trunk and may enhance use of the Balans chair (Fig. 5-36). EMG activity of the

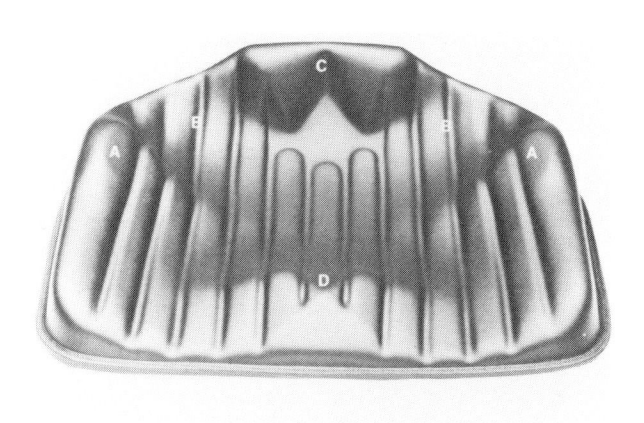

Fig. 5-34. Bottoms-Up. Support areas: **A**, A–Trochanteric; **B**, B–Ischial; **C**, C–Sacral; **D**, D–Pubic and Thigh. Reproduced with permission of Pleasing Patients Unlimited, 9348 Civic Center Drive, Suite 101, Beverly Hills, CA. 90210.

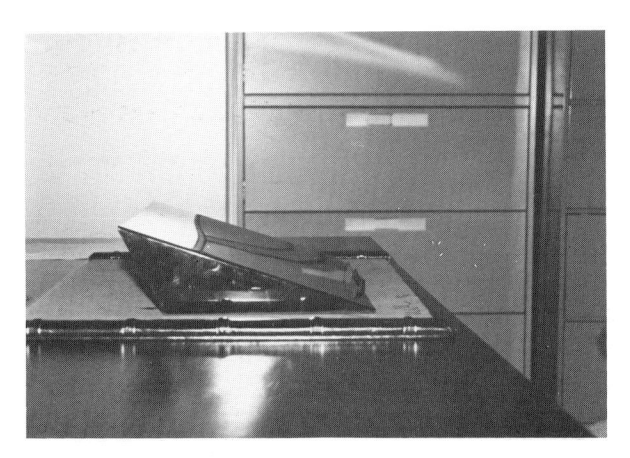

Fig. 5-35. Neck Correct. When placed on a horizontal desk, it provides for reading on an incline to allow for proper head position.

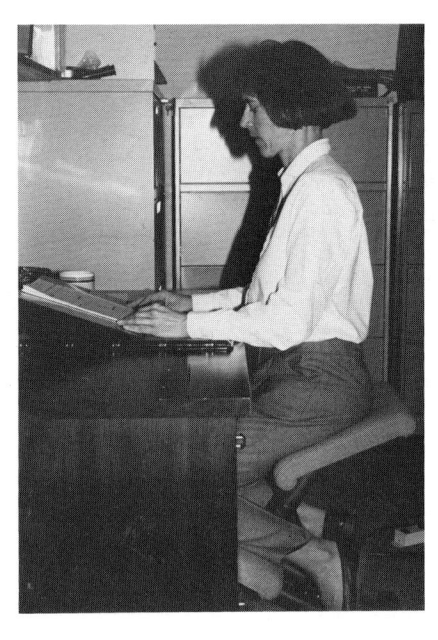

Fig. 5-36. Balons Chair with Neck Correct. Note improvement in head and neck posture as compared to Fig. 5-19. An increased degree of inclination would be more beneficial.

upper trapezius, deltoids, and erector spinae decrease when there is 25 degrees of shoulder flexion and 15-20 degrees of abduction. If a considerable amount of forward reaching is required from a seated position, an aid to extend the reach should be used. The critical distance is 15 inches in front of the body.[142,143]

Ergonomic chair design has become quite sophisticated within the past few years. Figures 5-37 to 5-40 illustrate various chairs that offer all or most of the of the requirements previously addressed. In addition, the incorporation of lordotic support for the cervical spine can be seen in figures 5-37 and 5-39. The most recent concept is the Ergomax Chair (Fig. 5-40) which offers a wide range of versatility for relaxed sitting, reading, typing, or artwork. The addition of a removable craniocervical support would enhance this chair when used in the reclining and traditional positions.

Video display terminal operators must not only utilize an ergonomically designed chair but should have a terminal that can tilt, swivel, and be raised or lowered. Glare must be avoided, and positioning away from windows is thus suggested. A source document holder is needed to eliminate the need to look down onto a flat surface. Figures 5-41 and 5-42 illustrate adaptive devices to maximize good head, neck, and low back posture while working at a video display terminal. Telephone operators and workers who perform deskwork as well as use the telephone for considerable periods of time should obtain a headset or speaker-phone.

The single most important requirement for the prevention of abnormal head and neck posture is maintenance of the lumbar lordosis when sitting and standing. Lumbar pillows are necessary whenever properly designed chairs are not available. Anyone that does prolonged driving or traveling in a seated position should utilize a lumbar pillow. The small pillows available on airplanes provide

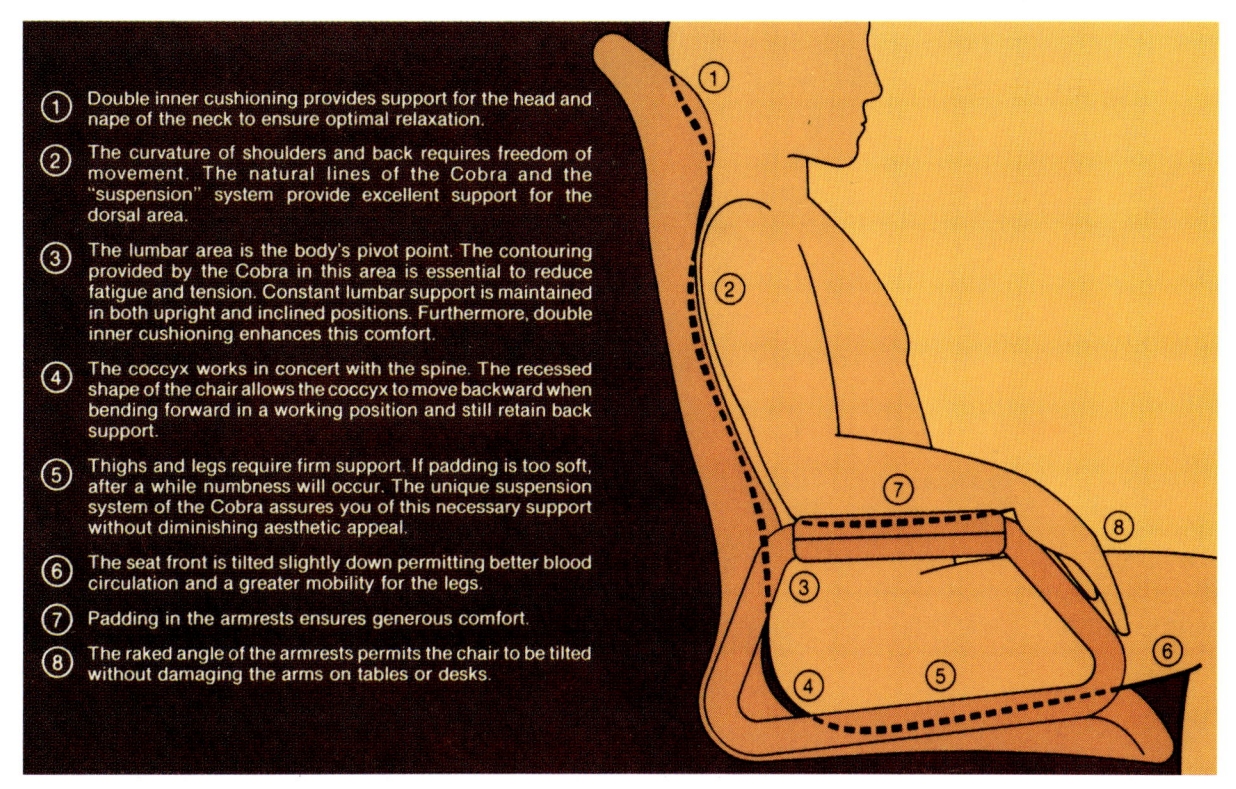

CHAPTER 5 Prevention and Restoration of Abnormal Upper Quarter Posture 131

① Double inner cushioning provides support for the head and nape of the neck to ensure optimal relaxation.

② The curvature of shoulders and back requires freedom of movement. The natural lines of the Cobra and the "suspension" system provide excellent support for the dorsal area.

③ The lumbar area is the body's pivot point. The contouring provided by the Cobra in this area is essential to reduce fatigue and tension. Constant lumbar support is maintained in both upright and inclined positions. Furthermore, double inner cushioning enhances this comfort.

④ The coccyx works in concert with the spine. The recessed shape of the chair allows the coccyx to move backward when bending forward in a working position and still retain back support.

⑤ Thighs and legs require firm support. If padding is too soft, after a while numbness will occur. The unique suspension system of the Cobra assures you of this necessary support without diminishing aesthetic appeal.

⑥ The seat front is tilted slightly down permitting better blood circulation and a greater mobility for the legs.

⑦ Padding in the armrests ensures generous comfort.

⑧ The raked angle of the armrests permits the chair to be tilted without damaging the arms on tables or desks.

Fig. 5-37. Artopex Cobra. Critical areas of support are outlined. Reproduced with permission of Artopex, Merchandise Mart. 1029 C & D, Chicago, Illinois 60654.

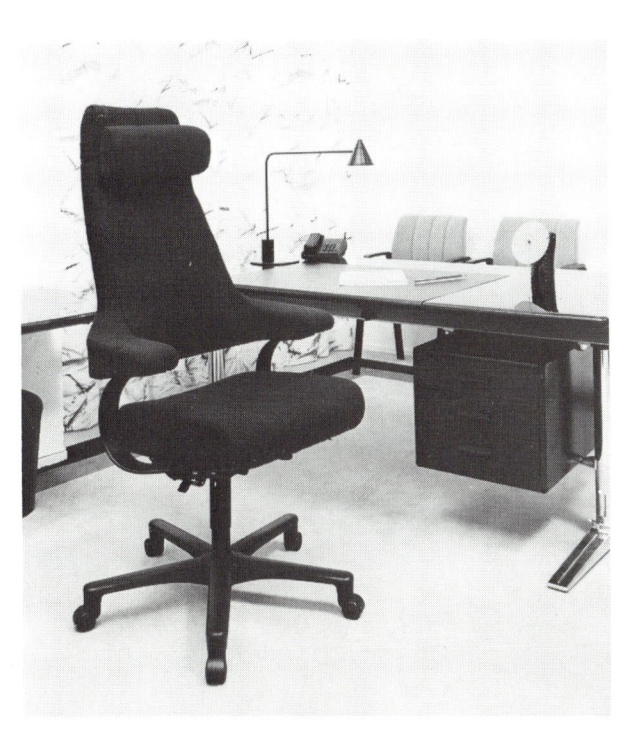

Fig. 5-38. Hag Anova. Note the presence of an adjustable cervical lordotic support. Reproduced with permission of HAG, USA, Inc. 108 Landmark Drive, Greensboro, NC 27409.

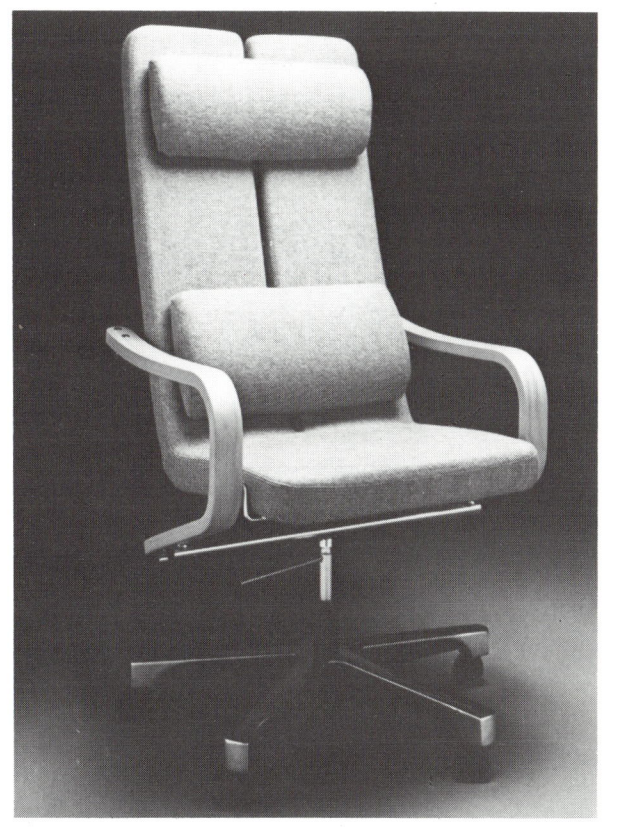

Fig. 5-39. Hag Split. Note the presence of cervical as well as lumbar lordotic supports that are adjustable. Reproduced with permission of HAG, USA, Inc. 108 Landmark Drive, Greensboro, NC 27409.

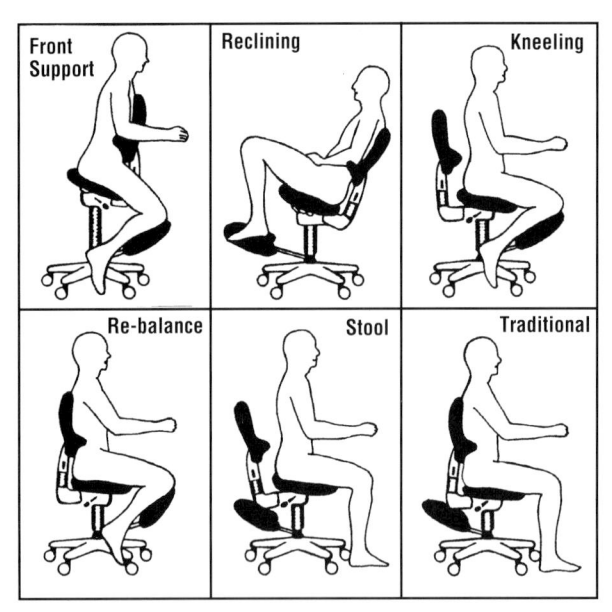

Fig. 5-40. Ergomax Chair. Reproduced with permission of American Ergonomics, 200 Gate Five Road, Sausalito, CA 94965.

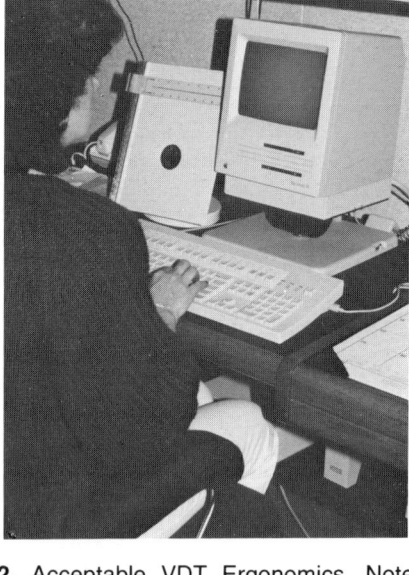

Fig. 5-42. Acceptable VDT Ergonomics. Note use of a lumbar support pillow, armrests, inclined detachable keyboard, tilting VDT, placement of feet under the work station, proper wrist angulation and head posture.

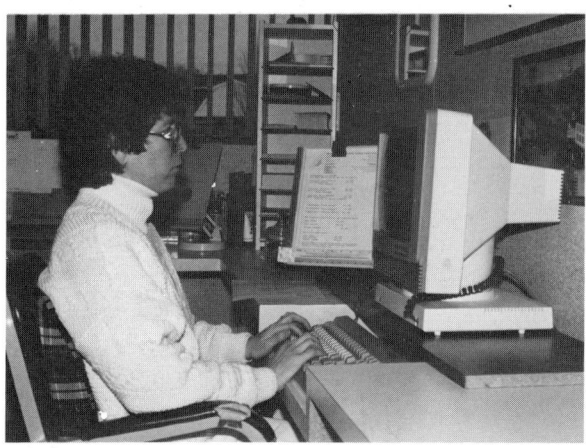

Fig. 5-41. Acceptable VDT Ergonomics. The center of the VDT is between 5-20 degrees below eye level and is equivalent with the source document holder. A lumbar support pillow helps to maintain proper trunk and head alignment. Forearm support is present but the keyboard should be moved slightly forward to minimize the degree of wrist extension.

Fig. 5-43. Correction of Lumbar Lordosis. Standing with palms of hands placed on the lumbar spine and head retracted. Backward bending or extension of the lumbar spine is performed with the hands acting as a counterpressure or fulcrum. The head should not posteriorly rotate upon the neck as the lumbar spine extends but remain in neutral position.

an acceptable lumbar support when placed between the airplane seatback and lumbar spine. Inflatable pillows which can be carried from place to place are now also on the market. Prolonged sitting in a transportation vehicle necessitates periodic correction of lumbar lordosis: Figure 5-43 illustrates the recommended standing backward bending exercise to perform periodically.

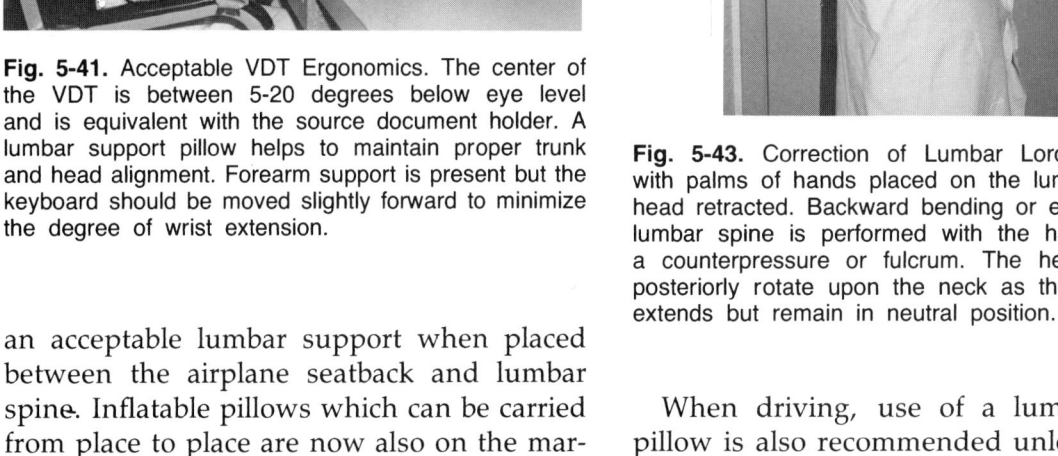

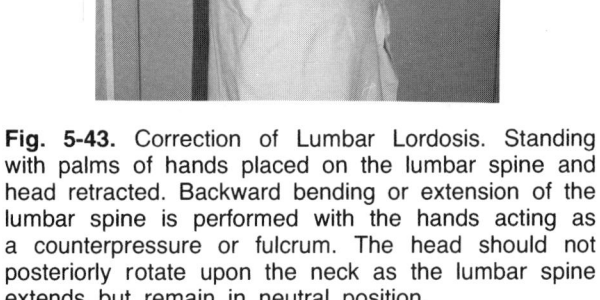

When driving, use of a lumbar support pillow is also recommended unless it is built into the car seat and adjustable. In addition, the adjustable head rest should be elevated so that it reaches a level equivalent with the top of the passenger's ears. The addition of an inflatable airbag in the steering wheel can

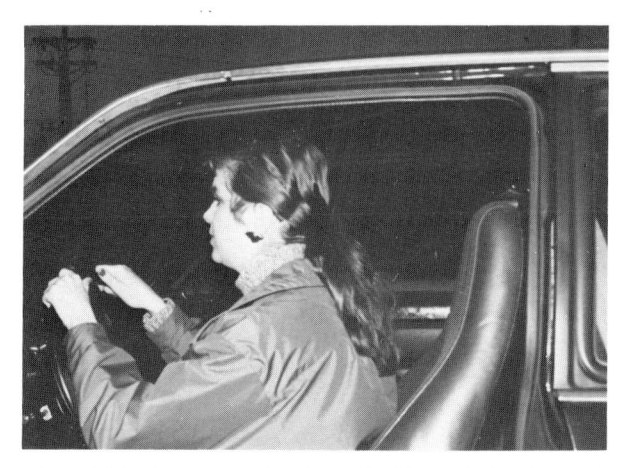

CHAPTER 5 Prevention and Restoration of Abnormal Upper Quarter Posture 133

Fig. 5-44. Improper Driving Position. Note forward inclination of the trunk and head resulting in loss of the lumbar lordosis and promotion of a FHP.

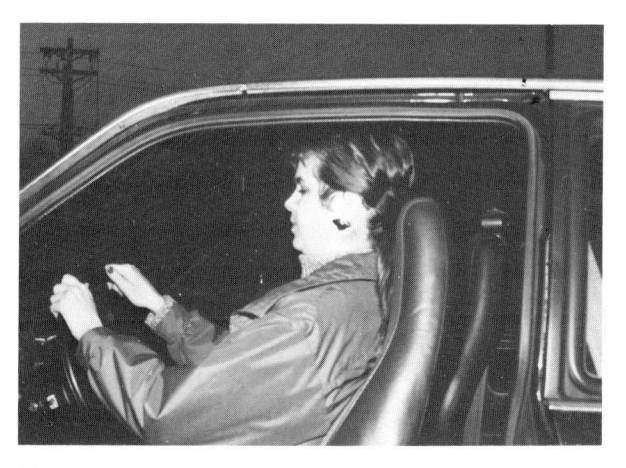

Fig. 5-45. Proper Driving Position. Note support of the craniocervical area by the posterior headrest. Optimal positioning would necessitate the addition of a lumbar lordotic pillow, a more upright inclination of the seat and an adjustable headrest.

significantly negate posterior cervical damage from a hyperflexion injury. Many car seats, however, do not offer seat adjustments relative to the angle of inclination and/or do not have a movable head rest. It thus may be impossible to adequately arrange the seat to minimize stress on the cervical spine.[53] Figures 5-44 and 5-45 illustrate proper and improper sitting postures when driving.

POSTURAL CORRECTIVE EXERCISE

Patient education is essential in obtaining sufficient compliance to reduce a postural abnormality or prevent one from occurring or progressing. It is immensely valuable to have each patient observe a Neck School videotape that emphasizes the FHP, its etiology, resultant pain and dysfunction, as well as corrective exercises.

The difference between normal and abnormal posture, when viewed by the patient, reinforces the discussion between patient and clinician. Various situations at work and home are shown, comparing proper and improper posture. Patients frequently realize that one or more of the situations presented relate directly to them, serving to foster an understanding of how their pain and dysfunction began and is perpetuated.

A FHP may also be perpetuated by the way in which a person gets out of bed from the supine position. Figures 5-46 A and B illustrate excessive contraction of the SCMs and other anterior cervical muscles due to arising from the bed by head, neck and trunk flexion against gravity. Instruction must be given to initally roll the body to the side while keeping the head supported on the bed, drop the legs over the edge and push up with the arms to an upright position. The head will thus be maintained in a neutral position.

Prevention of abnormal posture requires corrective exercises, especially when a prolonged seated posture cannot be avoided. Again, the starting point should be the lumbar spine. Figure 5-43 illustrates the backward bending exercise that serves to reduce intradiscal pressure and posterior nuclear migration as a result of a slumped posture.[21] It is common to observe individuals at ball games, concerts, and movies stand up and bend backward to reduce the discomfort from a prolonged flexed posture. Instruction on how to create lumbar lordosis actively in the seated position when support is not available is also recommended.

CORRECTION OF THE FORWARD HEAD POSTURE

HEAD RETRACTION

Education must emphasize the need for ongoing periodic performance of the home exercise program throughout the day. The number of repetitions may vary from 3 to 10 per set and the number of sets from 6 to 10 per

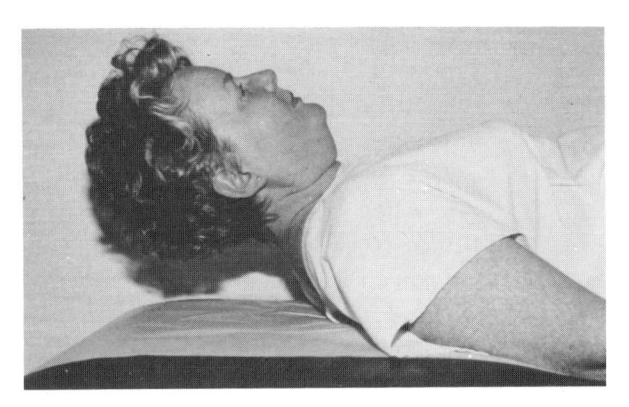

Fig. 5-46. Getting Out of Bed. **A**, Improper method which promotes strengthening of SCM and strain at the cervico-thoracic junction.

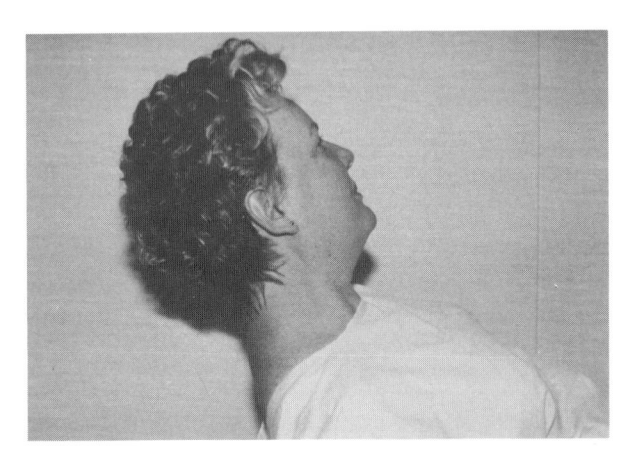

Fig. 5-46. B, Further progression into FHP as noted in Fig 5-12.

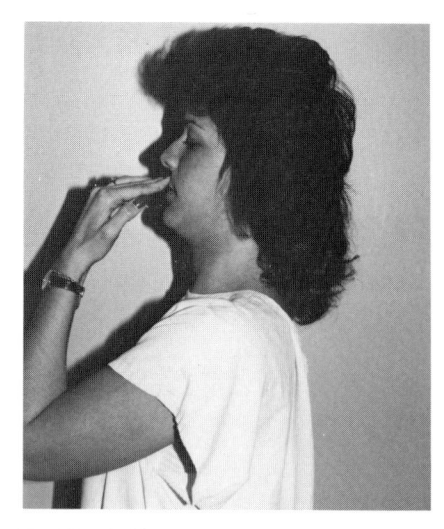

Fig. 5-47. Head Retraction. Patient placing finger tip on maxilla to assist in head retraction. The chin must be kept level so that posterior cranial rotation does not occur. The end range position is illustrated.

day, depending upon the patient. Rocabado, Kraus, McKenzie and others have been instrumental in the development of many exercises from which others have evolved. Patient handouts are now available that illustrate and discuss exercises as well as explain any necessary precautions.*

The initial exercise should be aimed at correction of FHP. In the presence of significant spondylosis, complete correction may be impossible, some reduction probable, and at the very least, education can prevent it from worsening. Head retraction, or dorsal gliding, is the first exercise which must be mastered.

Figure 5-47 illustrates a head retraction exercise, performed while either sitting or standing. The chin must be kept horizontal so that the posterior suboccipital extensors stretch. We do not encourage the patient to place one or more fingers on the chin to assist in movement as this may promote mandibular retrusion. If some form of hand assistance is needed, pushing against the maxilla is encouraged.

In the presence of any posterior cervical disc herniation, this exercise must be done with caution and guided by a physical therapist who should alter the movement dependant upon symptomatology. We recommend that the exercise be done only through midrange for the first week, thus minimizing the possibility of soreness.

Patients must be informed during the initial visit that they may develop increased pain or soreness in different areas as a result of the exercise program. Stretching of tight musculature and strengthening of antagonists may lead to discomfort. The explanation to the patient includes the scenario of a baseball player who does not have any pathology, but develops sore and achy muscles within the first week of spring training. Spring training consists of stretching as well as strengthening muscles that were somewhat dormant during the off-season. The sore and achy response is normal. The patient, on the other hand, has postural abnormalities and pathology, so even though only a very mild exercise program is initiated, soreness may still develop. The patient must be told to persist, although they can decrease the frequency or number of repetitions performed.

---

*"Treat Your Own Neck" Orthopedic Physical Therapy Products, P.O. Box Minneapolis, MN 55441.

Make sure that exercises are being properly performed. A patient who performs head retraction in conjunction with posterior cranial rotation, for example, may compress the suboccipital region and exacerbate the cause of his or her discomfort. Written and illustrated guidelines are always provided and periodic review of the home program should be done.

Shoulder Retraction and Depression

Shoulder retraction and depression is designed to reduce the round shouldered posture associated with FHP. An initial head retraction is followed by external rotation of the shoulders, and by scapular retraction and depression, also providing for a stretch of the scalenes and levator scapulae. Figure 5-48 illustrates the end position. A useful description of this exercise is "hitch hiking" with the arms at the side of the body, the elbows extended and the thumbs positioned appropriately.

Suboccipital Stretch

The last exercise that a patient is commonly instructed to perform during an initial visit is head retraction while lying. This is first done in the supine position, without a pillow or cervical roll, on the floor or a firm mattress. The exercise is basically a chin tuck with anterior rotation of the head, and is designed to stretch the posterior suboccipital area and provide a decompressive force.

Suboccipital stretching in the sitting. or standing position can also be performed by having the patient clasp both hands behind the neck with the most superior fifth finger placed on top of the spinous process of the axis. The hands must not pull the head forward, but are used to support the neck as the head is tilted forward on the upper cervical spine. The stretch is thus most pronounced in the suboccipital area. Figure 5-49 illustrates this exercise, which can be accentuated by placing a book or flat towel under the occiput to increase the stretch. I recommend the use of a towel roll to maintain cervical lordosis when this must be performed in the presence of a cervical disc herniation or bulge.

The patient is not instructed in any other exercises for the first week or two. These three

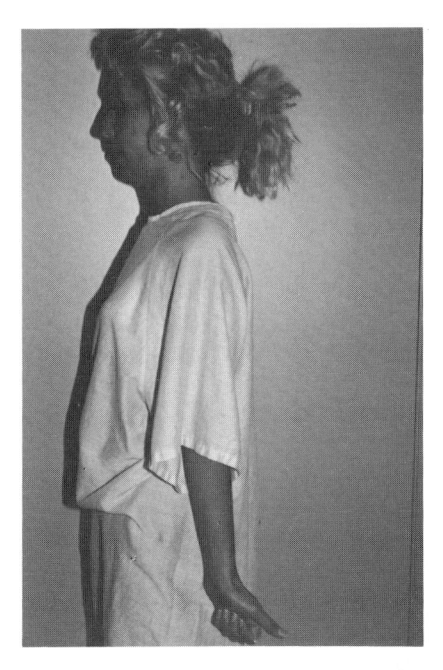

Fig. 5-48. Shoulder Girdle Retraction and Depression (Hitch Hiking). Patient standing with elbows extended and arms adducted. The thumbs are extended and abducted followed by posterior (external) rotation of the shoulders and scapular adduction plus depression. Head retraction should be performed first and maintained during the course of shoulder movements.

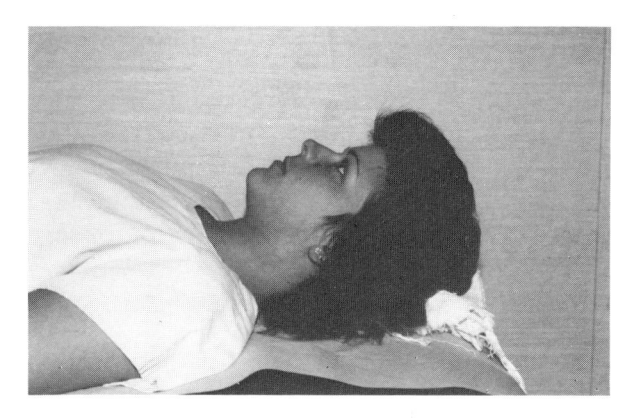

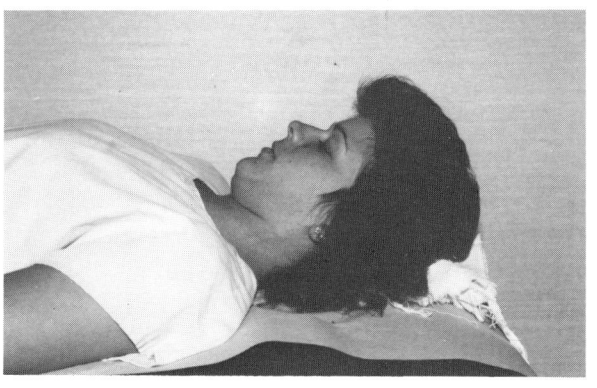

Fig. 5-49. Active Nodding In Supine. **A**, Patient lies in supine position without pillow. A flat towel my be placed under the occiput to enhance the degree of sub-occipital stretch. **B**, End position showing chin tuck and stretch of sub-occipital region.

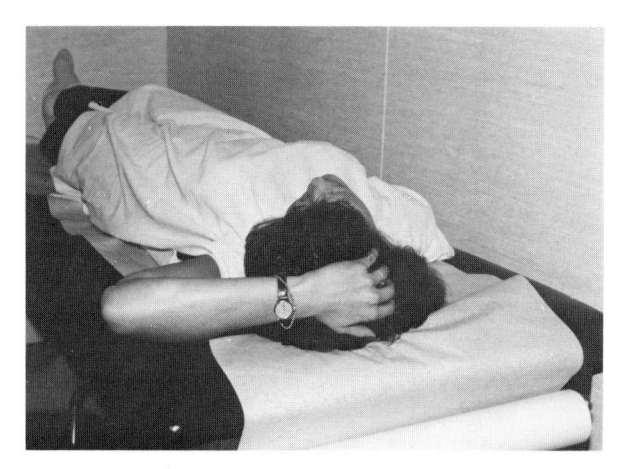

Fig. 5-50. Sidebending Stretch. Patient in supine position with right hand placed under lumbar spine to anchor shoulder girdle. The left hand grasps the right side of the head and sidebends the head to the left to stretch the right lateral cervical musculature.

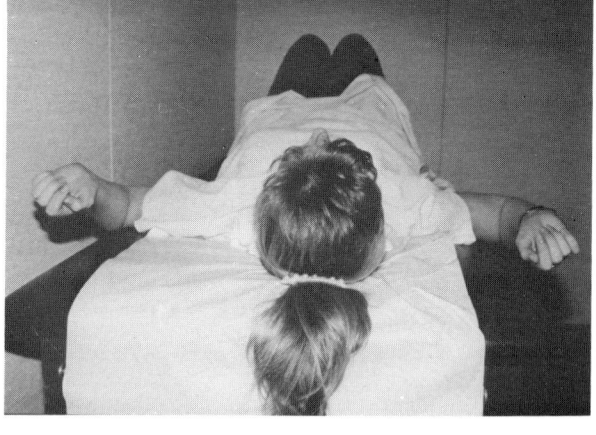

Fig. 5-51. Pectoral Stretching. Supine lying with external rotation of the shoulders. The effect of gravity and the weight of the arms promote a stretch of the pectoral region. Note placement of towel roll to support the cervical spine.

are usually sufficient, and more may only cause confusion. When the cervical musculature needs to be stretched, the patient must first assume the correct head position.

Sidebending Stretch

Sidebending of the head and neck is designed to stretch the tight scalenes and upper trapezius. This can be done while sitting, standing, or supine, but should only be done in the supine position if head retraction cannot be fully attained when sitting. Start by sidebending the head, without any significant rotation, away from the side on which the arm is hanging from the chair. This will provide a minimal stretch. Increase the stretch by holding the bottom of the chair while sidebending the head in the opposite direction. For the greatest stretch, use the opposite arm overhead and pull the head away from the anchored side.

Figure 5-50 illustrates use of the arm and hand to assist in sidebending in the supine position. The opposite hand may be used to either grasp the side of the bed or it may be placed under the low back or buttock to maximize stretch.

A further progression of this exercise involves rotation of the head from the sidebent position to the right and left to impart stretching specific for the anterior and posterior scalenes apart from the medial.

Caution must be used in the presence of a posterolateral disc bulge or herniation. Sidebending away from the side of a posterolateral herniated nucleus pulposus may result in widening of the intervertebral space or foramen, which can promote increased nuclear migration and referred pain. This exercise is also recommended for reduction and centralization of a cervical herniated nucleus pulposus when performed to the painful side. Research has demonstrated a reduction in cervical peripheral pain by abduction of the painful arm.[146]

Pectoral Stretch

Tight pectoral musculature is commonly associated with a prolonged FHRSP. The easiest way of initiating a stretch to the pectoral region in conjunction with external rotation of the shoulders and maintenance of good head and neck posture is in the supine postion.

Figure 5-51 illustrates this exercise, in which simple gravity and the weight of the arms are used to promote a mild passive stretch. This position may also be used to assess the degree of pectoral tightness limiting active shoulder external rotation. An active stretch can also be performed standing and facing a corner. Placing the hands at shoulder height is followed by active head retraction and forward inclination of the chest and trunk to provide a significant stretch (Fig. 5-52 A). An alternative

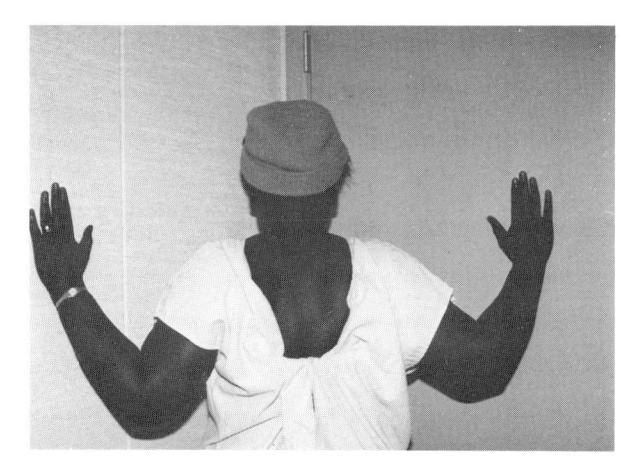

Fig. 5-52. Pectoral Stretch. **A**, Pectoral stretch with hands at shoulder level. Head retraction is initially performed followed by forward movement of the trunk towards the corner of the room.

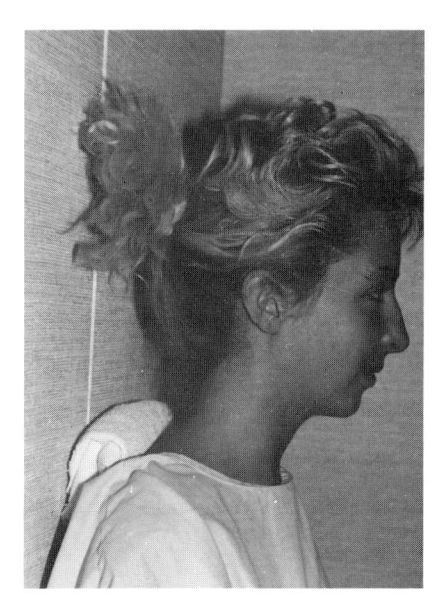

Fig. 5-53. Head Retraction in Standing with Towel Roll. Towel roll or wedge placed at level of the cervico-thoracic junction between wall and patient. Patient performs active head retraction in standing with counterpressure provided by the towel against the kyphosis. **A**, Standing position showing the FHP.

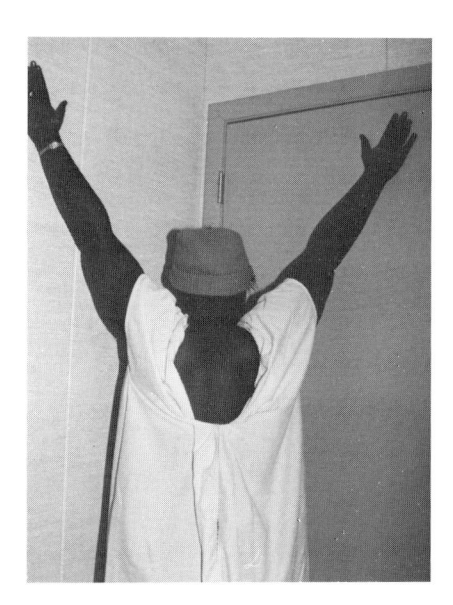

Fig. 5-52. B, Alternate method with arms extended and abducted overhead.

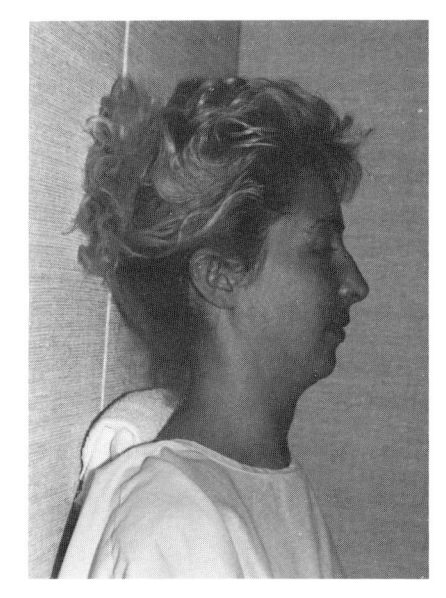

Fig. 5-53. B, End position of appropriate posture.

method, with the arms overhead, can provide a more profound stretch when shoulder elevation and abduction are not impaired (Fig. 5-52 B).

REDUCTION OF UPPER THORACIC KYPHOSIS

An associated dowager's hump or upper thoracic kyphosis is very difficult to reduce if present for a long time. To a certain degree, it will correct in the young individual as posture improves. Separate from the performance of manual techniques is the utilization of a towel roll or wedge in conjunction with active head retraction in the standing or supine positions. Figures 5-53 A and B illustrate this exercise, in which a towel is placed at the cervicothoracic junction to act as a compressive force as the patient actively retracts the head. The net result is similar to a posterior to anterior glide of the upper thoracic spine. A sustained

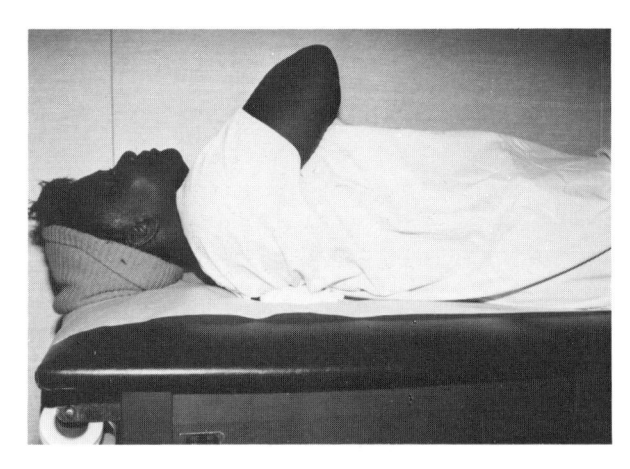

Fig. 5-54. Reduction of Thoracic Kyphosis. Patient lying supine on towel roll placed between treatment table and apex of thoracic curvature.

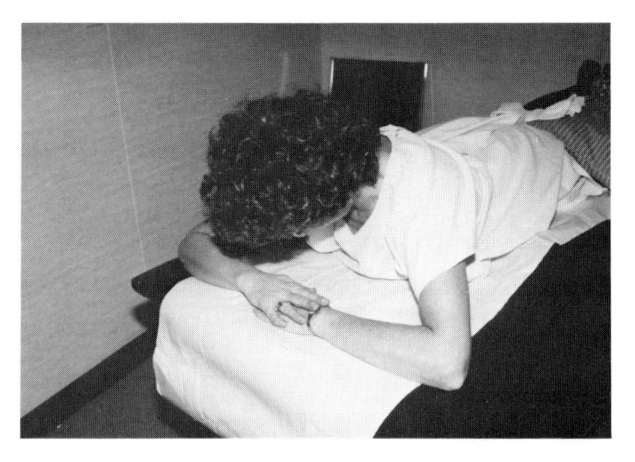

Fig. 5-55. Head Retraction Against Gravity. Patient rests prone on floor or table with forehead placed on dorsum of hands. The head is actively retracted without posterior cranial rotation thus strengthening the posterior cervical and upper thoracic musculature.

position as an alternative version is depicted in Figure 5-54 for a mid-upper thoracic kyphosis.

In addition to active stretching of the shortened musculature, strengthening of antagonistic muscles is needed to maximize postural correction. Strengthening exercises are usually not added for at least three weeks, and only when progress without increased pain is evident.

Many patients at this time begin to state that they can correct their posture but find it difficult to maintain. Strengthening of the scapular retractors, shoulder extensors, and head extensors is thus encouraged. The prone position is used to add the inherent weight of the head and arms as resistance.

Active head retraction without posterior cranial rotation is performed by actively lifting the head from the hands as high as possible (Fig. 5-55). This can be performed on a treatment table, bed, or floor. Upper cervical compression and contraction of the short suboccipital extensors is thus minimized. Strengthening of the scapular adductors and shoulder extensors can be accomplished by keeping the forehead on a towel roll and raising the arms toward the ceiling (Fig. 5-56). As this exercise becomes easier, wrist or hand weights can be added.

When patients are unable to assume a prone position for the necessary period of time, this exercise can be performed standing with elbows extended and shoulders abducted to 90 degrees. The hands may also be placed on

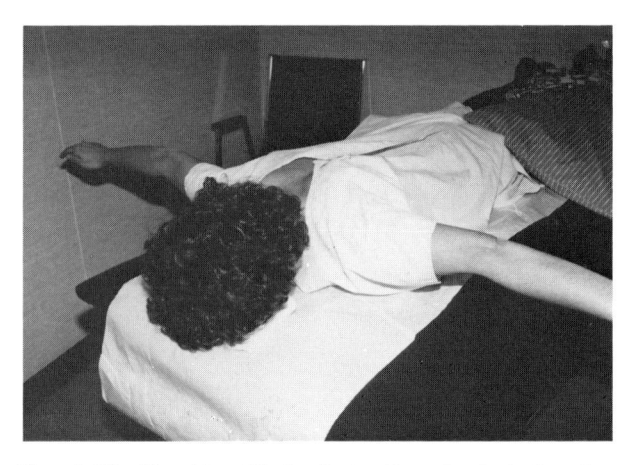

Fig. 5-56. Shoulder Girdle Retraction Against Gravity. Patient lies prone on table or floor with forehead resting on towel roll and shoulders abducted to 90 degrees with elbow extension. The arms are actively lifted from the table to maximal elevation to strengthen the scapular adductors, shoulder external rotators and extensors.

the hips, with the patient actively adducting the scapulae as the elbows approximate each other.

BIOFEEDBACK

For patients with difficulty grasping the exercise techniques, biofeedback can be used. Transcutaneous recording electrodes feed back information of increased activity (contraction) of posterior cervical musculature, usually during therapeutic sessions, with an electromyographic (EMG) biofeedback device.

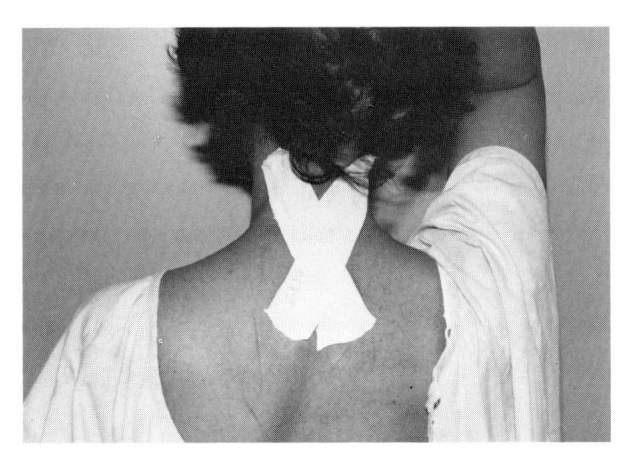

Fig. 5-57. Postural Correction with Tape. Two thick pieces of non-elastic adhesive tape are placed from the sub-occipital fossa to the contralateral scapular (superior medial angle). Tape is on slack when head retraction is maintained and pulls on the skin as forward inclination occurs.

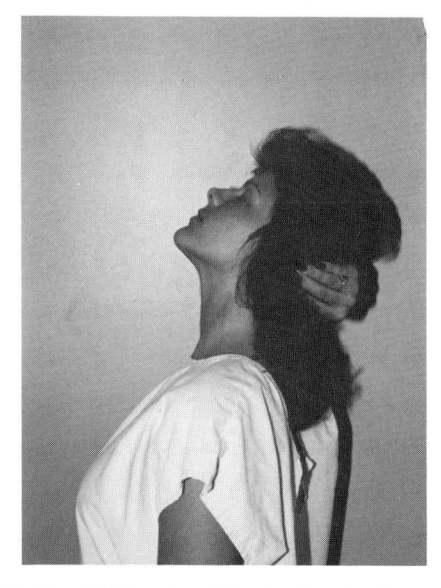

Fig. 5-58. Head Extension. Head retraction is performed first followed by placement of either hand on the occiput to guide backward bending and assist a return to the neutral position.

Increased patient awareness of postures or activities that cause significant motor unit activation, and corrected positions that decrease motor unit activity can also serve to convince the skeptical patient that posture is a prime etiological factor.[147]

The adjunctive use of EMG biofeedback should begin in the supine, nonweightbearing position and progress to sitting, standing, and working postures. A less expensive method of increasing postural awareness involves the use of tape patches. Figure 5-57 illustrates the use of a tape patch that provides feedback in the form of skin traction as the head migrates forward. The traction irritation of the tape thus reminds the patient to correct posture or perform head retraction. This method will not be as effective if an associated posterior cranial rotation also occurs. Placement of tape in the suprahyoid region may also be needed in such a situation.

REDUCTION OF POSTERIOR NUCLEAR MIGRATION

Whenever prolonged forward inclination of the head and neck occurs, the likelihood of posterior nuclear migration must be considered. A protruded head posture with loss of normal cervical lordosis and gapping of posterior intervertebral spaces is a prime cause of cervical disc bulging or herniation. This may be preceded by or associated with pain from overstretching of the nuchal, interspinous and posterior longitudinal ligaments.

When this occurs, the addition of a modified head and neck extension exercise, as a counterpart to backward bending to regain lumbar lordosis, is warranted. The patient should be cautioned not to perform this exercise without first performing head retraction to a comfortable position.

Figure 5-58 illustrates correct hand placement on the occiput, with backward bending of the head on the neck. This promotes a return of cervical lordosis and can reduce mild posterior annular bulging. Pinching of the disc upon the innervated outer annular fibers produces increased pain if the bulge is too large, negating the value of this exercise. Sustained manual traction, performed by the therapist, followed by backward bending of the head may produce reduction and is one of many techniques employed for the manual treatment of the cervical spine.

In the presence of a posterolateral herniated nucleus pulposus, the patient may need to first perform the sidebending excercise (Fig. 5-50) to the painful side in an attempt to obtain centralization.

Dependent upon the extent or deviation of the herniated nucleus pulposus, a therapist may need to perform manual cervical traction in conjunction with sidebending to the painful side, followed by backward bending and simultaneous distraction.

Sustained head extension may lead to suboccipital compression and related symptomatology: this can occur especially when backward bending of the head is done in the supine position over the edge of a bed and sustained for 30 seconds or more.

The exercises presented here are only the most common ones, but others may be needed to address individual variations. Additional exercises are also frequently needed to restore proper tongue position and to correct swallowing abnormalities such as tongue thrust. A discussion of these is beyond the scope of this chapter, but can be obtained from the reference list.[7,8,13,83]

When patients with minimal to moderate postural dysfunction and associated discomfort are referred early, education and instruction may be all that's needed. In such a situation, the patient is usually seen for three visits. That is the extent of the Neck School program, developed by Delaware Valley Physical Therapy Associates, adaptable not only to patients with mechanical disorders of the cervical spine but also to those with headaches, TMJ dysfunction and degenerative arthritis. An outline of each session follows:

FIRST SESSION

I. **EVALUATION:** History, structural and biomechanical analysis, joint mobility, neuromuscular function and pain assessment of the upper quarter, including the craniomandibular region.
  A. **Home environment:** Analysis of sitting and sleeping postures, type of mattress, pillows and chairs.
  B. **Work Environment:** Analysis of work habits, ergonomics, sitting, standing and lifting postures.
  C. **Recreational Activities:** Analysis of athletic, relaxation and other recreational activities engaged in.
  D. **Pre-Test:** Anatomy, posture, body mechanics, sitting, sleeping and reaching techniques.

SECOND SESSION

II. **INSTRUCTION:** Individualized for each patient or adapted to specific environmental or work situation after viewing neck school and body mechanics videotapes.
  A. **Instruction** in the anatomy of the spine, correct and improper posture or body mechanics, and causes of pain, headaches and associated TMJ dysfunction.
  B. **Instruction** in proper sitting, sleeping, and work habits, including lifting and reaching techniques. Preventative exercises, postural corrective techniques, as well as dietary suggestions about foods, additives or preservatives that may promote vascular headaches.
  C. **Instruction** and recommendations on special support pillows, chairs or suboccipital traction devices.
  D. **Written and illustrated** guidelines and exercises are taken home.

THIRD SESSION

III. **REVIEW:** A review of the specific techniques, exercises or life style changes suggested in session two.
  A. **Post-test:** Repeat of test in initial session and demonstration by patient of postural corrective techniques and exercises.
  B. **Report to physician, employer or insurance company:** A written report and summary of recommendations is prepared and forwarded to the appropriate party.

Each session lasts about between 1 and 1 1/2 hours, and the three-session program is usually presented over a two-week period. We recommend that the patient call 3-6 weeks after the last visit for a progress report. Modifications to the home exercise program may be warranted at that time.

FORWARD HEAD POSTURE AND ORAL APPLIANCES

Dentists need to be aware of postural factors when evaluating TMJ function and fabricating oral appliances. The position that a patient

Table 5-7. Postural comparison

STRUCTURE	NORMAL POSTURE	FORWARD HEAD-ROUND SHOULDER POSTURE
CRANIUM	Slight flexion on upper cervical spine	Forward inclination; extension on upper cervical spine (dependent upon degree of posterior cranial rotation).
MANDIBLE	Normal resting vertical dimension	Depressed and retruded (without significant posterior cranial rotation); elevated and retruded (with significant posterior cranial rotation).
TMJ	Loose packed position (Centric relation)	Posterior closed packed position
MAXILLO-MANDIBULAR RELATIONSHIP	2-4 mm freeway space; normal intercuspation and mandibular resting position	Decreased freeway space without posterior cranial rotation;* increased freeway space with significant posterior cranial rotation and increased posterior intercuspation.
HYOID	Posterior horn at level of C2-3 disc	Suprahyoids shorten and develop increased tension; lengthening of infrahyoids; elevation of hyoid proportional to loss and/or inversion of cervical lordosis
TONGUE	Against palate behind maxillary incisors	Drops to floor of mouth; increased activity of genioglossus may promote a tongue-thrust swallow
UPPER CERVICAL SPINE	Slight kyphosis	Suboccipital compression upon OA, AA, occipital nerves, trigeminal spinal tract and vertebral artery (all dependent upon degree of posterior cranial rotation); shortening of suboccipital muscles; proprioceptor alteration in favor of nociception.
MID-LOWER CERVICAL SPINE	30-35 degree lordosis; tripodism	Lordosis may become accentuated in presence of significant posterior cranial rotation; lordosis is decreased, may straighten or become inverted (kyphotic); alteration of tripodism; increased intradiscal pressure
UPPER THORACIC SPINE	Normal kyphosis	Increased kyphosis; decreased diaphragmatic excursion; increased use of accessory muscles of respiration.
SHOULDER GIRDLE	Clavicles horizontal and slightly posterior to first rib	Clavicles angulated and/or elevated; 60-90 degree SCM angulation; thoracic inlet compression; compression of AC and SC joints; internal rotation of GH joint; scapular abduction and protraction; shortening of upper trapezius and levator scapulae; lengthening of rhomboids and lower traps; shortening of pectorals

* Decreased freeway space equals increased occlusal contact and hyperactivity of masticatory muscles.

assumes when reclining in a dental chair may differ markedly from their normal daily posture, thus altering the resting position of the mandible. The study cast from which appliances are fabricated may then represent an occlusion that is not optimal for that patient. The appliance may even cause increased pain.

If appliances are fabricated without regard for posture, and the patient is forced to wear them, one factor can negate the other and progress may not occur. A reduction in the degree of anteromedial disc displacement by an anterior repositioning appliance may be accompanied by increased discomfort in the facial and cervical regions because the mandible is being forced down and forward by the appliance while the FHP promotes retrusion. The brunt of this is absorbed by the musculature being pulled in opposite directions simultaneously by the appliance and posture.

Patients with a FHP should be referred to a knowledgeable physical therapist for education, instruction, and reduction of the postural abnormality and use of a flat plane joint stabilization appliance without repositioning. In many instances, decompression of the TMJ's is sufficient to significantly relieve pain and promote increased function without repositioning. This, of course, is not feasible in every situation, but in the young patient with inherent tissue plasticity, a significant change in posture may occur in two to four weeks.[98] Revisions or alterations of the appliance will then be minimized. In the presence of acute pain and dysfunction from internal derangement, this sequence is not feasible. Use of an inexpensive temporary appliance, and fabrication of a better appliance as posture improves is suggested.

MANUAL THERAPEUTIC PROCEDURES AND TECHNIQUES

When education, instruction, ergonomic changes, and postural corrective exercises do not adequately correct abnormal posture, further treatment is indicated. This is usually the case in the presence of long-standing postural dysfunction with concomitant adaptive shortening of soft tissue (myofascial components) and associated joint hypomobility. Table 5-7 outlines the sequential events and progression of FHRSP. The forward head posture can lead to:

- Compression of the occiput on the upper cervical spine
- Occlusal alteration
- Increased posterior tooth contact
- Increased hyoid muscle tension
- Increased TMJ compression
- Upper thoracic kyphosis
- Shoulder impingement
- Scalene entrapment
- Thoracic inlet compression

Some common pain syndromes which occur as a result of FHP:

- Muscle contraction headaches
- Occipital neuralgia
- Temporomandibular joint dysfunction
- Degenerative joint disease
- Cervical disc herniation and nerve root impingement
- Neurovascular Compression Syndromes
- Scapulo-costal syndrome
- Shoulder impingement syndromes
- Shoulder tendonitis

A comprehensive rehabilitation program encompassing hands-on techniques and procedures is thus indicated. This is optimally performed in conjunction with dental management. An initial evaluation is first performed as outlined in the first session of the Neck School Education Program. The therapeutic objectives of the comprehensive rehabilitation program are outlined in Table 5-8.

Table 5-8. Therapeutic objectives

Reduction or correction of FHP to decrease compression, impingement, and entrapment forces
Correction of soft tissue restriction and muscle imbalance
Decrease pain and stress
Preserve or restore range of motion and strength to maximize functional activities of daily living
Increase patient knowledge on posture, activities, and home self-management techniques.

There are many useful manual and mechanical therapeutic procedures. Table 5-9 outlines the general variation of therapeutic procedures individualized to each patient.

Table 5-9. Therapeutic procedures

Joint and soft tissue mobilization techniques of the cranium, TMJ, cervical-thoracic spine and shoulder girdle
Manual or mechanical suboccipital traction
Soft tissue contract-relax stretching techniques
Myofascial release techniques
Trigger point desensitization
Biofeedback and relaxation training
Therapeutic and postural corrective exercise

Adjunctive Physical Therapy Modalities

These are used only as needed to obtain an increase in soft tissue viscosity, reduce capsular and collagen adhesions, eliminate retained metabolites, decrease muscle guarding, edema and pain. They will not be discussed, as the information is available elsewhere.[1,147]

Table 5-10. Physical therapy modalities

Moist heat
Ultrasound-plus stretch
Fluorimethane stretch and spray
High voltage galvanic stimulation
Transcutaneous Electrical Nerve Stimulation
Non-invasive electro-acupuncture techniques

A complete treatment session usually starts with 10-12 minutes of moist heat applied to the cervical spine with the patient supine and a pillow under the knees. A thin pillow or folded towel may need to be placed under the occiput to prevent posterior cranial rotation, depending upon the posture of the patient.

The manual techniques which follow have been adapted from participation in numerous post-graduate seminars given by Mariano Rocabado, Steven Kraus, Brian Miller, Barret Dorko, John Upledger, Robin McKenzie, Brian Mulligan, Ace Neame, Stanley Paris, Ola Grimsby, Wayne Rath, and James Cyriax.

Manual soft tissue release techniques are emphasised and not joint mobilization because joint and capsule hypomobility occur

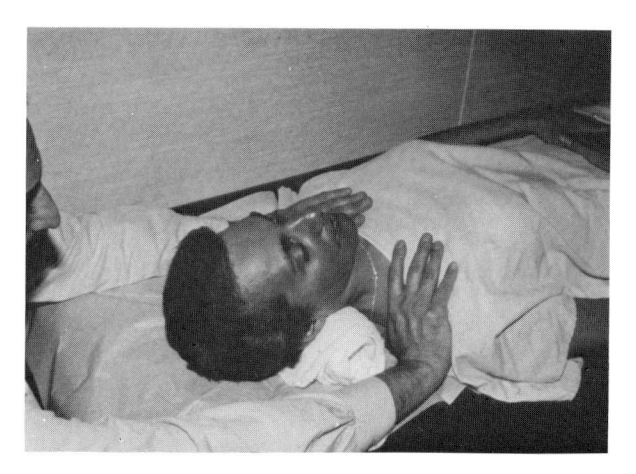

Fig. 5-59. Trager Alternate Rocking. **A**, Therapist sits facing the head of the supine patient. Hands are placed overlying each supraclavicular/upper trapezius region. Alternate rocking of each shoulder girdle is performed. A sidebending and rotation movement of the craniocervical region occurs without contact on the patient's neck simultaneously with mild stretching of the anterolateral cervical musculature.

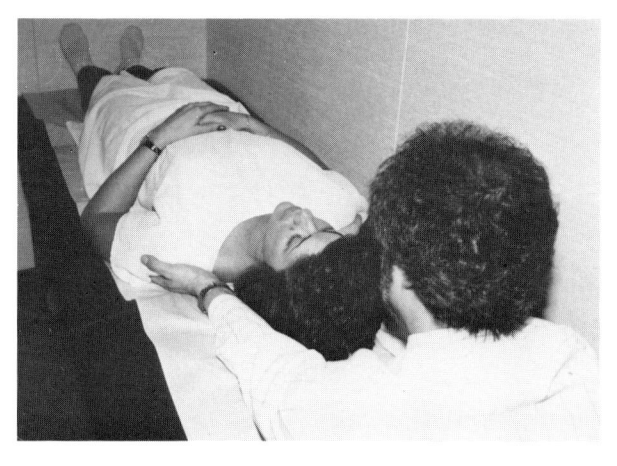

Fig. 5-59. B, Technique is the same except hand placement is now on the spine of each scapula. This changes the alternate rocking stretch to the levator scapulae and posterior scalene region.

primarily due to soft tissue restriction. This restriction which may be in the form of muscle contraction due to increased postural demands or contracture from physiological adaptation to a shortened position does not allow for full joint excursion or range of motion. Thus, if release or stretch of soft tissue helps to regain normal rest length and extensibility, joint motion will be restored with the aid of therapeutic exercise.

Mobilizing or manipulating joints in the presence of muscle guarding or contraction is similar to trying to drive a car while the

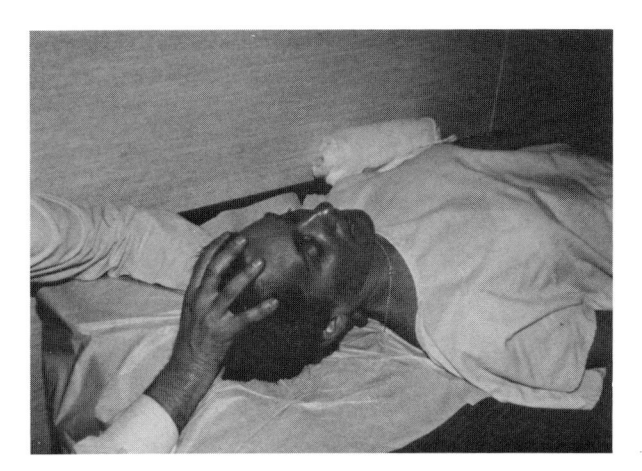

Fig. 5-60. Cervical Kneading with Cranial Rotation. Therapist sits facing the head of the supine patient. The thumb and/or fingers of one hand gently lift and knead the posterolateral cervical musculature as the other hand produces a small circular motion of the head. The soft tissue is gently lifted and stretched in short arcs as the head is rotated to the opposite side. Initiate at C7-T1, end at occiput.

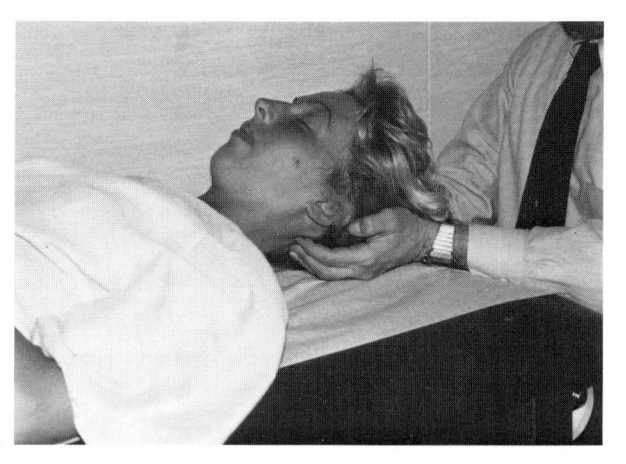

Fig. 5-61. Sub-Occipital Release. Therapist sits facing the head of the supine patient. The patient's occiput rest in the palms of the therapist's hands. Dorsum of hands remain in contact with treatment table. All fingers except thumb are placed in the sub-occipital fossa and finger or elbow flexion imparts a stretch or release of the occiput from the upper cervical spine. The patient's head and neck should not be lifted up into flexion. Sustain the stretch as tolerated for 10 seconds to 1-2 minutes and repeat periodically allowing for relaxation of the patient's head onto therapists fingertips.

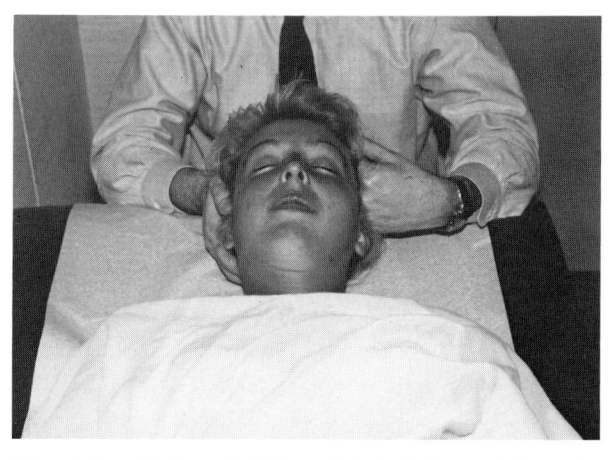

Fig. 5-62. Unilateral Sub-occipital Release. Therapist sits facing patient's head with second-fourth fingers of right hand in the sub-occipital fossa and the other hand stabilizing the head on the opposite side. In the presence of TMJ pain, the stabilizing hand can be placed solely on the temporal-parietal region with the fingers in 90 degrees of MCP flexion so as not to press against the painful area. When TMJ pain and tenderness is not a factor, stabilization of the head can occur from the cranium to the mandible. A unilateral circular stretch motion is performed at the sub-occipital area.

emergency brake is on. Joint mobilization is, however, indicated within a limited range of motion to specifically stretch restricted or adhered capsules, facilitate restoration of end-range motions, and correct positional faults. In many instances, the techniques to be illustrated produce soft tissue (muscle, fascia, and capsule) release and joint mobilization simultaneously.

Trager Oscillation

The following techniques represent a typical single treatment session geared to reduction of a FHRSP and restoration of normal function. After removing the moist heat, a Trager alternate rocking or oscillatory technique as shown in Figures 5-59 A and B is performed. This enhances mechanoreceptor input and produces sidebending/rotation of the craniocervical area with a concomitant alternate stretch of the lateral cervical myofascial structures. The constant oscillatory movement has a gating influence on nociceptive afferent input and therefore serves also as a form of pain modulation.[148]

It is helpful to instruct the patient to breathe diaphragmatically, keep the tongue up on the palate, teeth apart and lips together during most or all of these techniques. This is the "TMJ Mantra" which they can repeat to themselves (tongue up, teeth apart, lips together, breathe diaphragmatically).

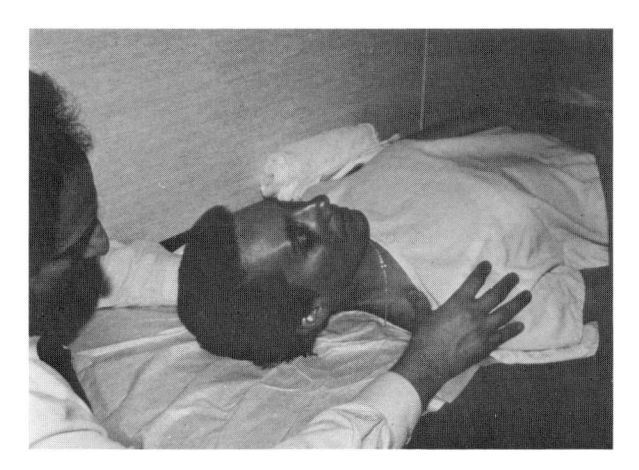

Fig. 5-63. Lower Arc Stretch. Therapist sits facing the supine patient with the thumb of the right hand maintaining light pressure in the supraclavicular fossa. The left hand is placed sub-occipitally. The left hand produces a circular motion of the head to the right with a stretch at the apex of the circle so that the chin and nose rotate to the same side. The head is not lifted off the table. Thumb position of the right hand determines the distribution of the soft tissue stretch. **A**, Placement of the thumb in the anterior.

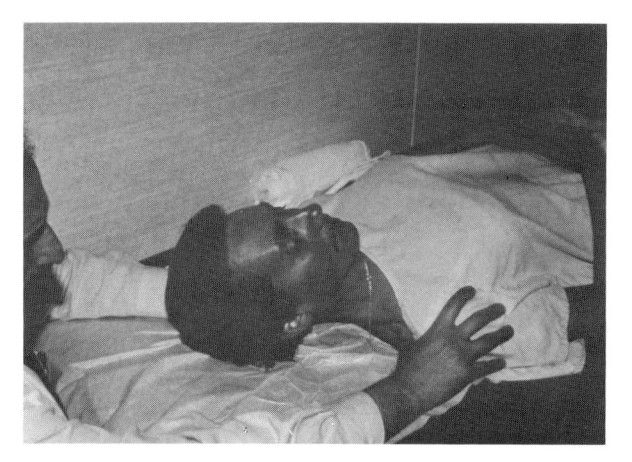

Fig. 5-63. B, Middle.

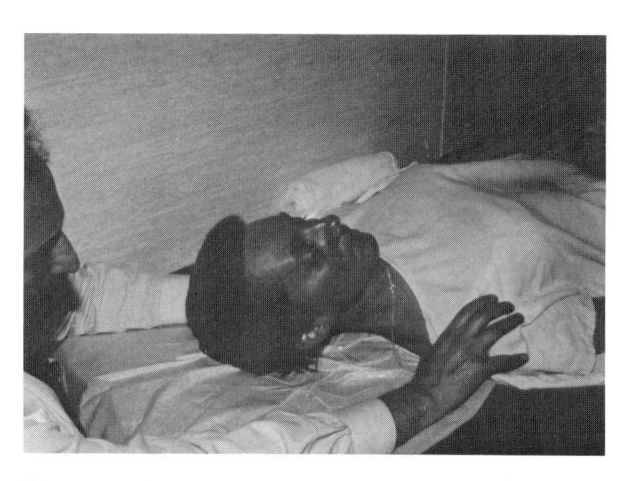

Fig. 5-63, C, Posterior supraclavicular regions respectively so that a stretch can occur throughout the supraclavicular musculature. The arcing is performed slowly for 15-20 seconds at each different thumb position and repeated on the opposite side. This is usually followed by upper arc stretching and/or the cross stretch.

Cervical Kneading with Cranial Rotation

A gentle kneading of the posterolateral cervical musculature from the cervicothoracic junction to the occiput (Fig. 5-60).

Suboccipital Release or Decompression Bilateral

This technique is frequently used before or after other procedures. It serves to decompress the trigeminocervical complex and thus decrease facial, occipital and occipital-frontal headaches (Fig. 5-61).

Suboccipital Release, Unilateral

When suboccipital release or decompression cannot be tolerated bilaterally, this variation allows for a unilateral release (Fig. 5-62).

Lower Arc Stretch

Light thumb pressure is used to delineate the distribution of the soft tissue stretch from the supraclavicular region to the upper cervical spine. Figures 5-63 A,B,C depict placement of the thumb in different locations of the supraclavicular fossa. Care must be taken not to impart a strong downward pressure against the underlying brachial plexus and vascular vessels.

Upper Arc Stretch

This technique uses the same contact points as the lower arc stretch, but the head is lifted off the table and rotated to the opposite side of the stabilizing thumb (Fig. 5-64, A and B).

Cross Stretch

The cross stretch is performed after completion of the arcing. One hand remains sub-

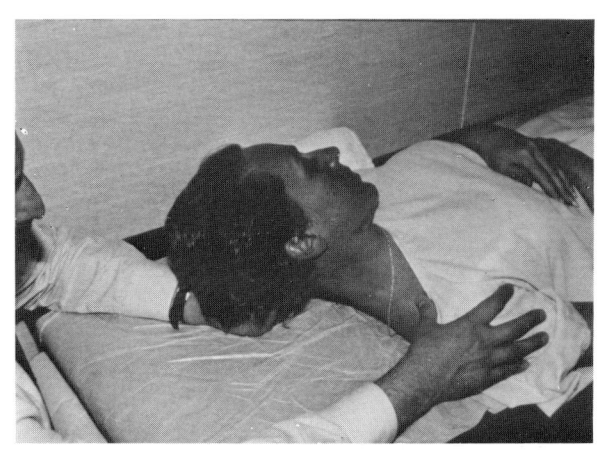

Fig. 5-64. Upper Arc Stretch. Therapist sits facing the supine patient with the thumb of the right hand maintaining light pressure in the supraclavicular fossa. The left hand is placed sub-occipitally. The left hand produces a circular motion of the head to the left. The head is held off the table to increase the degree of stretch. Thumb position of the right hand determines the distribution of soft tissue stretch which can vary within the supraclavicular region as shown in illustrations **A** and **B**.

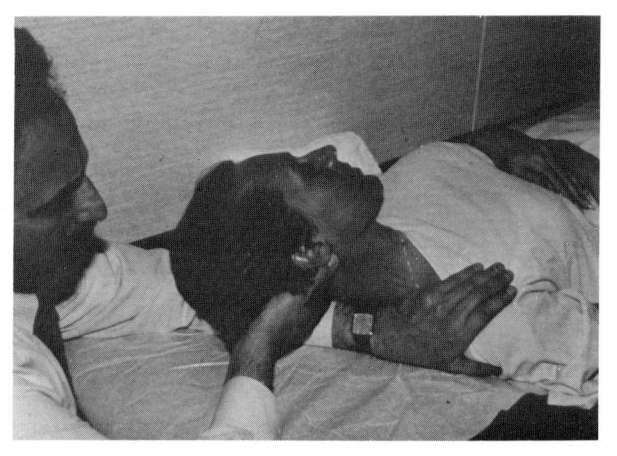

Fig. 5-65. Cross Stretch. Therapist sits facing the supine patient. One hand holds the head via the sub-occipital fossa while the other hand slides under the head and neck crossing onto the contralateral shoulder girdle. A sustained stretch is applied by simultaneous down and out pressure on the shoulder girdle with distraction and sidebending of the head in the opposite direction. This stretch is then repeated on the other side by switching hands.

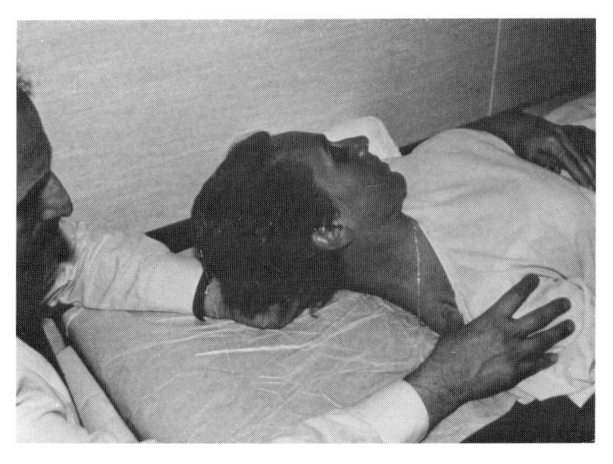

Fig. 5-64 B.

occipital while the other crosses under the patient's head to depress the shoulder girdle as the head is distracted and rotated to the opposite side (Fig. 5-65).

Sustained Release

When arc stretching is easily tolerated, treatment can progress to sustained release. Figures 5-66 A,B,C depict variations of head position and hand contact to stretch the anterolateral, lateral, and posterolateral myofascial tissue. The stretch is sustained for 15-120 seconds, as tolerated. Note the different distribution of tissue stretch in each position.

Bilateral Suboccipital Stretch

This technique not only decompresses the suboccipital region, but also stretches the suboccipital musculature (Fig.5-67). This technique alone often decreases or eliminates craniofacial and suboccipital pain. If relief is short-lived but dramatic, intermittent mechanical suboccipital traction (Fig. 5-80) is added to the treatment program. It is helpful to teach a family member how to perform this technique at home.

Anterior Release

This technique produces a sustained stretch of the infrahyoid region as well as the anterolateral, lateral and posterolateral regions. The distribution of the stretch is dependent upon the position of the patient's head and therapist's hand (Fig. 5-68 A,B,C,D).

Dorsal Glides

Passive head retraction with an associated stretch of the suboccipital tissue and facet

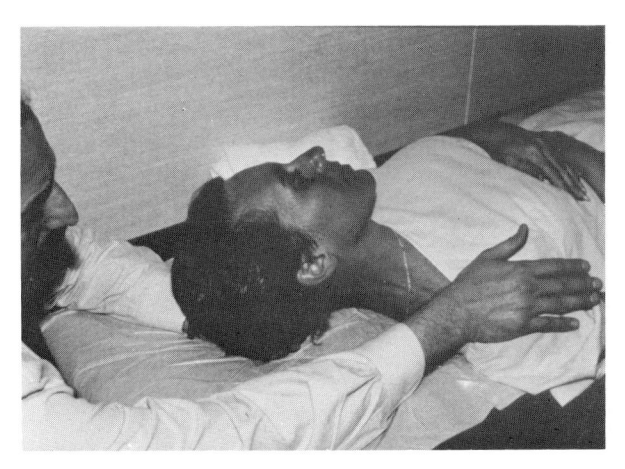

Fig. 5-66. Sustained Release. **A,** Anterolateral. Therapist's right hand is placed over the anterior acromial region and imparts a downward pressure in a lateral direction while the left hand distracts the occiput and rotates the head to the opposite side.

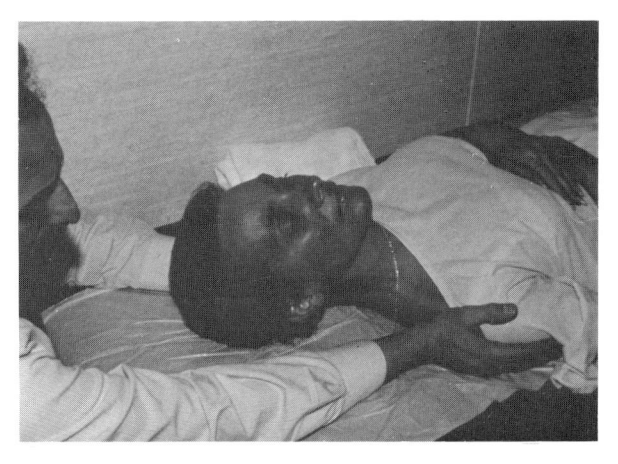

Fig. 5-66. C, Posterolateral. Therapist's right hand is placed behind the acromion on the superior aspect of the scapular spine. A downward pressure is performed while the left hand distracts the occiput and rotates the head to the same side.

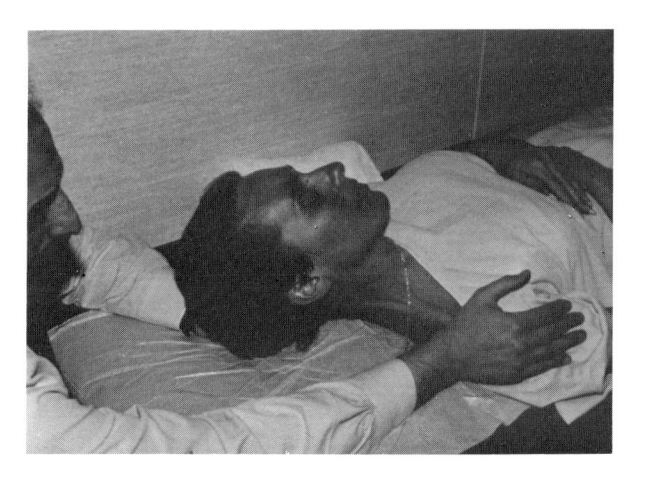

Fig. 5-66. B, Lateral. The therapist's right hand is placed over the acromion. The therapist then imparts a lateral pressure while the left hand distracts the occiput and sidebends the patient's head to the opposite side.

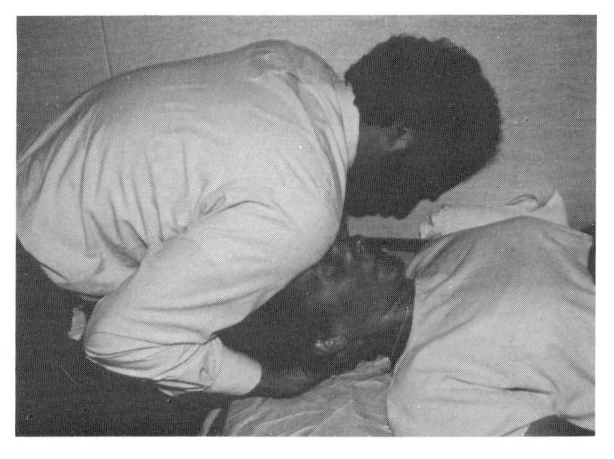

Fig. 5-67. Bilateral Sub-Occipital Stretch. Therapist stands with trunk in forward bending behind head of supine patient. Right hand is placed under the occiput with thumb contact in one sub-occipital fossa and second plus third finger in the other. The left hand is placed under the neck at the mid-cervical level distal to the right hand for stabilization. The therapist's right shoulder is placed on the patient's forehead so that the head is not lifted off the table into neck flexion. The right hand performs a forward tilt of the head on the neck to stretch the sub-occipital tissue.

joint capsules can be performed in the sitting position for the C2-T4 segments.

The therapist stands on the left side of the patient and cradles the head against his chest with the right arm. The arm is placed around the head above the nose to the suboccipital region. Care must be taken to avoid pressure on the patient's nose. The therapist's bicipital region is in contact with the patient's forehead. As counterpressure is applied by the therapist's left hand, a gentle distraction and posterior gliding motion is performed with the head. The chin must remain parallel with the floor (Fig 5-69 A,B). In the prone position with the forehead supported by the patient's hands, dorsal glides in a posterior-anterior direction can be performed by graded joint mobilization. Figure 5-70 illustrates this technique to reduce an upper thoracic kyphosis and promote restoration of normal posture.

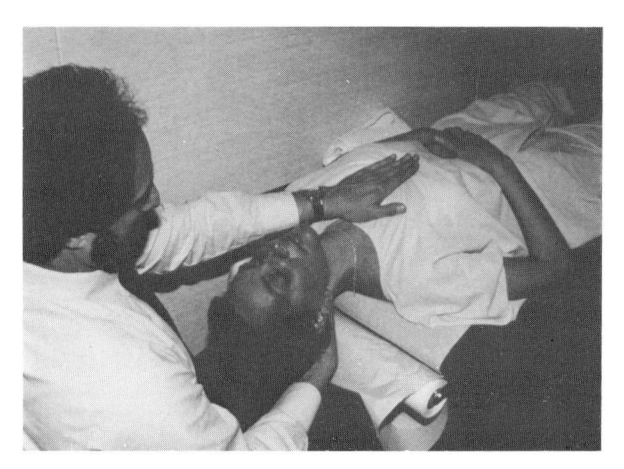

148 New Concepts in Craniomandibular and Chronic Pain Management

Fig. 5-68. Anterior Release. Therapist sits facing the head of the supine patient. One hand holds the patient's occiput in a position of extension over the edge of the table. The other hand imparts a sustained stretch upon **A**, sternal and infrahyoid.

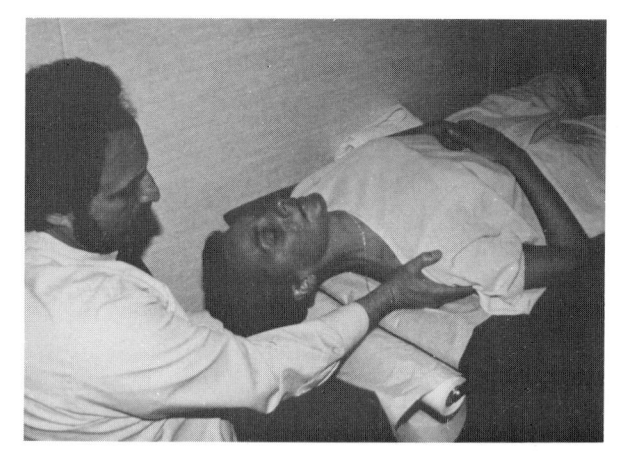

Fig. 5-68. D, Posterolateral regions respectively.

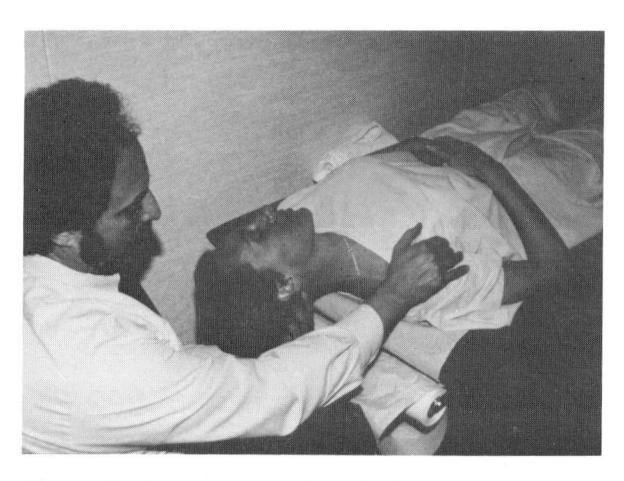

Fig. 5-68. B, Anterolateral cervical.

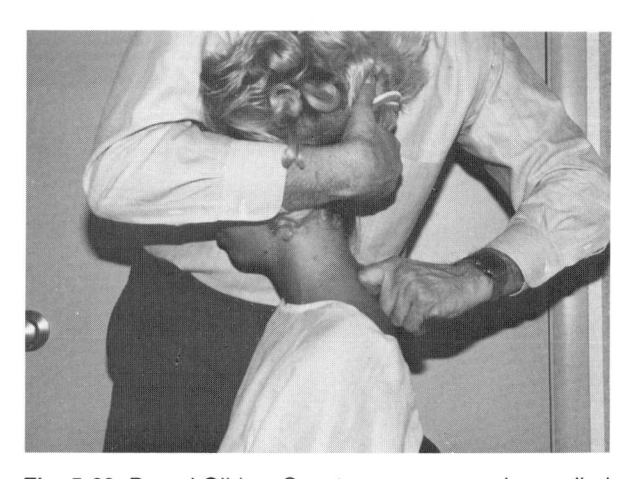

Fig. 5-69. Dorsal Glides. Counterpressure can be applied to the mid-cervical or cervico-thoracic junction. **A,** The technique can be isolated to a specific segmental level by placing the index finger of the stabilizing hand just below that of the index finger of the hand that cradles the head.

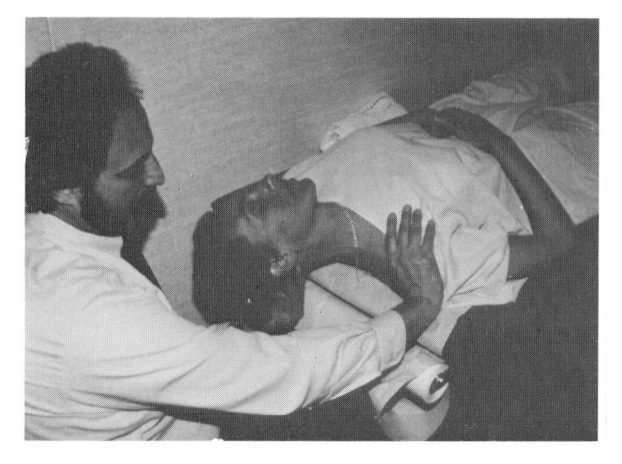

Fig. 5-68. C, Lateral cervical.

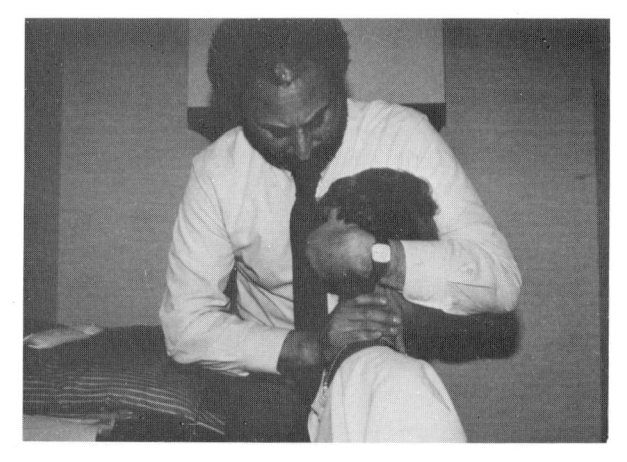

Fig. 5-69. B, An alternative method consists of contact on the lamina of a specific level with the spinous process between the flexed index finger and thumb.

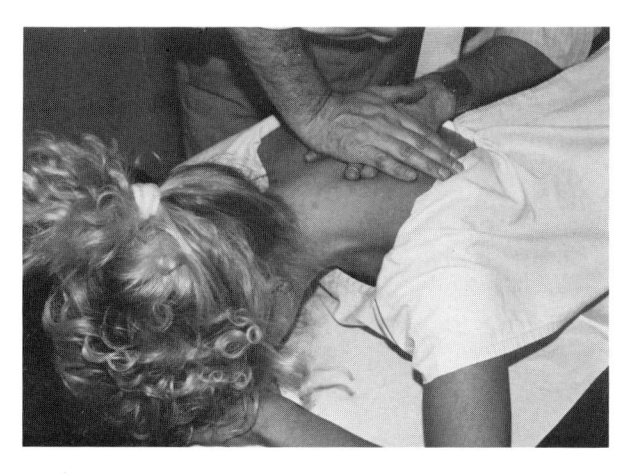

Fig. 5-70. Dorsal P/A Glide. Therapist stands to the side of the prone patient and places left hand and forearm along the spine. Volar surfaces of the second and third fingers are placed over the respective thoracic transverse processes. The wrist will need to be placed into radial deviation to compensate for the longer third finger. If this adjustment is not made the technique will cause rotation instead of a dorsal glide as the force will be directed to two different vertebral levels. The ulnar border of the right hand is placed over the distal phalanges of the left hand with the elbow at a 90 degree angle. Gentle graded oscillations are applied from the T3-4 to C6-7 levels.

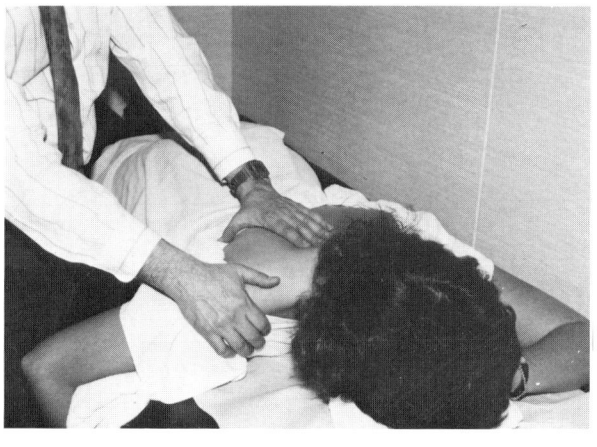

Fig. 5-71. Shoulder Girdle Technique. Patient lies prone with shoulder in 90 degrees of shoulder abduction and elbow flexion hanging over the edge of the table with a towel roll under the antecubital fossa. Various hand positions can be used to perform rotation as well as inferior and superior glides fo the scapula.

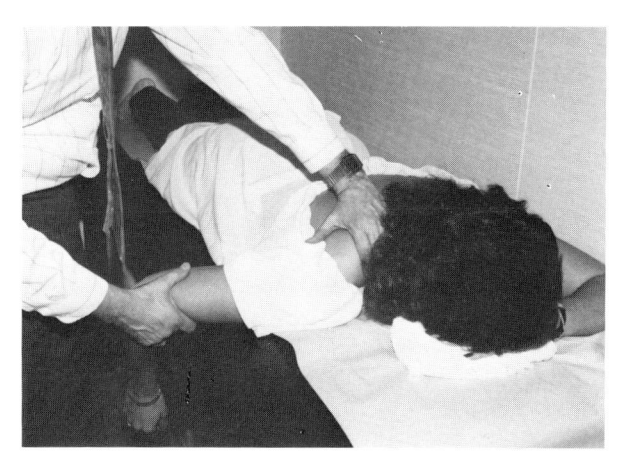

Fig. 5-72. Trager Shoulder Girdle Technique. Patient lies prone with arm over the edge of the table. Therapist stands alongside facing the patient with one hand over the supraclavicular area and the other under the antecubital fossa. A swinging oscillatory motion is provided to the arm within a range of 45 degrees into external and internal rotation. A downward stretch of the shoulder girdle can be performed simultaneously.

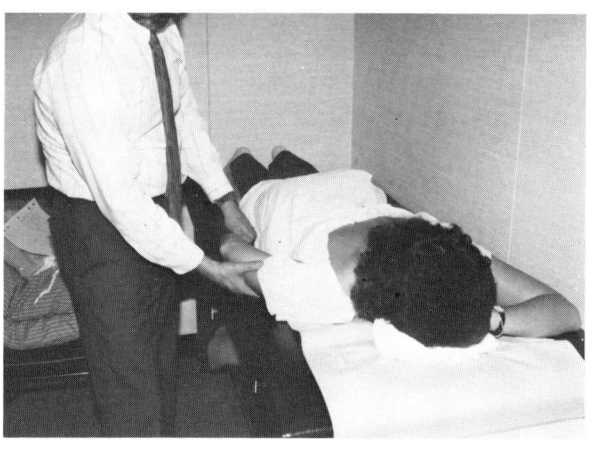

Fig. 5-73. Trager Shoulder Girdle Technique. Following the technique shown in Fig. 5-72, a progression to an increased stretch is now performed utilizing a swing and catch. The left hand is now used to catch the patient's forearm as the right hand swings it into internal rotation and then imparts a downward stretch or inferior glide. This is similar to a long axis distraction typically performed in the supine position.

SOFT TISSUE MOBILIZATION OF SCAPULA AND SHOULDER GIRDLE

Various mobilization techniques can be comfortably performed in the prone position to stretch or release the soft tissue of the shoulder girdle area. Inferior and superior glides as well as rotation of the scapulae can be easily obtained with various hand placements. The shoulder, inferior angle, vertebral border, and superior medial angle of the scapulae are typical points of contact, as illustrated in Figures 5-71 through 74. The constant Trager oscillatory motion can be used again to provide a pain modulating input to promote relaxation. These methods are tolerated much better than

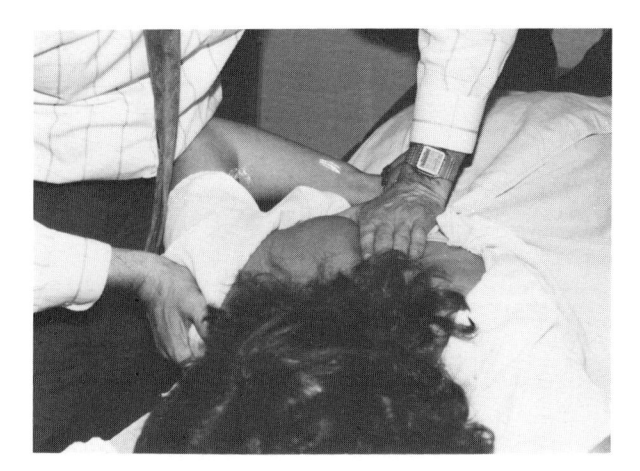

Fig. 5-74. Scapular Distraction. Patient lies prone with shoulder internally rotated and dorsum of hand placed in the lumbar region. This position promotes scapular winging and allows the therapist to place the radial border of the left index finger under the vertebral (medial) border of the scapula to distract it away from the thorax. The right hand can assist by simultaneously elevating the shoulder and oscillating the deltoid area. This technique also serves to stretch the rhomboids and middle trapezius.

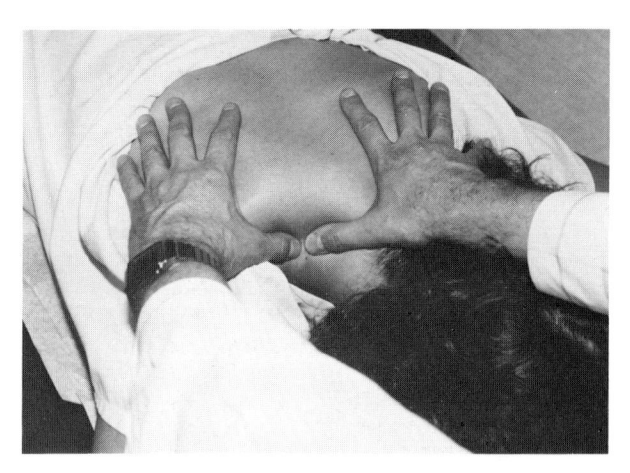

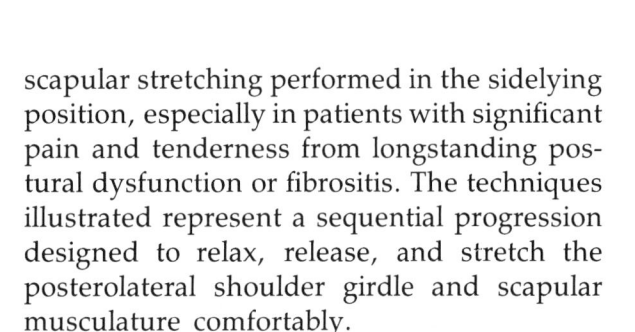

Fig. 5-75. Mobilization of First Rib. Patient lies prone with head slightly rotated to the opposite side or in neutral position in cupped hands. The therapist stands facing the patient on the side to be treated and places the volar surface of the thumbs on the first rib underlying the upper trapezius. The other fingers of each hand are spread out to stabilize. Gentle graded oscillatory pressure is directed towards the opposite foot. The force is produced by gentle rocking of the therapists body and not initiated by the thumbs.

scapular stretching performed in the sidelying position, especially in patients with significant pain and tenderness from longstanding postural dysfunction or fibrositis. The techniques illustrated represent a sequential progression designed to relax, release, and stretch the posterolateral shoulder girdle and scapular musculature comfortably.

Many other mobilization techniques can be performed on the shoulder complex: capsular stretching, distraction, and glides in all directions for the glenohumeral, acromioclavicular and sternoclavicular joints. These are excellently described and illustrated elsewhere.[148]

First Rib Mobilization

Soft tissue restriction of the anterior and medial scalenes can cause elevation of the first rib. In addition to scalene stretching, the first rib may at times need to be mobilized. The technique is shown in Figure 5-75.

Kneading of Upper Trapezius

Numerous variations of massage techniques can be performed: Figure 5-76 illustrates a soft tissue kneading technique for the upper trapezius.

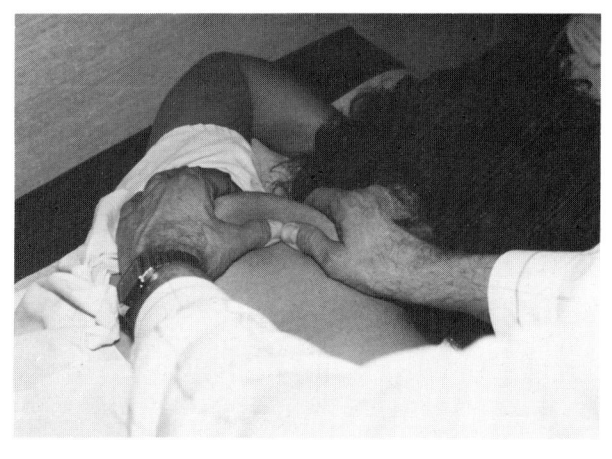

Fig. 5-76. Kneading of Upper Trapezius. Patient lies prone with upper trapezius on slack and forehead resting on hands. Therapist stands on the right side of the patient facing the left upper trapezius area. Therapist lifts the muscle and pushes it towards the thumbs by flexion of the second and third fingers. The thumbs then push the tissue forward as the wrists go into ulnar deviation to apply a stretch. The technique begins at the acromial area and proceeds to the occiput.

Contract-Relax Stretching of the Levator Scapulae

Stretching or release of the levator scapulae can be performed in the prone or supine positions, as previously illustrated, but is best isolated with the patient sitting, as shown in Figure 5-77. This technique should be per-

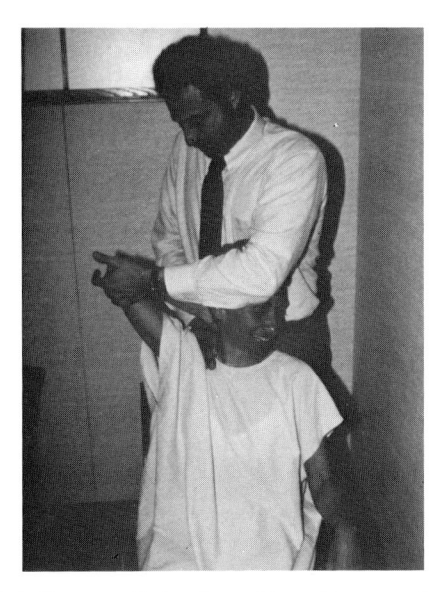

Fig. 5-77. Contract-Relax Stretching of Levator Scapulae. Patient sits in chair with therapist standing behind. Patient places the ipsilateral shoulder into external rotation with the hand holding the sub-occipital region. The therapist stabilizes the patient's head which is rotated to the opposite side by placing his arm around the forehead and holds the patient's arm in an abducted position. This promotes a downward rotation of the superior medial border of the scapula and imparts a stretch upon the levator scapulae. Rotation of the head to the contralateral side increases the stretch. The therapist places the thenar eminence of his other hand on the spine of the scapula and performs a downward movement as the patient goes into the expiration phase of breathing.

formed gently at first, as the stretch can be quite profound. Have the patient take a deep breath to impart a degree of contraction upon the muscle, and then depress the scapula during expiration. This is performed 3-6 times, followed by manual suboccipital traction in neutral position with the patient sitting.

STRETCH AND SPRAY TECHNIQUES

Travell and Simons have written the definitive text on myofascial pain and dysfunction.[42] Therefore, only one technique (Fig. 5-78) is shown with this procedure. Flouri-methane stretch and spray are used adjunctively in most treatment paradigms.

CERVICAL ROTATIONAL MOBILIZATION

After sufficient soft tissue release and pain reduction have been obtained, specific joint mobilization techniques may be indicated.

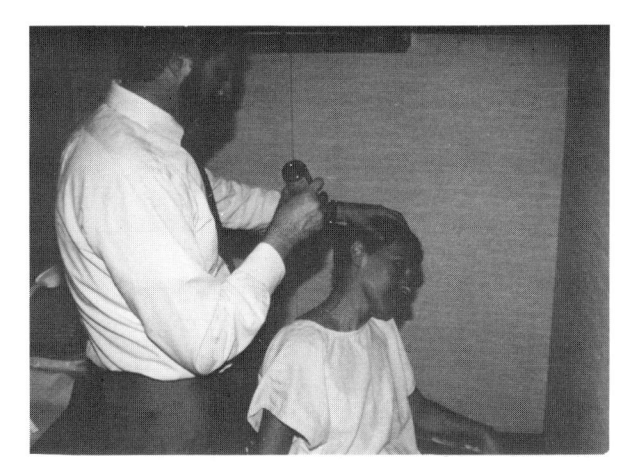

Fig. 5-78. Stretch and Spray of Scalenes. The patient is seated with the arm hanging over the side of the chair and the hand grasping the seat to stabilize. Stretch is initially performed by placement of the head in a sidebent position away from the anchored arm. The therapist, standing behind and/or to the side of the patient, increases the stretch on the scalenus anticus and medius by rotating the head to the opposite side. The spray is applied, while the stretch is maintained, from origin to insertion using the specific recommendations of Travell.

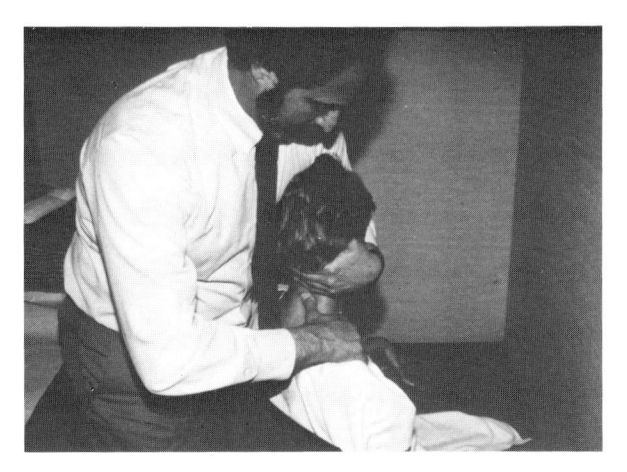

Fig. 5-79. Cervical Rotational Mobilization to the Left. The patient sits upright on a firm chair. The therapist stands behind and locates the level to be mobilized by flexion of the head on the neck and palpation of gapping between the cervical spinous processes. At the appropriate level, the head is sidebent to the painful side and rotated away until capsular and ligamentous tightening occur which indicates that the barrier has been reached. The patient's head is held against the therapist's chest by his left arm placed around the forehead with the hand at the sub-occipital region. The therapist's right thumb is positioned lateral to the appropriate spinous process to restrict it's movement towards the right as left vertebral rotation occurs. Gentle oscillatory (on and off) pressure is performed into left rotation to stretch the facet capsule on the right. If, for example, the spinous process of C-5 is blocked by the therapists thumb, mobilization of the C4-5 facet joint will occur. This technique can also be performed in the supine position.

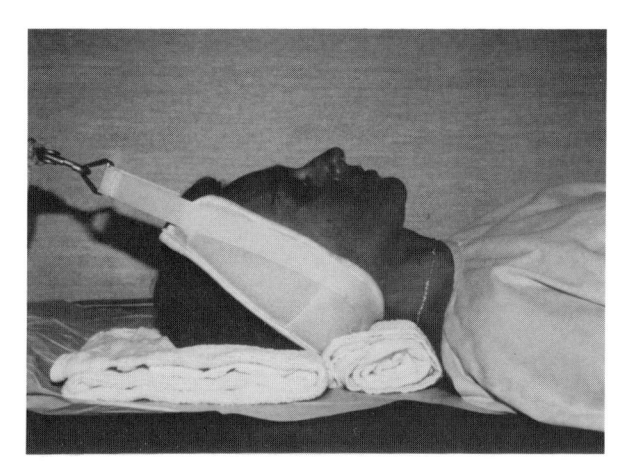

Fig. 5-80. Intermittent Mechanical Sub-Occipital Traction. The patient is positioned supine with a pillow under the knees. A towel roll supports the cervical lordosis and the halter is placed between the roll and the cervical spine just inferior to the occiput. An additional flat towel is recommended to negate any posterior cranial rotation. The tractional force generates a neutral pull on the occiput to distract the upper cervical region.

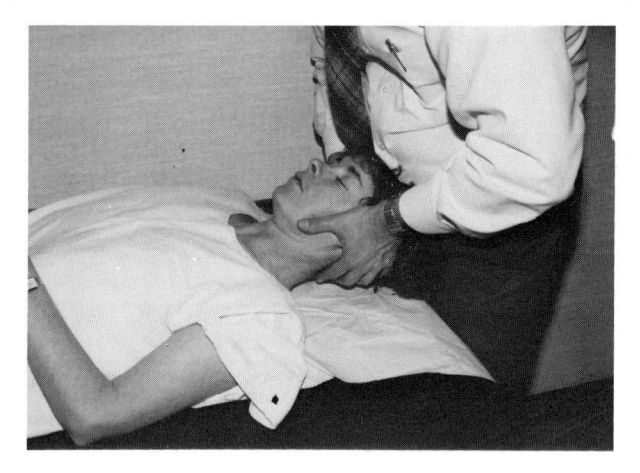

Fig. 5-81. Sidegliding of Occiput on Atlas. The patient lies supine with the therapist facing the patient's shoulders. The index fingers bilaterally are placed in the suboccipital fossa and the rest of the hand supports the cranium just above the table. The head is gently moved from side to side to apply a stretch at the occipito-atlantal joints while maintaining a neutral position of the head.

This is especially helpful in the presence of capsular adhesions which limit the last 25 degrees of rotation of a specific joint segment. Again, many different methods can be used, commonly in the sitting and occasionally supine positions, as illustrated in Figure 5-79. Manual suboccipital traction after this procedure is again used to decompress the region.

MECHANICAL TRACTION

In the presence of TMJ pain and dysfunction, only suboccipital traction is recommended. Chin straps should not be used, as the tractional force is then exerted upon the mandible, resulting in further TMJ compression and pain. Various suboccipital traction devices are available that can be added to conventional mechanical units. Intermittent mechanical suboccipital traction is added to the treatment paradigm when manual distractional techniques provide significant pain relief, but only of a transient nature. Prolonged traction usually proves beneficial in such situations as it provides a greater degree of decompression and release of the suboccipital region. Recent studies show that intermittent mechanical traction provides optimal improvement, compared to static or manual traction.[149]

A force greater than or equal to 20 pounds is needed to separate the vertebrae by 1-1.5 mm. The upper cervical segments do not distract as easily as the mid to lower segments, and the younger the subject, the easier it is to obtain separation. Zylbergold and Piper, in their study of supine mechanical cervical traction, concluded that rhythmic or intermittent traction produced twice as much separation as sustained or static traction.

The prime effects of traction are to increase movement, decrease pain and muscle spasm, promote relaxation of muscle and connective tissue (fasciae), and decrease nerve root irritation and compression due to foraminal encroachment, and facilitate an increase in tissue-fluid interchange.[150] Figure 5-80 illustrates the suggested method used with conventional intermittent traction and a suboccipital halter.

A force of 20-30 pounds is commonly used with a 15 second "on" phase and 10 second rest phase for 10-15 minutes, depending upon patient status. In certain situations, it is necessary to start with only 10-15 pounds and gradually increase over successive treatment sessions to develop tolerance and eliminate apprehension. It may be beneficial to also gradually increase the traction phase toward one minute, with the rest phase maintained at 10-20 seconds.

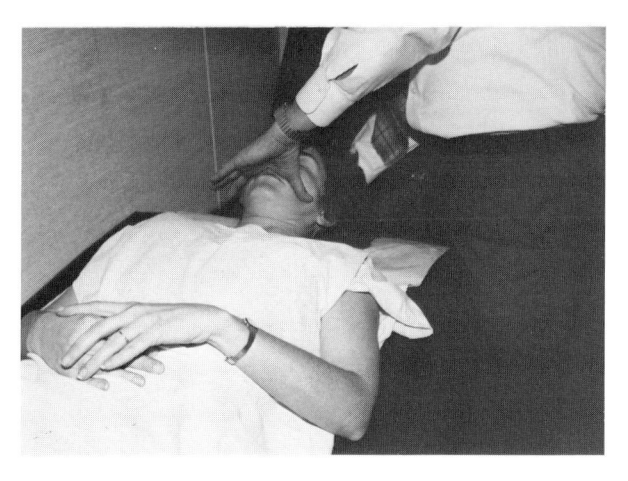

Fig. 5-82. Occipital-Atlanto Rocking. The patient lies supine and the therapist stands to the side of the patient. The therapist's right hand is placed under the occiput. The therapist's left hand applies on and off pressure via the web space through the maxillary region imparting a down and forward tilt of the head thus gapping the occipital-atlanto region.

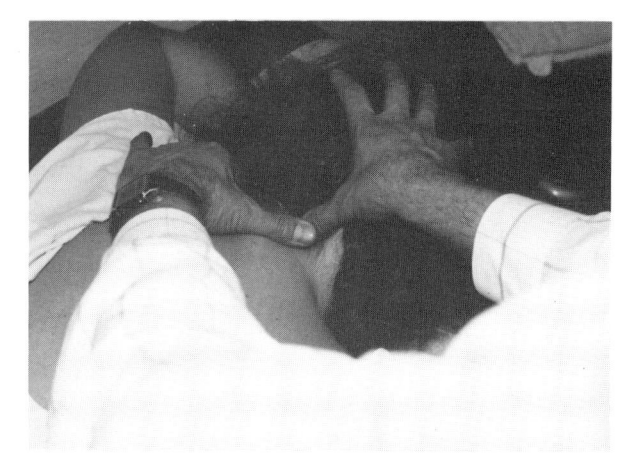

Fig. 5-83. Posteroanterior Unilateral Vertebral Pressure. The patient lies prone with the head rotated about 30 degrees to the right and positioned in slight flexion. The therapist's thumbs are placed one on top of the other overlying the right posterior aspect of atlas and oscillatory pressure is used to produce a rotation at C1-2. This provides a stretch to the right atlanto-axial joint and capsule which facilitates upper cervical rotation.

SPECIFIC MANUAL THERAPEUTIC TECHNIQUES

Additional techniques may be needed for some patients. The procedures illustrated in Figures 5-81 to 85 are examples of approaches used for a patient with hyperactivity of the left sternocleidomastoid and pain referral to the orbital region of the left eye with bilateral frontal headaches. Figure 5-13 shows the initial postural findings.

These techniques are used to reduce suboccipital restriction, release the shortened myofascial components of the left sternocleidomastoid, and gap or decompress the suboccipital area so as to decrease nociceptive input to the segmental innervation of the sternocleidomastoid (C2-3).

This patient was instructed to sit to the right of anyone that she is talking to, so as to require contraction of the right sternocleidomastoid. In addition, when watching television, she should gradually move the set to the left for the same reason. A home exercise program of resisted motions designed to increase the strength of the right and stretch the left sternocleidomastoid are also ongoing.

RADIOLOGICAL CONSIDERATIONS

A radiological analysis of skeletal posture and alignment may be helpful in certain situations to assist in the evaluative process. However, radiological findings are not considered until completion of the history plus subjective and objective assessment.

Many different positions are used for x-rays of the spine, but the posture that an individual assumes throughout most of the day is not commonly the position taken. Consequently, radiological findings may not relate well to an individual's pain complaints.

Gore and associates analyzed the roentgenograms of 200 asymptomatic people between the ages of 20-65. They found that 95 percent of the males and 70 percent of the females within the 60-65 year old group had at least one degenerative change. The most significant findings were posterior osteophytes at C5-6.[151] A decrease in cervical lordosis was associated with intervertebral narrowing in the older subjects. In a related study of 205 patients with cervical spine pain, they found that there was no significant relationship between degenerative changes, the sagittal diameter of the spinal canal, or the degree of the cervical lordosis to the severity of pain.[152] Of those injured patients who had normal x-rays at the time of injury, a greater tendency to develop degenerative changes (in comparison to the non-injured group) was seen. Trauma thus was considered likely to

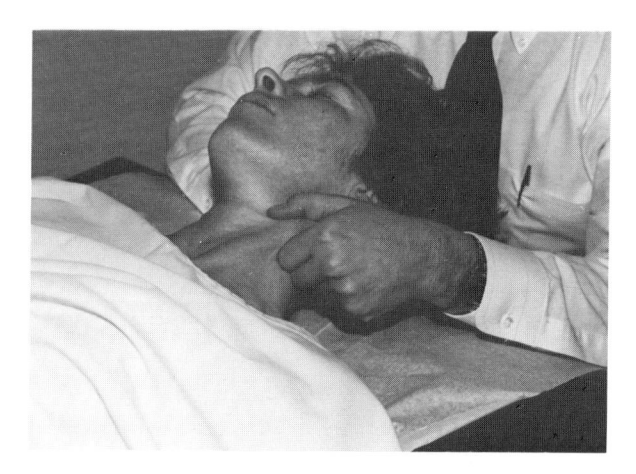

Fig. 5-84. Kneading of SCM. The therapist sits facing the supine patient. The left hand grasps the left SCM between the thumb and index finger. Care must be taken to ensure that the muscle rests on the radial surface of the left index finger and is gently held in place by the thumb. The therapist's right hand holds the patients occiput and slowly performs a circular motion of the head on the neck while simultaneously lifting and gently stretching the left SCM.

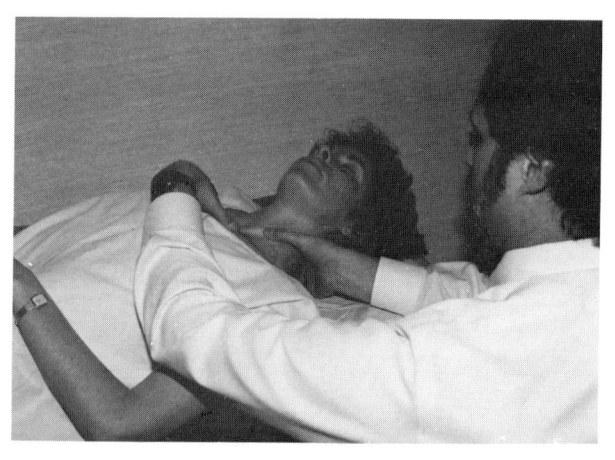

Fig. 5-85. Myofascial Release of Left SCM. The patient lies supine with head sidebent to the right and rotated to the left. This places the left SCM on stretch. The therapist sits facing the left side of the patient and places thumb opposite thumb with a gap of about one inch over the SCM. The starting point can be at the sternum or mastoid process. A slow sustained release is applied by thumb tension in opposite directions for 10-30 seconds. The technique should be specific for both the sternal and clavicular sections of the SCM. Care must be taken not to apply any significant anterior-posterior pressure against the patients cervical spine.

promote an increase in degenerative disc disease, but it was concluded that the radiographic data was of little value in predicting the outcome of a treatment program.[153]

Both of the aforementioned studies only analyzed lateral roentgenograms, and the exact circumstances in which they were taken were not known in every subject. If radiographic findings are to be of value in postural analysis, functional studies and additional means of evaluation are recommended to develop standardization. A functional roentgenogram analysis of the cervical spine should be performed in the sagittal plane and a comparison made between passive and active range of motion.[154] At the very least, a lateral view in neutral standing position, as well as full flexion and extension, should be taken to determine the degree of antero- or retrolisthesis of the vertebral segments.[154,155] In addition, a standing open mouth view must be taken to analyze the atlas-axis relationship. A study by Rocabado using a definitive radiological analysis revealed that 84 percent of the adult subjects that showed degenerative processes or hypomobility of the cervical spine also demonstrated a loss of cervical lordosis and tendency towards kyphosis.[154] A forward or backward vertebral displacement of 3.5 mm or more, associated with neurologic signs, is considered a clinically unstable segment.

The new concept of tripodism, as established by Rocabado, must be maintained between the anterior vertebral body, posterior third of the intervertebral disc, and the posterior aspect of the facet joints. A movable segment consists of two adjacent vertebrae and the related soft tissue components. Rocabado has updated this to what he terms a "functional spinal unit" consisting of anterior and posterior components. Stability of the cervical spine is thus dependent upon the anterior and posterior longitudinal ligaments plus the interverbral disc anteriorly, along with the yellow, intertransverse, interspinous and supraspinous ligaments, facet joint, and capsule posteriorly. Tripodism is necessary to maintain normal cervical lordosis, as well as pain-free motion through a normal range.[5,155,156]

A definitive standardized radiographic analysis can also determine the position of the hyoid bone in relation to the curvature of the cervical spine, as well as the degree of posterior cranial rotation. Rocabado has demonstrated by various tracing techniques that the hyoid bone increasingly elevates in the presence of a straight cervical spine to levels above the anterior inferior angle of C3. Hyoid elevation is even more pronounced with an inverted cervical lordosis. When the space between the occipital base and the posterior arch of atlas is less than 4mm (4-9mm is considered normal), suboccipital compression may occur. A combination of posterior cranial rotation and an inverted or kyphotic cervical spine results in the greatest degree of suprahyoid tension and corresponding hyoid elevation. The physiological ramifications of this objective data have been thoroughly discussed.

CONCLUSION

Here, the word "pain" surfaces again for final consideration. Myofascial pain dysfunction syndrome is frequently mentioned in the literature on upper quarter problems. It has numerous causes. Clinically, the trigger point can be considered a secondary manifestation of acute trauma or cumulative stress and strain of a postural or emotional nature.

The greatest concentration of trigger points and the related pain syndromes discussed in this chapter occur in areas of significant mechanical stress, such as the craniomandibular, cervical, shoulder girdle and lumbosacral regions.[42,157] Trigger points or the clinical entity of myofascial pain dysfunction syndrome can easily mislead the clinician into false diagnoses by mimicking symptom complexes indicative of postural dysfunction, as discussed in this chapter.

When myofascial pain dysfunction syndrome is considered, the terms fibrositis, myositis, fibromyalgia, and fasciitis may also be mentioned. Bonica states that myofascial syndromes have been described in terms of myalgia, myositis, fibrositis, fibromyositis, fasciitis, myofasciitis, muscular rheumatism, and muscular strain.[158] Thus any of the aforementioned terminology may represent myofascial pain dysfunction syndrome.

An individual with myofascial pain dysfunction syndrome commonly complains of deep, dull and achy muscular pain, a localized hyperalgesia at trigger points and concomitant pain referral. Prolonged presence of trigger points results in muscle spasm, loss of normal rest length, weakness, and even contracture due to fibrosis. Concomitant joint dysfunction occurs to compound the symptom complex, along with the possiblity of nerve entrapment. Associated autonomic nervous system signs of vasoconstriction, pallor, sweating and decreased skin resistance are commonly present.

It is proposed that myofascial pain dysfunction syndrome results from decreased muscular rest length and associated joint hypomobility. Muscle spasm leads to waste product liberation, vasoconstriction, and localized ischemia of adjacent muscle and nerve fibers. Ischemia further promotes waste product retention, and a decrease in the normal nutritional supply to the involved area.

The composite pattern leads to a continuous CNS bombardment of nociceptive impulses arising from mechanoreceptors and chemoreceptors of muscle, joint capsule and nerve of the involved area, all of which enter the dorsal horn of the spinal cord at related segments leading to the concept of facilitation.[33-38]

The most reliable and consistant changes in skin impedence occur as a result of segmental facilitation along the spine. Decreased skin impedence is considered to result from increased secretory activity due to sympathetic stimulation.[159] Stoddard states that a majority of adults develop one or more facilitated segments in the spine that may persist for months or years, usually as a result of postural deformities.[159] This is very evident in patients with a FHRSP. Patients who manifest this abnormality demonstrate a decreased threshold to vertebral spring tests, skin rolling, muscle palpation and joint mobility.

Figure 5-86 illustrates the concept of the facilitated segment, the proposed physiological basis behind myofascial pain dysfunction syndrome and trigger points. An individual with the postural abnormalities, pain and dysfunction described in this chapter will have multiple facilitated segments.[160] Sleep deprivation, fatigue, vitamin and mineral deficiencies or anemia all contribute to and enhance the composite picture of myofascial pain dysfunction syndrome.[42]

FACILITATED SEGMENT

SOMATIC INPUT
- SKIN
- MUSCLE
- JOINT
- TRIGGER POINTS

LAMINA 5

SYMPATHETIC INPUT
- VISCERA
- CIRCULATION
- SWEATING

CORTICAL REPRESENTATION
SOMATIC (DENSE INNERVATION)
VISCERAL (SPARSE INNERVATION)

SKIN REFERRAL CAN PREDOMINATE

CONVERGENCE
⇩
SUMMATION
⇩
PROJECTION
⇩
REFERRED PAIN
⇩
VISCEROSOMATIC/SOMATOVISCERAL REFLEXES (LAMINA 5)

.... Normal Proprioceptive Input Is Disrupted

.... Threshold to Noxious and Non-noxious Input Is Lowered

.... Subthreshold Stimuli of Somatic, Visceral, Cutaneous and Psychological Origin Result in Summation Mechanisms and Pain Projection

.... Skin Resistance is Decreased

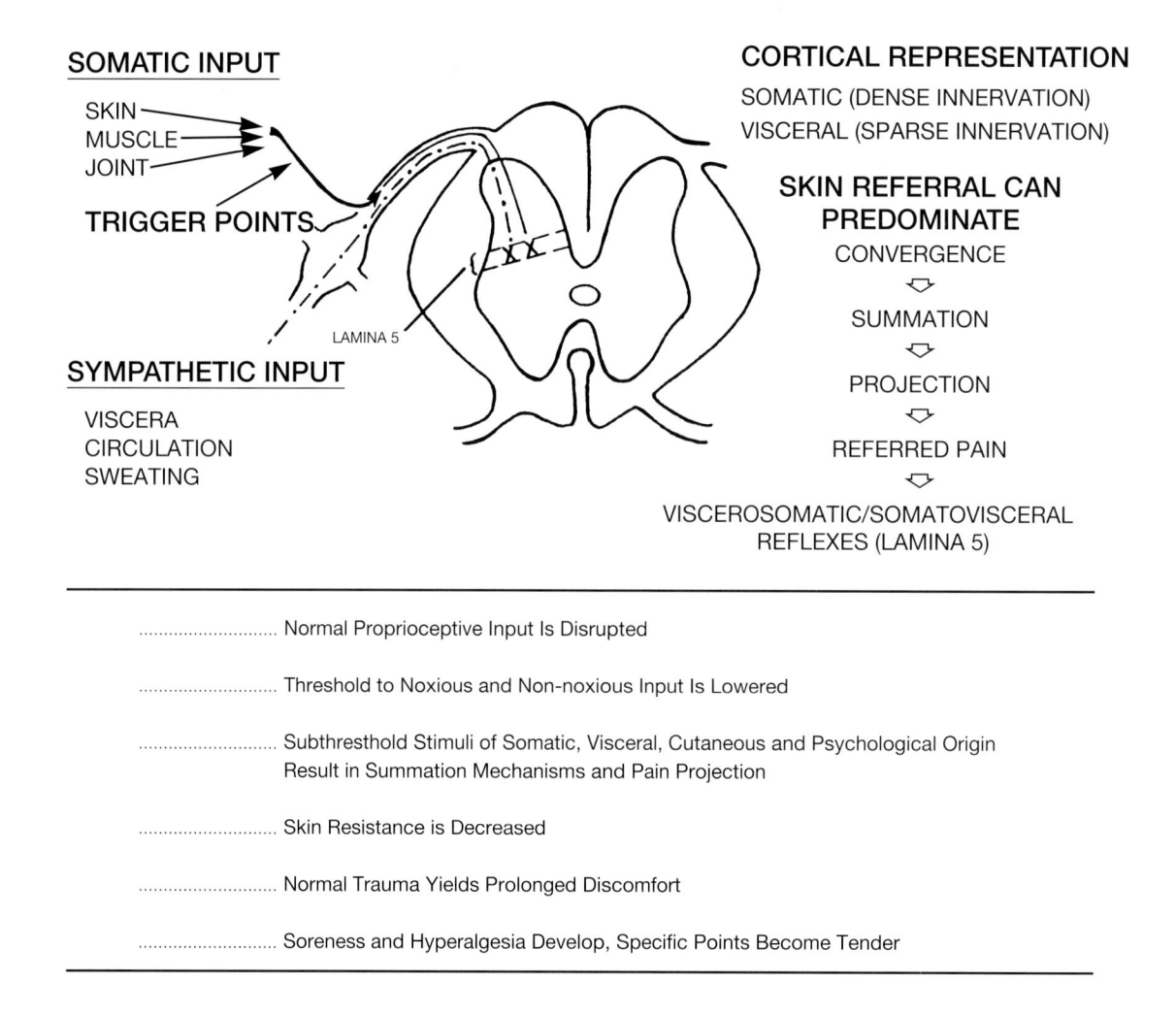

.... Normal Trauma Yields Prolonged Discomfort

.... Soreness and Hyperalgesia Develop, Specific Points Become Tender

Fig. 5-86. Facilitated Segment. Disruption fo the normal excitation threshold of a vertebral segment by abnormal physiologic input and resultant objective plus subjective associated responses. Reprinted with permission from Mannheimer, JS and Lampe, GN.[52]

The numerous etiological factors presented in this chapter promote the onset of abnormal posture with associated pain and dysfunction. Unless the multi-disciplinary interventional techniques (physician-dentist-physical therapist) that have been presented (along with patient compliance) are instituted, the pain and dysfunction will persist.

REFERENCES

1. Mannheimer JS. Non-medicinal and non-invasive pain control techniques in the management of rheumatic disease and related musculoskeletal disorders. *J Rheum*. 1987;14(suppl 15):26.

2. Driscoll DR. Anatomical and biomechanical characteristics of upper cervical ligamentous structures: a review. *J Manip and Physiol Therap*. 1987;10(3):107.

3. Kapandj IA. *The Physiology of the Joints*. Vol III The Trunk and Vertebral Column. New York, NY: Churchill Livingstone; 1974.

4. Panjabi M, Dvorak J, Duranceau J, et al. Three-dimensional movements of the upper cervical spine. *Spine*. 1988;13(7):726.

5. Rocabado M. Biomechanical relationship of the cranial, cervical and hyoid regions. *J Craniomand Disorders*. 1983;1(3):62.

6. Seemann DC. Center of gravity of the skull: A review of theories and a pilot study to determine location. *J Manip and Physiol Therap*. 1981;4(1):15.

7. Rocabado M. *Head, Neck and TMJ Joint Dysfunction, 1979.* Rocabado Institute for Craniomandibular and Vertebral Therapeutics. Course notes.
8. Rocabado M. *Advanced Upper Quarter, 1980.* Southfield, MI. Course notes.
9. Hesse JR, Hansson TL. Factors influencing joint mobility in general and in particular respect to the craniomandibular articulation: A literature review. *J Craniomand Disorders Facial and Oral Pain.* 1988;2(1):19.
10. Razook SJ. Nonsurgical management of TMJ and masticatory muscle problems. In: Kraus SL, ed. *TMJ Disorders: Management of the Craniomandibular Complex.* New York, NY: Churchill Livingstone; 1988.
11. Pal GP, Sherk HH. The vertebral stability of the cervical spine. *Spine.* 1988;13(5):447.
12. Worth DR. Movements of the cervical spine. In: Grieve GP, ed. *Modern Manual Therapy.* New York, NY: Churchill Livingstone; 1988.
13. Kraus SL. Cervical spine influences on the craniomandibular region. In: Kraus SL, ed. *TMJ Disorders: Management of the Craniomandibular Complex.* New York, NY: Churchill Livingstone; 1988.
14. Pertes RA. A review of vertical facial types and craniomandibular disorders. *NY State Dental J.* 1985;51(9):570.
15. Kendall WO, Kendall FF, Boynton DA. *Posture and Pain.* Huntington, NY: Robert E. Krieger; 1952.
16. Dieck GS, Kelsey FL, Goel UK et al. An epidemiologic study of the relationship between postural asymmetry in the teen years and subsequent back and neck pain. *Spine.* 1985;10(10):872-877.
17. Darlow LA, Pesco J, Greenberg MS. The relationship of posture to myofascial pain dysfunction syndrome. *JADA.* 1987;144:73-75.
18. Edeling J. *Manual Therapy for Chronic Headache.* London: Butterworth; 1988.
19. Edwards BC. Examination of the high cervical spine (Occiput-C2) using combined movements. In: Grieve GP, ed. *Modern Manual Therapy of the Vertebral Column.* New York, NY: Churchill Livingstone; 1986.
20. Magarey ME. Examination of the cervical and thoracic spine. In: Grant R, ed. *Physical Therapy of the Cervical and Thoracic Spine.* New York, NY: Churchill Livingstone; 1988.
21. McKenzie RA. *The Lumbar Spine: Mechanical Diagnosis and Therapy.* Waikanae, New Zealand: Spinal Publications; 1981.
22. Cyriax J. *Textbook of Orthopaedic Medicine. Vol. I: Diagnosis of Soft Tissue Injuries.* London: Bailliere Tindall; 1975.
23. Andersson GBJ. Epidemiologic aspects of low-back pain in industry. *Spine.* 1981;6(1):53.
24. Buchle PW, Kember PA, Wood AD, et al. Factors influencing occupational back pain in Bedfordshire. *Spine.* 1980;5(3):254.
25. Benn RT, Wood PHN. Pain in the back: an attempt to estimate the size of the problem. *Rheumatol Rehabil.* 1975;14:121.
26. Nachemson AL. The lumbar spine: an orthopedic challenge. *Spine.* 1976;1:59.
27. Wyke BD. Neurological aspects of back pain. In: Jayson M, ed. *The Lumbar Spine and Back Pain.* New York, NY: Grune and Stratton; 1976.
28. Botte RR. An interpretation of the pronation syndrome and foot types of patients with low back pain. *J Am Podiatry Assoc.* 1981;71:243.
29. Farfan HF. *Mechanical Disorders of the Low Back.* Philadelphia, PA: Lea and Febiger; 1973.
30. Frigerio NA, Stowe RR, Howe JW. Movement of the sacro-iliac joint. *Clin Orthop.* 1974;100:370.
31. Dontigny RL. Dysfunction of the sacro-iliac joint and its treatment. *J Ortho Sports Phys Ther.* 1979;1:23.
32. Yates A. Treatment of back pain. In: Jayson M, ed. *The Lumbar Spine and Back Pain.* New York, NY: Grune and Stratton; 1976.
33. Korr IM. Experimental alterations in segmental sympathetic (sweat gland) activity through myofascial and postural disturbances. *Fed Proc.* 1948;7:67.
34. Denslow JS. Pathophysiologic evidence for the osteopathic lesion. Data on what is known what is not known, and what is controversial. IN: Goldstein M, ed. *The Research Status of Spinal Manipulative Therapy.* Bethesda, MD: DHEW Publication No. (N/H) 76-998; 1975.
35. Korr IM, Thomas PE, Wright HM. Symposium on the functional implications of segmental facilitation. *JAOA.* 1955;54:265.
36. Denslow JS, Korr IM, Krems AD. Quantitative studies of chronic facilitation in human motoneuron pools. *Am J Physiol.* 1947;150:229.
37. Denslow JS, Hassett CC. The central excitatory state associated with postural abnormalities. *J Neurophysiol.* 1944;5:393.
38. Coote JW. Somatic sources of afferent input as factors in aberrant autonomic, sensory and motor function. In: Korr IM, ed. *The Neurobiologic Mechanisms in Manipulative Therapy.* New York, NY: Plenum Press; 1978.
39. Robinson MF. The influence of head position on temporomandibular joint dysfunction. *J of Prosth Dent.* 1966;16(1):169.
40. Sharp J, Druz W, Danon J, et al. Respiratory muscle function and the use of respiratory muscle electromyography in the evaluation of respiratory regulation. *Chest Suppl.* 1976;70:150.
41. Greenfield B. Upper quarter evaluation: structural relationship and interdependence. In: Donatelli R, Wooden MJ, ed. *Orthopaedic Physical Therapy.* New York, NY: Churchill Livingstone; 1988.
42. Travell JG, Simons DG. *Myofascial Pain and Dysfunction: The Trigger Point Manual.* Baltimore, MD: Williams and Wilkins; 1983.

43. Liebenson CS. Thoracic outlet syndrome: diagnosis and conservative management. *J Manip Physiol Therap*. 1988;11(6):493.
44. Tarsy JM. *Pain Syndromes and their Treatment*. Springfield, IL: Charles C. Thomas; 1953.
45. Finneson BE. *Diagnosis and Management Pain Syndromes*. Philadelphia, PA: WB Saunders; 1969.
46. Cailliet R. *Soft Tissue Pain and Disability*. Philadelphia, PA: FA Davis; 1977.
47. Grieve GP. *Modern Manual Therapy of the Vertebral Column*. New York, NY: Churchill Livingstone; 1986.
48. Grant R. *Physical Therapy of the Cervical and Thoracic Spine*. New York, NY: Churchill Livingstone; 1988.
49. Jeffrey's E. *Disorders of the Cervical Spine*. London: Butterworth; 1980.
50. Wyke B. The neurology of joints. *Ann R Coll Surg Eng*. 1977;41:25.
51. Cloward RB. Cervical discography: a contribution to the etiology and mechanism of neck, shoulder and arm pain. *Ann Surg*. 1959;150:1952.
52. Mannheimer JS, Lampe GN. Differential evaluation for the determination of TENS effectiveness in specific pain syndromes. In: Mannheimer JS, Lampe GN, ed. *Clinical Transcutaneous Electrical Nerve Stimulation*. Philadelphia, PA: FA Davis; 1984.
53. Mannheimer JS, Attanasio R, Cinotti W, Pertes R. Cervical strain and mandibular whiplash: Effects upon the craniomandibular apparatus. *Clin Prev Dent*. 1989;1:29.
54. Joseph J, McColl I. Electromyography of muscles of posture: Posterior vertebral muscles in man. *J Physiol (London)*. 1961;157:33.
55. Janda V. Muscles and cervicogenic pain syndromes. In: Grant R, ed. *Physical Therapy of the Cervical and Thoracic Spine*. New York, NY: Churchill Livingstone; 1988.
56. Baloh RW. *The Essentials of Neurotology*. Philadelphia, PA: FA Davis; 1984.
57. Jull GA. Headaches associated with the cervical spine. A clinical review. In: Grieve A, ed. *Modern Manual Therapy*. Edinburgh: Churchill Livingstone; 1986.
58. Goss CM. *Gray's Anatomy*. 29th ed. Philadelphia, PA: Lea and Febriger; 1973.
59. Baker EG. Alterations in width of maxillary arch and its relation to sutural movement of cranial bones. *JAOA*. 1971;70:559.
60. Magoun HI. The temporal bone: Trouble maker in the head. *JAOA*. 1974;73:825.
61. Upledger FE, Vredevoogd JD. *Craniosacral Therapy*. Seattle, WA: Eastland Press; 1983.
62. Upledger FE, Vredevoogd JD. *Craniosacral Therapy II: Beyond the Dura*. Seattle, WA: Eastland Press; 1987.
63. Retzlaff EW, Mitchell FL. *The Cranium and its Sutures*. Berlin, Germany: Springer-Verlag; 1987.
64. Hassler R, Walker AE. *Trigeminal Neuralgia*. Philadelphia, PA: WB Saunders; 1970.
65. Edmeads J. Headaches and head pains associated with diseases of the cervical spine. *Med Clin No Am*. 1978;62:533.
66. Elvidge AR, Li CL. Central protrusion of cervical intervertebral disc involving descending trigeminal tract. *Arch Neurol & Psych*. 1950;63:455.
67. Brodal A. *The Cranial Nerves: Anatomy and Anatomico-Clinical Correlations*. Oxford, England: Blackwell Scientific Pub; 1965.
68. Dubner R, Gobel S, Pierce DD. Peripheral and central trigeminal pain pathways. In: Bonica JJ, Albe-Fessard D, eds. *Advances in Pain Research and Therapy*. New York, NY: Raven Press; 1976.
69. Kerr FWL, Olafson RA. Trigeminal and cervical volleys: Convergence on single units in the spinal gray at C1 and C2. *Arch Neurol*. 1961;5:171.
70. Kerr FWL. Facial, vagal and glossopharyngeal nerves in the cat: Afferent connections. *Arch Neurol*. 1962;6:264.
71. Bogduk N. Innervation and pain patterns of the cervical spine. In: Grant R, ed. *Physical Therapy of the Cervical and Thoracic Spine*. New York, NY: Churchill Livingstone; 1988.
72. Bogduk N. Cervical causes of headache and dizziness. In: Grieve G, ed. *Modern Manual Therapy*. Edinburgh, NY: Churchill Livingstone; 1986.
73. Bonica JJ. Neurophysiologic and pathologic aspects of acute and chronic pain. *Arch Surg*. 1977;112:750.
74. Dugal GL, Anseman NE. The entrapped greater occipital nerve and internal derangement of the TMJ. *J Cranio Mand Pract*. 1983;2(1):52.
75. Steiger HJ. The anatomy of headache. *Manual Med*. 1987;3(2):37.
76. Kramer J. *Intervertebral Disc Diseases*. Chicago, IL: Yearbook Medical Publishers; 1981.
77. Hayashi K, Yabuki T. Origin of the uncus and of luschka's joint in the cervical spine. *Bone & Joint Surg*. 1985;67-A(5):788.
78. Pawl RP. *Chronic Pain Primer*. Chicago, IL: Yearbook Medical Publishers; 1979
79. Lous I. The cervicolingual syndrome. *Man Med*. 1987;3(2):63.
80. Gayral L, Neuwirth E. Oto-neuro-opthalmologic manifestations of cervical origin: Posterior cervical syndrome of Barre-Lieou. *NY State JMed*. 1954;54:1920.
81. Bogduk N, Windsor M, Inglis A. The innervation of the cervical intervertebral discs. *Spine*. 1988;13(1):2.
82. Oda J, Tanaka W, Tsuzuki N. Intervertebral disc changes with aging of human cervical vertebrae. *Spine*. 1988;13(1):1205.
83. Kraus SL. Influences of the cervical spine on the stomatognathic system. In: Donatelli R, Wooden MJ, eds. *Orthopaedic Physical Therapy*. New York, NY: Churchill Livingstone; 1988.

84. Solow B, Tallgren A. Head posture and craniofacial morphology. *Am J Phys Anthropol*. 1976;44:417.
85. Forrest EB. Astigmatism as a function of visual scan, head scan and head posture. *Am J Optometry and Physiol Optics*. 1980;57(11):844.
86. Kendall HO, Kendall FF. Developing and maintaining good posture. *J Am Phys Ther Assoc*. 1968;49(4)319.
87. Harmon DB. Vision, body mechanics and performance. In: Harmon DB, ed. *Dynamic Theory of Vision*. Duncans, OK: Optometric Extension Program Foundation Inc; 1958.
88. Daly P, Preston CB, Evans WG. Positional response of the head to bite opening in adult males. *Am J Orthod*. 1982;82:157.
89. Vig PS, Showfety KJ, Phillips C. Experimental manipulation of head posture. *Am J Orthod*. 1980;77:258.
90. Hellsing E, Forsberg CM, Linder-Aronson S. Changes in postural EMG activity in the neck and masticatory muscle following obstruction of the nasal airways. *Eur J Orthod*. 1986;8:247.
91. Solow B, Kreiberg S. Soft tissue stretching: a possible control factor in craniofacial morphogenesis. *Scand J Dent Res*. 1977;85:505.
92. Funakoshi M, Amano N. Effects of the tonic neck reflex on the jaw muscles of the rat. *J Dent Res*. 1973;52:668.
93. Funakoshi M, Fujiti N, Takehana S. Relations between occlusal interference and jaw muscle activities in response to changes in head position. *J Dent Res*. 1976;55:684.
94. Boyd CH, Slagle WF, MacBoyd C, et al. The effect of head position on electromyographic evaluation of representative mandibular positioning muscle groups. *J Craniomand Pract*. 1987;5(1):50.
95. Thompson JR, Brodie AG. Factors in the position of the mandible. *JADA*. 1942;29(7):925.
96. Mohl ND. Head posture and its role in occlusion. *NY State Dental J*. 1976; 42:17.
97. Darling DW, Kraus SL, Glasheen-Wray MB. Relationship of head posture and the rest position of the mandible. *J Prosth Dent*. 1984;52(1):111.
98. Ayub E, Glasheen-Wray HB, Kraus SL. Head posture: a recent study of the effects of the rest position of the mandible. *J Ortho & Sports Phys Ther*. 1984;5(4):179.
99. Goldstein DF, Kraus SL, Williams WB, et al. Influence of cervical posture on mandibular movement. *J Prosth Dent*. 1984;52:421.
100. Forsberg CM, Hellsing E, Linder-Aronson S, et al. EMG activity in neck and masticatory muscles in relation to extension and flexion of the head. *Eur J Orthod*. 1985;7:177.
101. Ricketts RM. Respiratory obstruction syndrome. *Am J Orthod*. 1968;54:495.
102. Hellsing E, Reigo T, McWilliam J, et al. Cervical and lumbar lordosis and thoracic kyphosis in 8, 11 and 15 year old children. *Eur J Orthod*. 1987;9:129.
103. Hellsing E, McWilliam J, Reigo T, et al. The relationship between craniofacial morphology, head posture and spinal curvature in 8, 11 and 15 year old children. *Eur J Orthod*. 1987;9:254.
104. Sicher H. Position and movement of the mandible. *JADA*. 1954;48:620.
105. Tallgren A, Solow B. Hyoid bone position, facial morphology and head posture in adults. *Eur J Orthod*. 1987;9:1.
106. Kraus SL. Physical therapy management of TMJ dysfunction. In: Kraus SL, ed. *TMJ Disorders: Management of the Craniomandibular Complex*. New York, NY: Churchill Livingstone; 1988.
107. Lowe A, Johnston W. Tongue and jaw muscle activity in response to mandibular rotations in a sample of normal and anterior open bite subjects. *Am J Orthod*. 1979;76:565.
108. Zacharkow D. *Posture, Sitting and Standing, Chair Design and Exercise*. Springfield, IL: Charles C. Thomas; 1988.
109. Kendall HO, Kendall FP. Developing and maintaining good posture. *J Am Phys Ther Assoc*. 1968;49(4):319.
110. Harms-Ringdahl K, Ekblom J, Schuldt K, et al. Load moments and myoelectric activity when the cervical spine is held in full flexion and extension. *Ergonomics*. 1986;29:1539.
111. Harms-Ringdahl K, Ekblom J. Intensity and character of pain and muscular activity levels elicited by maintained extreme flexion position of the lower cervical-upper-thoracic spine. *Scand J Rehab Med*. 1986;18:117.
112. Alexander CJ. Scheuermann's disease. *Skeletal Radiol*. 1977;1:209.
113. Fisk JW, Baigent ML. Hamstring tightness and Scheuermann's disease. *Am J of Phys Med*. 1981;60:122.
114. Nachemson AL. Disc pressure measurements. *Spine*. 1981;6(1):93.
115. Klein JA, Hukins DWL. Relocation of the bending axis during flexion-extension of lumbar intervertebral discs and its implications in prolapse. *Spine*. 1983;8(6):659.
116. Adams MA, Hutton WC. The effect of posture on the fluid content of lumbar intervertebral discs. *Spine*. 1983;8(6):665.
117. Kelsey JL, Githens PB, O'Connor T, et al. Acute prolapsed lumbar intervertebral discs. *Spine*. 1984;9:608.
118. Wilder DG, Pope MH, Frymoyer JW. The biomechanics of lumbar disc herniation and the effect of overload and instability. *J of Spinal Disorders*. 1988;1(1):16.
119. Rodgers SH. *Working with Backache*. Fairport, NY: Periton Press; 1984.
120. Bendix T, Jessen F, Krohn L. Biomechanics of forward reaching movements while sitting on fixed forward or backward-inclining or tiltable seats. *Spine*. 1988;13(2):193.

121. Steen B. The function of certain neck muscles in different positions of the head with and without loading of the cervical spine. *Acta Morphologica Neerlando Scandinavica*. 1966;6:301.
122. Grandjean E, Hunting W. Ergonomics of posture. A review of various problems of standing and sitting posture. *Appl Ergonom*. 1977;8:135.
123. Jones FP, Gray FE, Hannson JA, et al. Neck muscle tension and the postural image. *Ergonomics*. 1961;4:133.
124. Gray FE, Hansson JA, Jones FP. Some postural effects of neck and muscle tension. *Ergonomics*. 1966;9:245.
125. Maeda K. Occupational cervico brachial disorder and its causative factors *J Human Ecol*. 1977;6:193.
126. Hunting W, Grandjean E, Maeda K. Constrained postures in accounting machine operators. *Appl Ergonom*. 1980;11:145.
127. Westgaard R, Aaras A. Postural muscle strain as a causal factor in the development of musculoskeletal illness. *Appl Ergonom*. 1984;15:162.
128. Duncan J, Ferguson D. Keyboard operating posture and symptoms in operating. *Ergonomics*. 1974;17:651.
129. Bendix T, Hagberg M. Trunk posture and load on the trapezius muscle while sitting at sloping desks. *Ergonomics*. 1984;27:873.
130. Schuldt K, Ekblom J, Harms-Ringdahl K, et al. Effects of change in sitting posture on static neck and shoulder muscle activity. *Ergonomics*. 1986;29:1525.
131. Carlsoo S. The static muscle load in different work positions–an electromyographic study. *Ergonomics*. 1961;4:193.
132. Hunting W, Laubli TH, Grandjean E. Postural and visual loads at VDT workplaces. Constrained postures. *Ergonomics*. 1981;24:917.
133. Bendix T, Krohn L. Jessen F, et al. Trunk posture and trapezius muscle load while working in standing, supported sitting and sitting positions.. *Spine*. 1985;10(5):433.
134. Brunswic M. Ergonomics of seat design. *Physiotherapy*. 1984;70(2):40.
135. Lander C, Korbon GA, DeGood DE, et al. The Balans chair and its semi-kneeling position: an ergonomic comparison with the conventional sitting position. *Spine*. 1987;12:269.
136. Walpin LA. The role of orthotic devices for managing neck disorders. *Archives of Phys Med & Rehabil: State of the Art Reviews*. 1987;1(1):25-43.
137. Andersson GBJ, Murphy RW, Ortegren R, et al. The influence of backrest inclination and lumbar support on the lumbar lordosis in sitting. *Spine*. 1979;4:52-58.
138. Majeske C, Buchanan C. Quantitative description of two sitting positions: with and without a lumbar support pillow. *Phys Ther*. 1984;64:1531.
139. Williams MM, Hawley JA, Mckenzie RA, et al. A comparison of the effects of two sitting postures on back and referred pain. *Spine*. 1991;16:1185.
140. Nakaseko M, Grandjean E, Hunting W, et al. Studies on ergonomically designed alphanumeric keyboards. *Human Factors*. 1985;27:175.
141. Arndt R. Working posture and musculoskeletal problems of video display terminal operators–a review and reappraisal. *J Am Ind Hygiene Assoc*. 1983;44:437.
142. Grunstrom B, Kvarnstrom S, Tiefenbacher F. Electromyography as an aid in the prevention of excessive shoulder strain. *Applied Ergo*. 1985;16:49.
143. Mahlamaki S, Rauhala E, Remes A, et al. Effect of arm support on EMG activity of trapezius muscles in typists. *Acta Physiol Scand*. 1986;18A:126.
144. Occhipinti E, Colombini D, Frigo C, et al. Sitting posture: analysis of lumbar stresses with upper limbs supported. *Ergonomics*. 1985;28:1333.
145. Goetschell GE. A review of the development of an ergonomically balanced chair. *J of Manip & Physiol Therap*. 1987;10(3):65.
146. Davidson RI, Dunn EJ, Metzmaker JN. The shoulder abduction test in the diagnosis of muscular pain in cervical extradural compressive monoradiculopaties. *Spine*. 1984;6(5):441.
147. Mannheimer JS. Physical therapy concepts in evaluation and treatment of the upper quarter: therapeutic modalities. In: Kraus SL, ed. *TMJ Disorders: Management of the Craniomandibular Complex*. New York, NY: Churchill Livingstone; 1988.
148. Wolf SL. Neurophysiologic mechanisms in pain modulation: relevance to TENS. In: *Clinical Transcutaneous Electrical Nerve Stimulation*. Philadelphia, PA: FA Davis; 1984.
149. Wooden MJ. Mobilization of the upper extremity. In: Donatelli R, Wooden MJ, eds. *Orthopaedic Physical Therapy*. New York, NY: Churchill Livingstone; 1989.
150. Zylbergold RS, Piper MC. Cervical spine disorders: a comparison of three styles of traction. *Spine*. 1985;10(10):867.
151. Rath W. *Cervical Traction: A Clinical Perspective*. Minneapolis, MN: Lossing Orthopedic; 1984.
152. Gore DR, Sepic SB, Gardner GM. Roentgenographic findings of the cervical spine in asymptomatic people. *Spine*. 1986;11(6):521.
153. Gore DR, Sepic SB, Gardner GM, et al. Neck pain: A long-term follow-up of 205 people. *Spine*. 1987;12(1):1.
154. Dvorak J, Froehlich D, Penning L, et al. Functional radiographic diagnosis of the cervical spine: flexion/extension. *Spine*. 1988;13(7):748.
155. Rocabado M, Tapia V. Radiographic study of the craniocervical relation in patients under orthodontic treatment and the incidence of skeletal symptoms. *J Craniomand Pract*. 1987;5(1):36.
156. Rocabado M. The importance of soft tissue mechanics in stability and instability of the cervical spine:

a functional diagnosis for treatment planning. *J Craniomand Pract.* 1987;5(2):130.
157. Kraus H. Trigger points. *NY State J Med.* 1973;73:1310.
158. Bonica JJ. Management of myo-fascial pain syndrome in general practice. *JAMA.* 1957;164:732.
159. Stoddard A. *Manual of Osteopathic Practice.* New York, NY: Harper & Row; 1969.
160. Korr IM. Substained sympathicotonia as a factor in disease. In: Korr IM, ed. *The Neurobiologic Mechanisms in Manipulative Therapy.* New York, NY: 1978.

Chapter 6

Mandibular Rest Position: Relationship to Occlusion, Posture and Muscle Activity

Christine G Wheaton, MS, PT

INTRODUCTION

Dentists and physical therapists have found that they need to work together to resolve the problems of patients with Temporomandibular Joint Dysfunction. Postural rest position of the mandible and its relationship to a patient's overall posture are primary concerns for both professions. As Sherrington has stated, "Posture is the basis of movement and all movement begins and ends in posture."[27] Robinson[29] has demonstrated that placing a corrective lift in the shoe of a subject with a shorter leg produces a change in the firing sequence of the temporalis and masseter muscles during chewing. As he states: "A correction of pathologic intercuspation of the teeth is inadequate in the correction of Temporomandibular Joint Dysfunction without correcting the total posture of the individual."[29] Physical therapists' experience with musculoskeletal treatment should be combined with dentists' skill in occlusal restorations and mandibular orthodontics to achieve harmony within the stomatognathic system.[10]

Rocobado[30] has stated that mandibular position is altered in space in all planes as a result of occlusion, muscle activity, and head and neck posture. And Robinson,[29] as mentioned above, was the first researcher to investigate the relationship of leg length to masticatory muscle activity. The author of this chapter feels that further investigation into the relationships of occlusion, muscle activity, head position, and leg length with the position of the mandible is needed. Some clinical questions to be addressed are: 1) Does the mandible deviate toward the long or the short leg? 2) Will a shoe lift alter mandibular position and change a patient's pain symptomatology? 3) If muscle activity is a variable of rest position, is muscle dominance an additional variable to consider? For example, does the mandible normally deviate toward the preferred side of chewing or the hand-dominant side? And if so, can the midline position still be viewed as the goal in repositioning treatment?

In this chapter, information will be provided regarding the relationships of occlusion, posture, and muscle activity with mandibular position and masticatory muscle activity. This will be done first through a literature review, and then by presenting the results of a study done by this author. Mandibular measurement procedures and instrumentation are included and compared so that the reader can incorporate this knowledge into his or her clinical measurement techniques. A summary of the research results and potential clinical findings will lead us to treatment implications for both the dentist and physical therapist.

DEFINITION OF MANDIBULAR POSTURAL REST POSITION

The term "rest position" has generally been used to refer to the postural rest position of the mandible. Confusion exists in the dental literature, however, because the term has also been used to refer to the vertical dimension at rest, which is the position of the mandible in the sagittal plane only. The term "mandibular postural rest position" here refers to the postural position of the mandible from all planes of reference and should replace the term "rest position."

Atwood[3] defines "rest position" as the habitual postural position of the mandible when the patient is relaxing comfortably in the upright position and the condyles are in a neutral, unstrained position in the glenoid fossae. Additionally, there is no single absolute position that has been defined, but rather a normal range of positions which will vary between and within individuals at different times.[12,27] According to Mohl, the "rest position" of the mandible is present when the masticatory muscles are in equilibrium. The activity of these muscles is related to those of the neck and trunk and the direction of the gravitational forces acting upon the body. Consequently, an action or condition which alters the activity of a related muscle group should affect the masticatory muscles and theoretically alter the postural rest position of the mandible.[23]

A shoe lift or an injury such as cervical whiplash or low back strain can be considered as an action which could affect the masticatory muscles and therefore mandibular postural rest position. Any chronic spinal or other chronic orthopedic dysfunction anywhere in the body could also theoretically alter mandibular postural rest position over time due to structural and/or muscular imbalances which result in faulty posture and abnormal biomechanics. Conversely, the activity of the neck and trunk musculature may be related to that of the masticatory muscles such that an action or condition which alters the activity of the masticatory muscles could affect the muscles of the neck and trunk. For example, some patients with Temporomandibular Joint Dysfunction experience low back pain for the first time after receiving a mandibular repositioning appliance.

Mandibular postural rest position is defined as the habitual postural position of the mandible in all planes of reference, governed primarily by the activity of the temporalis and external pterygoid muscles, and is the result of occlusal, muscular, and structural interrelationships within the entire body.[6-8,11,16,20,21,23,25-30,33,36,40] The condyles of the mandible may or may not be in a neutral, unstrained position in the glenoid fossaè. Habitual posture may be considered to be orthostatic or pathologic. It represents one mandibular position, the others being the occlusal and centric position.[37]

LITERATURE REVIEW

Comparison of Instrumentation and Methodologies for Measuring Mandibular Postural Rest Position

"Anybody who has ventured upon rest position determinations by one method or another will have discovered that he has taken on a difficult task."[9]

Mandibular postural rest position has been measured with cephalometric radiographs, electromyography, kinesiography, and instrumentation using soft tissue markings between the subnasal point and the menton.[3,8,12,13,17,21,22,24,27,36] Clinical tools measuring facial markings are a caliper, a jaw relator, and the McMillan instrument.[12,22,24] To measure the transverse component of postural rest position, Rider[28] marks the dentition and Rocabado[30] utilizes the relationship of the lower lip frenulum to the upper lip frenulum with the mandible in the occlusal position.

Cephalometrics has been criticized as static and only two-dimensional, while the electromyograph has been felt to be clinically impractical.[12,13] Garnick and Ramfjord[12] found differences between clinical and electromyographic measurements. The mandibular kinesiograph does give a three-dimensional representation of the position of the mandible at rest and during motion. Given that fact, and the problems associated with other methods, the mandibular kinesiograph is felt by this author to be the best instrument for mandibular research. However, the time and financial investments required for this equipment do not make it readily available to every clinician. Niswonger[24] has recommended discarding the jaw relator, as edentulous patients found their previous rest position through what he termed tactile muscle sense. Additionally, measurements with the mandible in the occlusal position do not represent postural rest position even if they may be related to it.

McMillan, Barbenel, and Quinn[22] have found a high degree of reproducibility in mandibular measurements taken from soft tissue markings with the mandible in the occlusal position. But as they placed occlusal splints of differing widths intraorally to give increasingly greater vertical dimensions, they found measurements between facial marks to be unreliable. The invasiveness of an intraoral device and its effect on reproducible measurements must be considered in judging the validity of their results.

To facilitate the patient's placing his or her mandible in postural rest position, the clinician may use fatigue, phonetic, spontaneous relaxation, instructed relaxation, deglutition, and/or aesthetic appearance.[3,12,13,27] In comparison studies, no statistical difference was found between fatigue, phonetics, and relaxation techniques or between deglutition, phonetics and relaxation.[3,12] In contrast with those results, Eliasson found spontaneous or instructed relaxation to be more reliable than phonetics and swallowing.[13]

Traditional clinical analysis of the mandible is done with the patient sitting. But Shpuntoff and Shpuntoff[36] feel that the most accurate position for recording rest position is standing. However, if the patient is seated erect without a back support, they state that satisfactory readings can be obtained.

Factors to Consider in Mandibular Postural Rest Position

Many variables must be taken into consideration when conducting mandibular measurements. Posture, respiration, and stress have been described as short term variables, and edentulousness as a long term variable.[7] Fatigue, denture form, palatal thickness, tooth positioning, health, age, psyche, size, form and interrelations of the lips, and tongue size relative to the bony framework of the oral cavity have also been listed as factors in making mandibular measurements.[3] Shpuntoff and Shpuntoff[36] state that the major factors influencing the electromyograph of postural rest position are posture, pain, fatigue, and excitation of the central nervous system. One can begin to appreciate the difficulty an experimenter has in controlling so many variables in research and how challenging the mandible is to analyze and treat clinically. The ensuring literature review will be limited to a discussion of occlusion, posture, and muscle activity as variables in mandibular postural rest position.

Occlusion. Thompson[37] states that mandibular postural rest position is established before the teeth have erupted, and that it is constant regardless of the status of the dentition. Clinicians' experiences, however, would seem to belie this. However, some clinical relevance is found in his feeling that restorative and/or orthodontic procedures could not *permanently* alter postural rest position. The effect of postural imbalances on mandibular position is a possible reason for the inability of rest position to become permanently altered through occlusal treatment because posture is habitual and a result of compensatory mechanisms over time. Preiskel[27] has supported the concept of postural rest position as a learned site influenced by several factors. In contrast with Thompson, however, he states that the position of the mandible incentric occlusion is one factor in postural rest position.

An interrelationship between occlusion, masticatory muscle balance, and temporomandibular joint position has been described by Wentz.[17] Occlusion has been reported to influence patterns of neuromuscular activity.[17] In addition, occlusal imbalance has been said to mechanically change the relationship of the parts of the temporomandibular joint.[17] Occlusal interferences or premature contacts, as in Class II, Division I occlusion, have been related to muscle spasm associated with Temporomandibular Joint Dysfunction.[33]

Head Position and Movement and Its Effects on Mandibular Postural Rest Position and Upper Quarter Muscle Activity. Mohl[23] has stated that head posture appears to have the most significant and immediate effect upon mandibular postural rest position. Correction of forward head posture in patients with Temporomandibular Joint Dysfunctions has long been advocated by Rocabado.[30] Clinical research has supported this relationship (head posture/mandibular rest position) when physical therapy correction of a forward head posture on one subject was found to increase that subject's vertical dimension by eight millimeters.[4]

Studies have shown that the vertical dimension of postural rest position may vary with different head positions in the sagittal plane.[8,21,23,27,29,33,36] Cohen[8] has demonstrated cephalometric changes in the vertical dimension of rest position in edentulous subjects with three different head positions in the sagittal plane. Preiskel[27] has demonstrated electromyographically and clinically that vertical dimension at rest changes with different head positions in the sagittal plane. Schwarz[33] has found differences in occlusal wax forms with movements of the head in the sagittal plane. He theorizes that normal and abnormal development of occlusion may thus be related to chronic head posture. Posselt[23] has found changes in postural rest position when the Frankfurt plane of the head is altered.

Brill, Lammie, Osborne, and Perry[7] have stated that postural rest position will alter with changes in head position. The only study found investigating the transverse component of postural rest position was that done by Shpuntoff and Shpuntoff.[36] They found electromyographically that head movements produce a shift of the mandible, but they did not qualify their results.

The muscles of mastication and postural position have been found to be affected by head position.[6,11,16,20,29,36] Most of this electromyographical research has studied the effect of head rotation on upper quarter muscle activity and presents different results based on whether the sample had normal or abnormal occlusions. Funakoshi, Fujita and Takehana[11] have found that with right rotation of the head and neck, the right temporalis, masseter, and digastric muscles increase their activity in subjects with normal occlusions. In subjects with occlusal interferences, bilateral or contralateral muscles demonstrate increased activity. Halbert[16] has found increased activity in the right posterior cervical, left infrahyoid, right and left temporalis and masseter muscles with right rotation of the head and neck.

Latif[20] and Perry[26] found that the temporalis, particularly the posterior fibers, and the external pterygoid muscles are the fine working postural muscles of the mandible. Pruzansky found temporalis muscle activity with head rotation in a torticollis patient while there was no activity in the upright postural rest position in normals.[23]

Leg Length. Robinson's study[29] was the only one found relating the total posture of a subject to the function of the stomatognathic system. He established a relationship between leg length and masticatory muscle activity during chewing. A corrective lift for a shorter leg yielded a normal electromyographic firing pattern, while removal of the lift gave a firing pattern which was characteristic of malocclusion.

Leg length is a result of the structural relationships and muscle dynamics of the lower quarter. The position of the femoral head in the acetabulum is dependent on sacroiliac and pelvic positions/dysfunctions.[31] The pelvis is the key to good or faulty posture.[19] Iliosacral dysfunctions of posterior torsion or anterior torsion can produce an apparent shortening or elongation of the lower extremity, respectively.[31] Clinically, in standing, a relatively high iliac crest may be due to a long leg on that side or marked posterior torsion of the ilium. A sitting test of iliac crest levels would determine the cause. Standard ASIS to medial malleolus measurements of leg length were found to be reliable when the difference was 1/2 inch, but unreliable when the difference was 1/4 inch.[15] Differences of 3/8 inch with pelvic dysfunctions are most commonly found by this author.

Masticatory Muscle Activity During Chewing. In a study by Gibbs, Messerman, Reswick, and Derda,[14] eighty-six percent of the chews of subjects with normal occlusions showed a definite working side condyle with good closure repeatability in normal occlusions. They found that the first chews of a series indicated the working side condyle. In malocclusion subjects, repeatability of closure was poor. Perry[25] demonstrated that in both normal and abnormal occlusions, the greatest

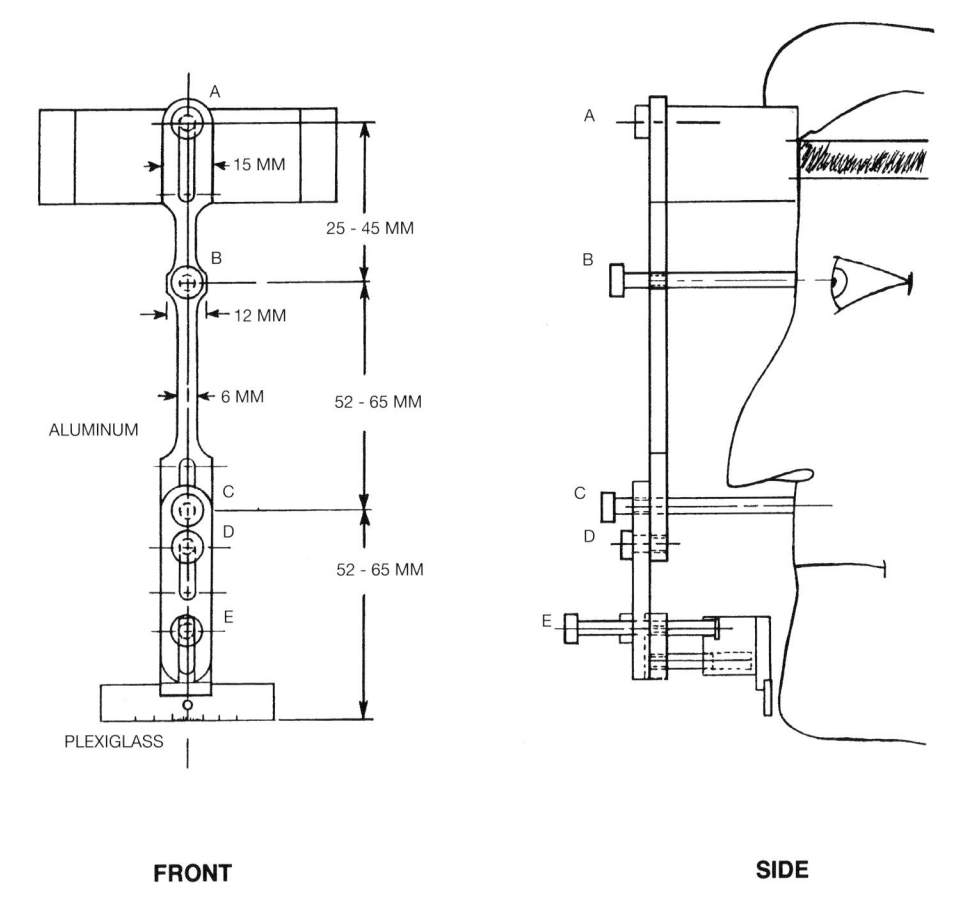

Fig. 6-1. The Mandibular Postural Locator (Patent pending, Wheaton, 1988).

synchrony and harmony of peak amplitudes occurred on the preferred side of the occlusion.

MANDIBULAR POSTURE AND ITS RELATIONSHIP TO OCCLUSION, POSTURE, AND MUSCLE ACTIVITY

It is necessary to expand the researcher's and clinician's point of view from the sagittal plane (vertical dimension at rest and forward head) into the transverse plane in order to compare left, right, and midline relationships between the mandible and occlusion, posture, and muscle activity. The mandibular postural locator was developed as a clinical tool for mandibular measurements in the transverse plane. Following the establishment of the instrument's reliability, it was used in a study to investigate mandibular postural rest position in the transverse plane to determine if correlations and intercorrelations exist with the longer leg, head tilt, incisive position, chewing dominance, and hand dominance.

The Mandibular Postural Locator (Wheaton, 1988)

For mandibular measurements, this instrument uses a reference line (nasion-subnasal), which is felt to be more reliable as a fixed reference than a single point (subnasal), as in previous soft tissue measurements.

Measurement Procedure. The nasion, subnasal point, and the mentonian symphysis are identified by soft tissue markings. The instrument is secured via the head band and adjusted for differing facial dimensions and mandibular positions (Fig. 6-1). The zero reading of the ruler is in line with the nasion-subnasal reference line. The mandible is measured by the vertical line drawn through the menton in reference to the horizontal millimeter ruler.

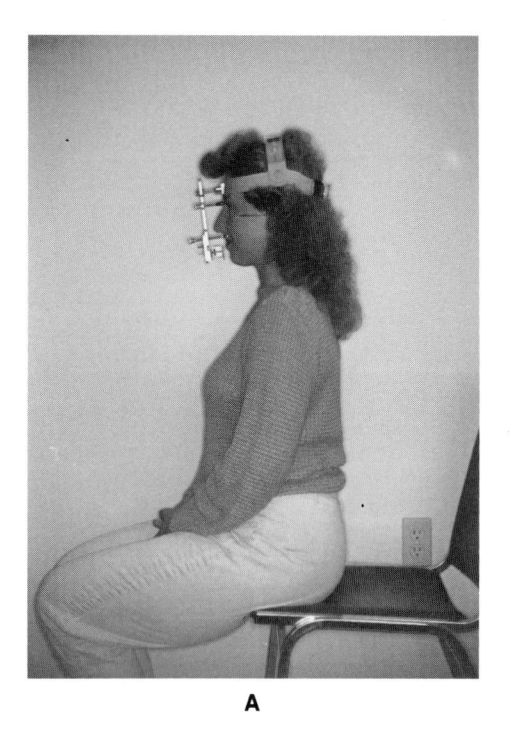

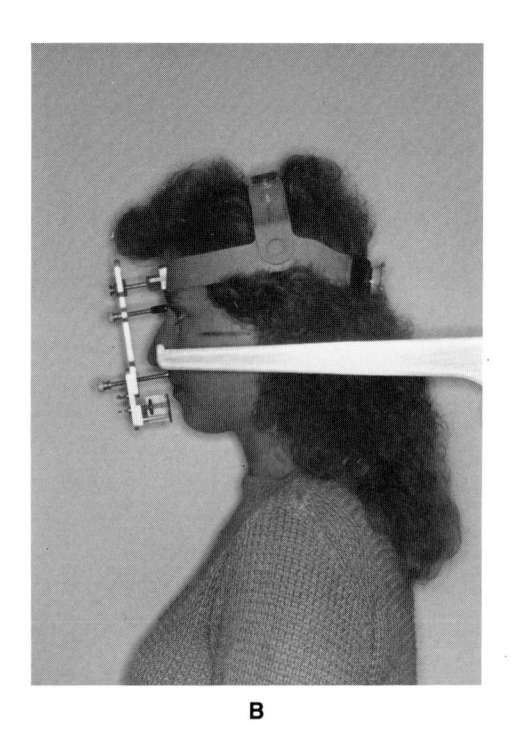

Fig. 6-2, A and B. Mandibular postural locator measurement controlled by Frankfurt plane.

Head and neck posture is controlled in the sagittal plane by maintaining the Frankfurt plane parallel to the floor when taking mandibular measurements.[12,23,24,27,34] An independent observer visually insures that the line drawn on the subject's face (Frankfurt plane) is horizontal to a reference bar at face height which is parallel to the floor during measurements (Figs. 6-2 A and B).

Spinal posture is controlled by having the subject sit erect at the edge of a chair, maintaining a normal lumbar lordosis.[36]

Since measurements should be taken on a relaxed subject, the subject is asked to relax, sitting for five minutes prior to testing with the instrument in place.[7,12,34]

In order to control for fatigue of the masticatory muscles, the subject is requested not to speak, masticate, or engage in parafunctional activities during the relaxation and measurement period.

The procedure for the subject to achieve mandibular postural rest position is deglutition and command relation with the lips contacting lightly, teeth apart.

Reliability. Intertester reliability was established by an analysis of variance comparing the means of three measurements on the same subject by four different testers. A non-significant difference in measurements among testers resulted.

A Spearman rank order correlation coefficient was computed to establish intratester reliability. The score for the test and retest was the means of three measurements taken on nine subjects by one tester. A moderately significant correlation (.721) was found between tests. Since the correlation was not high, a test for matched groups was applied as a double check of reliability. A non-significant difference between test-retest mean measurements was found.

The relative stability of the transverse component of postural rest position was supported. The average range of variation between each test of three measurements was .97 mm; the average variance, .1 mm; and the average standard deviation was .22 mm. In comparison to measurement studies done for the vertical dimension at rest using cephalometrics, these measurements had similar variations and a smaller standard deviation.[3]

A Study Done by Wheaton, 1988

Subject Selection. Fifteen Class I, Division I subjects (10 female and 5 male) who

Table 6-1. Normative criteria for subjects in the author's study, 1988.

1. Full teeth (third molars absent and one replacement tooth if functionally adequate occlusion)
2. No extensive restorations that were determined to have changed a subject's previous occlusion
3. No prior history of orthodontic treatment
4. No history of temporomandibular joint disturbance
5. No history of head or neck injury
6. A functionally adequate occlusion
7. No active periodontal disease or treatment
8. No history of bruxism in combination with headaches and extreme overclosure
9. No extreme overclosure
10. No present musculoskeletal pain
11. No present medications which would affect the neuromuscula

completed the Rieder questionnaire and met certain criteria[1,2,12,13,28,36] were randomly selected from a number of dental practices. A dentist determined the type of occlusion and if criteria 1, 2, 6, 7, 8, 9, and 13 were met (Table 6-1).

Measurement Instruments. Mandibular postural rest position was measured with the mandibular postural locator according to the previously described procedure. In order to measure head tilt, a plumb line was suspended from the head band assembly of this instrument at point A (Fig. 6-3) with its vertical component displaced away from the subject's face. The head tilt measurement was taken as the distance between the plumb line and the subnasal point. Leg length measurement was done by having the subject stand on two height and weight scales, one per leg, so that the level of the height scale could be placed at the greater trochanter and the measurement recorded for the entire supporting limb. Hand dominance was determined from the questionnaire. The first two chews of a 2 cm x 2 cm piece of hard bread indicated chewing dominance.[14,18] Comparison of the midline between the mandibular incisors with the maxillary incisors in the occluded position constituted incisive position.

Measurement Procedures. The sequence and number of testing was: 1) Mandibular postural rest position in sitting, three measurements; 2) Head tilt in sitting, three measurements; 3) Leg length in standing, two alternating measurements per leg; 4) Incisive position in sitting, one measurement; 5) Chewing dominance, first two chews.

A five minute relaxation period with the mandibular postural locator in place was given prior to mandibular measurements. A two minute standing relaxation period followed head tilt measurements. The subject was asked to stand equally on both feet with his/her midfeet six inches apart. Following leg length measurements and prior to the incisive position test, the subject relaxed in a sitting position for two minutes.

Subjects were asked if they were experiencing any pain or were on any medication prior to measurement. Those who answered positively were omitted from the study.

Speech, mastication, and parafunctional activities were not permitted from the initial relaxation period through the chewing dominance test.

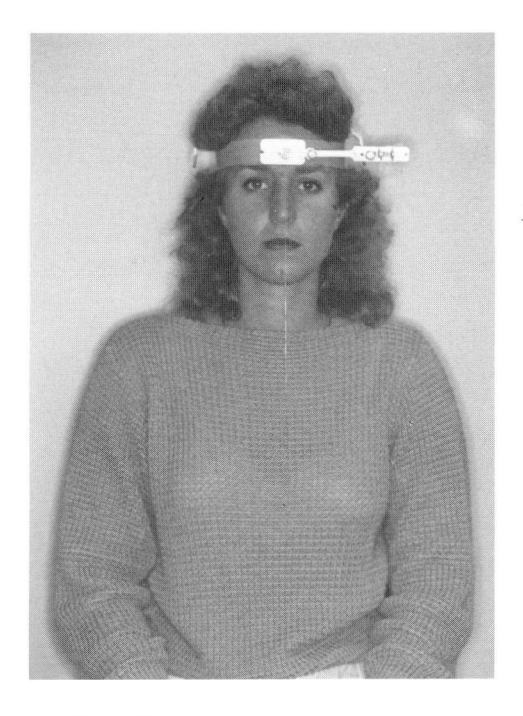

Fig. 6-3. Head tilt measurement.

Table 6-2. Correlations between mandibular postural rest position and incisive position, longer leg, chewing dominance, hand dominance, and head tilt, respectively, for combinations of magnitude and direction.

Class I, Division I Occlusion
Mandibular Postural Rest Position

Magnitude

	Direction r	Direction r	Magnitude r
Incisive position	.484	.755	*
Long leg difference	.430	.625	.165
Observed chewing dominance	.290	.505	*
Hand dominance	.220	.440	*
Head tilt	-.220	.103	.396

NOTE: *Magnitude tests were done only on continuous data. n = 15 for each group.

Analysis of Data. Measurable (continuous) data was obtained for mandibular postural rest position, the longer leg difference, and head tilt. A negative sign was assigned to all left-sided measurements and a positive sign to all right-sided measurements. Non-measurable (dichotomous) data constituted right, left, or midline position of the incisors, and right or left chewing and hand dominance. Left-sided determinations were rated as 0, midline as 1, and right-sided as 2. Three Spearman rank order correlations were computed to determine the magnitude and direction relationships and the directional relationships between sets of variables, and to represent the relationship of the magnitude of displacement of the mandible with the discrepancy between leg length and with the displacement of the head. The magnitude and displacement correlations were the only ones based on the raw measurable data without assignment of signs or numbers. A table of intercorrelations analyzed all relationships between all the variables.

Results and Interpretation of Results. In Class I, Division I occlusion, the variable with the strongest correlation to mandibular postural rest position was incisive position (.484, .755). The second strongest was the longer leg difference (.43, .625). The third strongest correlation was chewing dominance (.29, .505). The strengths of these correlations were considered to be low to moderate according to the broader significance levels of Sharp[35] since mandibular postural rest position has a normal range of values instead of a fixed position.

A weak correlation was found between mandibular postural rest position and hand dominance (.22, .44) while there was essentially no correlation with head tilt (-.22, .103, .396). Comparison of the results of the three Spearman rank order correlation coefficients is presented in Table 6-2.

In comparing the three rank order correlation analyses, it is important to note that the magnitude and direction correlations and the direction correlations support each other by demonstrating the same order or trend in variables with the highest to lowest correlations. Additionally, directional analysis presented the strongest correlations overall, supporting its use in the analysis of these variables.

The relationship between variables is presented in Table 6-3 for correlations of .4 or higher. The relationship between head tilt and hand dominance was the strongest among all variables.

On the basis of the results of statistical analyses, this author presents a conceptual

Table 6-3. Selected intercorrelations between mandibular postural rest position, incisive position, longer leg difference, head tilt, observed chewing dominance, and hand dominance.

Class I, Division I Occlusion

	Strength of r	Coefficient r_s*
Head tilt and hand dominance	Moderate Positive	.567
Incivise position and mandibular postural rest position	Low Positive	.484
Observed chewing dominance and hand dominance	Low Positive	.464
Longer leg difference and observed chewing dominance	Low Positive	.448
Longer leg difference and mandibular postural rest position	Low Positive	.430

NOTE: r_s = magnitude and direction Spearman rank order correlation.

*r_s > .4 only are listed

NEGATIVE CORRELATIONS   **POSITIVE CORRELATIONS**

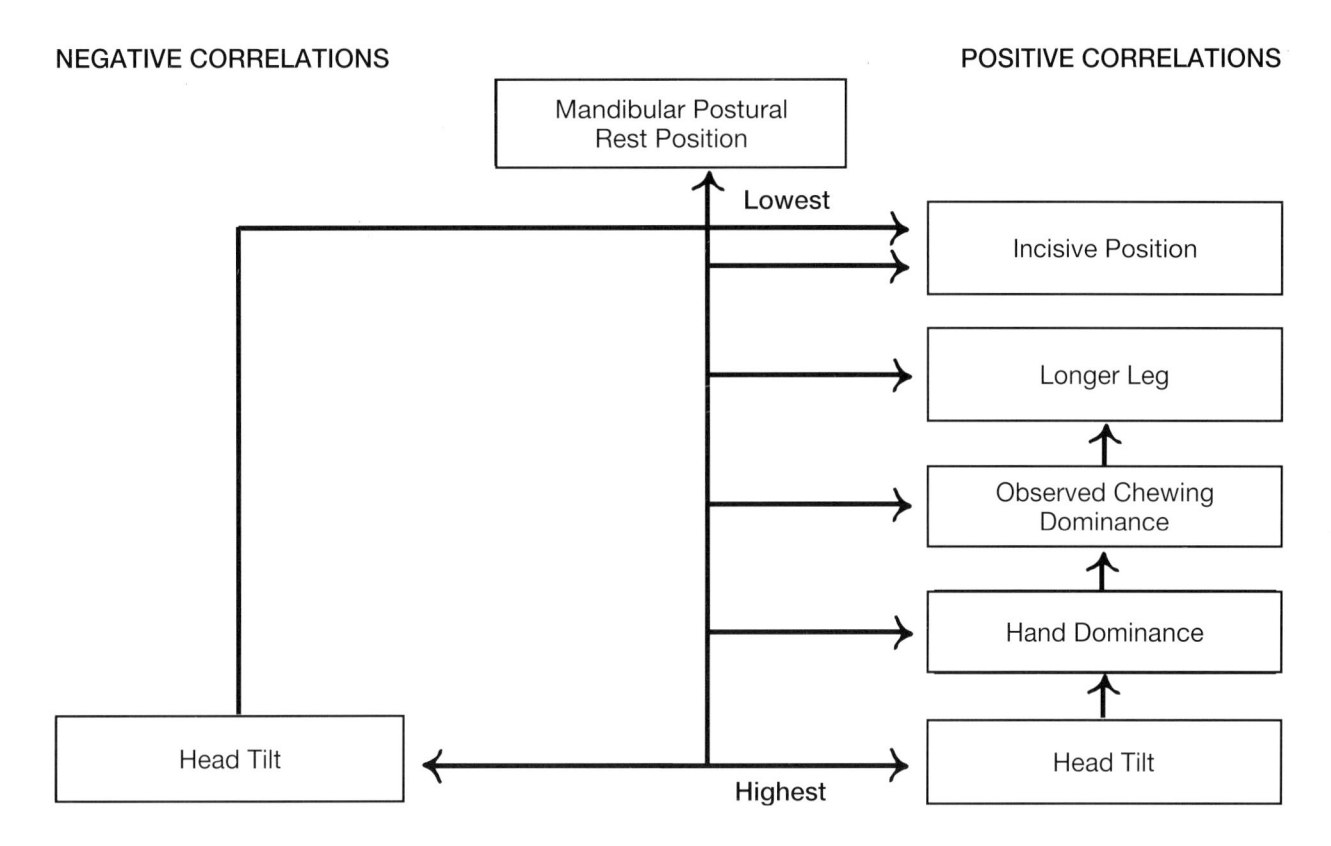

Fig. 6-4. Conceptual model for the relationship of the mandible to overall posture, occlusion, and muscle function of the upper quarter in Class I, Division I Occlusion.

model for the relationships between variables (Fig. 6-4).

Positive correlations would indicate that as one variable increases, the other would increase. When directionality is applied, one may possibly interpret a positive correlation as representing the two variables being toward the same side (a right sided mandible tends to deviate toward the longer leg, which is also right-sided). Conversely, a negative correlation would indicate that as one variable increased, the other would decrease with the possible result that each is on opposite sides (a right head tilt with a left incisive position).

Head tilt was the only variable to demonstrate both positive and negative directionality relationships with the variables. Head tilt demonstrated a negative relationship with the structural variables, mandibular postural rest position and incisive position (< .4). No correlation was found between head tilt and the longer leg difference, most likely because measurements were taken in a sitting position where the effects of leg length were eliminated. The positive correlations between head tilt and hand dominance, and hand dominance and chewing dominance may support the concept that masticatory muscle activity is modified by head position and that there is a dynamic component between head position and muscle activity of the upper quarter.[6,11,16,20,29,36] One may conclude that head tilt may have positive relationships with dynamic variables (muscle) and negative relationships with static ones (structural). To further understand the interplay between static and dynamic components of head tilt and the position of the mandible to the same or opposite side, the reader is referred to Figure 6-5.

Conclusions. The small sample size in this study can only suggest trends, but the fact that two statistical analyses demonstrated the same trend cannot be ignored. On the basis of the results of statistical analyses, one may conclude that in Class I, Division I occlusion, mandibular postural rest position has a

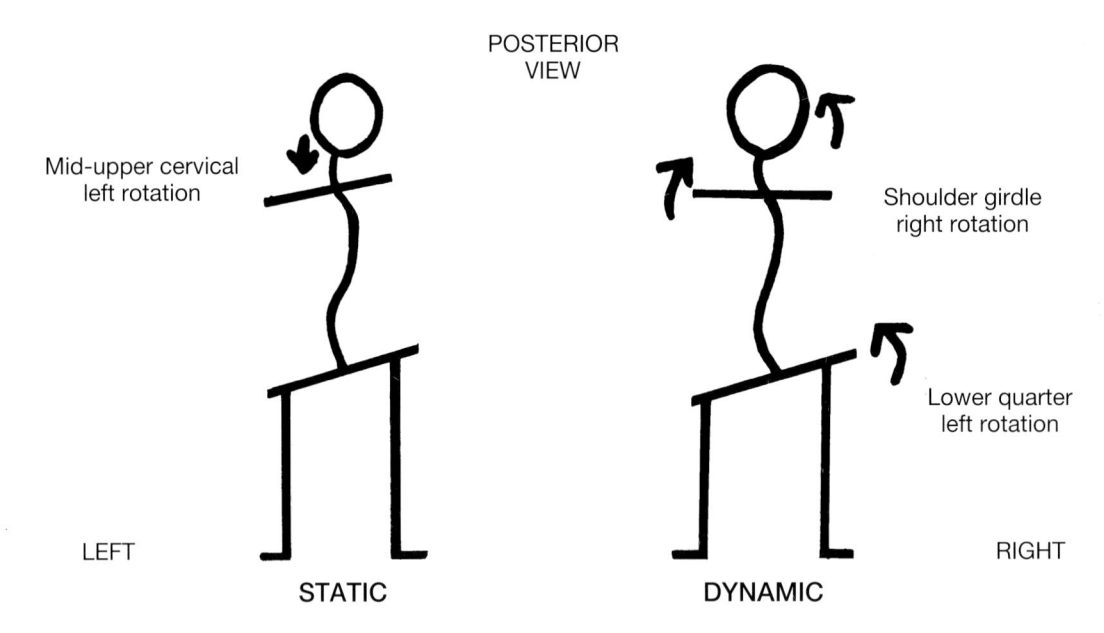

Fig. 6-5. Static and dynamic postural compensations of head tilt. Common static posturing with an elevated shoulder on the same side as the longer leg/higher iliac crest. At times the head tilt may tend to the right from increased right upper quarter muscle activity, but would be positioned left to maintain the eyes horizontal. The Dynamic figure represents total body compensation typically seen. Upper cervical spine left rotation to maintain the face forward position would result in a right head tilt. These examples, while not the only ones, help to explain why head tilt may have negative or static and positive or dynamic relationships. This may explain why upper cervical hypermobility is difficult to stabilize without treatment to the entire spine or body.

low-to-moderate positive correlation with incisive position, the longer leg difference, and chewing dominance; a low positive correlation with hand dominance; and no correlation with head tilt, although it was the only variable to present positive and negative directionality. Results suggest that since incisive position and the longer leg difference demonstrated the highest correlation with mandibular postural rest position, one may conclude that dental intervention and physical therapy treatment for total postural/spinal correction in temporomandibular joint patients is supported.

SUMMARY

Occlusion

Incisive Position has been found to be the variable with the highest correlation to mandibular postural rest position in Class I, Division I occlusion.[40] The teeth affect postural rest position through conditioned neuromuscular reflexes. Abnormal occlusion or articulation of the teeth can cause disturbances of the temporomandibular joint through muscle spasm and protective reflexes, resulting in an altered mandibular postural rest position.

Posture and Muscle Activity

The longer leg discrepancy had the second highest positive correlation to mandibular postural rest position in Class I, Division I occlusion.[40] An interrelationship between chewing dominance and the longer leg has been established by Wheaton and Robinson.[29,40] Leg length is a result of the structural relationships and muscle dynamics of the lower quarter. The measurements of the leg taken from the greater trochanter to the floor incorporate the entire supporting structure. The position of the femoral head in the acetabulum is dependent on sacroiliac and pelvic positions. The lumbar spine moves opposite to the sacrum through the iliolumbar ligaments. A right rotated sacrum would produce left rotation of the lower lumbar segments. The mid and upper lumbar segments would be in relative right rotation.[31] The biomechanical chain reaction throughout the entire spine is evidenced in the patient with a chronic lower quarter pain history which eventually spreads to involve the upper quarter, including headaches and facial pain.

Forward *head position* has been shown to affect the vertical dimension of postural rest position.[4,8,21,23,37,29,33,36] Head rotation has been shown to alter the electromyographic response of the muscles of mastication and postural position.[6,11,16,23] Head tilt has been shown to have weak positive and negative correlations with mandibular postural rest position in Class I, Division I occlusion.[40] On the basis of these findings, one may expect the mandible to be positioned opposite to the head tilt and toward the side of increased muscle activity of the temporalis muscle. A left head tilt would result in right rotation of the head with resultant increased activity of the right temporalis muscle, which would pull the right mandibular condyle toward a closed packed position. A right positional mandible may result. In abnormal occlusions or articulations of the teeth, the contralateral or bilateral muscle activity may result in different mandibular positions.[11,16,23]

Chewing dominance and hand dominance were shown to correlate positively to mandibular postural rest position and positively to each other (same-sidedness) in Class I, Division I occlusion.[40] Additionally, head tilt was found to correlate to the same side as the hand dominance. The importance of the relationship between upper quarter muscle activity and mandibular position has been supported. Muscle dominance must be considered as a variable in postural rest position when analyzing and treating the mandible.

TREATMENT IMPLICATIONS AND CONCLUSIONS

Rocabado advocates physical therapy treatment for the head, neck, temporomandibular joints, and for any dysfunctions within the upper quarter. He has claimed a seventy percent correlation between Class II malocclusion and an anterior head position, along with other postural changes of the upper quarter which result in facial pain.[32]

A recent study done by Darlow, Pesco and Greenberg[9] did not support the concept that posture is a primary etiologic factor in the evolution of Myofascial Pain Dysfunction (MPD) Syndrome. They found no significant difference between control and experimental groups among 19 static and 9 dynamic posture parameters. Head tilt and iliac crest measurements were not calculated in the statistical analysis because the groups did not present moderate or stronger grades of deficiencies. Chi square analysis was done on only one subject for trochanter height. Their result has raised concern among practitioners. Upon critical review of this study, one must consider that 1) the type of occlusion was not described for the samples; 2) there was a lack of controls; and 3) the grading procedure used is questionable since there were no measurements taken and mild discrepancies between variables within and between groups were not accounted for.

This author's determination of a positive correlation between mandibular postural rest position and the longer leg difference in Class I, Division I occlusion may support Rocabado's treatment approach for Class II malocclusion when one considers orthodontic treatment of Class II malocclusions to obtain a Class I relationship of the dentition and/or of the mandible. Although they are referring to two different classes of occlusion, both myself and Rocobado are advocating postural alignment and restoration of muscle equilibrium.

Treatment techniques for patients with Temporomandibular Joint Dysfunctions must expand from the limited viewpoint of upper quarter dysfunctions into a total biomechanical approach incorporating the entire body. John Barnes, P.T. and John Upledger, D.O. credit the fascial systema as the primary reason for interrelationships within the body. The fascia is a tough connective tissue which spreads three dimensionally throughout the entire body, surrounding every muscle, bone, nerve, blood vessel, and organ.[5,39] According to their beliefs, a restriction in the fascia in one area of the body may be the cause of pain complaints in another area. Additionally, the reason for the large percentage of patients with low back pain and dysfunctions who complain of head, neck, and facial pain and, conversely, the large percentage of patients with head, neck, and TMJ pain and dysfunctions who complain of low back pain may be attributed to the fascial system. While its role in integrating the body systems and pain symptomatologies is presently controversial, future treatment outcome studies will hopefully resolve this dispute. John Barnes' Myofascial Releases and John Upledger's Craniosacral Therapy address treatment of the fascial system to relieve pain and dysfunction with longer lasting results than other types of physical therapy techniques. According to both treatment concepts, altering the relationship of the glenoid fossa to the mandibular condyle through myofascial treatment adds another dimension to the present temporomandibular treatment approach.

Friedman and Weisberg state that "the experience that physical therapists have in dealing with muscles and joints in general should be combined with dentists' experiences in evaluating and modifying an occlusion."[10] Dentists and physical therapists should take into consideration the variables of incisive position, head position, leg length, pelvic base, and muscle activity and dominance of the upper quarter when analyzing and repositioning the mandible and when treating the musculoskeletal and myofascial systems in order to resolve Temporomandibular Joint Dysfunctions.

The mandible should be analyzed from all planes of reference, such as those done with the mandibular kinesiograph. The mandibular postural locator can be used for clinical measurements in the transverse plane in order to compare the position of the mandible with left and right postural and muscular findings of the patient. Standing mandibular measurements should be documented and compared with sitting measurements in order to examine the role of the longer leg. Finally, and most importantly, the differences in all measurements and finds must be described for each type of occlusal population since one should expect to find differences between groups.

A complete history, inclusive of past and present orthopedic dysfunctions, should be taken and followed by a thorough postural evaluation in order to understand the body's compensatory mechanisms over time. Some principles of biomechanics and some postural relationships, as clinically observed by this author, are presented in this chapter in order to stimulate other clinicians in thinking about the body as an integrated system. Every patient is different in terms of where the first dysfunction/injury occurred and how additional variables over time caused the patient to have the pain symptomatology and clinical findings that he or she is presenting upon examination. For example, a patient had sustained a motorcycle injury to his shoulder which went untreated and resulted in an osseous restriction in mobility and adaptive soft tissue shortening. He developed lower and upper quarter pain and dysfunctions over the years and was seen finally for a mandibular repositioning appliance because of headaches and facial pain. If the shoulder dysfunction were neglected in his treatment, a successful treatment result could not be expected in the long term, because the shoulder will always set up abnormal postural compensations and muscular imbalances which will spread.

Although the pelvic base must be restored to neutral, the author would caution against the use of a corrective shoe lift when apparent leg length differences may be due to pelvic, sacral, or lumbar dysfunctions. The patient's pain complaints may only be temporarily helped, or even worsened if treatment to correct those dysfunctions is not administered. The entire spine must be treated to undo long-standing compensatory mechanisms and change craniosacral relationships.

In summary, current research and treatment concepts and techniques for Temporomandibular Joint Dysfunctions are recommending that more variables be taken into consideration and treated in order to resolve the patient's pain symptomatology with longer lasting results. One must consider that we are dealing with an integrated system which requires a multidisciplinary approach.

REFERENCES

1. Alexander PC. Movements of the condyle from rest position initial contact and full occlusion. *J Am Dent Assoc.* 1952;45:282-293.
2. Atwood DA. A review of fundamentals on rest position and vertical dimension. *Int Dent J.* 1959;9:6-19.

3. Atwood DA. A critique of research of the rest position of the mandible. *J Prosthet Dent*. 1966;16:848-854.
4. Ayub E, Glasheen-Wray M, and Kraus S. Head posture: A case study of the effect on the rest position of the mandible. *J Orthop Sp Phy Ther*. 1984;4:179-183.
5. Barnes J. Myofascial Release Approach. Seminar presented in Boston, Mass. 1987: July 17-19.
6. Brennan HS. Postural effects on occlusion. *Dent Prog*. 4:47-51.
7. Brill N, Lammie GA, Osborne J, et al. Mandibular positions and mandibular movements. *Br Dent J*. 106:12;391-400.
8. Cohen S. A cephalometric study of the rest position in edentulous persons: influence on variations in head position. *J Prosthet Dent*. 1957;7:467-472.
9. Darlow LA, Pesco J, and Greenberg M. The relationship of posture to myofascial pain dysfunction syndrome. *J Am Dent Assoc*. 1987;114:73-75.
10. Friedman MH and Weisberg J. Application of orthopedic principles in evaluation of the temporomandibular joint. *J Am Phy Ther Assoc*. 5:597-603.
11. Funakoshi M, Fujita H, and Takehana S. Relation between occlusal interference and jaw muscle activities in response to changes in head position. *J Dent Res*. 1976;55:684-690.
12. Garnick J and Ramfjord SP. Rest position, an electromyographic and clinical investigation. *J Prosthet Dent*. 1962;5:895-910.
13. George JP and Boone ME. A clincial study of rest position using the kinesiograph and myomonitor. *J Prosthet Dent*. 1979;4:456-462.
14. Gibbs CH, Messerman DT, REswick JB, et al. Functional movements of the mandible. *J Prosthet Dent*. 1971;26:604-620.
15. Gogia PP and Braatz JH. Validity and reliability of leg length measurements. *J Orthop Sp Phy Ther*. 1986;4:185-188.
16. Halbert R. Electromyographic study of head position. *J Can DentAssoc*. 1958;24:11-23.
17. Jarabak JR. An electromyographic analysis of muscular and temporomandibular joint disturbances due to imbalances in occlusion. *Angle Orthod*. 1956;26:170-190.
18. Jemt T, Hedegard B. Reproducibility of chewing rhythm and of mandibular displacements during chewing. *J Oral Rehabil*. 1982;9:531-537.
19. Kendall FP and McCreary EK. Muscles: Testing and Function, 3rd ed. Baltimore: William and Wilkins; 1983.
20. Latif A. An electromyographic study of the temporalis muscle in normal persons during selected positons and movements of the mandible. *Am J Orthod*. 1957;43:577-591.
21. McLean LF, Brennan HS, and Freidman MGF. Effects on changing body position on dental occlusion. *J Dent Res*. 1973;5:1041-1045.
22. McMillan DR, Barbenel JC, and Quinn DM. Measurement of occlusal face height by dividers. *Dent Pract Dent Rec* 1970;5:177-179.
23. Mohl ND. Head posture and its role in occlusion. *NY State Dent J*. 1976;42:17-23.
24. Niswonger ME. The rest position of the mandible and the centric relation. *J Am Dent Assoc*. 1934;21:1572-1582.
25. Perry HT. Functional electromyography of the temporal and masseter muscles in class II, division I malocclusion and excellent occlusion. *Angle Orthod*. 1955;1:49-58.
26. Perry HT. Facial, cranial, and cervical pain associated with dysfunctions of the occlusion and articulations of the teeth. *Angle Orthod*. 1956;3:121-128.
27. Preiskel HW. Some observations on the postureal position of the mandible. *J Prosthet Dent*. 1965;4:625-633.
28. Rieder CE. Development of a simplified system for clinical evaluation of occlusal relationships, Part IQ Acquisition of information. *J Prosthet Dent*. 4:264-441.
29. Robinson MJ. The influence of head position on temporomandibular joint dysfunction. *J Prosthet Dent*. 1966;1:169-172.
30. Rocabado M. Head, Neck and Temporomandibular Joint Dysfunction. Seminar presented in Boston, Mass. 1980: March 3-5.
31. Rocabado M. Pelvic Girdle. Seminar presented in Keystone, Colo. 1983: February 11-13.
32. Rocabado M. Physical therapy and dentistry: an overview. *J Craniomandib Prac*. 1983;4:46.
33. Schwarz AM. Positions of the head and malrelations of the jaws. *Int J Orthod*. 1928;14:56-68.
34. Shanahan TEJ. Physiologic vertical dimension and centric relation. *J Prosthet Dent*. 1956;6:741-747.
35. Sharp VF. Statistics for the Social Sciences. Canada: Little, Brown, and Co.; 1979:320.
36. Shpuntoff H and Shpuntoff W. A study of physiologic rest position and centric position by electromyography. *J Prosthet Dent*. 1956;5:621-628.
37. Thompson JR. Concepts regarding function of the stomotognathic system. *J Am Dent Assoc*. 1954;48:626-637.
38. Thompson JR and Brodie AG. Factors in the position of the mandible. *J Am Dent Assoc*. 1942;7:925-941.
39. Upledger JE and Vredevogd JD. Craniosacral Therapy. Seattle, Wash: Eastland Press; 1983.
40. Wheaton CG. Mandibular posture and its relationship to occlusion, posture, and muscle activity. Thesis, Northeastern University, Boston Bouve College of Human Development Professions, Boston, Mass: 1988.

Chapter 7

The Essentials of the Alexander Technique

Stanley Knebelman, DMD
Patricia Ralston Dressler, MSEd
Mary Mathews Brion, MSW
Lynn Buono, BA

INTRODUCTION

An individual is in the best of health only when the body is so used that there is no strain on any of its parts. The Alexander work is about changing misuse of the body that causes strain to good use of the body that promotes health. It was discovered by F.M. Alexander in the 1890's. He was in his early twenties and enjoying the prospects of a very successful acting career. Unfortunately, he was plagued with recurring sore throats and loss of voice that did not respond to conventional medical treatment. He took it upon himself to study and observe in mirrors how he was using his body while speaking and reciting. After close to nine years, he found out what he was doing to injure himself and how to correct it. His pupil, George Bernard Shaw, wrote "he set himself to discover what it was that he was really doing to disable himself in this fashion by his efforts to produce the opposite result. In the end, he found this out and a great deal more as well. He established not only the beginnings of a far-reaching science of the apparently involuntary movements we call reflexes, but a technique of correction and self control which forms a substantial addition to our very slender resources in personal education." The painstaking, step-by-step observations that Alexander made are documented autobiographically in his *Use of the Self*.

Upon speaking or reciting, Alexander found he used unnecessary muscle tension. The unnecessary muscle tension involved pulling down his head in the back, gasping for breath, and depressing the larynx; loss of voice was the result. In addition, as he misused his head and neck to speak, he also noticed that he lifted his chest, and in his words "shortened his stature." He then concluded that the way he used his head, neck and torso affected the way his larynx functioned.

At this point, he thought that all he had to do to cure himself was to stop the bad habits he'd discovered. He could stop pulling down his head, as well as the other misuses individually, but as he started to speak, all of the misuse of his head, neck and torso returned. He could not do what he thought he could do to stop the misuse, nor could he depend on what he felt to help himself. His conclusion was that his sensory appreciation was not "trustworthy" and could not be used as a guide to correct faulty habit patterns in the use of himself to speak or recite on stage.

After many more months of observation, he realized that it was the very thought of speaking that established the pattern of misuse of his head, neck and back in the act of speaking. Up until now, the emphasis had been on the physical aspect of voice production that he was trying to control. At this point, controlling thinking about the act became a critical factor. It was now necessary to unite mind and body in an effort to stop the faulty habit pattern in producing the misuse; the problem now needed a psychophysical solution. He decided to refuse to speak and at the same time project thoughts as to the relationship his head, neck and back were to assume to one another as he spoke. These thoughts in Alexander's work are called *orders*. The refusal he called *inhibition*, not to be confused with Freudian inhibition. The relationship of his head to his neck to his back he called the *Primary Control* of his use. The orders were: Let the neck be free to let the head go forward and up; Let the back lengthen and widen. The inhibition and ordering were used to learn a new way of speaking. At first, he broke down words and pronounced a syllable; inhibited the desire to speak; got his orders to his head, neck and back going again; and gave permission to pronounce a second syllable. This process was repeated and repeated with thinking, inhibition, and ordering accompanying the act of speaking first syllables, then words, and sentences. Finally, he was able to speak with his neck free to allow his head to go forward and up, to allow his back to lengthen and widen. This personal clinical research spanned a period of at least nine years. During this time, he found out the cause of his functional disorder, and discovered how to correct it.

After becoming well, he did not return to the stage; instead, he chose to teach others what he had learned. Alexander became known as a teacher of breathing and voice production. By 1899, he was recognized by the medical profession in Australia, who sent him patients. The Alexander Technique had become a method for changing and controlling reaction to stimuli. The present day definition of stress in Dorland's Medical Dictionary is, "the sum of the biological reactions to any adverse stimulus, physical, mental or emotional, internal or external, that tend to disturb the organism's homeostasis; should these compensating reactions be inadequate or inappropriate, they may lead to disorders." Alexander was diagnosing and successfully treating stress disorders long before Selye's scientific work on stress; and although Alexander never conducted any scientific research to satisfy the medical community, he helped thousands to gain relief from headache, backache, respiratory illnesses, indigestions, constipation, and various kinds of nervous disorders.

In 1934, Alexander delivered a lecture at the Bedford Training College for physical therapists in England. He explains the rationale of his Technique. "Those of you who have read the *Use of Self* will know how after long experimentation on myself, when I was trying to overcome my own difficulties, I found that a certain control of the use of my neck and head in relation to my back brought about a more satisfactory working of the musculature, and not only relieved my special difficulty, but improved conditions generally. In working with my pupils, I have used this experience and have found that as soon as you can establish this 'primary control,' as we call it, a satisfactory control of the rest of the workings of the organism can be expected to follow in due time, according to the conditions present." Alexander goes on to say, "If anything is wrong with a person's use of himself, the first thing is to find out what he is doing that is causing the trouble and to get him to stop doing that."

In a pamphlet entitled *The Brain and Its Mechanism* (Cambridge University Press, 1937), Sir Charles Sherrington wrote, "I may seem to stress the preoccupation of the brain with muscle. Can we stress too much that preoccupation when any path we trace in the brain leads directly or indirectly to muscle? The brain seems a thoroughfare for nerve action passing on its way to the motor animal. It has been remarked that Life's aim is an act, not a thought. Today the dictum must be modified to admit that to refrain from an act is no less an act than to commit one, because inhibition is coequally with excitation a nervous activity."

In Alexander's fourth book, *The Universal Constant in Living*, 1941, he wrote, "The carrying out of the procedures in my technique is just this preoccupation of the brain with the thought responsible for the nervous activity involved in the passing on of messages, whether these result in the prevention or in the carrying out of the act."

THE ALEXANDER LESSON

The object in neuromuscular re-education (The Alexander Lesson) is to teach the pupil the inhibitory technique while he learns to send messages for the carrying out of an act without engaging in motor activity. The teacher provides the motor activity in a gentle fashion, the pupil allows this to take place.

There has to be an understanding and acceptance of the principles involved in the Alexander Technique by the pupil. Inhibition, stopping, non-doing all mean refusal to react to stimuli, i.e., the idea to sit, stand, talk, walk, write, etc. are refused. Guiding orders to neck, head and back relationship are thought by the pupil. These orders are repeated and repeated and at the same time, the pupil allows the teacher to free the neck, guide the head forward and up (in the standing position) to allow the back to lengthen and widen.

As a rule, lessons should start with the pupil flat out, preferrably on an examining table. The table should be suited to the requirements of the teacher's stature when he or she is in good use. Usually, support under the head is needed so that unnecessary tension in the suboccipital region is able to be released with gentle guidance by the teacher. One or both knees should be pointed up to the ceiling with one or both feet flat on the table. The arms should be able to rest on the table, elbows out, palm surfaces down. Initially, it may be necessary to brace hands, arms, legs, and feet with sand bags or pillows to allow them to assume a position of release without strain. With both the pupil and teacher ordering (the pupil to himself, the teacher sometimes out loud to help the pupil learn the process), the teacher may now guide the head, free the neck, widen and lengthen the back, lengthen and move an arm, a hand or leg, release the shoulders, the fingers, the toes. Now, repeat the process with pupil non-doing while ordering the head, neck and back pattern. The body is treated as a whole by the teacher, who is coordinating tension-free movement of all parts with his and the pupil's primary control in good use.

Once the principle of inhibition is learned and appreciated by the pupil, new experiences in tension-free movement may be had. The pupil may now be ready to be taught good use in standing, walking, sitting, getting in and out of the chair, etc., the teacher's hands gently releasing, guiding without undue force. The touch is one of a physical suggestion to the pupil; the pupil's decision to allow release and movement at the behest of the teacher's touch and guidance causes the new experience in movement by the pupil. A lesson usually lasts 30-40 minutes. The number of lessons required is usually 10-15 minimum. One is learning a new lifestyle, not getting therapy. To truly benefit from the Alexander Principle and Technique, there should be a willingness to apply this re-education to daily living. Once the commitment to inhibition, ordering, and thinking in activity is made a daily routine, bodily use will get better and better. All physiological processes will improve and the environment for good health will be promoted.

The Harvard University Chart for Grading Body Mechanics

A—Excellent mechanical use of the body

1. head straight above chest, hips and feet;
2. chest up and forward;
3. abdomen in or flat;
4. back, usual curves not exaggerated.

B—Good mechancial use of the body (compare with A)

1. head too far forward;
2. chest not so well up or forward;
3. abdomen, very little change;
4. back, very little change.

C—Poor mechancial use of the body (compare with A)

1. head forward of chest;
2. chest flat;
3. abdomen relaxed and forward;
4. back curves exaggerated.

D—Very poor mechanical use of the body (compare with A)

1. head still farther forward;
2. chest still flatter and farther back;
3. abdomen completely relaxed, "slouchy;"

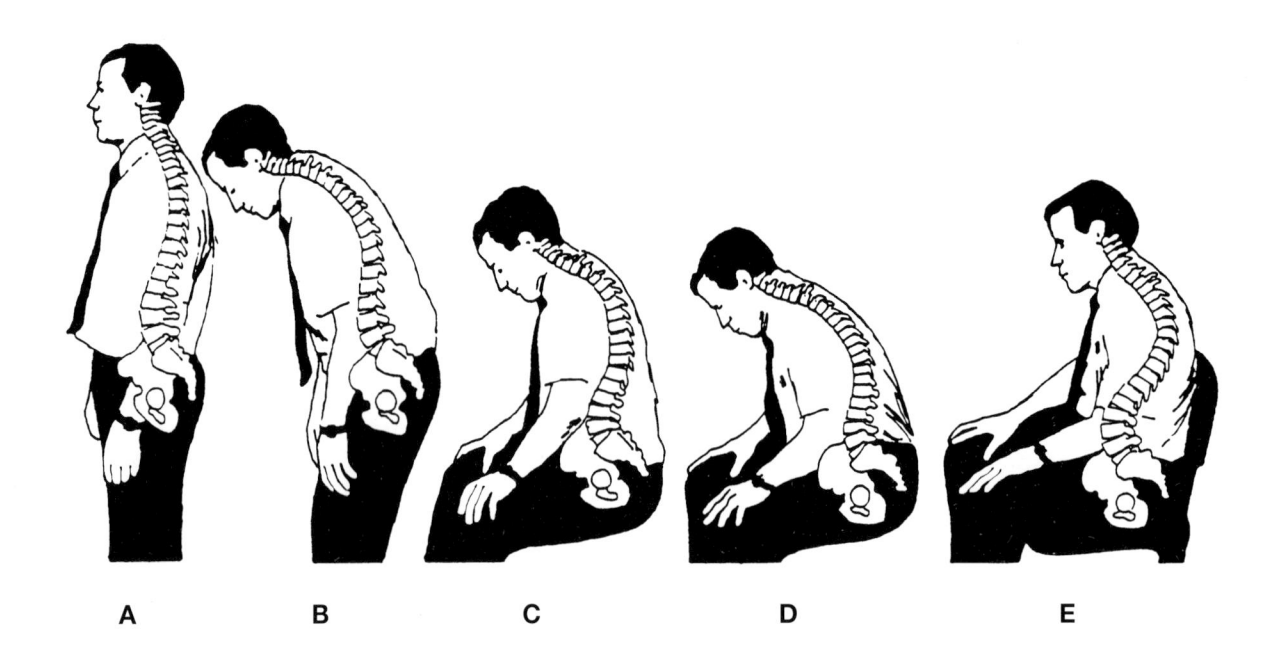

Fig. 7-1. Misuse in standing and in the act of sitting down. **A,** Misuse in standing—the head held forward with the neck being pulled down in the back—early kyphosis of the thoracic spine. **B-C,** In the act of sitting down the forward head position is not being supported properly by the cervical spine and its unsupported weight causes an increase in the kyphotic curve with concomitant unnecessary strain on all of the vertebrae, their joints, ligaments and associated muscles, nerves and blood vessels. **D,** The hands and arms are now used to brace the weight of the thorax, head and neck assuming the role that the cervical thoracic and lumbar spine should play. **E,** Getting situated "comfortably" in the slumped position in the chair. In this position, all physiological processes associated with the head, neck, thorax and abdomen are compromised by this habit in the act of sitting down.

4. back, all curves exaggerated to the extreme.

With permission from: Goldthwaite E, Brown T, Swaim T, Kuhns G. *Essentials of Body Mechanics in Health & Disease.* 5th ed. Philadelphia, PA: JB Lippincott Co; 1952.

If someone is standing in a slumped position, they are causing an exaggeration of the spine, dropping of the chest, crowding of the viscera and all the sequela of visceroptosis. The approach should not be to medicate for back, respiratory or digestive problems, but rather to make the patient aware that his lack of control and conscious direction in the use of himself in the act of standing is a prime consideration.

Since the patient's response to the idea of standing is to slump, it is the thought and habit of standing that has to be changed. Trying to stand straight from a slump that is habitual is like asking a crooked man to walk a straight mile. The point is that the kinesthetic sense that has been used as a guide for standing with strain cannot be depended on to establish standing with physiological balance and ease. The Alexander teacher gives the patient the new experience of standing with ease and balance with gentle manipulations of the tense anatomical parts. It is interesting to note that Goldthwaite et al. said, "The first requirement for use of the body as a whole in proper poise is that the curves of the spine from the sacrum to the occiput shall not be exaggerated. For example, in the habitual standing or sitting position, the lumbar curve, particularly at the lumbo sacral junction, must have further motion in extension as well as flexion. In the common faulty standing position (with the pelvis in a forward position and the lower abdomen prominent), the lumbo sacral joints are used in the position of complete extension. This applies to the other parts of the spine as well."

Table Lesson

Preparation: Light, loose-fitting clothing is preferred. If the pupil wears glasses, he or she should keep them on to maintain orientation in space. The pupil is aligned in the middle of the table, equally distant from side to side so the midline of the table corresponds to the pupil's spinal column, and the top of the head is on line with the top edge of the table, knees up. This position provides the basis for the teacher's corresponding optimal muscle tonis, optimal use of self, optimal synchrony of verbal instructions, and interactions between structural relationships of teacher to pupil and pupil to teacher (Fig. 7-2).

Chair Lesson

As the understanding between pupil and teacher grows, they become more of a synchronized unit, the teacher thinking in activity—the pupil thinking in activity, inhibits and directs allowing the subtle body learning of good use to take place (Fig. 7-3).

CONCLUSION

In teaching the Alexander work to help people suffering from stress disorders, it is essential to enlist the aid and cooperation of the pupil to assume responsibility for their misuse. Unfortunately, willingness to want to correct poor habit patterns is not sufficient to change automatic responses to stimuli. "Patterns of all movement by voluntary muscle are dictated by cortex function and stored memory engrams." The principle of inhibitory nervous function applies to changing habit and re-education of the faulty reflex patterns.

A well poised body in activity without unnecessary muscle tension or rigidity means better health through tension-free organic functioning. When the body is working without strain, there is an improved energy level and all ailments due to stress will be lessened. Lessening of head, neck and back pain occurs concommitant with a series of lessons, since there is a return to normal range of motion and proper anatomical spacing of all parts. Cailliet in *Neck and Arm Pain* states, "the early manifestations of neck pain and the significance of limited motion are frequently overlooked because of ignorance of normal functions and abnormal deviations. In later life, neck pain and its sequelae are attributed to aging or to the wear and tear of life. Sufferers from these effects would have benefitted from earlier recognition and a more physiological approach to treatment."

After a successful series of lessons, the pupil will have learned how to consciously control his own reaction to stimuli and be able to return to a balanced resting state after reacting to a given situation. This is truly a psycho-physical phenomenon. It is important to note that one must continue the discipline of working on oneself in daily life. It may be necessary to take refresher lessons.

"Learning how to learn" is what distinguishes the Alexander Technique from all other "ways to grow." Thinking, directing, giving orders, or however you wish to describe it, is not an end in itself. It has value, and meaning only as it is applied to the pupil's own life. As Marjorie Barstow, an American teacher who was in Alexander's first training course put it, "giving orders is a procedure that turns into activity, not (into) fixed positions; the teacher is only a guide to help the student learn to think and do for himself—it is the teacher's job to help the student carry 'the work' into daily activities."

Professor Raymond Dart, anatomist, anthropologist, paleontologist and discoverer of the skull which was called "The Missing Link," had this to say: "The validity of Alexander's work has been proven. In fact, one might say it is self-evident. Therefore, do not waste any more time trying to prove it. Get on and teach it."

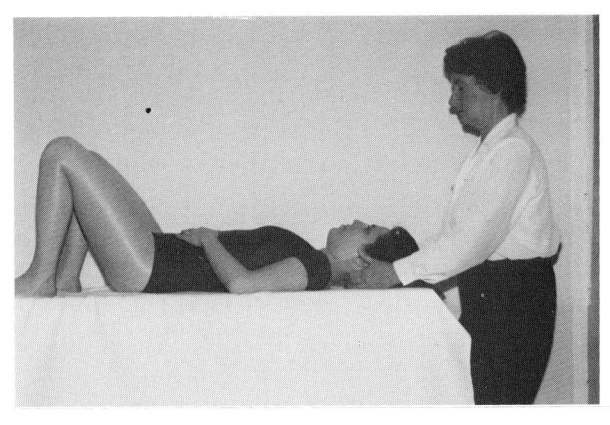

A. The teacher's hands give gentle, precise directions. This contact produces a minimal stretch and resultant release.

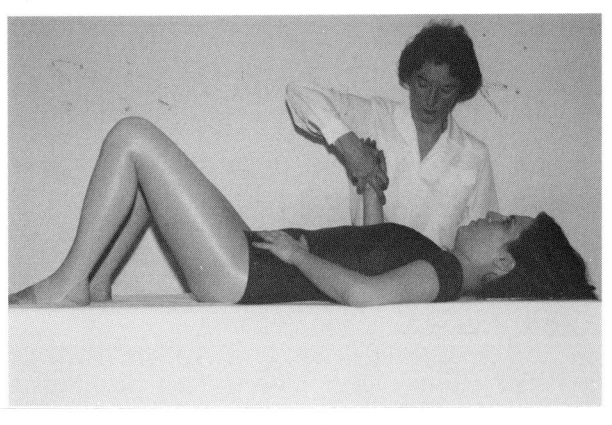

B. The teacher lifts an arm by bridging the wrist joint and keeping the forearm on its center of gravity. This permits a natural stretch. Conscious constructive use of gravity is an integral part of the lesson.

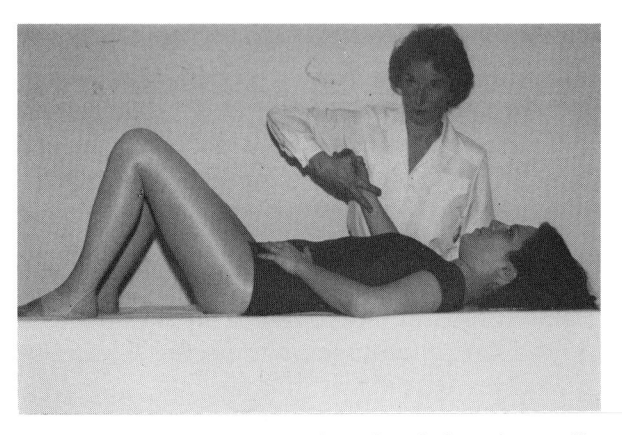

C. With both the teacher and pupil ordering, the pupil's arm is gently supported and moved away from the torso. This gives the pupil the experience of movement through the normal range of motion with the relief of any tension and restriction in the shoulder girdle.

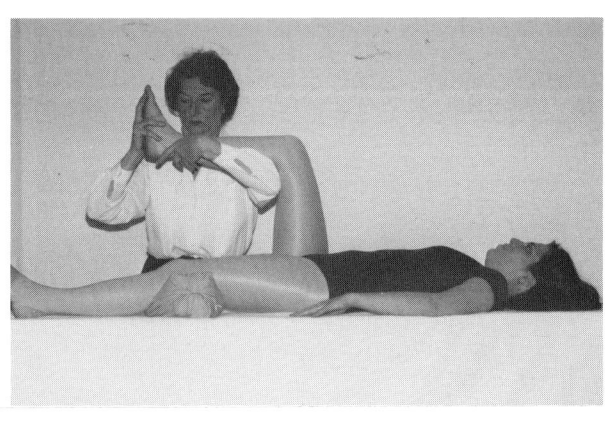

D. The teacher emphasizes the natural patterns of good movement and gives the experience of "relationings" of weights, leverage and differences in angles of lower leg to upper leg and leg to pelvis.

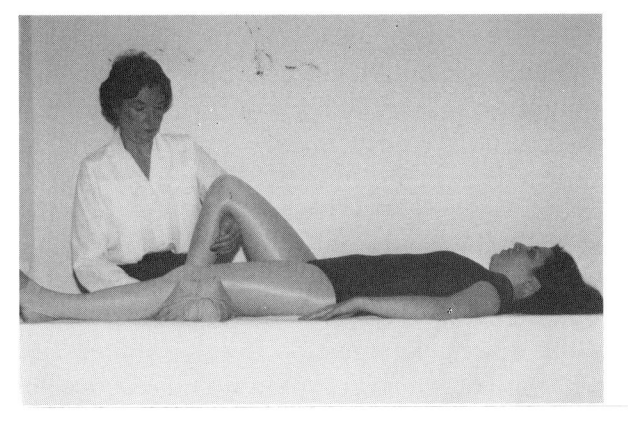

E. The pupil, feeling her body supported by the table, is encouraged to release any tension and allow the teacher to give her the experience of tension-free movement. She thus may discover the existence of tension patterns of which she was not previously aware.

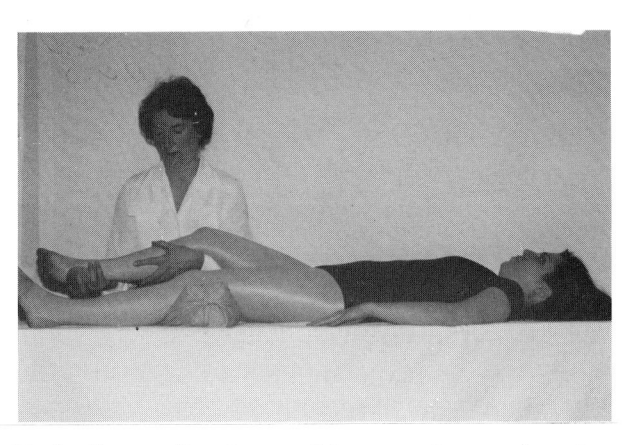

F. As the pupil gains confidence and can allow the teacher to move a leg without anticipating the move or helping, learning can take place.

Fig. 7-2, A-F. The Alexander Table Lesson.

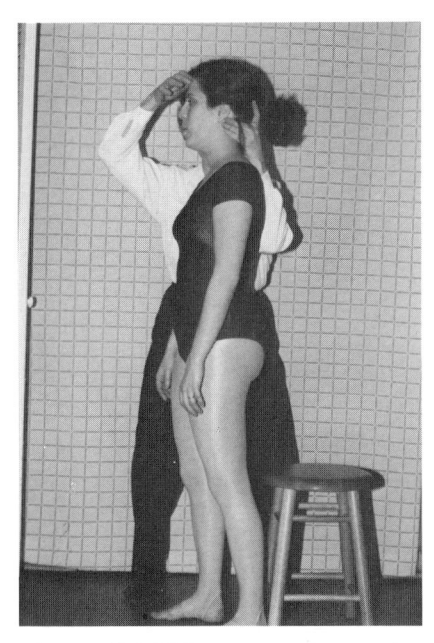

A. Here the pupil inhibits, responding to the stimulus to sit down. "Inhibition is a positive, not negative force. Some degree of inhibition is essential not only for a good life, but for any life at all. Inhibition maintains the integrity of the responding organism so that a particular response can be carried out economically without involving inappropriate activity in unrelated parts."

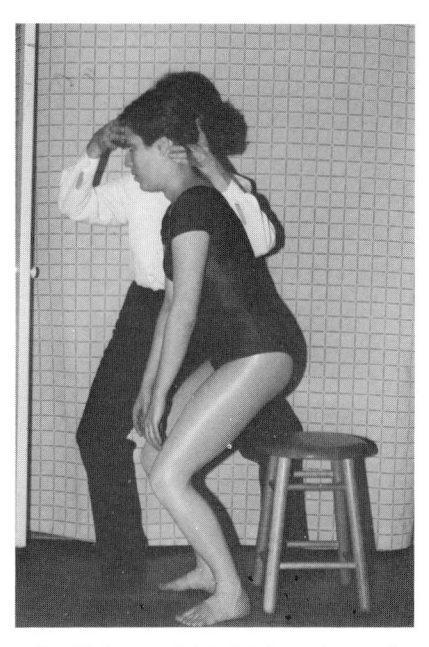

B. The pupil with her weight distributed equally on each foot, stands with them apart, the same distance as the width of her shoulders. She then allows the teacher to guide her head forward and up with her neck free, to allow the knees to bend forward and out and the back to go back.

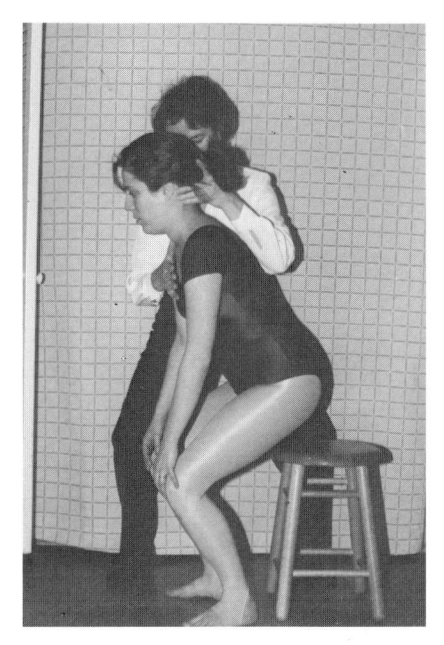

C. The pupil is moving down on her center of gravity with the spine lengthening in both directions (up and down).

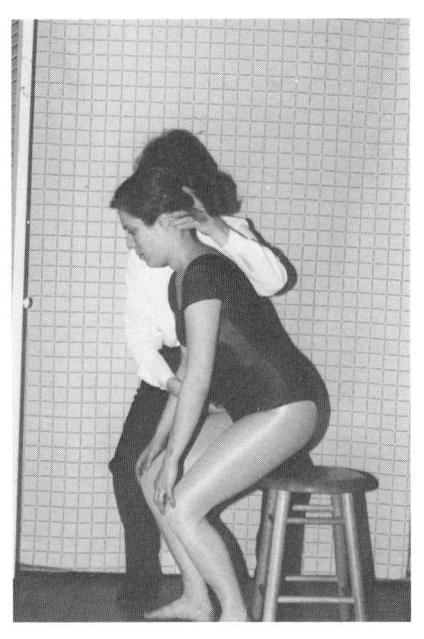

D. The teacher makes certain that there is no unnecessary tension at the atlanto occipital junction, so that flexors and extensors of the neck and head are balanced in their "pulls."

Fig. 7-3, A-F. The Chair Lesson.

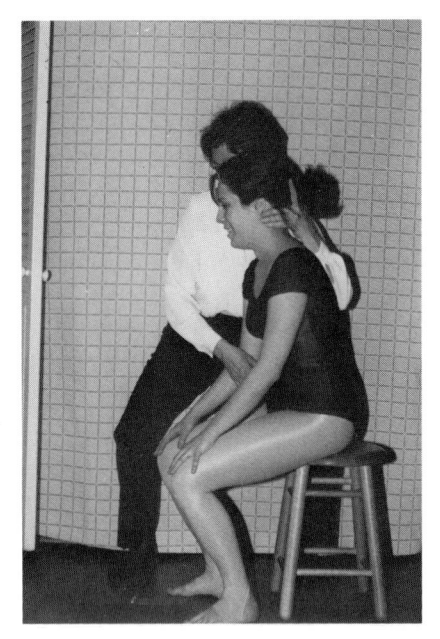

184   New Concepts in Craniomandibular and Chronic Pain Management

E, The pupil registers surprise and pleasure at the ease with which contact is made with the chair. The improved motor performance is appreciated.

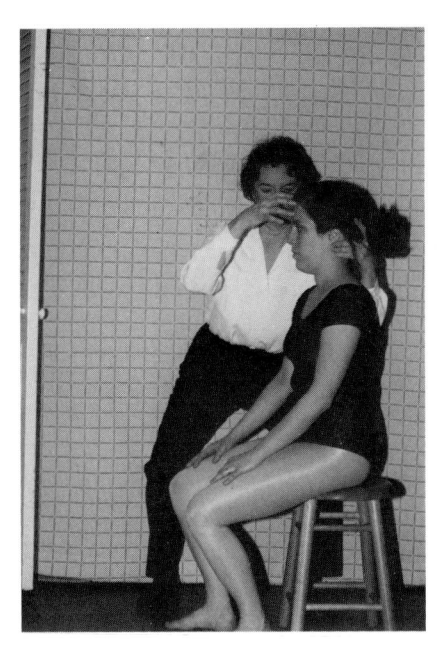

F, Pupil is seated on her ischial tuberosities, erect breathing enhanced, level gaze. She experiences a pleasurable sense of expansion and lightness throughout the body.

Fig. 7-3. The Chair Lesson (continued)

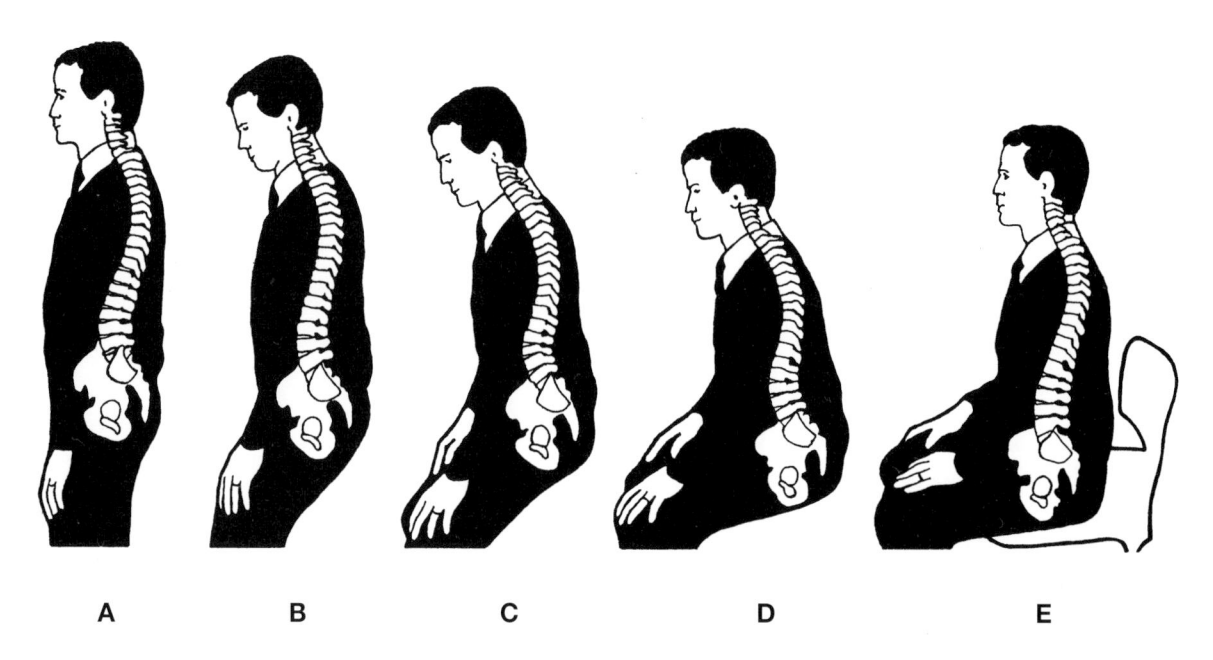

  A   B   C   D   E

Fig. 7-4. How someone "can work on himself" after a successful series of Alexander lessons. **A,** In standing— a moments hesitation—refusing to react to the idea of sitting down—orders to the neck, and back are started; while still ordering, permission is given to sit down—"means whereby orders" are started—knees forward and out, bend forward from the hips—continue both sets of orders all through **B, C and D,** finally to be seated. **E,** This is thinking in activity, and the method should be used in daily life: standing, sitting down, walking, talking, eating, driving, etc. Notice that in this sequence that the spine is not shortened nor are the curves exaggerated.

SUGGESTED READING

Alexander FM. *Constructive Conscious Control of the Individual*. London: Methuen; 1924.

Alexander FM. *The Use of the Self*. New York, NY: Dutton; 1932.

Alexander FM. *The Universal Constant in Living*. New York, NY: Dutton; 1941.

Barlow W. *The Alexander Technique*. New York, NY: Knopf; 1941.

Cailliet R. *Neck and Arm Pain*. 2nd ed. Philadelphia, Pa: FA Davis Co; 1981.

DePeyer E. *The Encyclopedia of Alternative Medicine and Self-Help*. New York, NY: Shocken Books; 1979.

Dorland's Illustrated Medical Dictionary. 26th ed. Philadelphia, Pa: WB Saunders Co; 1981.

Goldthwaite JE, Brown LT, Swaim LT, Kuhns G. *Essentials of Body Mechanica in Health and Disease*. 5th ed. Philadelphia, Pa: JB Lippincott; 1952.

Guyton AC. *Textbook of Medical Physiology*. Philadelphia, Pa: WB Saunders Co; 1981.

Jones FP. *Body Awareness in Action*. Rev. ed. New York, NY: Shocken Books; 1979.

Maisel E. *The Resurrection of the Body. The Essential Writings of F. Matthias Alexander*. New York, NY: A Delta Book; 1978.

Mathews A. *Development and Education in the Alexander Technique*. Bank Street College of Education, Institute for Research; 1984. Thesis.

Westfeldt L. *F. Matthias Alexander—The Man and His Work*. Westport, Conn: Associated Book Sellers; 1964.

Selye H. *The Stress of Life*. New York, NY: McGraw Hill; 1976.

Chapter 8

A Biophysical Model for Craniomandibular Management

Richard Koritzer, DDS, PhD
Lucile St. Hoyme, PhD

INTRODUCTION

We will use a three-part approach to present our model here: first, we will give an anatomic overview, stressing clinically important functional relations; second, a discussion of biomechanical phenomena reflected in bone will be presented; and finally, a clinical case report that demonstrates the applied model will be presented.

Any patient management system should be based on parsimonious and satisfying hypotheses formed in terms of the clinician's observations. We advocate a treatment philosophy based upon such hypotheses: further, the propositions used should be structured in a dynamic, functional model. We seek a rational therapy even as we depart from a wholly empirical method.

While striving to recognize what we do know, understanding what we do *not* know is also essential. We seek to guard against overinterpreting our observations. The primary objective is efficacious improvement of each patient's health.

The largest body of patients needing management in the general dental office for craniomandibular disorders may be treated simply. Such a patient sample usually includes few serious or complex deviations from normal function. An objective and reasonably limited diagnostic approach is most useful in terms of both time and money.

The specialty office sample of craniomandibular patients, however, will include more severe, even bizarre, cases. The level of knowledge for case identification should be high for all practitioners involved. This does not mean, however, that all general dentists should possess the most complex treatment skills.

What does seem reasonable is that the general dentist be capable of involvement in early diagnosis and management of craniomandibular disorders. This segment of the dental discipline—the general dentist—is destined to contribute significantly to future treatment of craniomandibular disorders. It is not inconceivable that failure to diagnose patient problems in this area may become as imposing as failure to diagnose periodontal disease.

AN ANATOMIC OVERVIEW

The most important distinction to be made about craniomandibular pathology is that it is systemic. Internal derangement, myofascial phenomena, and skeletal remodeling cannot be separated. They form a continuum.

The dynamic, functional heart of the craniomandibular articulation is the "disc-capsule assembly." The term *assembly* defines the complex that includes the dense fibrous connective tissue disc, the capsule, and the synovial lining. A blending of the connective tissue into the periosteum is demonstrable in gross dissection. Into these fibrous, connective, disc-capsule tissues blend muscle perimyseum and epimyseum.[1]

The muscles associated directly with the disc include the lateral pterygoid; the upper head extends medially and variably an-

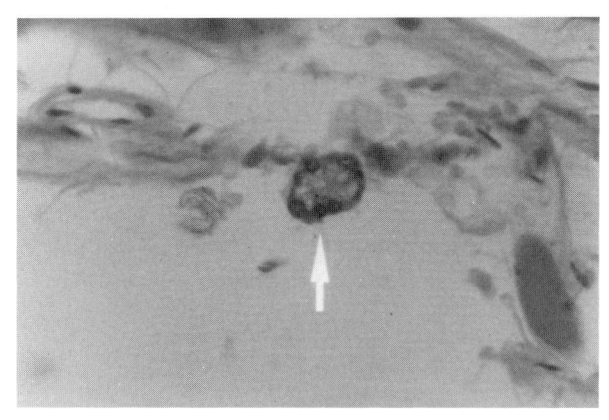

Fig. 8-2. Parotid strand cross-section in thin connective tissue and muscle area peridiscally.

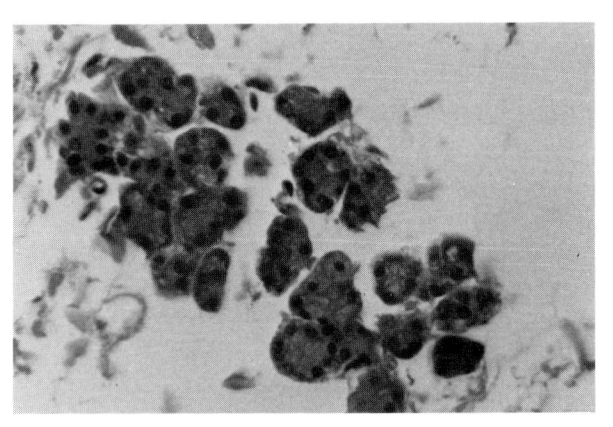

Fig. 8-3. Morphologically distinct parotid elements in the medial peridiscal-capsular area.

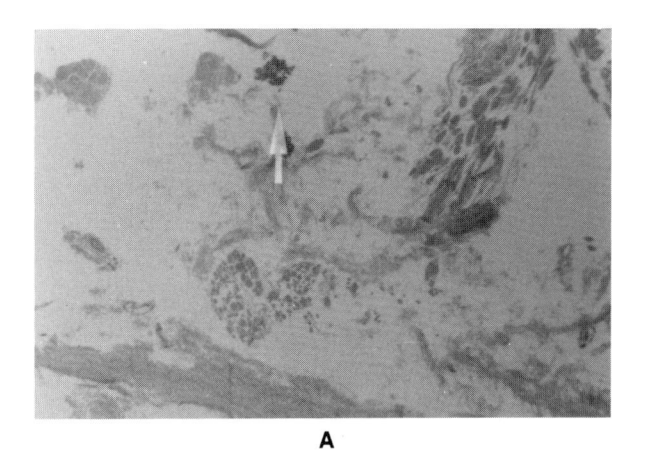

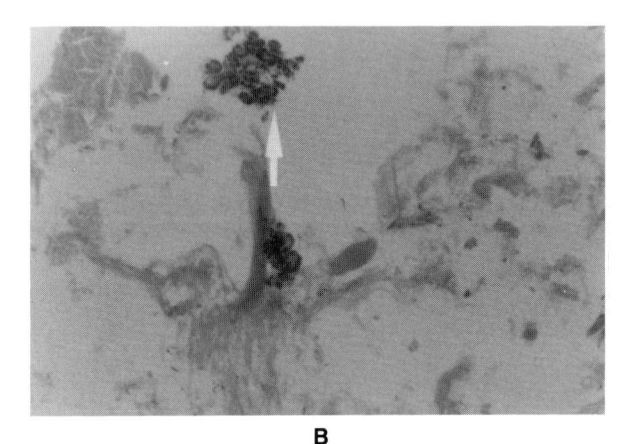

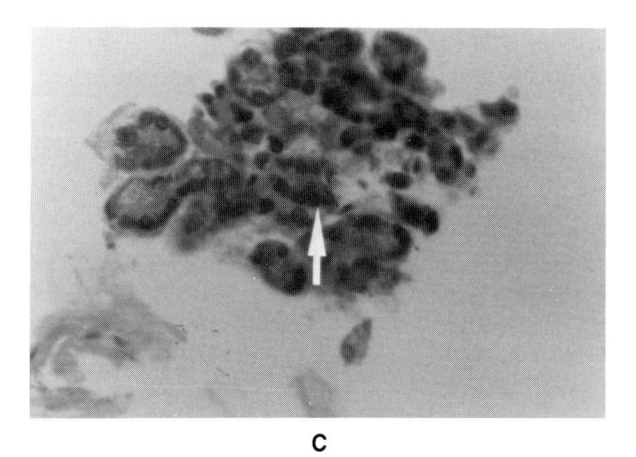

Fig. 8-1 A, B, and C. Successively increasing power magnification of peridiscal salivary strand showing typical parotid acinar structure.

teriorly.[2(pp 148-149)] We occasionally observe slight extension on the medial posterior. The mandibular-capsular muscle is lateral, and the temporal muscle is anterior.[3]

The central, thin, bearing portion of the disc against the articular eminence posterior slope is comprised of densely woven collagen. The fiber orientation is syncytial and multidirectional, and the fiber is compactly layered. This central area, when thick, is almost avascular inferiorly. When thin, little or no vascularity is found. The fiber orientations suggest a gyroscopic force pattern developing as alternating stresses fluctuate dynamical.

The remaining disc and capsule is richly supplied with vessels and nerves. Into the peripheral medial and anterior capsular tissue, elements of the parotid gland blend (Figs. 8-1 through 8-4).

The potential for parotid pathology affecting the joint tissue and surrounding musculature does exist. Extrinsic infectious processes may follow the parotoid connective tissue, as may occur in any space compartment. Lymph glands and ducts may also be seen in this area. It might be important, clinically, to note this anatomic potential for disc-capsule inflammatory reaction that would respond to antibiotic therapy. This anatomic hypothesis, while inviting, must be clinically tested.

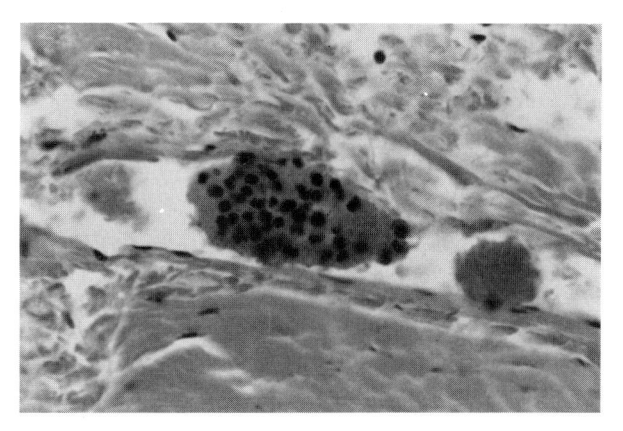

Fig. 8-4. Perdiscal salivary tissue in oblique section at high magnification showing proximal bearing on synovium.

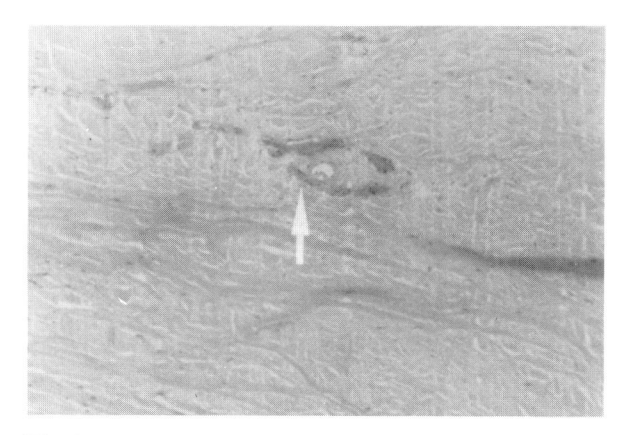

Fig. 8-5. Low power view of vessels in disc for orientation.

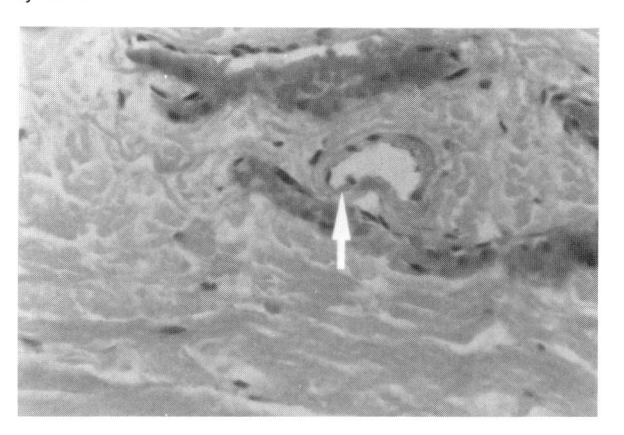

Fig. 8-6. High power view clearly identifies disc collagen morphology and multiple vessels.

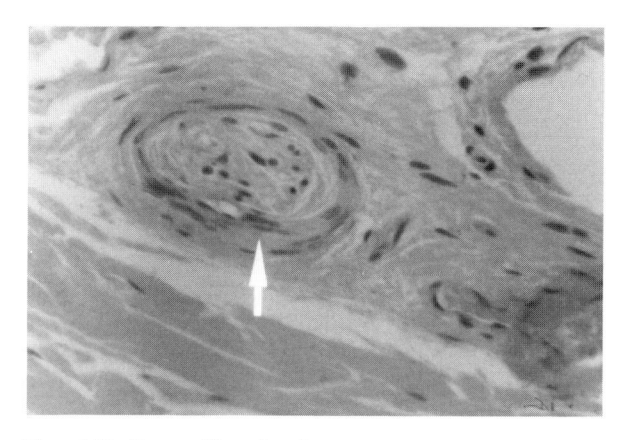

Fig. 8-7. Nerve fiber in disc.

The presence of medial peridiscal parotid elements when malignancy is present could pose an unanticipated risk. Furthermore, complete excision of the parotid seems unlikely, so that surgery ought certainly to be followed by radiation therapy. It also follows, unfortunately, that shielding of the disc-capsule is impossible and scarring would be a serious complication.

In examining serial microscopic sections of the disc-capsule assembly, nerve trunks of significant size were seen entering the inferior anterior disc surface, which is transitional with the capsule. The observed nerve trunks were oriented anterior-posteriorly. These entities were then identified in gross dissection. It is an inescapable anatomic conclusion that there is a highly developed proprioceptive feedback from the disc-capsule assembly. In addition, the rich intracapsular and discal vascular network signifies a high level of metabolic activity (Figs. 8-5 and 8-6).

One might postulate that there is a "trampoline-like" action apparent when the central disc collagen orientation is microscopically viewed. The central disc seems to mirror the proprioceptive feedback to the muscles blending into the capsule and disc (Fig. 8-7). It follows that the disc and capsule are far from passive elements.

Nutrition for these central-bearing tissues may indeed come from the synovium, but the greatest source is vascular. The intercellular fluid is probably pumped to the cells and fibers by the "trampoline-like" activity in the relatively avascular stress-bearing area.

Our anatomical observations imply resilience during energetic function and relative physiologic balance. When the physiologic limits are exceeded, the potential for complete or partial repairing activity over time is present. If surgical intervention is required, the anatomical tissue potential will be a factor in procedure design and prognosis. With care, gross anatomical derangements may be surgically corrected without sacrificing delicate proprioceptive mechanisms.

Here is an excellent area for emphasizing what we do not know. We have observations from serial microscopic sections and from gross dissections. We have, as yet, no clinical trials of the speculations about surgical compromise. Nevertheless, we have generated a novel model, hopefully with explanatory power, that may be used to expand our knowledge and improve techniques. They should then be sequentially modified.

Often artificial anatomic distinctions are made that describe limited or local disease in the disc-capsule, myofascial or skeletal components of the articular system. In fact, the joint components represent a systemic, functional whole. The muscles are essentially leashed to the disc-capsule assembly. Internal derangement, for example, must have myofascial, proprioceptive, and metabolic effects.[5]

The often glibly-used conceptual term "myofascial" tends to subordinate the importance of the fascial functional contribution. While the fascia is fixed at many points, it still may be visualized as one large sheet, with varying densities and displays, packaging anatomical contents.[6(pp 32-41)] The fascial system stores potential and discharges kinetic energy. It transmits or dampens force. This model provides an inviting explanation for the actions of otherwise unrelated muscle groups synchronously. This direct mechanism will operate in addition to central neural feedback.

The lateral pterygoid upper head has a continuous origin on the infratemporal fossa medial roof, and extends anteriorly to the infraorbital fissure edge. The infraorbital fissure is bridged by the orbitalis muscle.[7-9] This diaphragm-like muscle, which is nonstriated, is responsible for exophthalmia. The lateral pterygoid upper head and orbitalis blend so that pterygoid spasm may produce exophthalmia. This anatomic relation may be the source of pain behind the eye often reported by clinical patients.[10]

Following the origin posteriorly, we find the lateral pterygoid, upper head, associated with the pterygospinale ligament near the foramen ovale. This ligament is an embryonic component of the lateral pterygoid upper head.[11(p 204)] The ligament wraps intimately around the elements emerging from the foramen ovale. The nerve sheath may shield some of the effects of pterygoid muscle spasm on the neural trunk produced by the tensing ligament, but only within limits. Exceeding these limits may mimic trigeminal neuralgia. This is another hypothesis that needs clinical verification in scientific trials.

Laterally, the lateral pterygoid upper head on the infratemporal fossa roof blends with the temporal muscle. The muscles are not separable.[12] As described above, the upper head inserts consistently into the disc-capsule assembly on the medial and inserts variably on the anterior superior. In the anterior relation, it underleaves the temporal muscle-disc insertion. Not infrequently, we have seen extension of this muscle for a short distance onto the medial posterior. The muscle, anteriorly, is found in horizontaly displayed levels which fuse inferiorly, with little or no fascial plane definition into the lateral pterygoid lower head on the condylar neck.[2(p 148)]

The temporal fossa, on the skull, lateral aspect, and the infratemporal fossa beneath it, align approximately at right angles. The infratemporal fossa roof is perpendicular to the lateral pterygoid plate. The pterygoid plate is inferior and medial to the temporal origins[13(p 13-15)] (Figs. 8-8, 8-9).

All the bone surfaces are covered with periosteum, which is a continuous sheet. Muscle, with perimyseum blending into the periosteal surface, arises from these areas. The greatest temporal muscle surface of origin is the temporal fossa. However, the greatest temporal muscle bulk is in the lateral infratemporal fossa.[3] In addition, we have recently identified temporal muscle origin from the post orbital, zygomatico-frontal bone. This area forms a long shallow, somewhat more narrow, fossa. The most lateral fibers project posteriorly, inserting into the body of the temporal muscle as a thin, right-angled fan. The major and medial fibers descend to the anterior coronoid slope and represent the most anterior pull during contraction. We might suggest a relation to the production of "the convenience bite" or "centric occlusion." Interestingly, in this relation longer

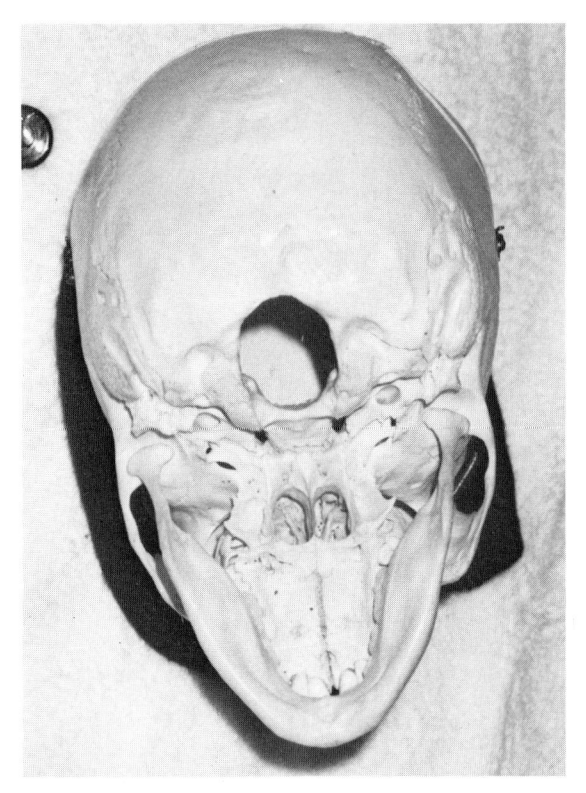

Fig. 8-8. View of skull base and inferior mandible allows observation of the infratemporal fossa roof oriented by condylar position. Temporal fossa is vertical at a right angle. As one looks into the pterygoid fossa medially, the flaring lateral pterygoid plate is appreciated, oriented to the condyle.

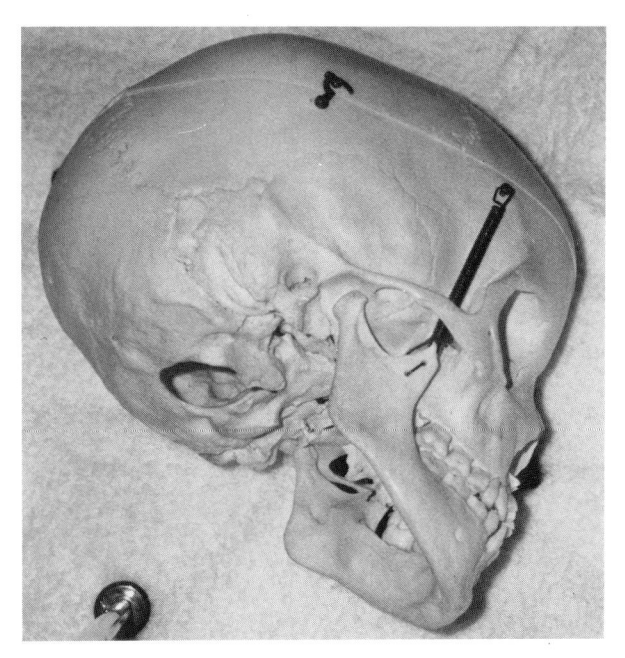

Fig. 8-9. Oblique view of skull allows appreciation of temporal and infratemporal fossa relation. The insertion area of the temporal muscle onto the coronoid process and retromolar location can be visualized. The continuous surface for muscle origin is apparent.

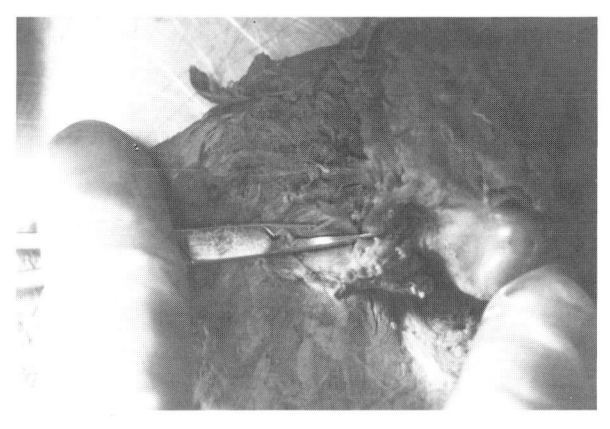

Fig. 8-10. Relying on the orientation of the previous two figures, the change of plane and rotation of the temporal muscle into the disc is seen. The impression of the articular eminence in the disc is clear, and extension in a "school-boy's peaked cap effect" (as described by Rees) into the infratemporal fossa is apparent.

fibers passing superficialy over the fibers originating post-orbitaly and bound by muscle connective tissue may contribute to torsion biomechanically.

We have also consistently observed origin of temporal muscle from the superior surface of the posterior zygomatic rampart. Similarly to the anterior origin situation, these deep fibers are overlain by longer superficial fibers that could contribute to torsion. As the anterior fibers are the shortest going to the coronoid, the posterior fibers are the shortest going to the lateral of the anterior disc insertion. The complexity of the temporal muscle continues to unfold and represents multifunctional activity.

The temporal muscle, part of what is a contiguous muscle mass, includes three insertions: the anterior disc-capsule assembly,[3] the coronoid process, and the retromolar mandible and ramus[14(p 534-535)] (Fig. 8-10). While the ramus is parallel to the temporal fossa and pterygoid plate, the mandibular retro-molar area is parallel to the infratemporal fossa roof.[15] Thus the conditions for force translation and mechanically balanced, dynamic articulation are established.

Classically, the fan-shaped flat muscle in the temporal fossa is divided into anterior, middle, and posterior segments. A functional model is then designed around this muscle display. Fiber length and direction are related vectorially about the coronoid insertion.[16-18]

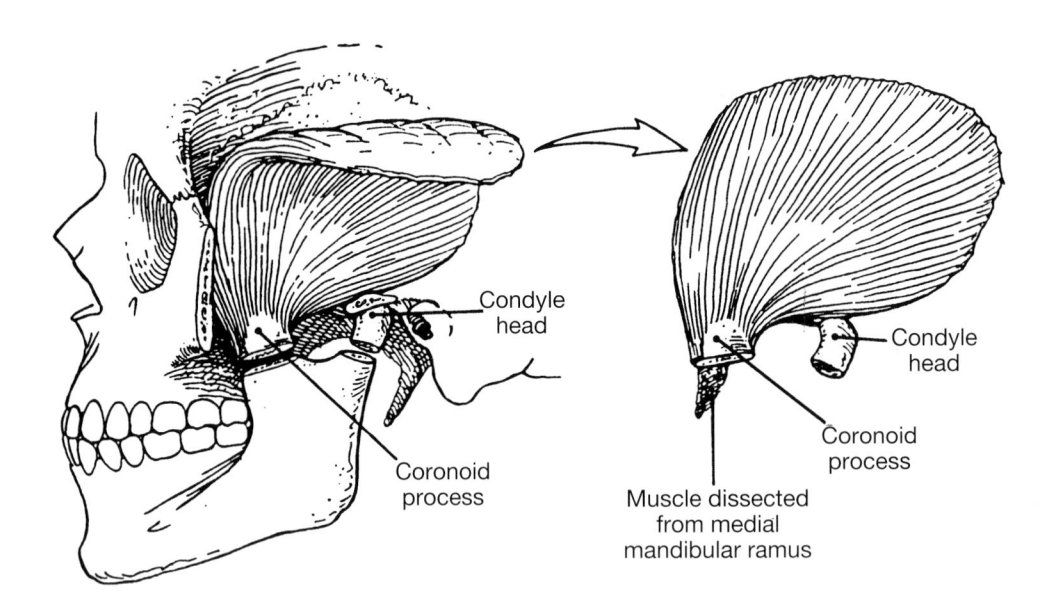

Fig. 8-11. *Left*, orientation of temporal muscle elevation from the temporal fossa. Separation of condyle and coronoid process is depicted. *Right*, the temporal muscle excised in-toto.

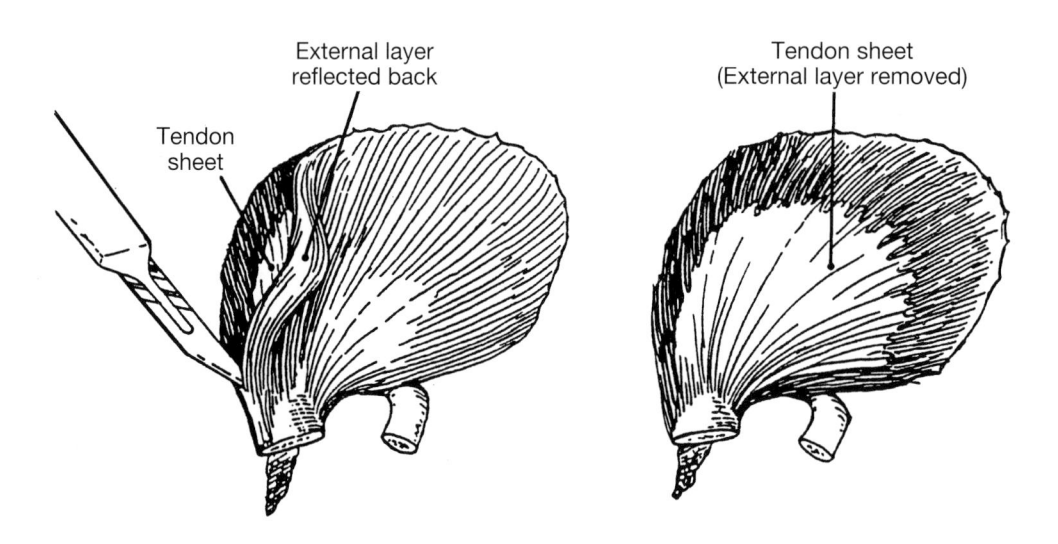

Fig. 8-12 A. Separation, by a fascial plane, of the lateral muscle-connective tissue sheet is represented. The solid muscle margin is seen and the fan-shaped central tendon intimately fixed to the deep sheet.

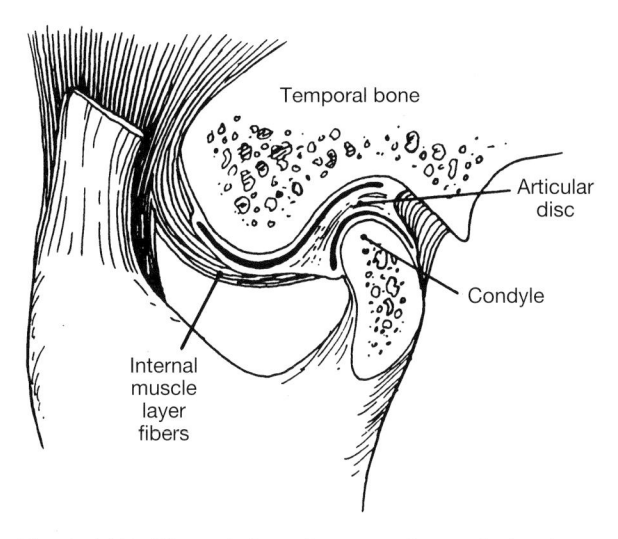

Fig. 8-12 B. The relation of temporal muscle is shown schematically to the disc. The medial muscle sheet rotates from the vertical temporal fossa to the horizontal infratemporal fossa roof and invests the disc anteriorly.

We suggest a more complex model based on the lateromedial dissection of the temporal muscle levels. Beginning at the temporal line, the first several centimenters are a single muscle mass (Fig. 8-11). Below this level, a broad, flat, fan-shaped tendon occupies the internal of the muscle (Fig. 8-12 A and B). The anterior and posterior borders are solid muscle for a width of about 1 cm. The muscle sheet, deep to the tendon, is the heaviest, and the fibers blend into the central tendon. In a gross dissection, the deep temporal muscle sheet must be flayed from the tendon. The superficial muscle sheet is easily separated by a fascial plane.

While the deep temporal muscle is displayed about the anterior disc, the component converging about the central tendon passes inferiorly and just anterior to the disc-capsule, giving off fibers to the unit and proceeding to the coronoid process, The relation is complex and suggests an intricate biomechanical interplay.

The retromolar temporal muscle is divided. The lateral part is contributed by the thin muscle superficial to the central tendon. The heavy medial part of the muscle contributes the retromolar internal insertion (Fig. 8-13). Functionally, we suggest that the latero-medial temporal insertions generate the dental trituration power stroke. The lateral insertions bilaterally execute the return stroke (Fig. 8-14). This mechanical function may be likened to the power and return stroke of a hand saw. The temporal muscle system may now be visualized translating and coordinating disc gyroscopic action with dental trituration with central coronoid balance.

The temporal muscle, originating on the lateral infratemporal fossa roof, blends medially with the lateral pterygoid upper head. The lateral-inferior temporal muscle, just below the zygomatic process, fuses with the masseter muscle's medial aspect. This area is about 1 cm in diameter and is called the zygomatico-mandibular muscle.[2(p 143)] Near the hamulus, the medial pterygoid muscle and temporal may fuse.[17] Anteriorly, at the infraorbital fissure edge, as mentioned above, the temporal muscle blends longitudinally into the orbitalis muscle.

The articular disc is described as having "a school-boy's peaked cap" effect by Reese.[18] The anterior attachment of the disc may be likened to the "bill" on the cap. In this location, the disc is anterior of the articular eminence and in the posterior infratemporal fossa. It should not be surprising, therefore, that the temporal medial sheet, rotating onto the infratemporal fossa roof, invests the disc anteriorly (Fig. 8-10).

In serial microscopic sections, the perimyseum and epimyseum of muscle are seen to blend with fascial-type capsular tissue and into collagen that is clearly disc. This zone is transitional in appearance (Figs. 8-15 through 8-20), with no sharp interface. The zone is also rich in large vessels and nerves.

In reptiles, the tooth-bearing, horizontal "mandible" is the dentate bone. Phylogenetically, the post-dentate bones, comprising the craniomandibular articulation, were rotated upward to become the ear ossicles.[19] The post-dentates were replaced by the ramus. Thus, the original transmission system between teeth, mandible, and skull was lost.

We postulate that the temporal muscle, including the complex facial-muscular relations described here, has replaced the original force distribution and discrimination system. Force is transmitted from the vertical, superior to the horizontal, inferior both posteriorly at the disc and also anteriorly at the retromolar area.

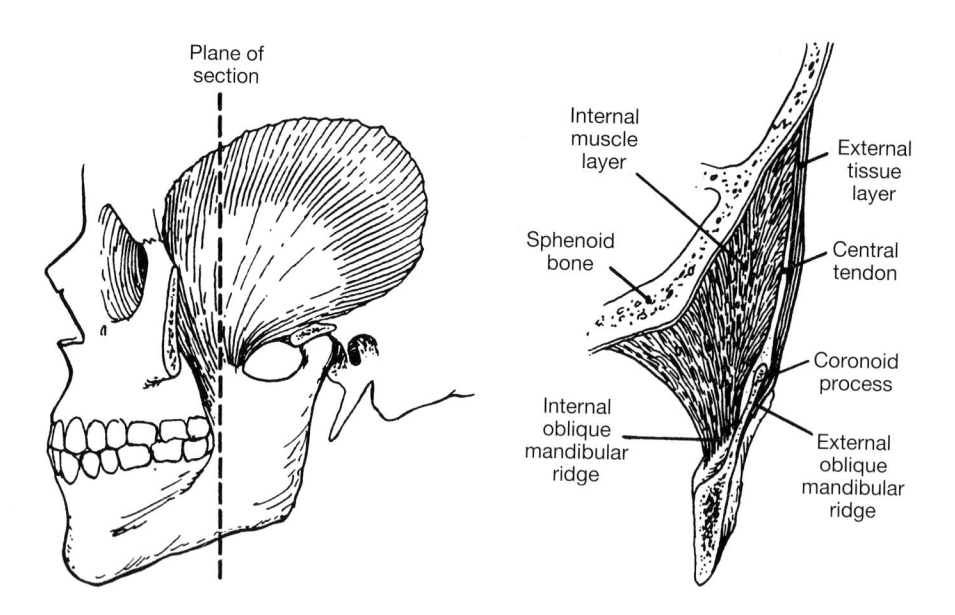

194 New Concepts in Craniomandibular and Chronic Pain Management

Fig. 8-13. The plane of section on the right gives orientation for the somewhat graphic explanation of the retromolar separate insertions of the temporal muscle.

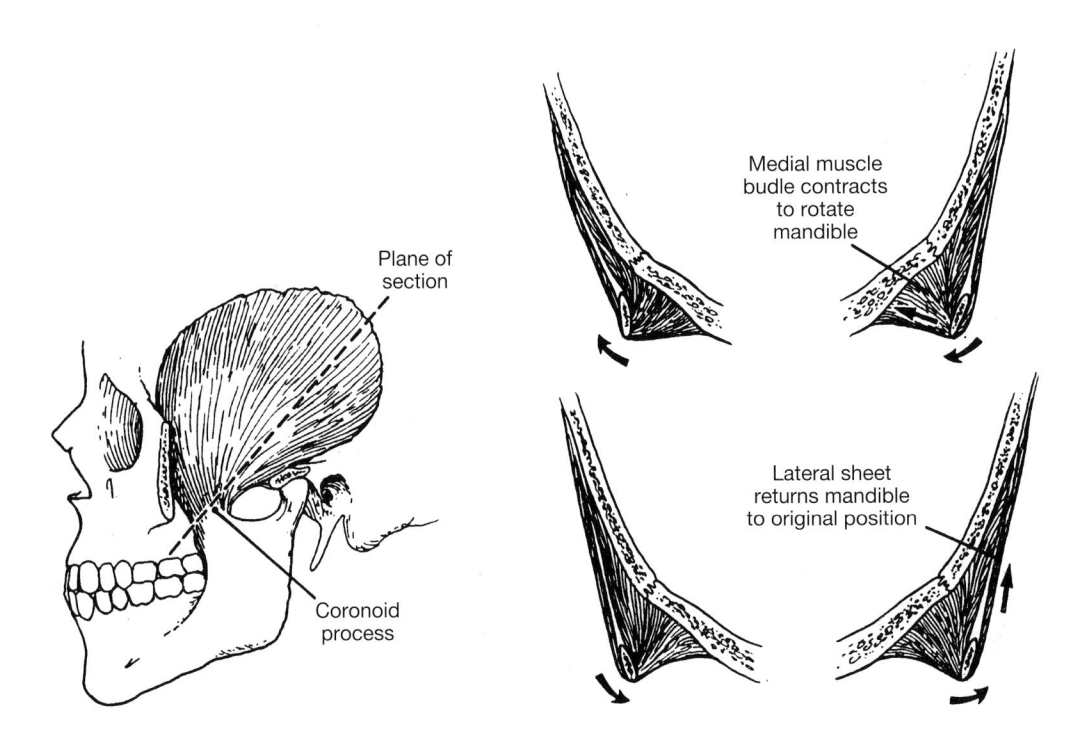

Fig. 8-14. The plane of section relates the transmission mechanically to the retromolar plane. The functional interpretation of trituration by the retromolar temporal muscle is displayed.

CHAPTER 8 A Biophysical Model for Craniomandibular Management 195

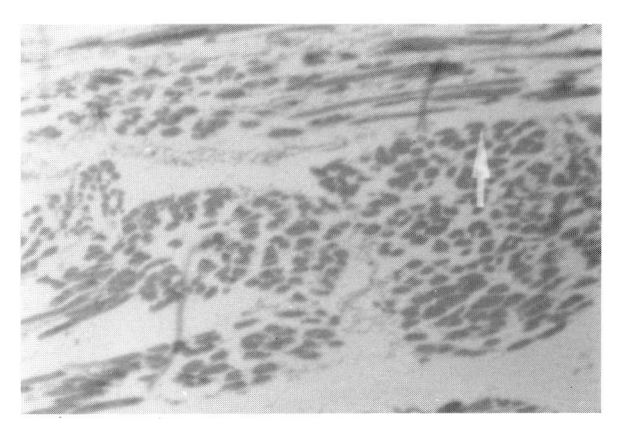

Fig. 8-15. Muscle fibers varying from cross-sectional to longitudinal. There is connective tissue binding the muscle fibers and bundles like a fine network.

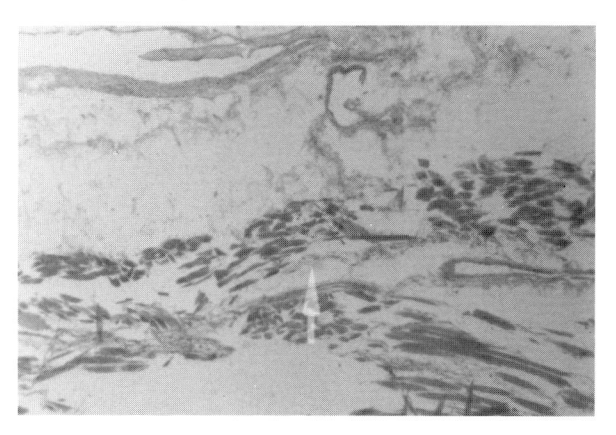

Fig. 8-16. Muscle bundles contributed multidirectionally are inferior to light connective tissue that begins to show more condensed sections. This is posterior to Fig. 8-15.

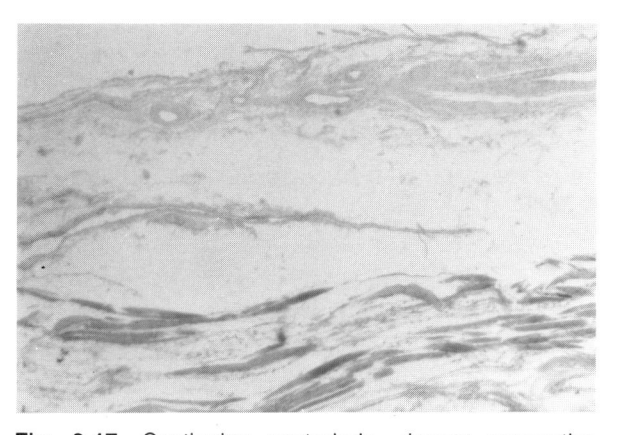

Fig. 8-17. Continuing posteriorly, denser connective tissue richly supplied with vessels (note arterioles) is superior. Mainly longitudinal muscle fibers are inferior. The light connective tissue binding the developing disc capsule to muscle in this sagittal section can be appreciated.

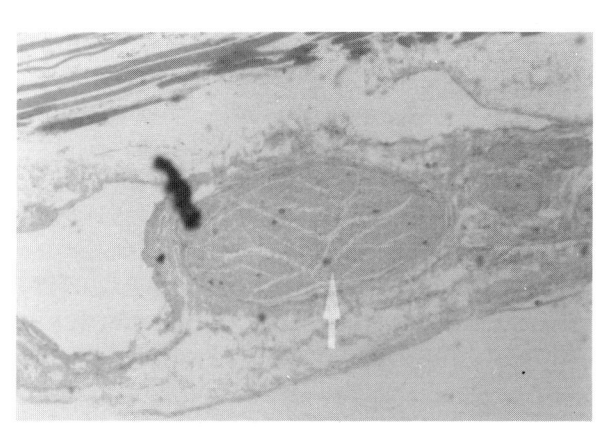

Fig. 8-18. The transitional disc capsule connective tissue zone now includes large nerve trunks. The area where tension may best be recorded by proprioceptors is supplied. The relation of muscle and transitional anterior disc joined by connective tissue seems physiologically functional.

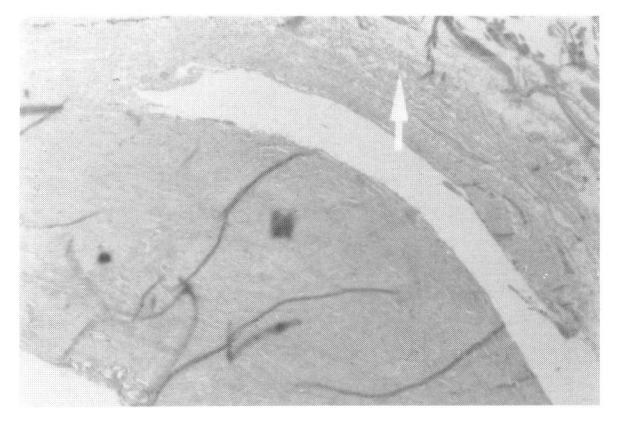

Fig. 8-19. The muscle relation to dense connective tissue as we proceed posteriorly in this sagittal section is now intimate. The dark lines in the disc proper represent artifacts due to folding when cutting a more resistant material. Note that vessels may be seen in this dense disc.

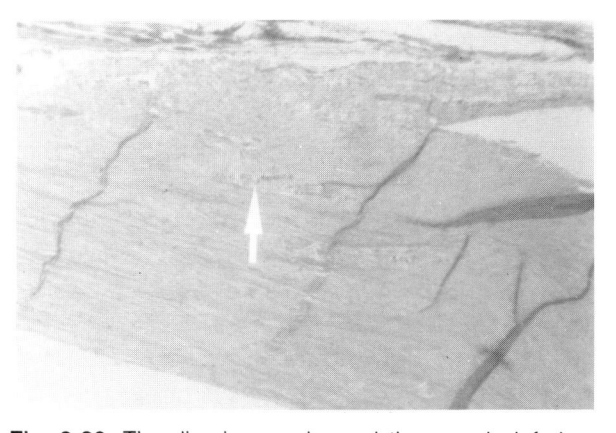

Fig. 8-20. The disc is superior and the muscle inferior. There are still vessels in this part of the disc. The concept of transition should now be clear.

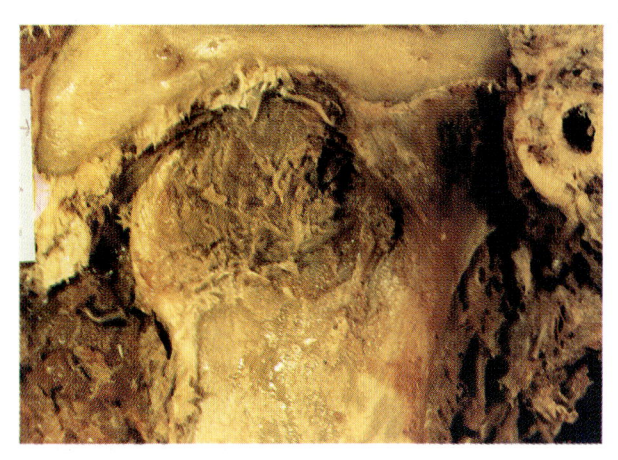

Fig. 8-21. Cut section of the area of fusion of masseter and temporal muscles. Note that the zygomatic arch is intact, but the tendinous insertion on the coronoid process is seen. Remnants of the mandibular-capsular muscle are also apparent. To orient this view note the external earhole from which the zygoma extends anteriorly. The zygomatic mandibular muscle is above the mandibular ramus.

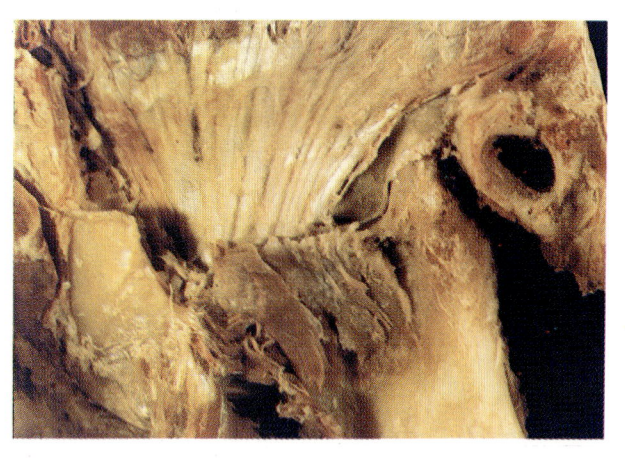

Fig. 8-22. The mandibular-capsular muscle is seen originating in the mandibular notch and inserting on the anterior-lateral disc. The disc is seen to extend well in front of the condyle. The disc has been elevated and then dropped inferiorly so that the impression of the articular eminence is obvious. This relation also demonstrates how the anterior disc is actually in the infratemporal fossa.

The coronoid process, in this context, is an insertion that balances centrally and stabilizes functionally. This becomes particularly reasonable in light of the total muscle networking with fusions, blendings, and connective tissue relations. The system may be interpreted as one comprised of flexible beams (bones) operated by pulsing energetic sources (muscles) absorbing and transmitting force complexes in XYZ planes per time. The exotic biophysical system implied by this model should not be lost on the reader.

The masseter muscle is extensively described in available literature.[20] The zygomatic process is its origin, and the insertion is onto the lateral mandibular surface. The muscle is broad and quadrilateral. There is a wide anterior superficial component and a narrower deep posterior part. The area of fusion with the temporal muscle has been mentioned above (Fig. 8-21).

An additional muscle unit, sometimes heavy is present in about 80% of individuals. It arises in the mandibular notch and inserts into the lateral disc-capsule assembly. Koritzer and Suarez have labelled this muscle "mandibular-capsular" after a series of dissections in collaboration with Robert Kenyon[3] (Fig. 8-22). When viewed microscopically, it is evident that the perimyseum and epimyseum of muscle blend into the capsular connective tissue (Figs. 8-15 through 8-20). Since independent innervation was not identified, this muscle segment is most likely part of the masseter complex embryologically.

From a functional viewpoint, however, the mandibular-capsular muscle must be considered a separate entity. The origin must be the more fixed point, the mandible. The insertion is the lateral disc-capsule. Dynamically, an origin on the mandible in motion delivers continuous stabilization to a gyroscopically fluctuating disc. Reciprocal function is synergistic with unilateral lateral pterygoid upper head and the anteriorly inserted temporal. Bilateral synergism is even more complex. While the usually heavier lateral pterygoid upper head and temporal activate force strokes, the lighter mandibular-capsular may function to restore midline alignment more passively.

A lateral surgical or cadaver dissection separates this entity. Any attempt to artificially function the mandible under these conditions will convince the observer of fallacious disc position and activity.

The lateral pterygoid lower head arises from the lateral surface of the lateral pterygoid plate, which is superiorly and roundly confluent with the infratemporal fossa roof. The upper and lower pterygoid heads are actually blended supero-inferiorly and so fused that dissection from the medial aspect in a hemi-sected skull displays them as one.

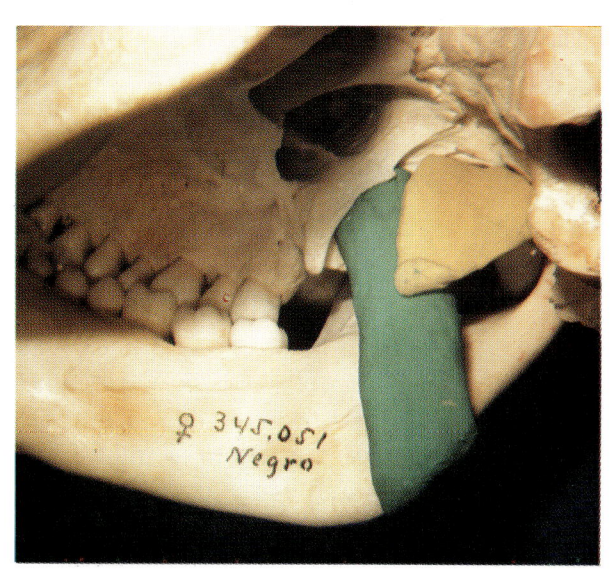

Fig. 8-23. Green moulding clay represents the internal pterygoid muscle originating in the pterygoid fossa. The pterygoid hamulus is visible, as is the maxillary tuberosity. The relation of the medial pterygoid plate and the palate can be well understood. This view is from the medial, and the one edge of the internal surface of the lateral pterygoid plate is seen. The insertion area on the lingual surface of the mandibular angle actually extends about an equal width of clay further forward. The accessory medial pterygoid muscle (yellow clay) is inserting on the medial superior of the medial pterygoid just below the tendinous part of the muscle as it merges from the fossa. The broad triangular shape originating from the skull base is demonstrated.

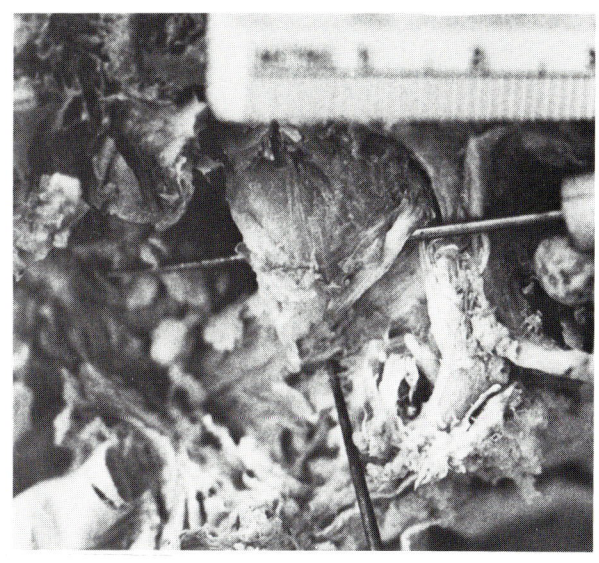

Fig. 8-24. The accessory medial pterygoid muscle is indicated, originating on the skull base. The dendritic insertion into the medial pterygoid is also demonstrated.

Dissection from the lateral picks up the "Y" configuration and may inadvertantly result in completing an artificial separation.

The lateral pterygoid lower head is inserted into a fovea on the anterior mandibular neck just below the condyle.[21] Taken alone, lower head contraction is directed medially, anteriorly, and slightly superiorly. As will be noted below, the thin pterygoid plate is plastic under functional stress. Reciprocal force is distributed as bone flexion at the origin, and mandibular excursion occurs via the insertion.

The medial pterygoid muscle origin is the pterygoid fossa, which is the recess between the lateral and medial pterygoid plates.[22(p 402)] The muscle is generally heavy, and for the first centimeter after exiting the fossa of origin is tendinous. Descending laterally and posteriorly, insertion is into the medial mandibular angle. Passing the hamular area, the muscle may blend with the temporal. Placement of a prosthesis at the hamular notch may impinge on this muscle complex and cause unexpected effects on mandibular excursion.

The accessory medial pterygoid muscle originates on the skull base, beginning at the superior edge of the lateral pterygoid plate and continuing to the edge of the carotid foramen (Figs. 8-23, 8-24). This thin triangular muscle descends until the apex inserts into the medial pterygoid muscle's superomedial aspect. Dissection of the muscle insertion exposes a dendritic invasion of the medial pterygoid muscle middle fascicle.[23]

The accessory medial pterygoid muscle is independently innervated and may be considered, anatomically, an independent entity. It most probably belongs to the primitive pterygoid muscle complex described by Barghusen. The insertion into the medial pterygoid muscle is a common location of muscle spasm.

The digastric muscle is a particularly interesting complex. Two bellies, with a tendon interposed, are supplied by different nerves (Fig. 8-25). The posterior belly, supplied by the facial nerve, originates in the digastric groove medial to the mastoid process. The muscle descends anteriorly and laterally and inserts into the tendon under cover of the mandible. The anterior belly supplied by the trigeminal nerve, mandibular division, arises from the medial inferior mandible and passes posterolaterally and inferiorly to insert into the tendon. The tendon is encased in fascia, much like a carpal tunnel. The description

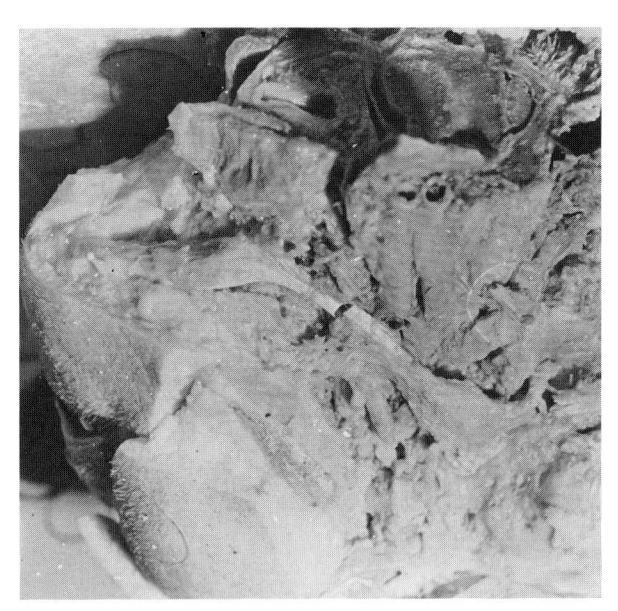

Fig. 8-25. The digastric tendon is cut close to the middle. The anterior muscle belly is seen originating near the center of the chin to the right. The posterior belly originates from the digastric groove medial of the mastoid process. The mastoid bone has been sectioned for this preparation so that the entire length of the origin can be appreciated.

most often seen in the literature is of a strong, well-defined, ligamentous band securing the tendon to the hyoid bone.

The cervical fascia is a single connective tissue sheet that encases the neck contents. Although it is possible to expose the ligamentous band described above, a more careful dissection reveals the fascial tunnel within which the tendon slides freely. The functional result of the fascia being around the tendon is limitation of digastric muscle directionality and discrimination.[24]

The action of each digastric belly occurs in XYZ planes, a 3x3 system. Each belly may either contract or relax, a 2x2 system. The total potential 4x9 digastric action complex yields 36 possible resultant vectors. This large activity range indicates significant function.

It may be useful to inquire about this tendon located in such a novel relation in the neck. In fact, the digastric system is homologous to the gill of a fish. It controls the terminal swallowing position. This is the dental centric relation.

The neck and skull muscle relations, by way of connective tissue, both fascial and intramuscular, form a functional systemic model. The masticatory muscles originate from a single muscle evolutionarily, the adductor mandibulae of fish. This may well account for the muscle fusions and blendings described here.[25]

Attempts at clinical management using a model of separate, discretely defined, masticatory muscles require central neural feedback coordinating four or more independent units. The orchestration, however, is much more complex. Systematic intermeshing connective tissue activity yields great potential to coordinate and fine-tune energy distribution.

The articular disc, for example, may function gyroscopically, advancing over the articular eminence guided by three muscles intimately related with the disc-capsule assembly. Proprioceptive monitoring and feedback per time constantly facilitates functional adaptation. Finally, the connective tissue relatedness and the muscle fusions suggest group function.

THE CIRCUMCERVICAL FUNCTIONAL COMPLEX

It is quite common to observe concomitant craniomandibular and posterior cervical musculo-skeletal pathology. The most frequent explanation, when connectedness is conjectured, is neurophysiologic feedback. Without negating this mechanism, there is also the necessity of considering mechanical factors.

Most anatomies depict the medial pterygoid muscle at the mandibular angle, separated quite clearly, and at some distance from the sternocleidomastoid (SCM) muscle.[13] However, we have found the SCM anterior border tucking under the mandibular angle where it underlies the medial pterygoid muscle at its insertion (Fig. 8-26 A). The head position affects this relation so that when turned to the left the muscles relate less intimately on the right, and on the left when the head is turned to the right. The two muscles are clearly separated by a dense fascial plane which, as part of the cervical fascial sheet, binds rather than separates these functional units. Langenbeck[20] depicts this relation, and it is also apparent in Bradley et al's text, *Magnetic Resonance Imaging*.[30]

The proximity of these two muscles on one side is greatest when the head is turned to that

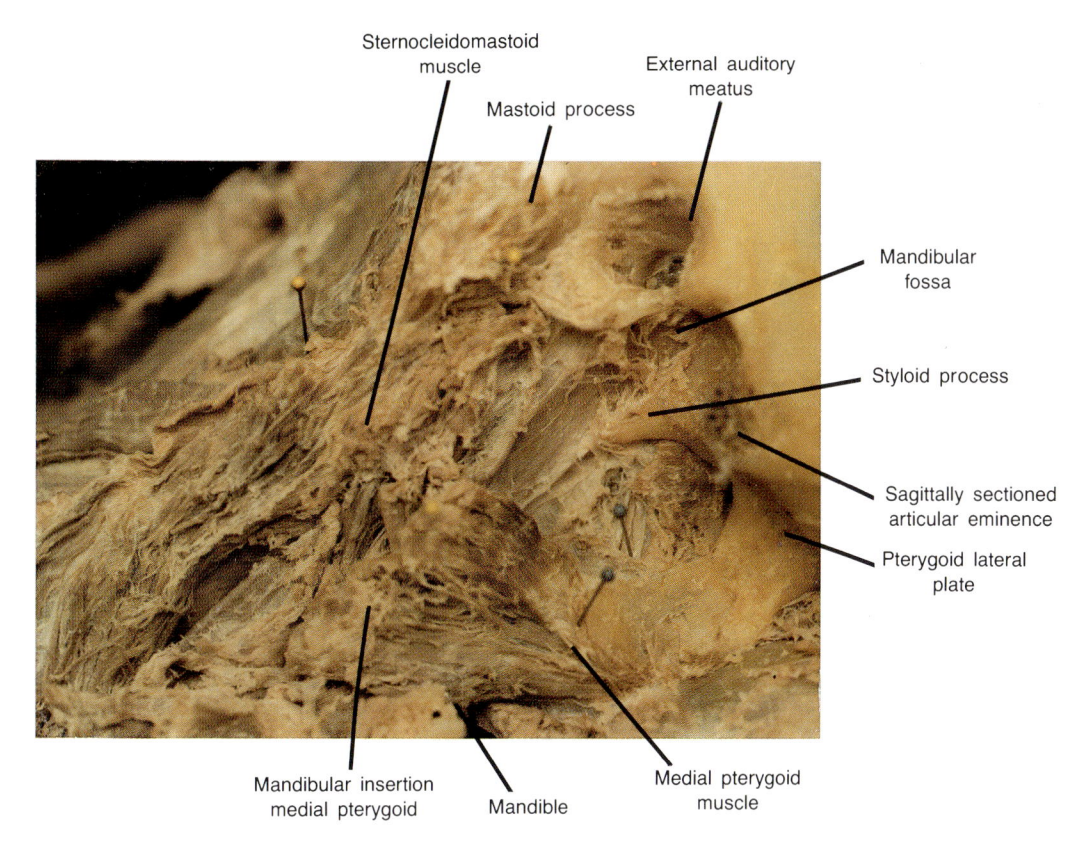

Fig. 8-26 A

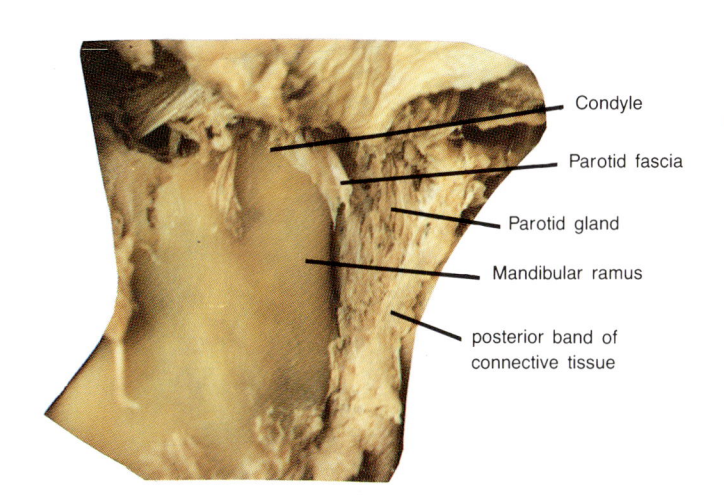

B, A clear plane can be created between the mandibular ramus and the parotid gland, but the condylar relation is much more secure. The posterior dense connective tissue band attaches to the external ear cartilage almost inseparably.

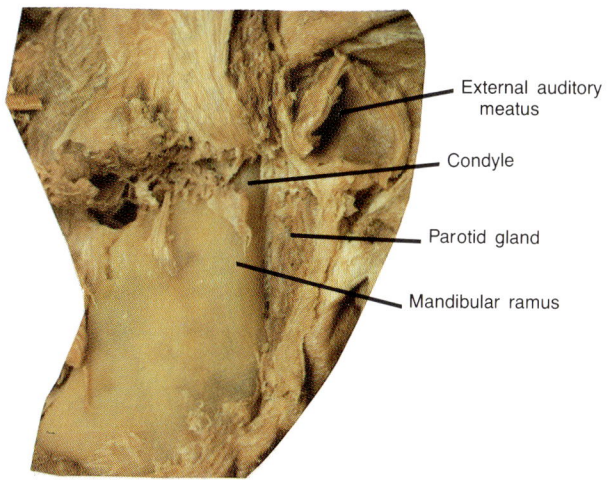

C, The relation and orientation of the mandible and retromandibular parotid gland and fascia with the articular disc and cartilaginous part of the external auditory meatus is integral and systematic.

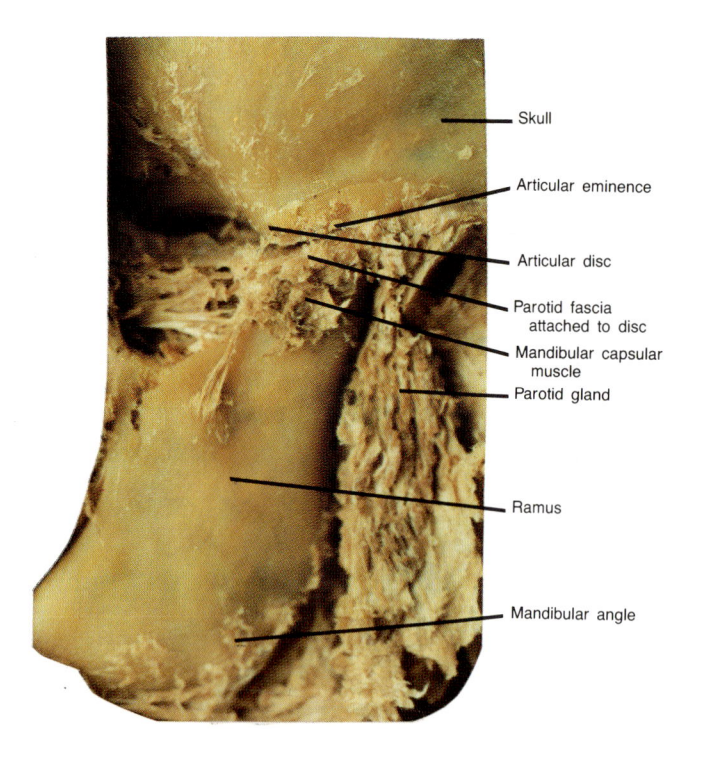

D, The sagittal bony section allows visualization of the disc eminence relation. The anteriorly attached discal tissues have been elevated from the periosteum and dropped inferiorly so that the nature of the attachment and the relation anterior to the eminence in the infratemporal fossa is seen. The posterior attachment to the parotid fascia and confluently to the cartilaginous external auditory meatus is displayed. Orientation of the skull and mandible aids conceptualization.

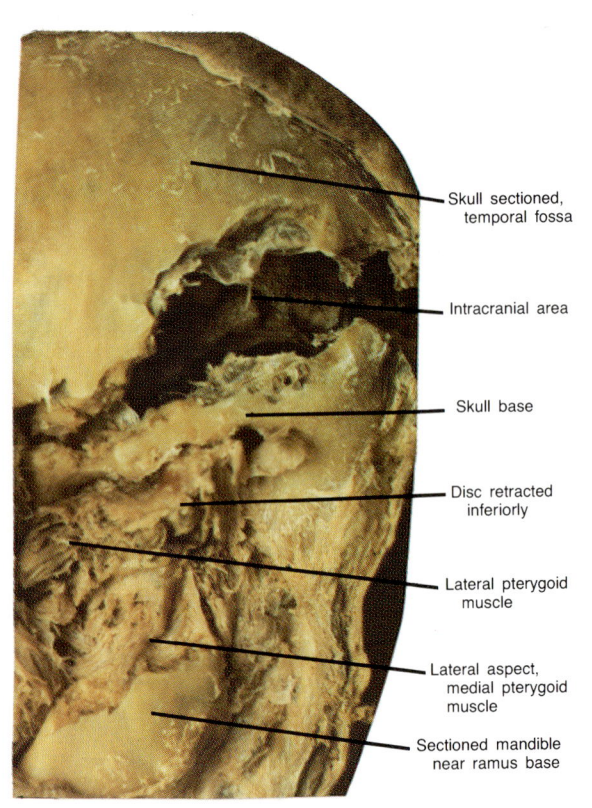

F, Note thickness of cranial base in this sagittally sectioned joint. The relation of disc and eminence is clear. The retrodiscal area is integumentary to the disc. The relation of the medial pterygoid is seldom seen in a dissection, and better orients this muscle with the masticatory group.

E, Note the parotid fascia, ligamentous in texture, densely bound to the cartilage of the external ear posteriorly and retrodiscally anteriorly. The lateral mandibular capsular muscle is quite clear.

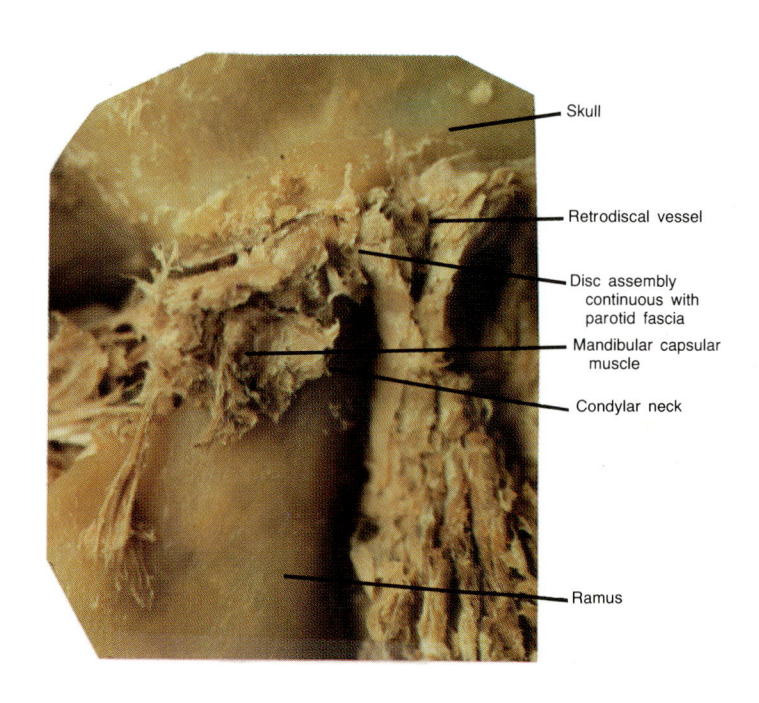

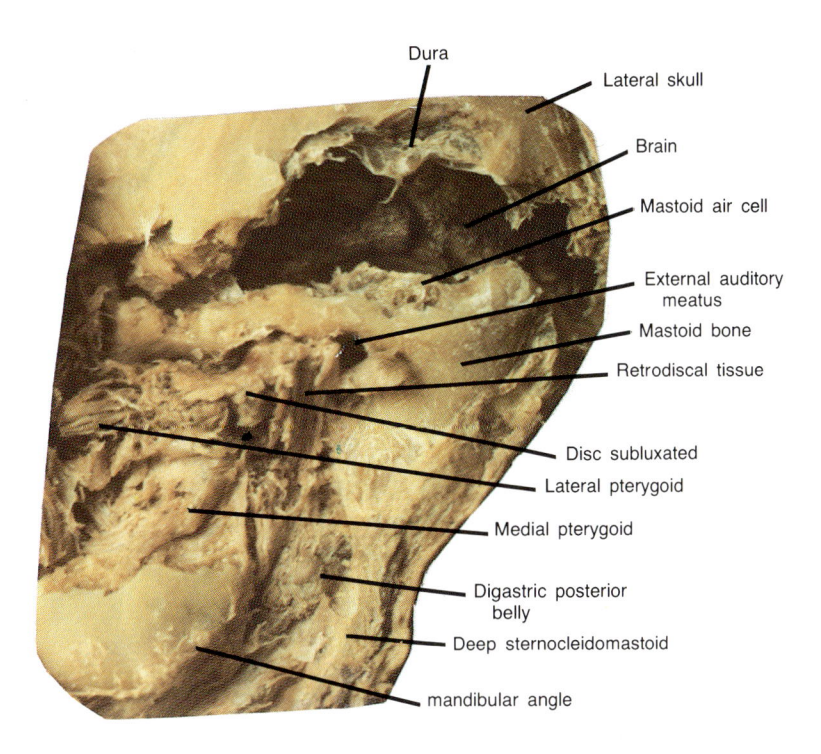

CHAPTER 8   A Biophysical Model for Craniomandibular Management   201

G, Overview of relations between functionally integrated elements of the dental articulation. The meticulously cleaned and isolated anatomic entity lacks the reality of this view. The closeness of the dental articulation and the brain and the mastoid areas suggest the potential for concomitant pathologies.

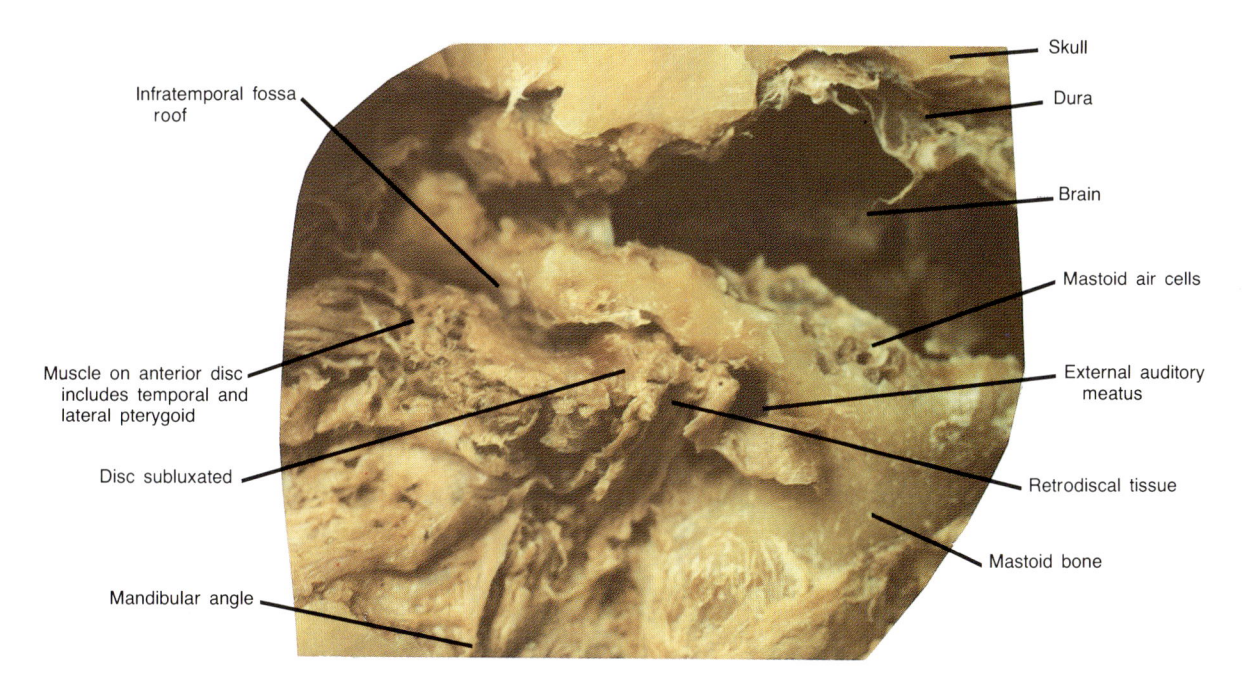

H, Close-up view of the previous photo shows more clearly the relation of ear, retrodiscal tissue, disc, and surrounding musculature. The location of the disc anterior to the eminence is here made obvious. It becomes clear that the continuous sheet of the temporal muscle onto the infratemporal fossa roof would invest the disc anteriorly.

side. The largest distance apart occurs when the head is turned to the opposite side. When the head is depressed anteriorly, proximity is great. When the head is flexed dorsally, separation increases. The forward head posture seen in MPD patients places these muscles in closer proximity. Lateral head movements in this posture have greater circumcervical mechanical potential. Contrarily, when the head is flexed dorsally with great kinetics, as in discus throwing, the tensile properties of the connective tissue are most severely tested when circumcervical function occurs. The inescapable functional activity involves the entire myofascial skeletal complex.

The relationship of TMD and aural symptoms has been a subject anatomically obscure, but often clinically troubling. Figures 8-26 A through H depict the intimate relations of dense connective tissue to the disc-capsule assembly and the cartilaginous ear tube. The tensile qualities of connective tissue result in greater or lesser densities of fibers in response to forces distributed per unit area. In addition, fiber orientation will be directional with vectorial distribution. Where dense bands of connective tissue develop, function has concentrated.

The disc-capsule assembly, with its attendant muscular units described above, is seen to be anchored about the cartilaginous ear tube, participating in the lateral aspect to the posterior and onto the mastoid bone where there is intermingling with the tendinous insertion of the SCM. Transmission of wave-like forces in function may now be seen to readily contribute to the potential for ear fullness, wave-like sounds and tinnitus. While these causes are not the only ones for these frequently observed symptoms, they may explain the relief obtained occasionally by orthotic therapy. This portion of our study was in collaboration with Anthony Schwartz and Robert Harris.

In *Gray's Anatomy*, 36th British edition,[24(p 523)] under the description, *deep fascia*, it is noted that the deep fascia is often indistinguishable from aponeurotic tissue. Wherever the deep fascia comes in contact with periosteum, it fuses and is thus well able to accept the attached muscle pull. In the neck, laminae continuous with the deep fascia pass between muscle groups. These septa often serve to connect rather than separate muscles, and may function as intermuscular aponeuroses. This description, which I have abbreviated from Gray, applies well to the relation of the medial pterygoid and SCM. It should be noted that this dense cervical fascia also invests and sheaths the carotid as well as the entire arterial system of the neck: thus the vessels are bound functionally to the muscle system. This phenomena is being considered currently by Meyers.[31]

The relation of the circumcervical muscle elements at the skull base is depicted in many anatomies.[30(pp 58-67), 2(pp 250-261)] If one visualizes the artistic spaces as fascial sheets, as described above, binding functional groups and transmitting tensile forces, complex MPD symptoms are explicable.

It is not by accident that the plane of an orthotic, interposed dentally, changes mandibular posture and incidentally alters cervical group function. Is the oral physician, then, treating a stomatognathic system attached to the body? Or is he rather treating a patient with a view to stabilization in the unique area of dental opportunity? Does this dental approach in fact enhance and support management by physicians concerned with other anatomical regions? It should. Our place on the health-care team will continue to be redefined.

BIOMECHANICS REFLECTED IN BONE

Previously unappreciated lateral pterygoid plate distortion patterns aroused our curiosity. It appears that the lower head of the pterygoid muscle bends and shapes the bone directionally, with the resultant shape reflecting the net effect of the habitual function. Anatomic descriptions of the masticatory muscles usually describe a fixed origin and movable insertion. We now suggest that bone is plastic, and should be treated as a non-rigid structure distributing normal, energetic stress in predictable patterns.[26]

The entire pterygoid fossa bone is thin. It is moulded by the muscles originating from its surfaces. The zygomatic arch, the masseter muscle origin, is a readily flexed bone,

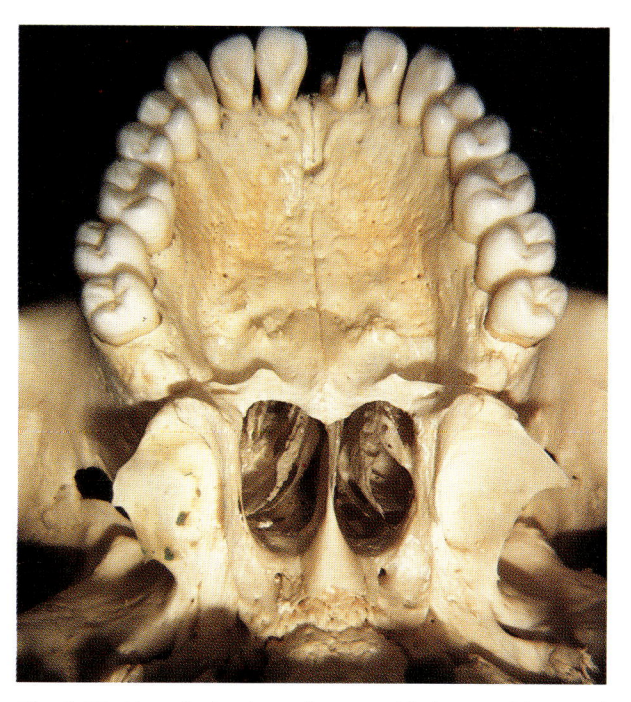

Fig. 8-27. Note flaring lateral pterygoid plate and fossa of origin for the medial pterygoid muscle. The lateral plate is directed laterally, posteriorly, and somewhat inferiorly by the functional tension of the lateral pterygoid muscle on the lateral surface plastically deforming the bone.

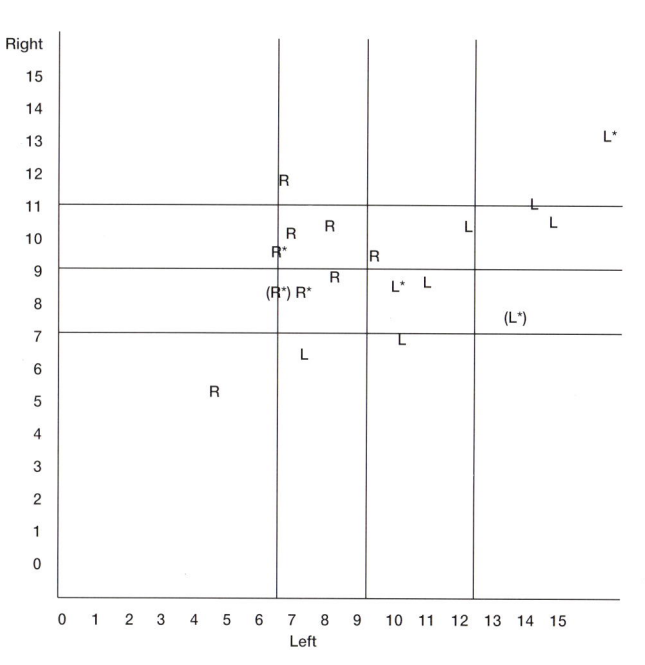

Graph 8-1. Lower head lateral pterygoid muscle algorithm, including greater and lesser dimensions of the lateral pterygoid plate and the measurement from the center of the plate to the medial pole of the mandibular condyle. *Illinois Amerindian, Arkansas Amerindian.** () includes one estimate.

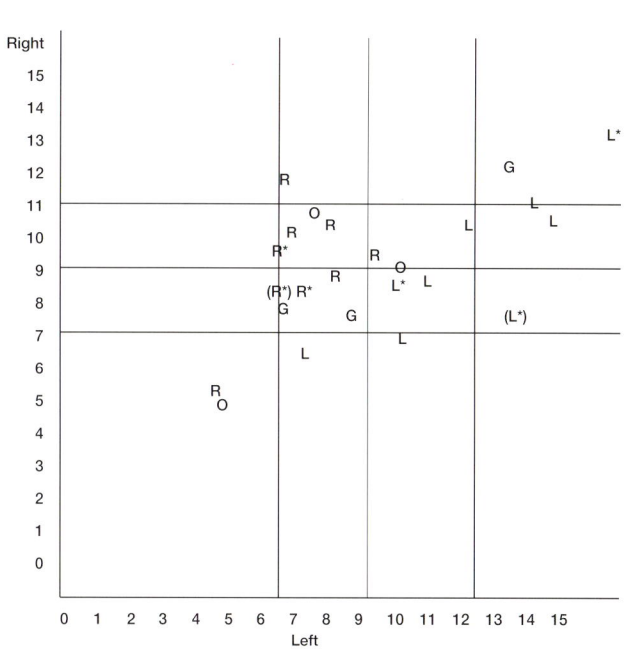

Graph 8-2. Lower head lateral pterygoid muscle algorithm, including greater and lesser dimensions of the lateral pterygoid plate and the measurement from the center of the plate to the medial pole of the mandibular condyle. *Illinois Amerindian, Arkansas Amerindian.** () includes one estimate. Orangutan and Gorilla added.

centrally, although its anterior and posterior roots are well buttressed. The equilibria of bone are dynamic rather than rigid and static. Reciprocal movement occurs between muscle origin and insertion.

We have also observed frequent variation of pterygoid plates and fossa shapes and dimensions (Fig. 8-27). Testing of systematic variation intra-individual and by population was undertaken to validate and quantify our conceived hypothesis.

The lateral pterygoid plate length and width was measured. This gave a rough approximation of origin area of the lateral pterygoid lower head. The pterygoid lateral plate center was found and the distance from this point to the resting position, medial, anterior condyle pole was recorded. Assuming a roughly uniform quadrilateral muscle, the multiple of the three dimensions represents an algorithm for volume.

Using the same principle, for the medial pterygoid muscle, the greater and lesser dimension of the pterygoid fossa was found. The distance from fossa center to gonial angle was the third multiplier.

For the masseter muscle, the greater and lesser ramus dimension was determined. The muscle length was estimated as the dis-

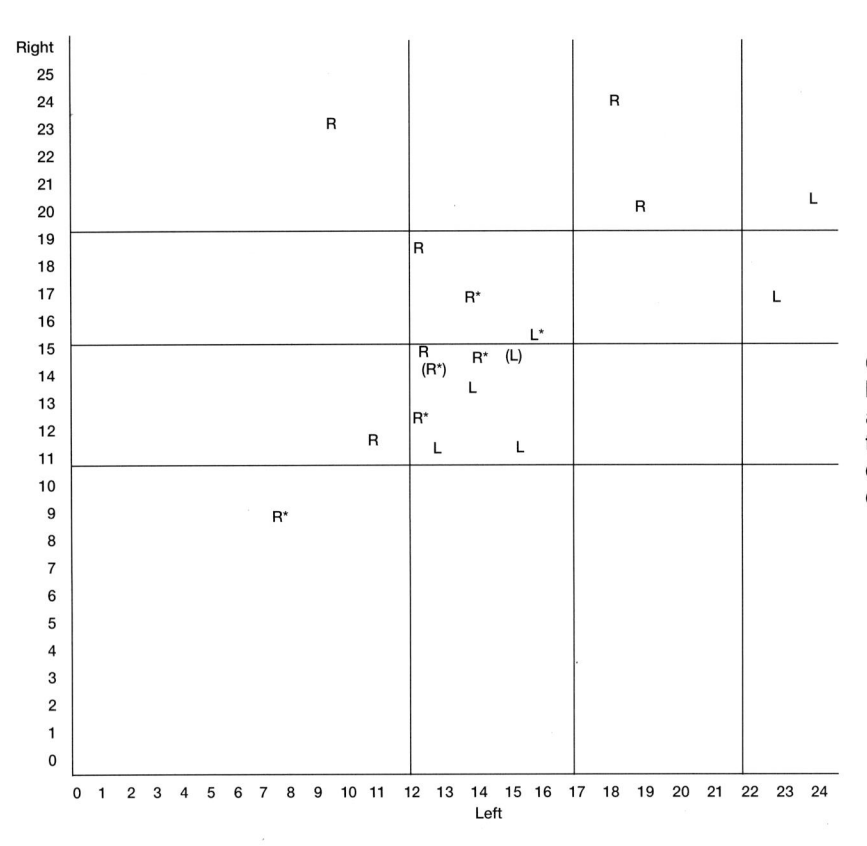

Graph 8-3. Medial pterygoid and lesser dimensions of pterygoid fossa and length from center of fossa to gonial angle. Illinois standard deviation, Arkansas Amerindian,* () dimension estimated.

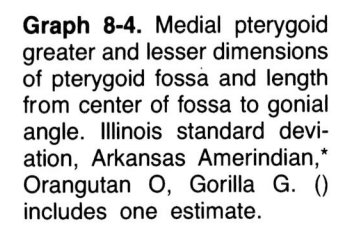

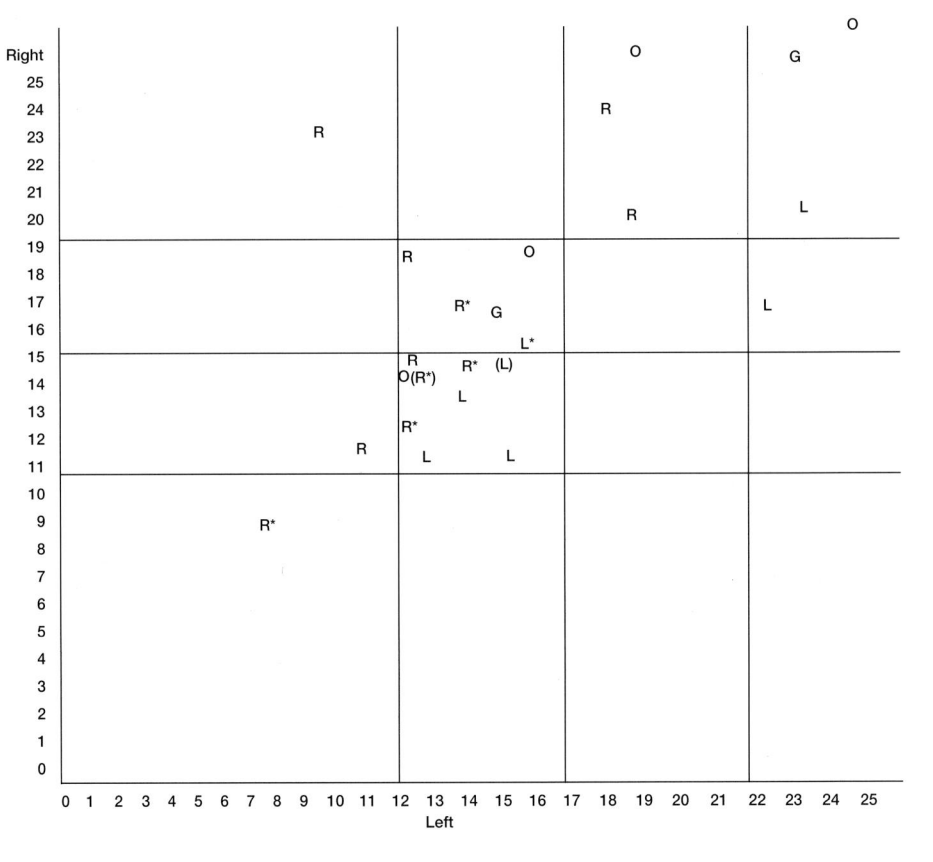

Graph 8-4. Medial pterygoid greater and lesser dimensions of pterygoid fossa and length from center of fossa to gonial angle. Illinois standard deviation, Arkansas Amerindian,* Orangutan O, Gorilla G. () includes one estimate.

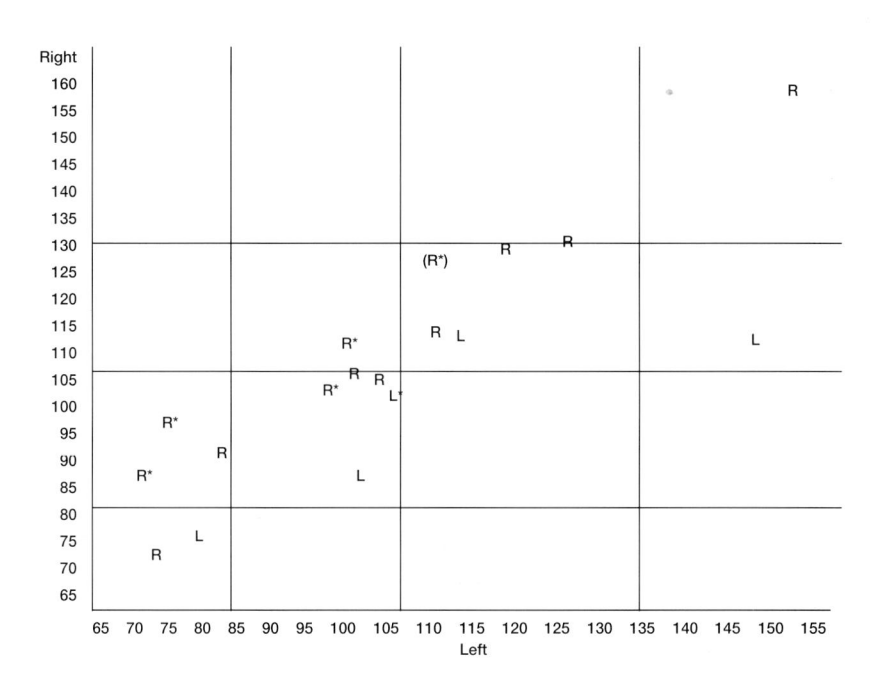

Graph 8-5. Masseter muscle includes ramus height and minimum width and length from zygomatic arch to mandibular inferior border. Illinois standard deviation, Arkansas Amerindian,* ( ) includes one estimate.

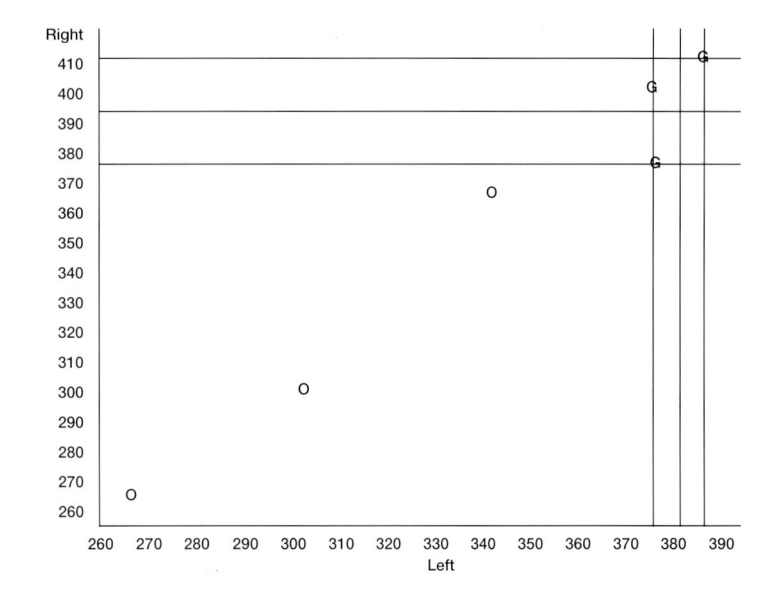

Graph 8-6. Masseter muscle includes ramus height and width and length from zygomatic arch to mandibular inferior border. Gorilla standard deviation and Orangutan.

tance from the zygomatic arch to the inferior mandibular border.

Amerindian skulls stored at the Smithsonian Institution, Washington, D.C., were used in this study. A series from Southern Illinois and another from Arkansas were selected. To assess comparative variation, three orangutans and three gorillas were also used.

A posterior dental "field" was defined as the plane bounded by a line between the mesials of the right and left first premolars and a line between the distals of the right and third molars. These lines were connected by an approximation of the buccal arcade derived by interarch width measurement at the premolars and third molars. The area of this plane was determined for both the upper and lower dentition. The question asked is, if long-term dynamic bone and muscle distortion relates to occlusal plane dimension, mirroring the displayed forces.

The Arkansas group has considerable skull flattening due to the cradle-boarding of infants. The Illinoisans lacked this effect.

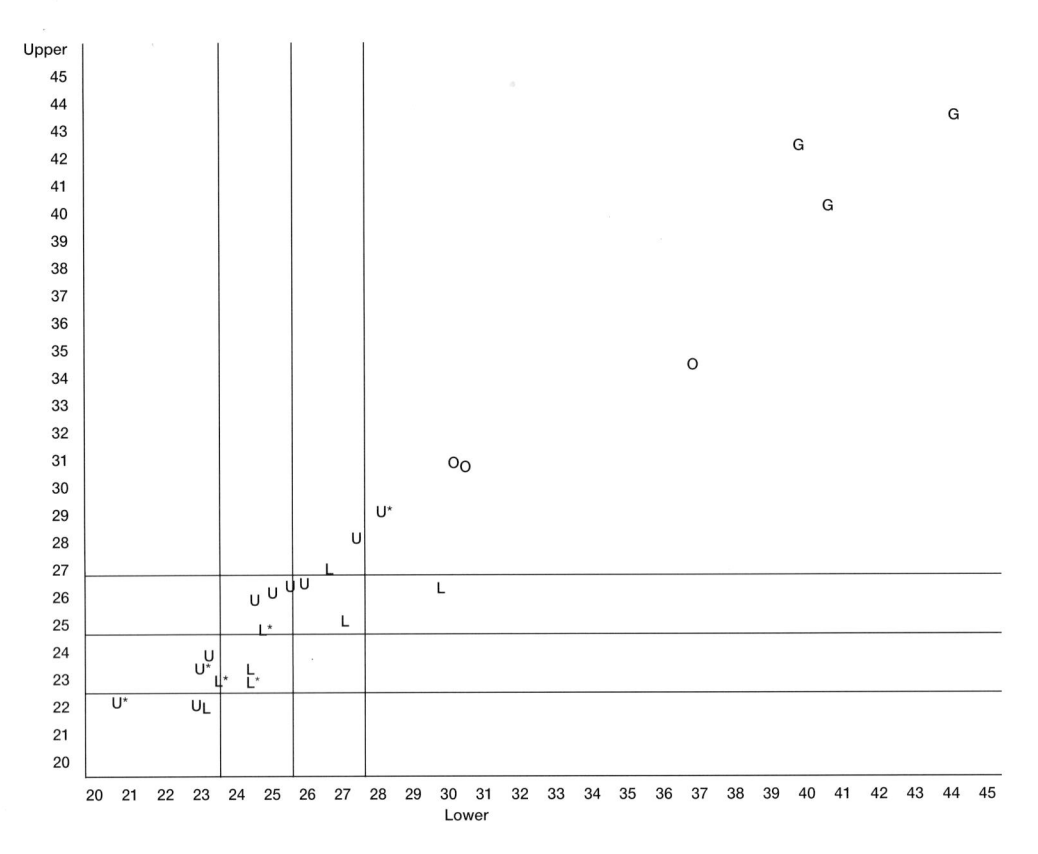

Graph 8-7. Mean arch length and breadth multiplied to give intradental posterior arch "field" for upper and lower. Illinois Amerindian mean and standard deviation, Arkansas,* Gorilla G, Orangutan O, () one estimated value.

Orangutans have a very powerful build, but are not oversized compared to humans. The gorilla is the biggest primate, and because of great sexual dimorphism, we used only females.

It is interesting that the orangutan and gorilla lateral pterygoid lower head and medial pterygoid algorithms are within the human range (See Graph 5). Only the masseter muscle algorithm, for both non-human primates, is markedly greater than that for humans. For this feature, the difference between orangutan and gorilla is marked as well. Thus, from an evolutionary view, the more central and older muscles are more stable than the masseter, which dates to the reptilian-mammalian interface (according to Barghusen).

The dental posterior arch area, stated as field or plane where force is applied, associates best with the masseter muscle algorithm distribution. The greater mass and power of the non-human primates' jaw function is most attributable to the masseter. The pterygoids are not greatly different from those in humans.

If one examines the plot for the lateral pterygoid muscle, it is readily apparent that when the right side is greater, asymmetry also is likely to be great. When the left side is greater, overall size tends toward the upper end of the range. This separation is not complete, but represents a visually apparent trend for humans not joined in by the gorillas and including only one orangutan.

The asymmetrical individuals for the medial pterygoid are striking, graphically, as is the preponderance of the right side as the greater dimension. On the other hand, symmetry is the overwhelming norm for the masseter algorithm, regardless of absolute size. The right side is dominant, but by insignificant dimensional difference.

The bilateral pterygoid muscles' difference suggests a greater torsion role than with the masseter muscle. On the other hand, the masseter and dental field symmetry suggests

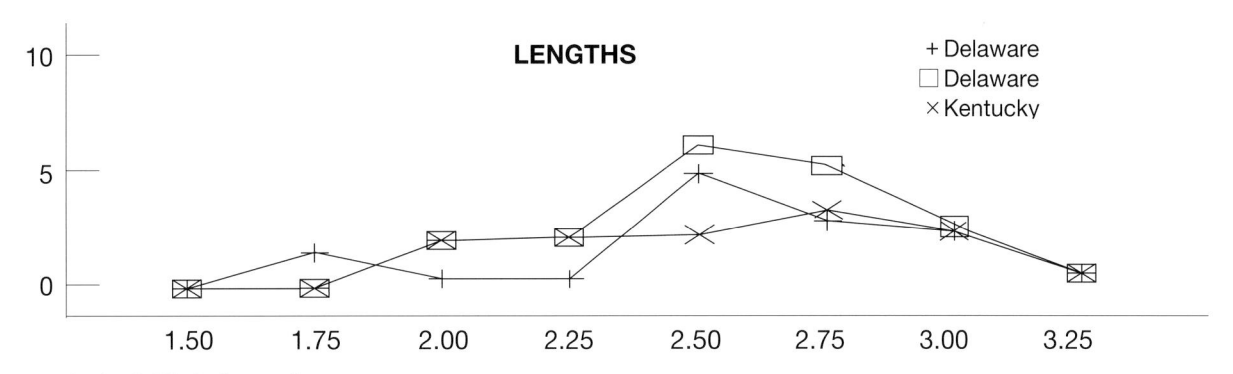

CHAPTER 8 A Biophysical Model for Craniomandibular Management

LENGTHS

+ Delaware
□ Delaware
× Kentucky

1. Left Male Lengths

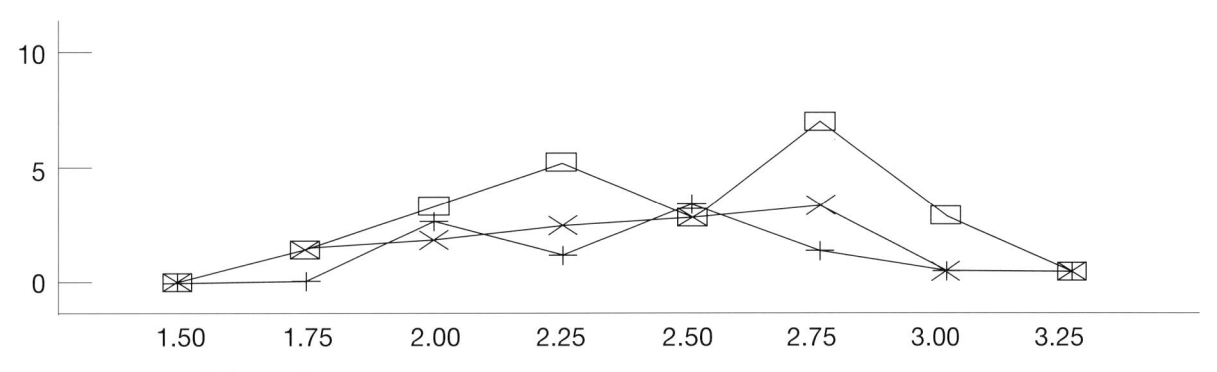

2. Right Male Lengths

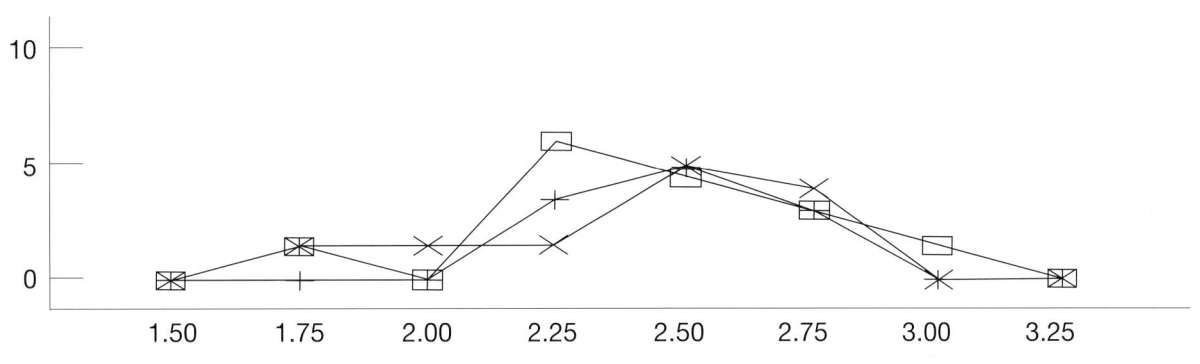

3. Left Female Lengths

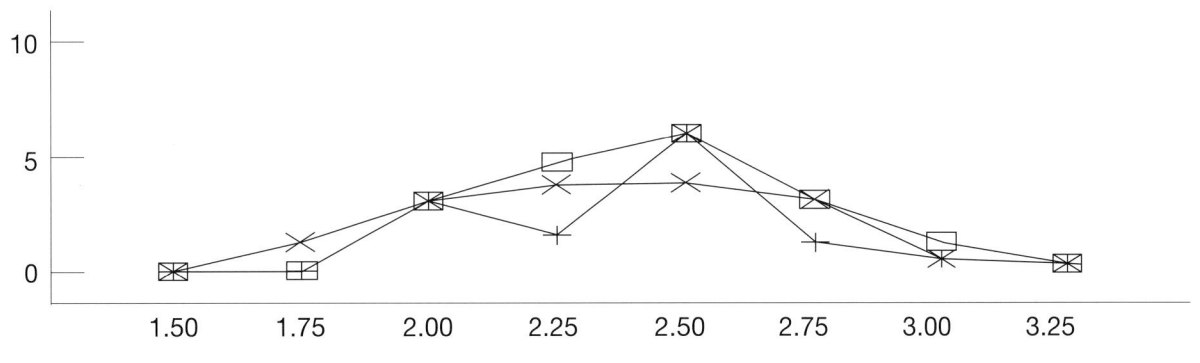

4. Right Female Lengths

Graph 8-8 A. Digastric groove characterics obtained from three Amerindian skull series at the Smithsonian Institution.

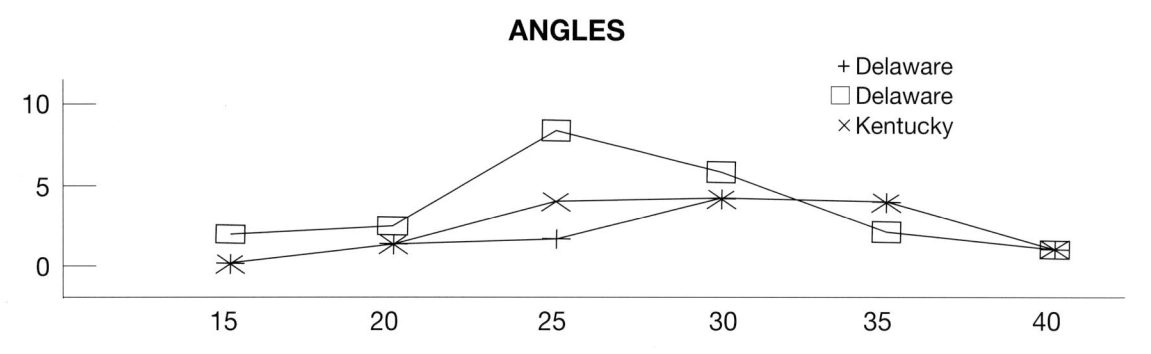

ANGLES

5. Left Male Angles

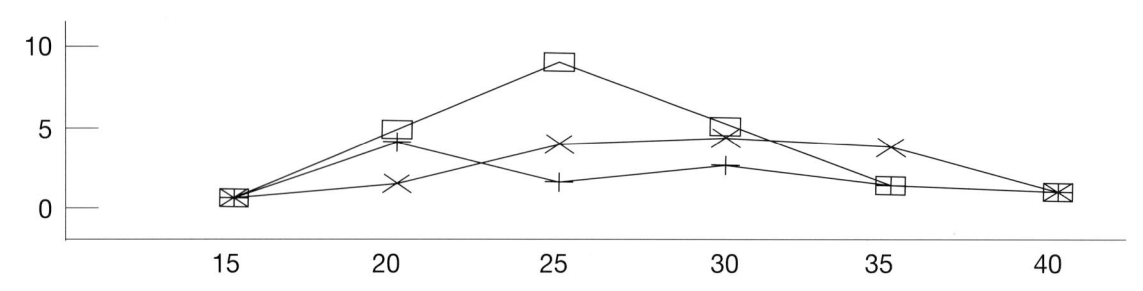

6. Right Male Angles

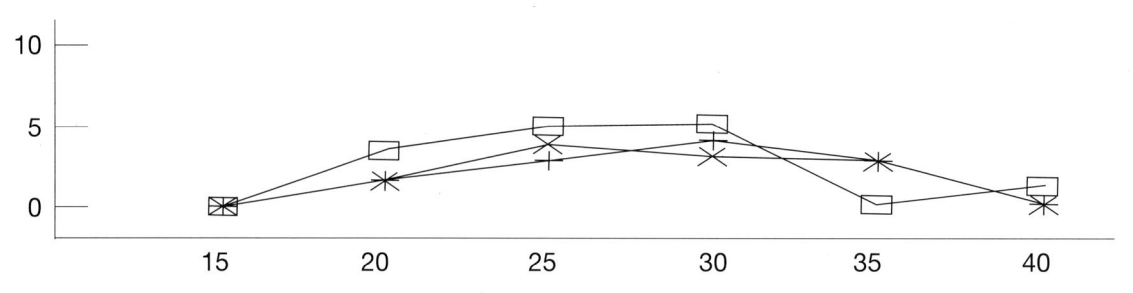

7. Left Female Angles

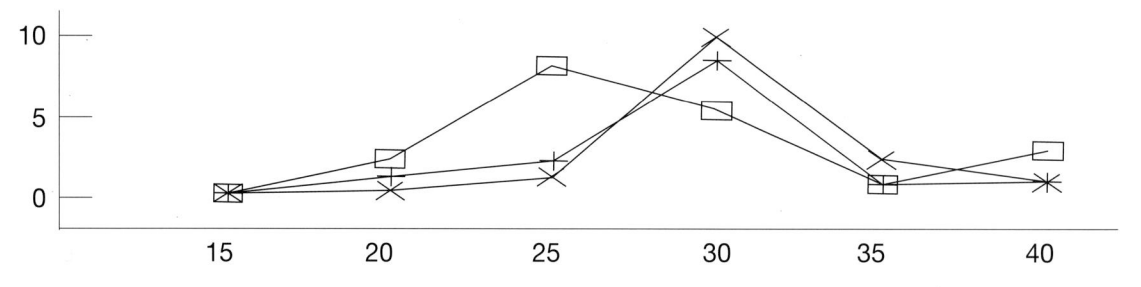

8. Right Female Angles

Graph 8-8 B. Digastric groove characterics obtained from three Amerindian skull series at the Smithsonian Institution.

mass action centrally directed. It appears that spasm is more likely to result in the pterygoid group from torsion and in the masseter from absolute force when it does occur. The treatment modality for patients may differ on this basis.

The digastric groove is found medial of the mastoid process.[27] The groove length is a robusticity indicator. The angles, bilaterally, we use as a measure of asymmetric torsion. Digastric energetics translate dynamically to the entire craniomandibular system. At death, a record of functional quantity and direction remains in the bone. The interplay of genetic and cultural differences may be seen. Specific occupational or other modifiers of function are then open to speculation.

Our study of digastric groove characteristics was done using skulls stored at the Smithsonian Institution. Indian Knoll, Kentucky Indians (ca. 3,000 B.C.); Mound 50, Jersey County, Illinois Indians (ca. 600 A.D.); and New Jersey, Delaware Indians (ca. 1400 A.D.) were included (Graph 8-8).

Remarkably, the digastric groove cranial base area is highly stable over time and intrapopulation. Sub-adult short digastric groove lengths and high angles with the sagittal plane continue into the 18-to-35-year-old group. This is more than likely a growth phenomenon. In the combined groups, left grooves are significantly longer than right groves. This might be akin to right-handedness, reflecting chewing habits.

Female digastric groove length difference, due to short right grooves, contributed most of the side difference for the entire population. Sexual dimorphism in size ought to be bilateral. Furthermore, the left side female length is in the male range. The most likely explanation for the observed variation is cultural.

Greater left-side length occurs in those over 35, but not in the young. The effect is largely the result of long older-male left sides and the younger female short right sides. The 40- to 50-year-olds' left sides are most markedly long, but the right sides seem stable in length over time. Changing dynamics with increasing age develops longer left sides and shorter right sides of the digastric groove. The biomechanical interpretation is that left sides are sweeping in a long arc and pivoting against the right sides.

Sub-adult angle means are greater on the left. Male left angles are greater, but female angles are similar bilaterally. The effect is due to small right angles with the mid-sagittal plane.

The 18-to-35-year-olds show marked angle difference, while the 36-to-50 group shows none. The effect seems to be a carryover of the sub-adult difference, so that the 18-to-35 group's left sides are high and right sides low compared to the 36-to-50 age group. There seems to be a tendency for angles to level with time, and they may even reverse slightly.

The digastric groove develops into a record of biomechanical activity because of bone plasticity under muscle stress. The clinical application of this model will emphasize pertinent history and seek to identify any cultural etiologies for craniomandibular dysfunction. Management modalities should include correction of habitual and parafunctional damaging activities. Over time, efficacious bone remodeling may occur.

We undertook a further study trying to verify the relation of tooth and face shape. The gorilla was chosen as the original primate subject with a plan to later include orangutans, and then several human groups. The gorilla sample available at the Smithsonian Institution was small and biased. The Cleveland Museum of Natural History, however, has 300 gorilla skulls. An initial sample of about 200 from both sources was examined. In addition to the original study intent, observation of the craniomandibular articular areas was included. Bone remodeling was striking, and a model applicable to the human situation emerged.

A distinct mandibular fossa, articular eminence, and anterior disc imprint in the posterior infratemporal fossa could be seen. The bony imprint of anterior extension of the disc beyond the articular eminence fits the "peaked cap" shape described by Rees. In the young, the extension anterior of the eminence is only a few millimeters.

Progressively with age, the eminence height reduces. The mandibular fossa fills with bone. The eminence tends, as it flattens, to become wider. Initially, the infratemporal fossa, roof,

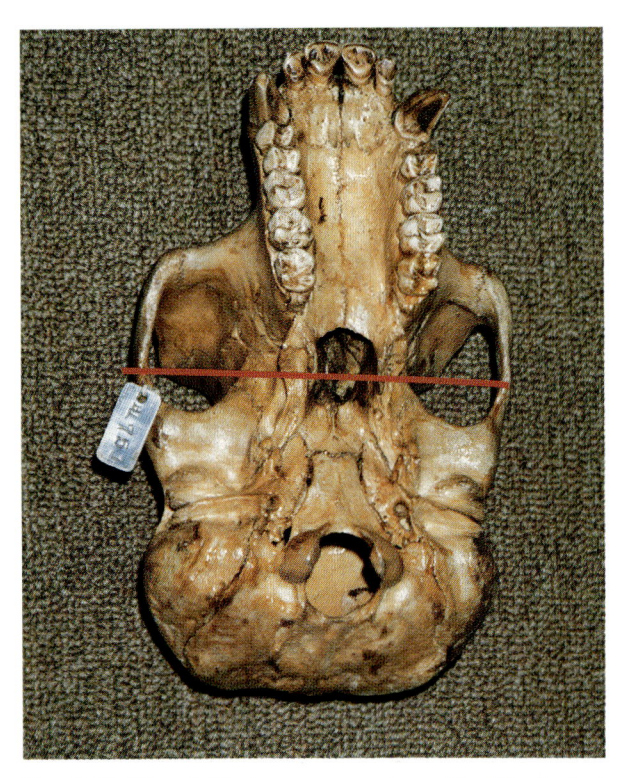

Fig. 8-28. The skull of a young male gorilla. The typical wear pattern involves the incisor tips lingually. Prehensile chewing is the preferred mode. The posterior teeth are virtually unworn, and the third molar is at the occlusal plane. Approximate age is 12, based on gorilla third molar eruption age. The line marks the bizygomatic dimension. The mandibular fossa and eminence area is shiny, partially due to the lighting but also because of the bone quality. In this young individual, there is little or no evidence of plastic remodelling.

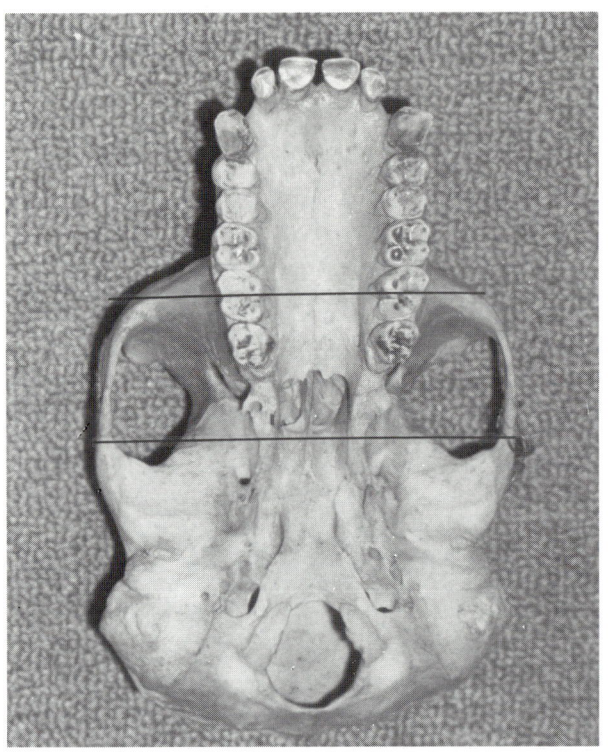

Fig. 8-29. The incisor wear pattern has progressed in this individual and is now clearly lingual on the centrals. A progressive molar wear pattern from first to third is typical, reflecting different lengths of time in the mouth. The anterior line is the bijugal, and the posterior is bizygomatic. At this stage, the changes in fossa and eminence become apparent. Lighting is different, but bone quality is also different. The impression of "pitted type" remodelling of bone is given. The bony functional imprint of disc-periosteal tension is migrating anteriorly.

and disc area is well behind the sphenotemporal suture. By the age of 18 to 20, the suture is usually obliterated. The disc "imprint" advances anteriorly. In some older adults fully half of the infratemporal fossa roof is included (Figs. 8-28 through 8-30).

At the later adult stage, there is little or no remaining articular eminence. The bone imprint of disc suggests that function is very broad. We interpret our observations to mean that periosteum, under functional stress, hypertrophies and is included in the disc mechanism. This occurs without full separation of the periosteum from the bony base. The effect is bony plastic imprinting.

This natural experiment shows that, functionally, with advancing age, but within physiological range, the disc can extend well in front of the articular eminence. Plastic bone remodelling, within reasonable limits, is probably adaptive. Finding the disc in front of the articular eminence is quite normal.

Biomechanical principles dictate that bone, connective tissue, and muscle must satisfy dynamic equations. None of these components are static. Adaptive remodelling is ongoing in all tissues. This is a model that allows rational alteration of clinically presented anatomic relations that are outside normal bounds.

CASE REPORT

The application of our model to the clinical management of craniomandibular dysfunction is our logical objective. It is clear that the state of our art is imperfect. But the patient seeking care cannot wait for our perfection: we must treat with the knowledge at hand to the best of our abilities.

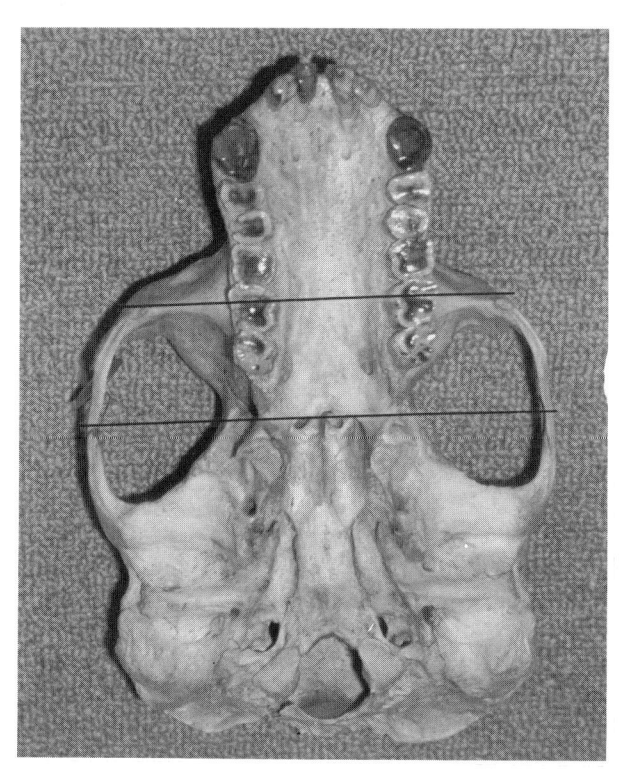

Fig. 8-30. This older gorilla has heavy incisor wear with supereruption. The prehensile pattern exposes the lingual roots more than the labial. The successive molar wear pattern is continued. Preferential right side use is most clearly seen in the premoiars. The lines indicate zygomatic arch shape that may represent response to stress. The anterior edge of the disc-periosteum imprint ont the right is exophytic bone, not a suture line. At this age, the spheno-temporal suture has long been obliterated. The functional area extends laterally to include the posterior zygomatic root. Habitual prehension and heavy wear over time results in physiologic remodeling of the disc-periosteum and plastic bone.

In this spirit, and restating our earlier premise that we proceed from the empirical to the rational, we present one case report. The sole objective is to display method.

The patient is a 15-year-old white female in no physical distress. At her regular 6-month check-up, she complained of an audible craniomandibular joint click when eating. Her mother corroborated the statement. A diagnosis of "clicking" in the joint had been suggested 18 months before, but without patient interest in follow-up.

Transcranial radiographs revealed no bony pathology or other abnormality. Lateral excursions were notably beyond the normal envelope of movement. There was a faint sound at the midpoint of lateral excursion on both the right and left sides.

The patient evidenced mild acute necrotizing gingivitis. Microscopic examination of a gram-stained sample from a flattened dental papilla revealed numerous fusiform bacillus. The patient was nervous and of pubertal age, suggesting hormonal imbalance.

Tetracycline therapy was instituted and continued until follow-up gram-stained preparations returned to limits compatible with a normal oral flora. Repeated Stim-u-dent tests were done until, on the fifth 6-week cycle, the number of bleeding points on touch was 5 in the upper arch and 3 in the lower.

In the subsequent 6-month check-up visits, no significant pathology was noted. At the current examination, a Stim-u-dent test revealed no bleeding points on touch and no new carious lesions. However, the click had become marked and audible on the right side.

Electromyography was undertaken. Resting values were never achieved. The electrode placed in the anterior temporal region on the right side recorded a mean of 5.6, compared to a maximum expected resting value of 2.5. The right posterior temporal was 12.6 rather than an expected 2.5. After repeated testing, the posterior temporal was still 10.3 on the right. The left anterior temporal was 4.5 and the right anterior digastric was 4.3. The other values were within acceptable normal limits.

Testing in function (clenching), the masseter muscles were equal, as were the anterior digastrics. The right anterior temporal was twice that of the left. The occipital musculature was measured, with no marked elevation. However, the anterior sternocleidomastoid muscle gave a 5-to 7-fold higher reading on the right compared to the left.

Study casts were made and related on a simple centric frame. The lower jaw appeared moderately overdeveloped compared to the upper in the premolar to premolar segment anteriorly. The upper right lateral incisor was in distal torsion, but the overall dental relation interdigitated. The lower center deviated to the right about 1.5 mm and both first molar relations were about 2 mm class III. The lower anteriors were crowded.

An extensive history was then taken with mother and child present. The patient was alert and intelligent and noted that clicking occurred when eating and on arising in the morning, persisting for 1-1.5 hours and then subsiding. Her mother said she "radiates" heat at night, which might be suggestive of elevated BMR. The patient was hypoglycemic. She had had a concussion at age 3 due to falling down steps. She had had several incidents of broken arms and ankles. She expressed the fear that the clicking might hurt her jaw permanently.

There was a history of headache equal in the forehead and predominantly in the right temple and behind the right eye only. Strabismus had been corrected surgically. There were some moderate occlusal and postural habits. Most notably, there was heavy lifting, gum chewing, and nail biting.

The patient was 5'10" and weighed 170 pounds. The history of medications included aspirin PRN for headaches and muscle pain. It was noted that the young lady had recently gone out for track and been assigned to shot-putting. Since she was right-handed, it seemed most likely that the acute exacerbation of what was previously a minor clicking was associated with the athletic activity. The patient and her mother were reluctant to discontinue the shot-putting for social reasons.

The patient is now being managed with a flexible mouth guard, custom fabricated at "centric" fully engaging upper and lower dentitions. The objective is to prevent torsion or dislocation of the craniomandibular components during stressed unbalanced function. We have here a case of full body function bordering on the traumatic, resulting in localized disc displacement exacerbation in a patient with pre-existing symptoms. The patient was clearly predisposed.

When the physical activity is discontinued, a total re-evaluation of the occlusion will be undertaken to attempt stabilization of the supporting structure for the acceptance of equitable full-body forces.

Surface myography does not measure the intended muscles as suggested. Any electrode placed on the neck will measure the platysma much more preferentially than the digastric anterior belly, for example. The region of the anterior temporal is overlain by the obicularis oculi and the frontalis muscle. To place an electrode over the posterior temporal without shaving the hair results in recording the muscle groups originating around the mastoid process.

Nevertheless, the regional record of muscle activity has utility, as is seen in this case. This is another area where we should recognize what we do not know. All tissue will give off some electrical activity. In another case, for example, a recording was made over a carotid artery immediately beneath the surface. The patient had had radical neck surgery 20 years previously. The carotid artery record synergistically equalled the anterior sternocleidomastoid muscle of the opposite side.

The pain behind the eye in this patient could well be a "red herring", with concern over previous ocular muscle surgery possibly accounting for the phenomena. Conversely, via the orbitalis muscle relation, the surgery could actually have contributed to the pain behind the eye. The question is open. Any surgical procedure may elicit varying amounts and qualities of scar tissue, and via the connective tissue system, alter myofascial responses.

The history of headache in the frontal region implicates the frontalis muscle. However, the EMG of the occipital muscle showed minimal activity. Generally these two muscles, with the intervening galea aponeurosis, should act together. The right anterior temporal area electrode recorded at a level two times greater than resting norms and two-times greater than the left side's functional activity. This coincides with a headache area. This evidence militates in favor of muscle connective tissue etiology rather than vascular etiology.

The failure at EMG to achieve resting norms suggests hypertonus. This activity is compatible with elevated BMR. To the extent that acute necrotizing gingivitis mimics the common cold, attacking the "run down" vitamin-deficient individual who may concomitantly be "nervous", the picture is compatible with a hyperactive, hypoglycemic state. There is the additional possibility of iron deficiency anemia associated with heavy menstrual bleeding.

The extremely high resting and disproportionate functional activity of the posterior temporal actually is registering over the mastoid sternocleidomastoid origin, and the anterior sternocleidomastoid belly elevated activity is compatible with this observation. All of this ocurring on the right side strongly supports the diagnosis of muscle connective tissue derangement as the etiology of the patient's symptoms. The effect produced by the physical exercise (throwing) is torsion, which is also compatible with a mid-line deviation. These observations are also associated with the elevated activity of the digastric suprahyoid area on the right side.

The point of the study of this patient is to demonstrate the utility of the biomechanical model we have presented. It also shows an application of the progression from speculation to hypothesis-building. We have attempted to set limits on what is certitude. Finally, we show the progression from the empirical toward the rational, from art to science.

REFERENCES

1. Shore Na. *Temporomandibular Joint Disfunction and Occlusal Equilibration*. Philadelphia, Pa: JB Lippincott Company; 1976:84.
2. Sicher H. *Oral Anatomy*. St. Louis, MO: CV Mosby Company; 1965:148,149.
3. Koritzer RT. The biology of muscle physiology in occlusion and TMJ pain and dysfunction. Chicago, Il; (Lecture).
4. Koritzer RT, Hyatt J, Levy B, Tarpley T, Neff P. Peridiscal parotid elements. (in preparation).
5. Howell DS. Etiopathogenesis of osteoarthritis. In: Mc Carty DJ, ed. *Arthritis*. 10th ed. Philadelphia, Pa: Lea and Febiger; 1985:1400-1407.
6. Warwick R, Williams PL. *Gray's Anatomy/* 35th ed(British). Philadelphia, Pa: WB Saunders Company; 1973:39-41.
7. Bo WJ, Meschan I, Krueger WA. *Basic Atlas of Cross-Sectional Anatomy*. Philadelphia, Pa: WB Saunders Company; 1980:Plates 1-16 to 1-19.
8. McMinn RMH, Hutchings RT, Logan BM. *Head and Neck Anatomy*. Chicago, Il: Year Book Medical Publishers; 1981:121.
9. Helmut E, Staubesand J. *Sobotta Atlas of Human Anatomy*. Vol 1. Baltimore, Md: Urban and Schwartzenberg; 1983:225.
10. Bell WE. *Oralfacial Pains*. 3rd ed. Chicago, Il: Year Book Medical Publishers; 1985:266-268.
11. Breathnach AS. *Anatomy of the Human Skeleton*. 6th ed. Boston, Ma; Little Brown and Company; 1965:204.
12. Ledley RS, Huang HK, Mazziotta JC. *Cross-Sectional Anatomy: An Atlas for Computerized Tomography*. Baltimore, Md: Williams and Wilkins; 1977:50,51.
13. Ferner H, Pernkopf E. *Atlas of Topographical and Applied Human Anatomy*. Philadelphia, Pa: WB Saunders Company; 1963:13-15.
14. Langenbeck CJM. *Icones Anatomicae; Osteologiae et Syndesmologiae*. Goettingen, Electorate of Hanover: Sumptibus Auctoris; 1826-1841.
15. Morgan DH, House LR, Hall WP, Vamvas SJ. *Diseases of the Temporomandibular Apparatus*. 2nd ed. St. Louis, Mo: CV Mosby Company; 1982:93,94.
16. Ramfjord SP, Ash MM. *Occlusion*. Philadelphia, Pa: WB Saunders Company; 1966:5-7.
17. Stanton Dh, Shackleford LS. Further evaluation of the superficial and deep tendons of the human temoralis muscle. *Anat Rec*. 1982;202:537-548.
18. Reese LA. The structure and function of the mandibular joint. *Br Dent J*. 1954;96:125-133.
19. Barghausen HR. On the evolutionary origin of the Therian tensor veli palatini and tensor tympani muscles. In press.
20. Langenbeck CJM. *Icones Anatomicae; Osteologiae et Syndesmologiae*. Goettingen, Electorate of Hanover: Sumptibus Auctoris; 1826-1841.
21. Allen H. *A System of Human Anatomy*. Philadelphia, Pa: Henry C Lea's Son and Company; 1883:255,256.
22. Cunningham DJ. *Textbook of Anatomy*. 3rd ed. New York, NY: William Wood and Company; 1909:402.
23. Koritzer RT, Suarez F. Accessary medial pterygoid muscle. *Acta Anat*. 1980;107:467-473.
24. Williams PL, Warwick R. *Gray's Anatomy/* 36th ed(British). Philadelphia, Pa: WB Saunders Company; 1980:523,539,540.
25. Piersol GA. ed. *Human Anatomy*. 8th ed. Philadelphia, Pa: JB Lippincott Company; 1923:477.
26. Koritzer RT, Hoyme LE. *Primate craniomandibular relations*. Presented at 55th Annual Meeting, American Association of Physical Anthropologists; April 1986 New York City.
27. Koritzer RT, Hoyme LE. *Cranial base variations; the digastric groove*. Presented at 53th Annual Meeting, American Association of Physical Anthropologists; April 1984: Philadelphia, Pa.
28. Koritzer RT, Hoyme LE. *Correlation between facial and incisor dimensions in gorilla and man*. Presented at 57th Annual Meeting, American Association of Physical Anthropologists; April 1988 San Diego, Calif.
29. Toldt C. *An Atlas of Human Anatomy*. Vol 1. 2nd ed. New York, NY: The Macmillan Company; 1919:302.
30. Bradley WG Jr, Adey WR, Hasso AH. *Magnetic Resonance Imaging*. Rockville, Md: Aspen Systems Corporation; 1985:72.
31. Meyers L. Personal communication, 1988.
32. Vidic B, Suarez FR. *Photographic Atlas of the Human Body*. St. Louis, Mo: CV Mosby Company; 1984:58-67.
33. Symposium on TMJ sponsored by The American Dental Association. Chicago, Il; 1988.

Chapter 9

An Orthopedic Approach to the Diagnosis and Treatment of Craniocervical Mandibular Disorders

Harold Gelb, DMD
Michael Gelb, DDS, MS

At the outset of our approach to the vexing problem of posture maintenance and chronic pain, it is appropriate to quote two famous individuals whose statements may provide food for thought. Winston Churchill once said: "Out of intense complexities intense simplicities emerge." George Bernard Shaw stated: "All progress is initiated by challenging current conceptions and executed by supplanting existing institutions."[1]

The basic problem to be faced in this area is that we in the dental profession are still focusing on teeth, not the jaws and surrounding structures which are integral parts of the whole, namely the total person. We must focus on the jaws, head, and neck to fulfill our role as doctors, and in the final analysis, we must treat people instead of teeth and their investing structures.

As dentistry matures as a profession, and as we gain the increasing recognition we so richly deserve from our medical colleagues and other professionals, we must accept the responsibility of increasing educational standards. The disciplines of physiology, pathology, anatomy, and psychology, in fact the entire spectrum of medical understanding, must be integrated into our diagnostic and treatment planning. Dentists must also have some basic understanding of mandibular movement, tooth form, temporomandibular articulation, and how these factors relate to the functioning of the other neuromuscular components.[2]

In addition, knowledge of neuromuscular function and dysfunction, and of the effect of environmental stimuli is necessary in order to treat the chronic pain patient successfully.

A more scientific approach to this problem has emerged in recent years. Increasing information is helping us to cope more successfully with many symptoms not originally believed to be of dental etiololgy (Fig. 9-1). Modern research and newer diagnostic devices and techniques such as the kinesiograph, telemetry, electromyography, sonography, thermography, advancements in radiographic techniques, computerized axial tomography and magnetic resonance imaging have enabled us to explore the etiology of craniocervical mandibular disorders in greater depth.

The knowledge, experience, and training needed to recognize the symptoms produced in the head, neck, and jaw area must be obtained from graduate and continuing education programs; these areas are not usually covered in sufficient depth at the undergraduate level. Then, perhaps, such oral conditions as dental malocclusion with or without malposition of the jaws, loss of posterior teeth, decrease in vertical dimension, poorly fitting dental prostheses, abnormal swallowing, noxious and stress-induced oral habits, postural irregularities, unilateral mastication, and diseases of the craniomandibular articulation will be recognized and treated properly.

Clarification of joint structures, neuromuscular function, and psychosomatic influences is necessary in order to treat craniocervical mandibular malrelationships successfully. The temporomandibular joint is freely moving and subject to a wide range of movement. This movement allows for change in vertical dimension, shifts and rotations to the right and the left, horizontal and vertical tilting, and protrusions and retrusions in the sagittal plane.[3]

There is not one physiologic characteristic of the body—including weight, height, red and white blood cell count, blood pressure, calcium phosphorous level, and so on—that does not exist in a range which is considered normal. It is in its normal range of activity, then, that the physiological relationship of the jaws, head and neck must be studied, so as to be able to discern deviations therefrom.

One must always bear in mind that malposition of the jaw does not necessarily result in pain or other disturbances. Whether or not such conditions develop depends not only on the presence of abnormal stresses or strains, but also on the adaptive capacity of the individual. This potential varies from one person to another, and also varies with age, health, emotional status, and other factors. This accounts for malocclusions of considerable dimension in some persons not causing any symptoms, while the slightest deviation in others results in extreme discomfort.

Etiology

The etiologic factors involved in craniomandibular disorders are multiple, including genetic, developmental, physiologic, traumatic, pathologic, environmental, mental, and behavioral factors.[4] At one meeting the entire presentation was devoted solely to fatigue. The Moderator, Emanuel Cheraskin, M.D., D.M.D., showed the following slide at the outset:

$$R + S \times E = \text{Health or Disease}$$

In other words, resistance, coupled with susceptibility (both factors involving genetic tendencies), multiplied by environmental factors, constitute either health or disease. This helps to explain the adaptive capacity which we all possess, and why some of our patients develop pain symptoms while others do not.

The American Academy of Craniomandibular Disorders has divided the causative agents as follows: "Predisposing factors include structural (size and/or shape) discrepancies with any of the tissues of the masticatory system. In addition, physiologic disorders such as neurologic, vascular, nutritional, or metabolic disorders can predispose the patient to craniomandibular problems. Pathologic factors include systemic disease and infections, neoplasias, and orthopedic imbalances. Behavioral factors related to the personality profile of the patient and how that patient responds to stress, which can be expressed as noxious habits such as bruxism and tooth clenching."

"Perpetuating (sustaining) factors are manifested primarily by the myospasm-pain-spasm cycle and can be related to any one or a combination of the above predisposing or precipitating factors."

In their manual on myofascial pain and dysfunction, Travell and Simons[5] devote an entire chapter to perpetuating factors. They highlight the following: mechanical stress, nutritional inadequacies, metabolic and endocrine inadequacies, psychological factors, chronic infections, and other factors, such as allergy, impaired sleep, radioculopathy, and chronic visceral disease, all of which prolong the treatment time needed for recovery. The routine screening laboratory tests that are most useful in identifying perpetuating factors are serum vitamin levels, a blood chemistry profile, complete blood count with indicies, the erythrocycte sedimentation rate, and thyroid hormone levels (T3 and T4 by radioimmunoassay).

The continued search for other etiologic factors in cranio-mandibular disorders has brought us back to an investigation of form and function. The adequacy of the nasopharyngeal airway and the postural relations of the head and neck are two physiological fac-

CHAPTER 9 An Orthopedic Approach to Craniocervical Mandibular Disorders

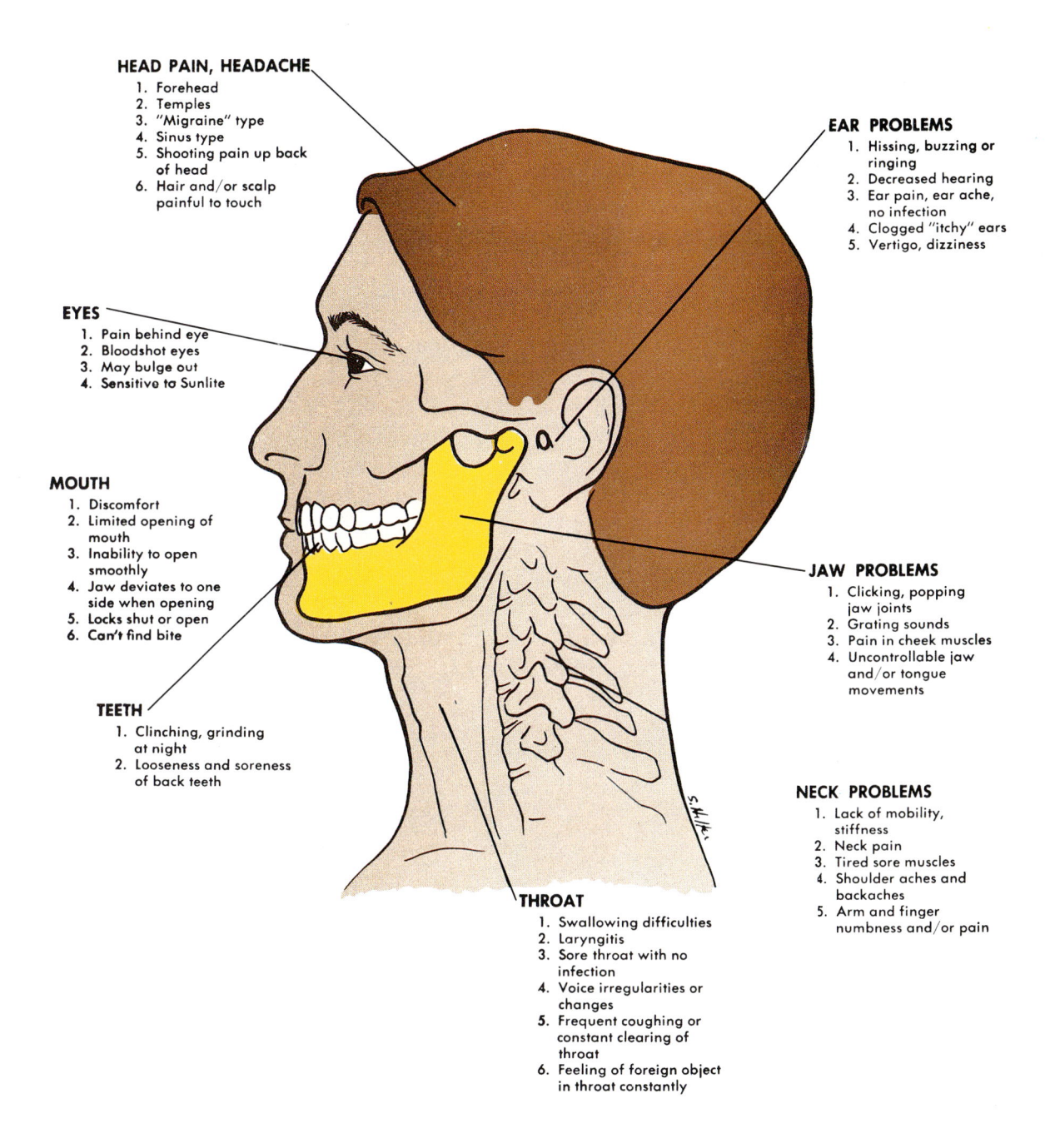

HEAD PAIN, HEADACHE
1. Forehead
2. Temples
3. "Migraine" type
4. Sinus type
5. Shooting pain up back of head
6. Hair and/or scalp painful to touch

EAR PROBLEMS
1. Hissing, buzzing or ringing
2. Decreased hearing
3. Ear pain, ear ache, no infection
4. Clogged "itchy" ears
5. Vertigo, dizziness

EYES
1. Pain behind eye
2. Bloodshot eyes
3. May bulge out
4. Sensitive to Sunlite

MOUTH
1. Discomfort
2. Limited opening of mouth
3. Inability to open smoothly
4. Jaw deviates to one side when opening
5. Locks shut or open
6. Can't find bite

JAW PROBLEMS
1. Clicking, popping jaw joints
2. Grating sounds
3. Pain in cheek muscles
4. Uncontrollable jaw and/or tongue movements

TEETH
1. Clinching, grinding at night
2. Looseness and soreness of back teeth

NECK PROBLEMS
1. Lack of mobility, stiffness
2. Neck pain
3. Tired sore muscles
4. Shoulder aches and backaches
5. Arm and finger numbness and/or pain

THROAT
1. Swallowing difficulties
2. Laryngitis
3. Sore throat with no infection
4. Voice irregularities or changes
5. Frequent coughing or constant clearing of throat
6. Feeling of foreign object in throat constantly

Fig. 9-1. The KFS Temporomandibular Joint Visual Index. A visual, clinical index correlated from the most frequently seen symptoms documented in craniomandibular pain patients by Dr. Bruce H. Kinnie (Columbia, South Carolina). Dr. Lawrence Funt (Bethesda, Maryland) and Dr. Brendon C. Stack (Falls Church, Virginia) and patterned after the F-S Index of the Craniomandibular Pain Syndrome.

tors which have a great impact on craniofacial growth and development.

This chapter will attempt to further explore the relationship of posture to craniomandibular disorders. Head posture, mandibular posture, tongue posture, and lip posture can all contribute to myofascial and skeletal pathology.[6] Certain postural variants play an important regulatory role in growth and development, while others appear in adulthood and are often occupationally or traumatically induced.

Orthodontists and general dentists are fascinated by the concept that craniofacial morphology can be at least partially determined by postnatal environmental influences. By controlling respiration, posture and other variables, growth modification and regulation can be achieved.

Breathing obstruction has been associated with both craniocervical angulation and craniofacial morphology. The craniocervical angulation of a forward head posture and the craniofacial morphology of retro-gnathism are correlated with temporomandibular joint (TMJ) dysfunction,[27,28,29] condylar morphology,[27] and mandibular posture.[15] Certain craniocervical mandibular disorders may then be traced back to childhood through a mechanism described by Solow and Krieborg,[27] as follows. With extension of the head, the soft tissue environment of the ligaments, capsules, and muscles is stretched to produce a downward traction on the cervical fascia and a retrusive force on facial morphology. This is a hypothesis which helps to simplify the complex series of events which result from forward head posture (Fig. 9-2).

Children with airway obstruction and enlarged adenoids have been observed to have a reduced facial prognathism and a larger mandibular plane inclination in relation to the anterior cranial base and the palatal plane.[11,13,15] When the adenoids were removed, the average craniofacial morphology of these children approached that of a control group. A lowered tongue posture was suggested by Linder-Aronson as the causal mechanism.[13] Others have confirmed these results.

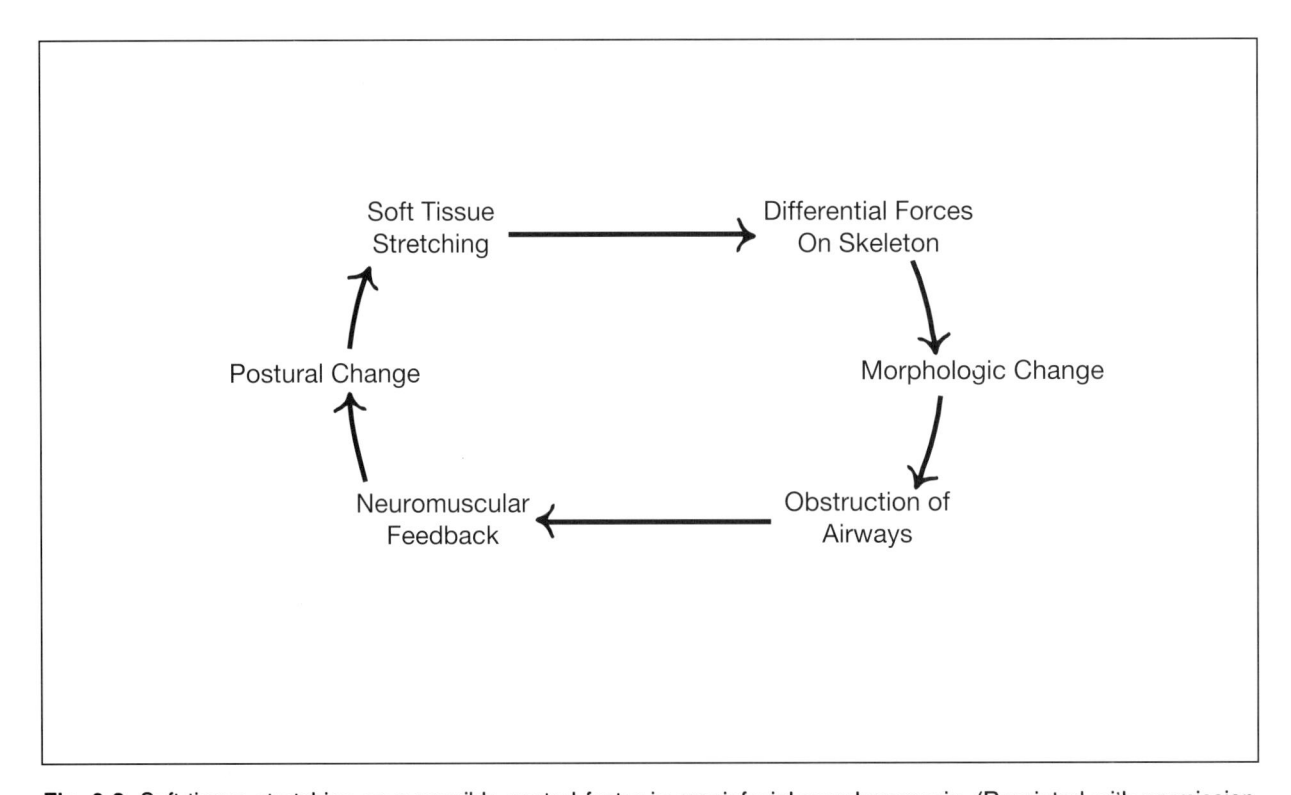

Fig. 9-2. Soft tissue stretching as a possible control factor in craniofacial morphogenesis. (Reprinted with permission from Solow, B, and Kreiborg, S. Soft tissue stretching: a possible control factor in craniofacial morphogenesis, *Scand. J. Dent. Res.*, Munksgaard, Denmark, 85:507,1977.)

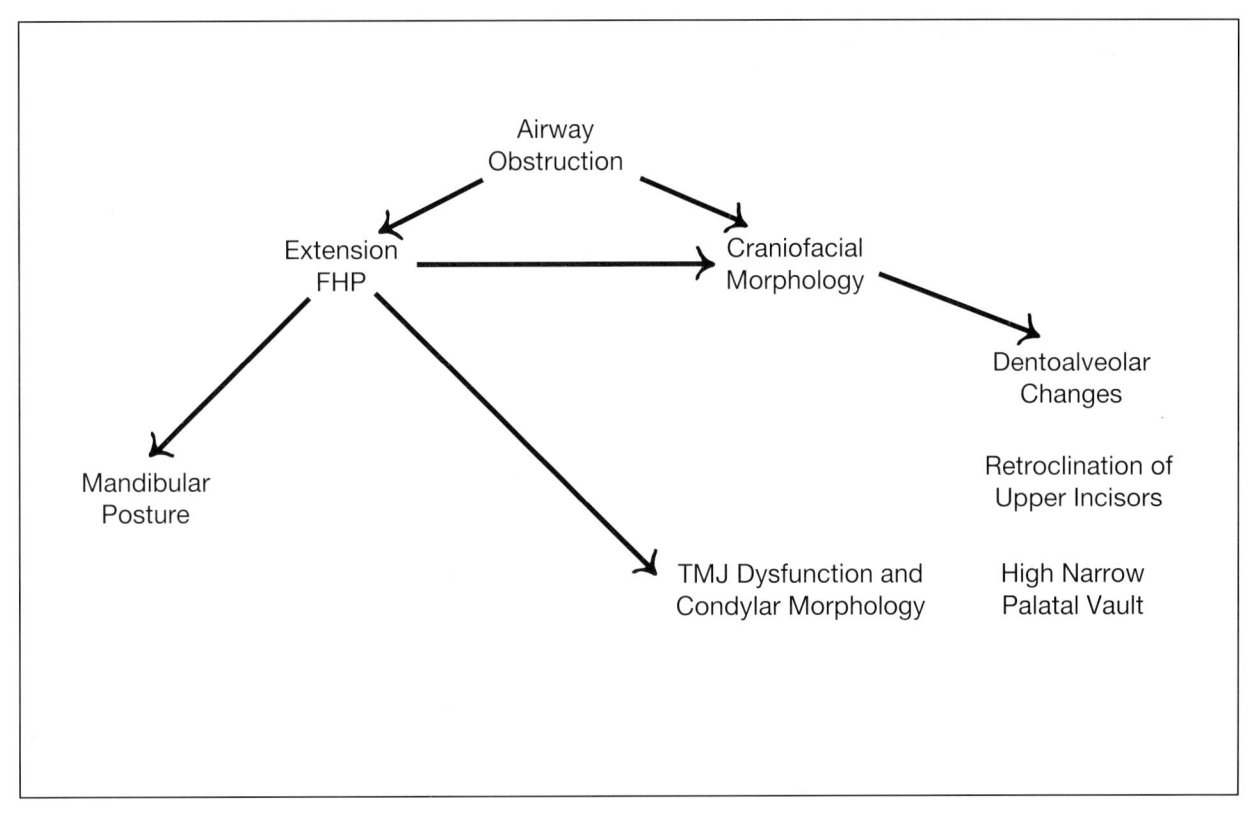

Fig. 9-3. Clinical correlations supported by current literature.

Schwarz, in 1926, attributed the development of a Class II malocclusion to hyperextension of the head relative to the cervical column during sleep.[17] Marcotte[16] and Bjork[30] found a high head posture significantly correlated with a retrusive mandible in subjects with a flat cranial base. Solow and Tallgren have added a great deal to the literature on head posture and craniofacial morphology. Subjects with a large craniocervical angulation had reduced facial prognathism, a large mandibular plane angle and a large lower anterior face height.[11,12,13] The similarity of morphological characteristics in subjects with obstructed airways and extended heads led Solow and Krieborg to their hypothesis, seen in Fig. 9-3.

The hypothesis would predict an extended head posture in children with enlarged adenoids and airway obstruction. This was independently tested by two laboratories that examined children hospitalized for adenoidectomy.[13] Presurgically, a positive correlation was found between craniocerivcal angulation and nasal respiratory resistance. The head was 2° higher in the adenoid children. But four months post surgery, this difference had disappeared.

The relationship between craniofacial morphology, craniocervical posture, and airway adequacy (Fig. 9-3) has been demonstrated in pathologic and nonpathologic populations. The results indicate that a general control mechanism is present in craniofacial development, related to posture and respiration. Is the resultant craniofacial morphology related to temporomandibular disorders, or do head posture and respiration have primary effects on the craniomandibular complex?

Temporomandibular disorders have received much attention in the past few years. Recent research indicates that children with TMJ dysfunction have specific growth patterns, and that head posture is intimately related to temporomandibular disorders both in children and adults.

Dibbets[27] examined children in a longitudinal study begun in 1969. He divided the children into four groups: 1) those with objective symptoms, 2) those with subjective

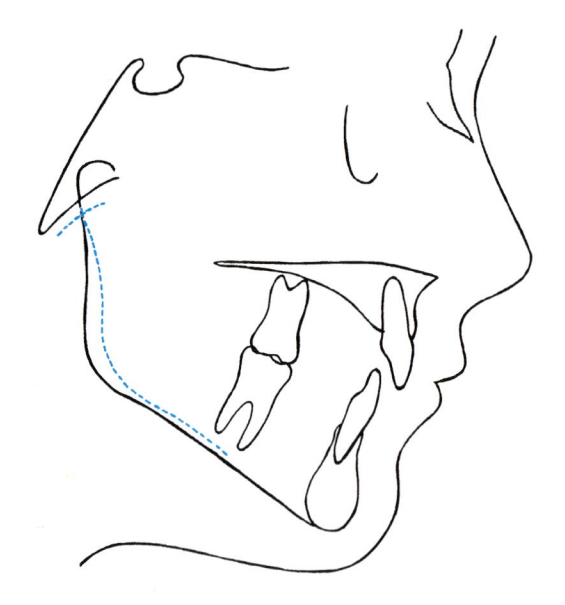

Fig. 9-4. Tracing of the "average" or "reference" patient (solid) and the subjective symptom group (dotted). The dotted parts are derived from the reference by assimilating the relevant results of the regression analyses. The soft tissue profiles are estimates. The ramus appears to "lean backwards" with articulare in a more inferior position.

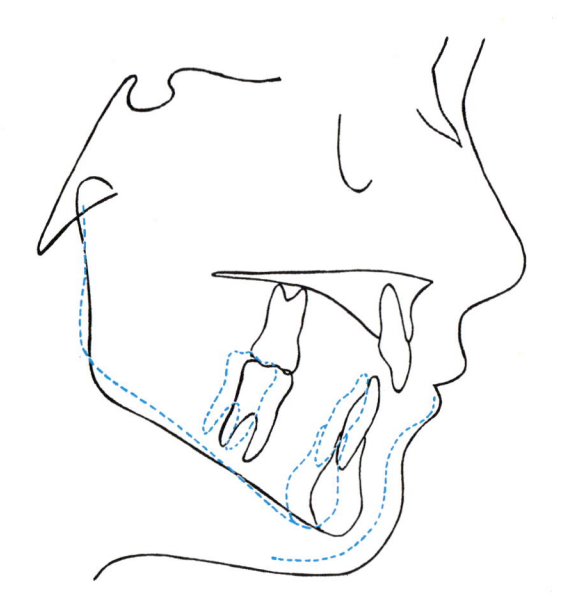

Fig. 9-5. Tracing of the "average" or "reference" patient (solid) and the X-ray deformity group (dotted). The dotted parts are derived from the reference by assimilating the relevant results of the regression analyses. The soft tissue profiles are estimates. The problem is mainly a shorter Corpus and consequently a smaller mandible. The profile is more Class II. Articulare occupies a higher position. *(Figs. 9-4 and 9-5 reprinted with permission from Dibbets, J., VanDerWeele, L. and Uildriks, A. Symptoms of TMJ dysfunction: indicators of growth pattern? Journal of Pedodontics. 9:276, 1985.*

symptoms, 3) those with radiographic conylar deformation, and 4) a control group.

Children with subjective symptoms formed a morphologically distinct group based on cephalometric x-ray (Fig. 9-4). The profile was more Class II with a larger gonial angle, shorter corpus, shorter ramus, and smaller posterior face height.

The children who had a deformed condylar projection, called Arthrosis Deformans Juvenilis (ADJ), also had a typical profile distinct from the subjective group (Fig. 9-5). There was a greater degree of retrognathism, dominated by a shorter corpus, although articulare was positioned superiorly. The growth pattern was also different from the other children, with linear deposition of bone under the gonial angle forming a prominent antegonial notch.

This was the first study which morphometrically linked TMJ dysfunction with mandibular posture. Mouth breathing and nasal obstruction have been clinically implicated with an anterior open bite and a high narrow palatal vault. Vig[10] has proposed the following sequence of biological events to explain these dentoalveolar changes:

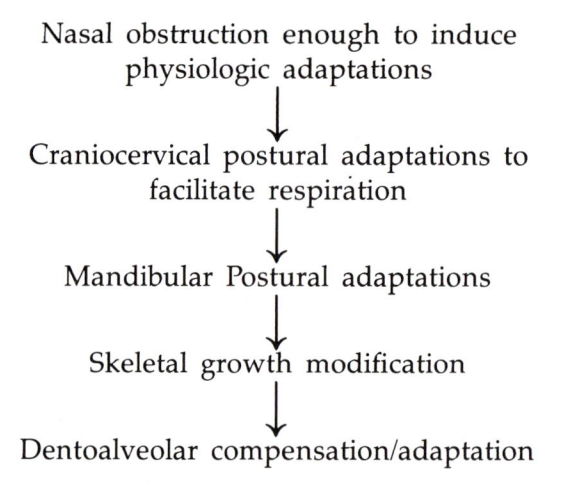

Nasal obstruction enough to induce
physiologic adaptations
↓
Craniocervical postural adaptations to
facilitate respiration
↓
Mandibular Postural adaptations
↓
Skeletal growth modification
↓
Dentoalveolar compensation/adaptation

An obstructed airway with extended head posture has also been associated with facial retrognathism and retroclination of the upper incisors (Fig. 9-6). This is defined dentally as a Class II Division 2 malocclusion. Many clinicians have found this occlusal relationship to be associated with temporomandibular disorders. The relationship of a Class II Division 2 malocclusion on myofascial disease and intra-

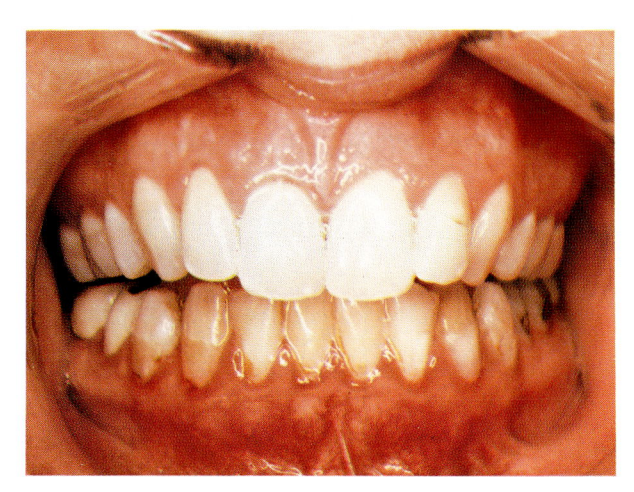

Fig. 9-6. Class II Division 2 malocclusion.

capsular pathology will be discussed later in the chapter.

Extended head position is seen clinically as forward head posture (FHP); the individual attempts to maintain a horizontal and parallel relationship of the bipupilar, otic, and occlusal planes with the ground. This relationship allows the visual gaze to be horizontally oriented. Rocabado[28] has demonstrated a direct relationship between, FHP, craniovertebral abnormalities, and craniomandibular dysfunction.

Mouth breathing has been shown to produce a forward head posture, with accessory neck muscles facilitating respiration. FHP may also develop, however, due to a genetic predisposition, or from prolonged daily activities with the upper extremities in front of the body. Darnell[29] has proposed a chronology of events of forward head posture (Fig. 9-7).

The development of myofascial pain syndromes of the head and neck has been divided into two basic concepts[6]

1. Repetitive microtrauma from poor postural habits and parafunctional oral habits.
2. Factors that weaken and predispose a muscle to the problem, such as structural disharmony or the presence of other intercapsular disorders.

Fricton[6] found 96% of a myofascial pain syndrome population to have poor sitting/standing posture. A forward head tilt was observed in 84.7%, and rounded shoulders seen in 82.3% of the group. The retrognathic percentage was 89.6, either Class II Division 1 (58.5%), or Class II Division 2 (31.1%). Howard[8] also found the retrognathic mandibular posture of Class II malocclusion to be twice as common in TMJ patients as in controls.

Structural disharmony, such as vertical condylar and ramus height asymmetry, plays a role in the pathogenesis of craniomandibular disorders. Williamson[9] found an average difference of 2.8 mm between the heights of the right and left ramus of the same mandible. The range was 0 to 8 mm, measured from the top of the condyle to the menton. The short side was always the Class II side. The right and left corpus of the mandible showed a mean difference of 2.67 mm with a range of 0-11 mm. Again, the dentition was always more Class II on the short side.

Bezuur,[18] in a recent Ph.D. thesis, found the mean condylar asymmetry (9.10 mm + 7.8 mm) to be greater in a myogenous pain sample than in an arthrogenous sample (4.83 + 4.63). Habets[19] had already established that condylar asymmetry was more common among craniomandibular disorders patients than among general dental patients.

Bezuur[18] has proposed the following speculations on pathogensis of a craniomandibular disorder, based on his findings.

A slight condylar asymmetry might trigger muscular hyperactivity.
↓
Muscular hyperactivity contributes to overloading in specific intraarticular areas.
↓
Compensatory reactions take place in the articulating surfaces, increasing the soft and hard tissues.
↓
Condylar asymmetry increases.
↓
At the exhausted level of adaptation, the increased asymmetry starts to decrease (deterioration of articulating surfaces).
↓
With time and no intereruption of the pathogenesis, the symmetry tends to return, i.e. in the final stage of craniomandibular disorder, osteoarthrosis.

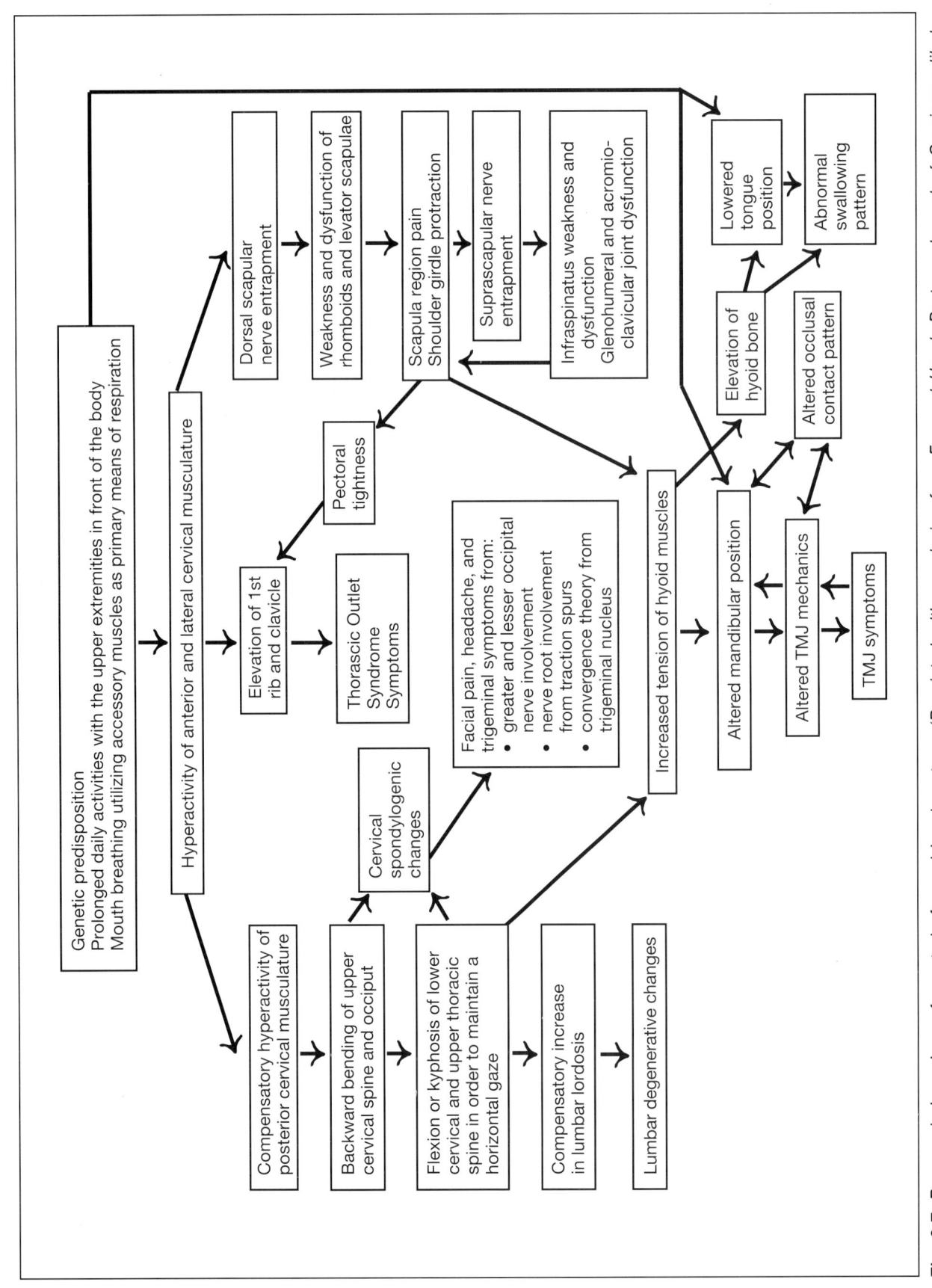

Fig. 9-7. Proposed chronology of events in forward head posture. *(Reprinted with permission from Forward Head Posture, Journal of Craniomandibular Practice, Chroma, 1977, p.53.)*

Individuals with mandibular asymmetry will usually chew on the short, low, or Class II side. Lagaida and White[25] found that 20 of 20—or 100%—of the children studied chewed on the more collapsed side. This was also the side of the highest eye in 100% of the cases.

Dentoalveolar morphology was found to be correlated with facial morphology in all of the children studied. Condylar flattening was often seen on the opposite side.

Any structural disharmony which leads to a retrognathic mandibular posture will predispose to craniomandibular dysfunction. Respiration, head posture, loss of teeth, dental equilibration, and iatrogenic orthodontic therapy, including unnecessary or poorly performed 4-bicuspid extraction technique can all exacerbate structural disharmony of the mandible.

Condylar retroposition or retursion is often associated with a Class II or retrognathic mandibular posture. Posterior condylar position occurs more frequently in women, and more frequently on the right side.[22]

According to Moss's functional matrix concept,[32] genetic factors provide only the possibility of condylar cartilage growth, but it is environmental factors which primarily regulate skeletal unit form and growth. Therefore, it appears that joint morphology is merely a secondary response to altering functional demands. "The major factors determining the development of the bone form is genetic. The extension of the full genetic potential of any form of life also depends on both optimal environment and functional states." In essence, functional matrices "stimulate," whereas skeletal units "respond."[31]

To quote Sicher and DuBrul:[34] "The growth of the mandibular condyle, removing, as it were, the mandibular body from the bases of the skull, creates a space between maxilla and mandible into which the alveolar processes of both of these bones grow and into which upper and lower teeth erupt. However, there are many cases known in which, for some unknown reason, the alveolar processes, crudely speaking, seem not to be able to take advantage of the space that is provided for their growth and thus do not grow to their full height. This development is characterized by an abnormal increase in the free-way space or interocclusal clearance; the mandibular ramus grows to a normal height, therefore, the elevators of the mandible, masseter, medial pterygoid, and temporal muscles grow to their normal length, and thus the rest position of the mandibular body is normal. But since mandibular and maxillary alveolar processes have not grown to their full height, too wide a space remains between upper and lower teeth."

A traumatic deep bite can also be the result of the tongue resting between the buccal segments. As it rests between the buccal teeth, the tongue introduces an apical vector, preventing full eruption of those teeth.[35] Further, if the tongue rests between the dental arches, or if it is thrust bilaterally between the posterior teeth during deglutition, it can prevent those teeth from erupting, although the jaws will continue in their normal growth pattern. If we check a normal swallow with EMG, we get powerful contraction of the masseter muscle, whereas an atypical swallow exhibits marked circumoral muscle contraction. There are eight different atypical swallowing patterns.

In "Nutrition and Physical Degeneration,"[36] Weston Price, D.D.S., clearly shows that members of primitive races all over the world, while staying on their native diets, have no cavities and maintain broad arches, normal facial form, and excellent occlusions. This all changes for the worse when the diet is altered to include modern foods. The faces become narrowed, the nostrils pinched, the cuspids outside the arch line, and the laterals depressed.

Generally speaking, it is possible to find good correlations between mandibular morphology and an individual's diet.[37] Of interest, one notes that sites of mandibular muscle attachments are decidedly affected by changes in consistency of diet. Furthermore, muscle structure itself alters when the consistency of the diet does.[38] As the "hardness" of the diet increases, a concomitant increase in the force of contraction of the masticatory muscle takes place. This factor alters the loadings transmitted through the skeleton and is followed by observed compensatory skeletal adaptations.[33] Such a causal chain of events has been observed both in man[39] and in monkeys.[40] Therefore, it is not unreasonable to suggest that cranial muscles have a functional design well correlated with their function.[36]

As we observe youngsters, especially at night, we find that they clench and brux their teeth, resulting in depressed and worn down deciduous posterior teeth. These worn down and depressed deciduous teeth influence the eruption potential of the first permanent molars.

If one were to assess the aforementioned material, would it be any wonder that so many patients do present with reduced vertical support posteriorly and concomitant displacement of condyles posteriorly and superiorly in their fossae?

To quote Rocabado: "The condyle has a major area of trabecular bone in the anterior joint surface; the disk, which is a biconcave structure, is highly innervated and highly irrigated in the anterior and mainly the posterior edges. The middle portion where the biconcave surfaces meet is avascular and noninnervated. One surface of the disk (inferior) relates to the anterior portion of the condyle. The opposite surface (superior) faces the middle third of the eminentia articularis temporalis, which has the major area of trabecular bone at that point. There are three surfaces—The anterior portion of the condyle, the biconcave joint surface of the disk, and the middle third of the eminentia articularis—which face each other in maximal intercuspation of the teeth."[42]

The condyle disc assembly should be in firm contact with the articular eminence of the glenoid fossa at all times. To quote Sicher and DuBrul:[34] "One point cannot be overstressed. Strong contact between articulating bodies is found in all movable joints because muscles are always arranged to pull across joints. This means that condyles, discs, and eminences are in close contact at rest, in all movements, and in all positions." When this contact is lost, it may be considered a dislocation of the joint.

A retruded condyle might biomechanically predispose to an internal derangement of the TMJ. A concentric or 4-7 position would keep the disc in close apposition with the condyle and eminence (Fig. 9-8, A and B).

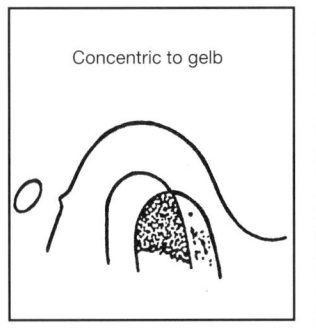

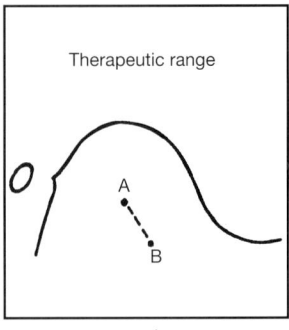

Fig. 9-8. *(Left)* Comparison of a concentric condyle (light dots). The concentric position is the posterior limit of acceptability, and the anterior limit of acceptability is the 4-7 position. *(Right)* (A) Concentric; (B) 4-7 position. On or between these two limits is the therapeutic zone, which should be the treatment goal for condylar positioning. Condyles posterior to the concentric position are retruded and may lead to posterior capsulitis or anterior disk displacement. Condyles anterior to B may bring about anterior resorption, bruxing, or other problems. *Reprinted with permission from Owen, A.H. Orthodontic/Orthopedic treatment of craniomandibular pain dysfunction. 1. Diagnosis with transcranial radiographs. J. Craniomand. Pract. 2(3):245, 1984.*

A diagnosis of dysfunction cannot be based solely on mandibular asymmetry or retruded condylar position, because asymmetric individuals with all condylar positions are found in a "functionally" normal position.

If one were to view the position of the condyle in the closed, rest, and open positions, it would soon become apparent that the condyle in the rest position comes close to the position where the corrected centric position would be in those cases where a loss of posterior support was obvious using our present diagnostic procedures (Fig. 9-9).

At this time it is appropriate to study the picture of a patient with no symptoms, a Class I occlusion, and optimum condylar position (Fig. 9-10, A-D). Note the amount of tooth structure visible anteriorly as well as posteriorly.

Looking at three individual faces, one with a full complement of teeth, then one that is partially edentulous, and finally one that is completely edentulous, we see three different types of lip contours and faces in both profile and frontal views (Fig. 9-11). In an article published several years ago,[43] we found that approximately 55% of our sample were fully complemented, with no caries or periodontal disease, but had multiple craniomandibular symptoms. It became apparent to us on

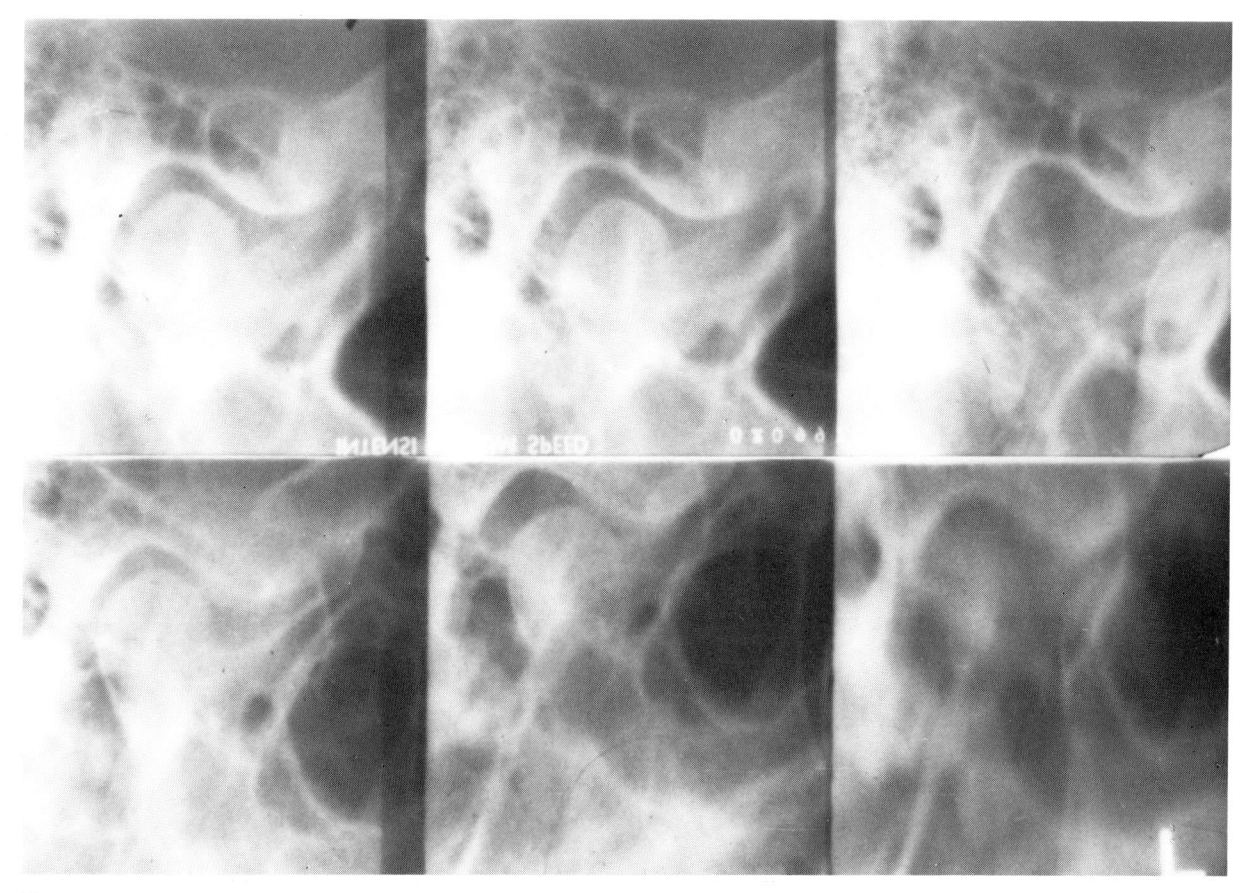

Fig. 9-9. The condyle in closed, rest, and open positions.

visual examination that there was a correlation between facial contours and lip asymmetries seen clinically and the position of the condyle in the fossa on x-ray, as well as felt by palpation of the condyles through the external auditory meatus, and the particular type of malocclusion present with or without mid-line deviation, phonetics, and muscle palpation and testing.

Postural Dental Assessment

Movement of a body part about a joint is not limited only to the parts directly affected: other muscles and joints are influenced by the initial actions. With strong or sustained contraction of the temporalis muscle necessary to retract the mandible, the balance or homeostasis of the suprahyoid muscles is disturbed. These muscles then become activated as the mandible moves, and thus the hyoid bone moves also.

Any relationship of the mandible to the maxilla which would result in a faulty posture of the skull upon the first and second cervical vertebrae could result in the displacement of the cervical vertebrae and in a repositioning of the spine, pelvis, shoulder girdle, and head, as well as symptoms referable to the mouth, ear, face, or even the thoracic or abdominal cavities. Furthermore, faulty curvature of the cervical spine, for whatever reason, with the strains it produces, often is responsible for pain and other symptoms in the head, neck, shoulder, chest, arms and legs.[44]

In the correct standing posture, the different segments of the body, head, neck, chest, and abdomen are balanced vertically one upon the other so the weight is borne mainly by the bony framework, with minimum effort and strain on muscles and ligaments. In profile, the long axis of the segments form a vertical line instead of a zigzag. The chest is held high, scapulae in moderate eduction, pelvis tilted forward normally, and the lower limbs are in full extension with the body's weight poised over the arch of the foot[45] (Fig. 9-12).

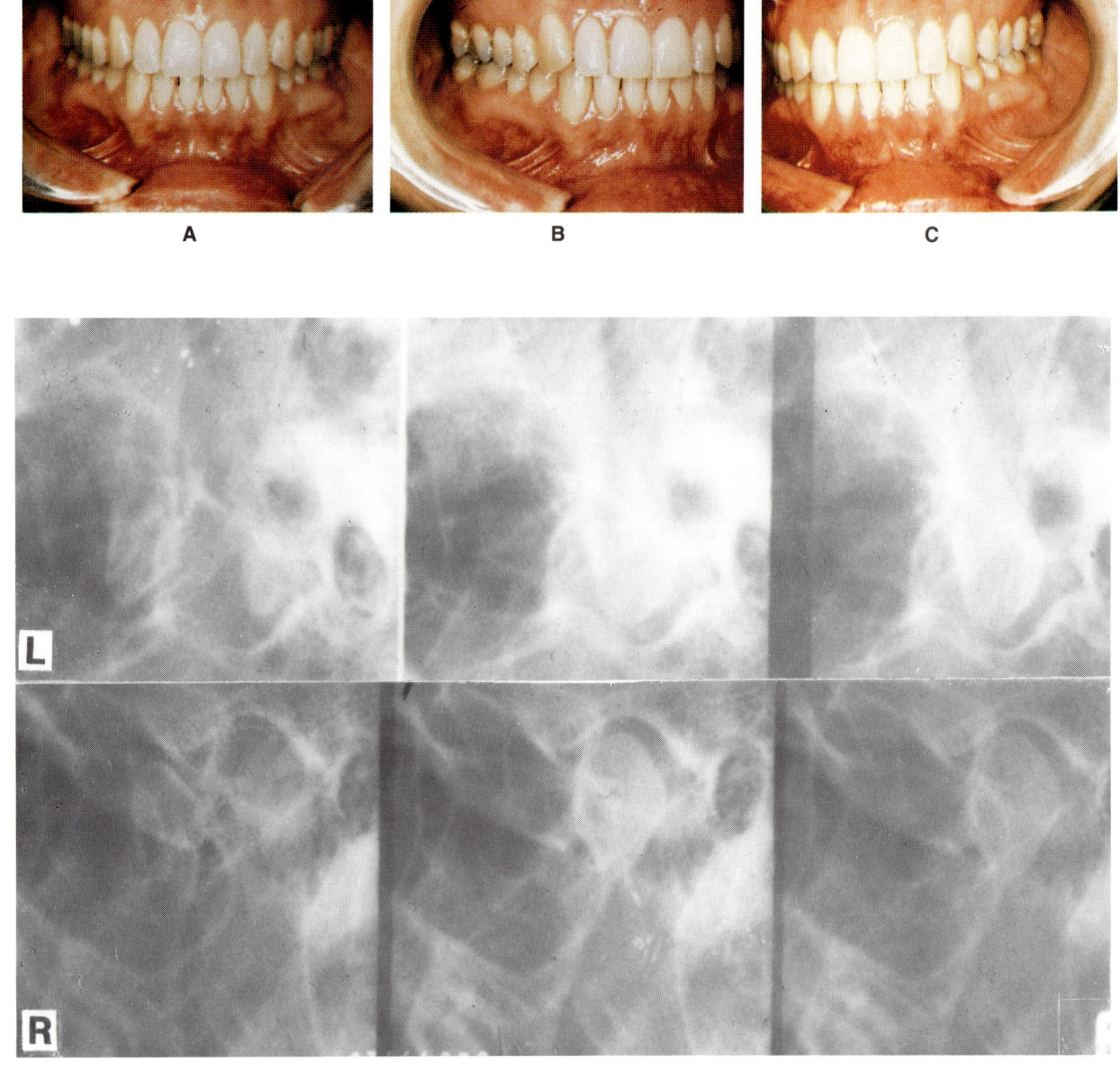

Fig. 9-10. A, Frontal view-centric occlusion-Class I jaw relationship. **B**, Right lateral view. **C**, Left lateral view. **D**, Transcranial x-rays of patient in closed, rest, and open positions.

Many of the patients we see exhibit a forward head-neck posture (Fig. 9-13), with an abnormal curvature of the cervical vertebra, and an associated abnormal craniocervical relationship. The correlation between Class II occlusion and forward head posture is as high as 70%, and is probably the strongest evidence observable of the relationship between head posture and malocclusion.

Several recent articles by Rocabado, a well-known physical therapist, will help bring into focus some points which should be emphasized. In one of these, he states,[46] "Temporomandibular Joint problems begin early in life even though the symptoms are not present until the adult years. Physical therapy in collaboration with dentistry provides an increasingly successful approach to longer lasting treatment. A correlation between Class II occlusion and forward head posture provides further evidence that the team approach is essential. Many TMJ headaches and referred

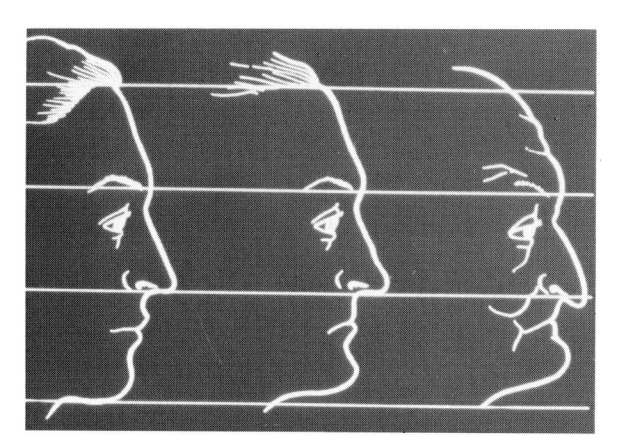

Fig. 9-11. Facial contour alterations from the young adult with an adequate dentition through intermediate middle age with a less adequate dentition to the aged with an inadequate dentition. *(Reprinted with permission from Grieder A., Cinotti, W.R. Periodontal Prostheses, C.V. Mosby Co., St. Louis, 1968, p. 288.)*

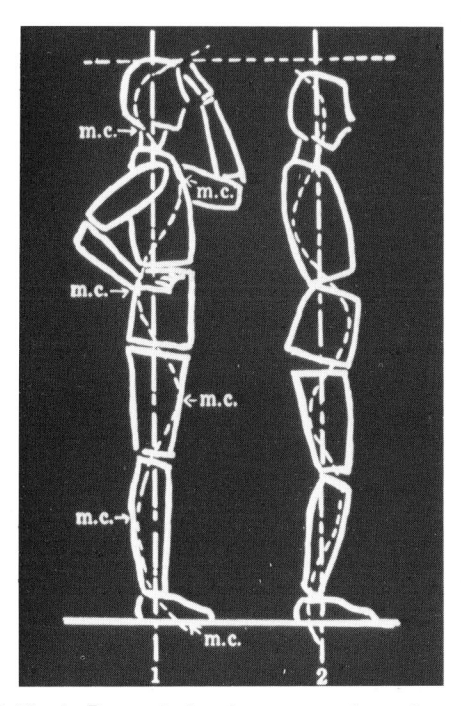

Fig. 9-12. 1. Power balancing power through opposed muscle centers. Muscle centers coordinate cross line of gravity in movement when bones are balanced. 2. Bones opposing bones. When bones are unbalanced, weight opposes weight across line of gravity, thus throwing muscle centers under tension. *(Reprinted with permission from Gelb, H.; Clinical Management of Head, Neck, and T.M.J. Pain Dysfunction, Ishiyaku EuroAmerica, St. Louis, 1991, p. 37.)*

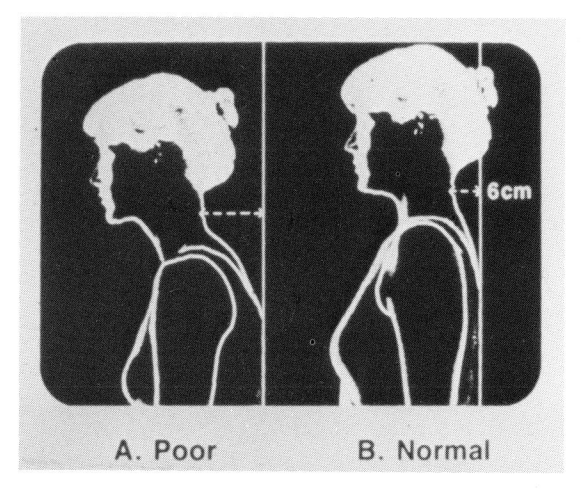

Fig. 9-13. A. Forward Head-Neck Posture (abnormal). **B.** Normal Head-Neck Posture. *(Reprinted with permission from Rocabado, M. Biomedical relationship of the Cranial, Cervical and Hyoid Regions, J. Craniomandibular Practice 1:61, June 1983.)*

pains to the neck and shoulders are caused by compression of the cervical joints. The proper orientation of four planes—the vertical plane, the bipupillary line, the plane of the otic system, and the occlusal plane—is necessary for case success. Treatment involves the proper body mechanics, overcoming parafunctional oral habits, and instruction to restore mobility of the spine. The coordinated approach to treatment involves dental and medical professionals and physical therapists to intercept many serious conditions." In still another article,[28] he goes on to say that, "The relationship between the cranial, cervical, and hyoid regions can be modified by removable orthopedic repositioning appliances installed by the dentist and by manual orthopedic techniques applied to the cervical spine by the physical therapist. However, each of these disciplines evaluates and treats according to the patient's symptoms and various objective criteria that are primarily limited to that specialized field."

Rocabado suggests that these two approaches to normalizing those relationships must be coordinated. He presents an objective method of evaluating x-rays to determine the impact of both disciplines, and suggests that this can help determine the normal biomechanical relationship of these structures (Fig. 9-14).

He also discusses the importance of the following points as they relate to his method:

1. The position of the hyoid bone in determining the appropriate curvature of the cervical spine.
2. The distance between the occiput and the atlas, and its relevance to the headache syndrome.

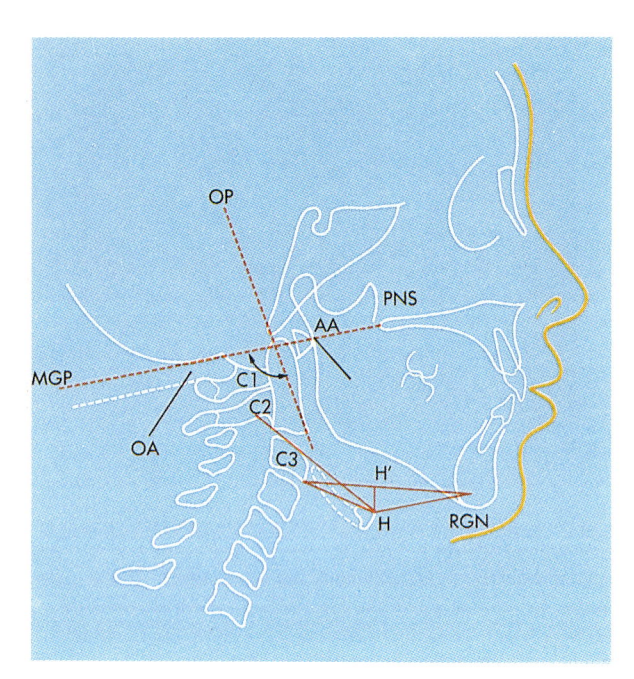

Fig. 9-14. Cephalometric tracing of normal head and neck posture. *(Reprinted with permission from Rocabado, M. Biomedical relationship of the Cranial, Cervical and Hyoid Regions, J. Craniomandibular Practice 1:61, June/August 1983; p. 64.)*

3. The angular relationship of the cranium and the cervical spine.

Baseline for Cephalometric Tracings:[28]

1. Trace McGregor's (MGP) plane.
2. Trace the Odontoid plane (OP).
3. Measure the posterior angle of the intersection of the MGP and OP planes.
4. Measure the distance between the basi-occiput and the posterior arch of the atlas (C1 vertebra).
5. Trace the hyoid triangle. Draw lines from C3 to RGN, from C3 to H, and from H to RGN.

Pertinent Measurements:

1. The normal distance from the basi-occiput to the posterior arch of the atlas (C1 vertebra) averages between 4 and 9 mm. When it is less than 4 mm, mechanical suboccipital compression may be induced; this is a source of posterior headaches.
2. Craniovertebral positions may be evaluated by using the posterior angle produced by the intersection of the MGP plane and the OP plane. This angle is an average of 101 degrees and can vary 5 degrees in either extension or flexion.
3. The analysis of the hyoid triangle gives the position of the hyoid bone fixed in space in three directions without the use of cranial reference planes. In normal head-neck posture we usually see a positive hyoid triangle.
4. Normal cervical lordosis with a normal craniovertebral relationship.

This technique permits the clinician to determine normal and abnormal curvatures of the cervical spine, as well as normal and abnormal craniocervical relationships.

The Concept of Oral or Maxillofacial Orthopedics

The term oral, or maxillofacial, orthopedics gained prominence in the 1950's. Dorland's Medical Dictionary[48] defines orthopedics as "pertaining to the correction of deformities of the musculoskeletal system." It also defines functional jaw orthopedics as "the correction of malformations of the face and jaws." The Group for Orthopedic Research in Dentistry has defined oral orthopedics as "the concept of dental science and art concerned with postural relationships of the jaws, both normal and abnormal, analysis of the harmful influence of improper relationship of the mandible to the maxilla on dental and other related structures; the diagnosis and correction (as far as possible) of such malrelationship; and the treatment or prevention of disturbances resulting therefrom." It is sad that the profession has not yet expanded its horizons sufficiently to truly understand the impact of the craniocervical mandibular articulation as it relates to chronic pain states.

Posselt defined orthopedics as the treatment of inherited or acquired deviations from normal form and position of some extremity or joint: i.e., the mandible, including its muscles. His treatment included orthopedic treatment with respositioning of the condyle; muscle relaxation with physical therapy; and adjustment of the occlusion by means of grinding, biteplates, splints, orthodontic treatment, and permanent prosthetic reconstruction.[49]

The Orthopedic System of Classification of Malocclusions[53]

Class A - Correct occlusion
Class B - Structural Malocclusions
Class C - Functional malocclusions
Class D - Structural-functional malocclusions

Class A

Correct occlusion may be said to occur when the following elements are harmoniously developed and related for optimal functional efficiency:

1. Dental elements
   a. Structural components
      1. Teeth
      2. Jaws
      3. Temporomandibular joint
      4. Dento-facial relationship
   b. Functional components
      1. Muscles of mastication
      2. Tongue muscles
      3. Lip muscles
      4. Cheek muscles
      5. Neck muscles
      6. Back muscles
2. Non-dental elements
   a. Role of posture
   b. Related functions (structures involved)
      1. Respiration
      2. Swallowing
      3. Speech

Malocclusion is said to exist when the structures or the functions described above are inharmoniously developed or related.

Class B

Structural malocclusion (the result of inharmonious development) may be due to:

1. Incorrect relations of basic structures
   a. Correct maxillary development with mandibular underdevelopment
   b. Correct maxillary development with mandibular overdevelopment
   c. Correct mandibular development with maxillary underdevelopment
   d. Correct mandibular development with maxillary overdevelopment
   e. Bimaxillary underdevelopment
   f. Bimaxillary overdevelopoment
2. Incorrect relations of teeth due to aberation in
   a. Size
   b. Form
   c. Number
   d. Position

(The above mentioned may occur either in correctly related basic structures or in any of the incorrectly related basic structures in Class B)

Class C

Functional malocclusions: incorrect relations of properly developed basic structural-postural malrelations:

1. Retrusions
2. Protrusions
3. Lateral displacement
4. Rotations
   a. Vertically
   b. Horizontally
5. Incorrect intermaxillary space
6. Combinations of any of the above

Class D

Structuro-functional malocclusions (various combinations of Class B and Class C)

Patient Evaluation

Going back to the 1950's, Posselt[51] and a group of European investigators treated patients with joint symptoms, ear symptoms, head symptoms, and nasopharyngeal symptoms. They did not include cervical, back, or other symptoms in their assessment of the patients at that time.

```
NAME _____          REFERRED BY _____
AGE _____ SEX _____ DATE _____       ADDRESS: _____
                                       TELEPHONE: _____
ADDRESS _____           PATIENT'S PHYSICIAN _____
_____            ADDRESS: _____
TELEPHONE (HOME)                       _____
          (BUS.)                       TELEPHONE _____

I.   CHIEF COMPLAINT _____
_____
_____
_____
_____
_____
_____
_____
_____
_____
_____
_____
_____
_____
_____

II.  HISTORY OF PRESENT ILLNESS _____
_____
_____
_____
_____
_____
_____
_____
_____
_____
_____
_____
_____
_____
_____
                                       Medications _____
III. PAST MEDICAL HISTORY
          Allergy to Medications _____
_____
_____
_____
_____
_____
_____
```

Fig. 9-15. Figures 9-15 through 9-18 show complete Medical/Dental patient history and evaluation forms. (continued)

CHAPTER 9 An Orthopedic Approach to Craniocervical Mandibular Disorders **231**

IV. TRAUMA (Date, Location, Type) (Breech/Forceps Delivery) _____

V. ENDOCRINE (Skin, Nail, Hair, Temperature Tolerance) _____

VI. PAST DENTAL HISTORY _____

    A. Oral Conditions
        1. Full complement
        2. Full Upper and Full Lower
        3. Partial Upper and Partial Lower
        4. Partially Edentulous

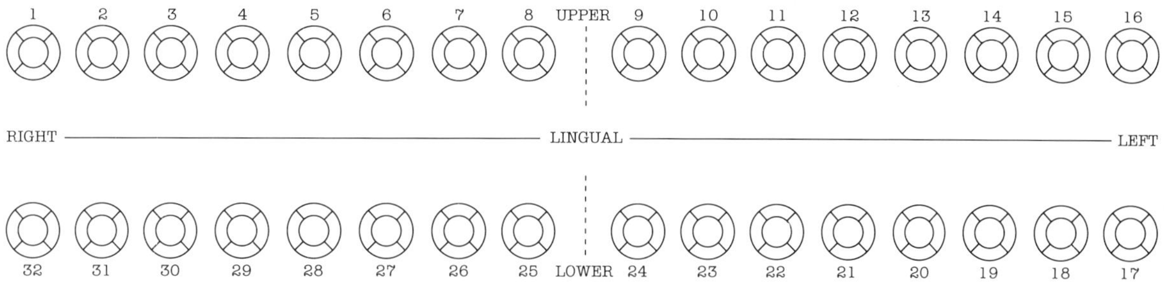

1 2 3 4 5 6 7 8 UPPER 9 10 11 12 13 14 15 16

RIGHT ————————————————— LINGUAL ————————————————— LEFT

32 31 30 29 28 27 26 25 LOWER 24 23 22 21 20 19 18 17

    B. Remarks: (Extractions, Orthodontic Care) _____

    C. Occlusion:
        1. Class _____
        2. R working – Cuspid Rise: _____ Balancing contacts
            Group Function
        3. L working – Cuspid Rise: _____ Balancing contacts
            Group Function
        4. Miscellaneous: (Molar support, tooth inclination) _____

        5. Midline Deviation to the: _____

VII. PERIPHERAL FINDINGS/HABITS
    1. Jaws clenched upon awakening   7. Nail biting
    2. Clenching & grinding while asleep   8. Gum chewing
    3. Clenching & grinding while awake   9. Tongue thrust
    4. Wear facets   10. Phone habit
    5. Scalloped tongue   11. Other work related
    6. Singer/Musical Instruments   habits or parafunction.

VIII. SOCIAL HISTORY/OCCUPATION _____

Fig. 9-16. (continued)

IX. CLINICAL EXAMINATION   DATE   DATE
   a. Objective Pain
      1. Temporomandibular Joint   (R) (L)   (R) (L)
      2. Upper back   (R) (L)   (R) (L)
      3. Middle back   (R) (L)   (R) (L)
      4. Lower back   (R) (L)   (R) (L)
      5. Scapula area   (R) (L)   (R) (L)
      6. Shoulder   (R) (L)   (R) (L)
      7. Arm   (R) (L)   (R) (L)
      8. Fingers   (R) (L)   (R) (L)
      9. Chest   (R) (L)   (R) (L)
      10. Iliac crest   (R) (L)   (R) (L)
      11. Calf   (R) (L)   (R) (L)
      12. Occipital area   (R) (L)   (R) (L)

   b. Regional Examination (tenderness & pain on palpation)
      1. Temporalis
         a. anterior fibers   (R) (L)   (R) (L)
         b. middle fibers   (R) (L)   (R) (L)
         c. posterior fibers   (R) (L)   (R) (L)
      2. Masseter
         a. zygoma   (R) (L)   (R) (L)
         b. body   (R) (L)   (R) (L)
         c. lateral surface of angle of mandible   (R) (L)   (R) (L)
      3. Internal pterygoid: insertion   (R) (L)   (R) (L)
      4. External pterygoid: insertion   (R) (L)   (R) (L)
      5. Sternocleidomastoid
         a. body   (R) (L)   (R) (L)
      6. Trapezius   (R) (L)   (R) (L)
      7. Posterior cervicals   (R) (L)   (R) (L)
      8. Splenius Capitus   (R) (L)   (R) (L)
      9. Mylohyoid   (R) (L)   (R) (L)
      10. Hyoids   (R) (L)   (R) (L)
      11. Coronoid process   (R) (L)   (R) (L)
      12. Stylomandibular ligament   (R) (L)   (R) (L)
      13. C spine (Transverse process)   (R) (L)   (R) (L)

C. TMJ Examination (anterior wall tenderness)   (R) (L)   (R) (L)
           lateral pole tenderness   (R) (L)   (R) (L)
D. TMJ Symptoms (other than pain)
   1. Noises (stethoscopic exam and/or
        digital palpation)
      a. crepitation   (R) (L)   (R) (L)
      b. rubbing   (R) (L)   (R) (L)
      c. sagittal opening click: (R) (L)   (R) (L)
         immediate   (R) (L)   (R) (L)
         intermediate   (R) (L)   (R) (L)
         full opening   (R) (L)   (R) (L)
      d. sagittal closing click:
         inmediate   (R) (L)   (R) (L)
         intermediate   (R) (L)   (R) (L)
         terminal closure   (R) (L)   (R) (L)
   2. Audible click
   3. End feels _____

Fig. 9-17. (continued)

CHAPTER 9 An Orthopedic Approach to Craniocervical Mandibular Disorders   233

    4. Sagittal Pattern of Mandibular Movement
        a. Deviation from straight-vertical-opening-closing
            movement to the   (R)   (L)   (R)   (L)
        b. Widest interincisal opening
        c. Lateral excursions:

          (R) 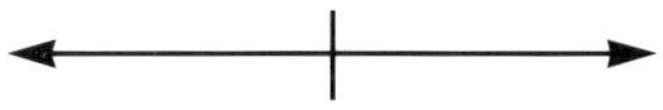 ←———|———→ (L)

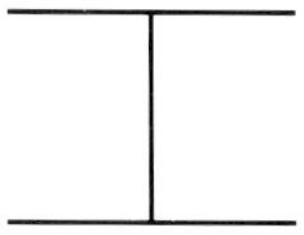

    5. Remarks _____

E. Clinical Postural Observation:
    1. Higher eye   (R) (L)   (R) (L)
    2. Lower shoulder   (R) (L)   (R) (L)
    3. Lower breast   (R) (L)   (R) (L)
    4. Lower hip   (R) (L)   (R) (L)
    5. Forward head posture yes_____   no_____
    6. Vermillion Boarder   (R) (L)   (R) (L)
    7. Cervical ROM (limited/pain)
COMMENTS _____

X.   RADIOGRAPHIC FINDINGS _____

XI. SUMMARY OF GENERAL EXAM (Impression/Diagnosis) _____

XII. RECOMMENDED THERAPY _____

XIII. PROGNOSIS (Duration/Frequency of Visits) _____

Fig. 9-18.

It should be stated that a distinction must be made between signs, symptoms, and dysfunction. According to Mongini[52] in a recent article, the result of clinical, anatomic, and experimental studies in the last few years have opened new vistas in the treatment of patients with craniomandibular disorders. The data acquired about the functional and structural relationships among the three components of the three components of the stomatognathic apparatus, namely, the jaws, temporomandibular joints, and the muscles, should encourage the clinician to do a careful examination of them, with all diagnostic means at his or her disposal. The so-called asymptomatic case frequently shows, at the subclinical level, signs of dysfunction or a beginning lesion. These should not be overlooked, and the treatment plan should be modified accordingly.

Since we are dealing with a multifactorial problem requiring a multidisciplinary approach, it is necessary to evaluate craniomandibular disorders under three major categories: 1) general systemic disease, 2) local pathology, and 3) abnormalities of the masticatory mechanism. Before we focus on the latter, we must first rule out 1) and 2) by investigating these areas:

A. Aural, nasal and nasopharyngeal diseases
B. Adenopathy
C. Neural Disorders
D. Collagenous Diseases
E. Bone Dyscrasias
F. Traumatic Disorders
G. Neoplasm
H. Arthridities
I. Psychogenic Factors

At this time, the use of base line records can help the clinician assess the physiological requirements of the patient's stomatognathic system in relationship to the other skeletal and soft tissue systems in the body.

Both correct and incorrect mandibular positions are related to and influence neuromuscular function. Long-standing abnormal patterns of behavior sometimes will not respond rapidly to treatment. Time is required for reconditioning in such cases, depending upon the length of time the faulty mechanism was in operation, the rate of its development, the extent of the deviation from normal, and the pathologic changes that have been produced. The contributing factors can be neuromuscular, psychological, structural, hormonal, or dietary in nature.

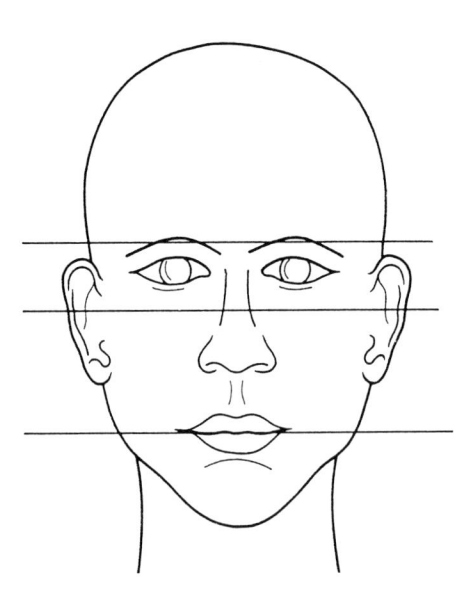

Fig. 9-19. Facial symmetry.

Fundamentally, instead of trying to find the patient's given relationship at the time of presentation, the previously mentioned dental and non-dental elements are analyzed and related to each other.

1. **Complete Medical/Dental History and Evaluation:** Patients should be screened for organic and psychogenic pathology before dental procedures are begun. (See Figs. 9-15 through 18.)

2. **Visual Examination:** Discrepancies in facial symmetry and head posture, indications of mouth discomfort, noxious oral habits, stress-induced as well as swallowing habits, speech difficulties, and deviations of the mid-line on opening and closing should be noted (Fig. 9-19).

Note that the following habits can contribute to the cause of craniocervical-mandibular disorders:[47]

A. Habit neuroses
   1. Lip-biting
   2. Cheek-biting
   3. Toothpick-biting
   4. Abnormal occlusal habits resulting from nervousness
   5. Occlusal and incisal grinding
      a. During sleep
      b. As a nervous habit
      c. From delayed dentition
   6. Abnormal tongue pressure against teeth
   7. Fingernail-biting
   8. Pencil and fountain pen-biting
      a. By bookkeepers, typists, stenographers and others who place a pencil between their teeth
      b. By school children
   9. Biting on the bow of eyeglasses
   10. Playing with artificial bridges and dentures in the mouth.
   11. Clenching the teeth when under emotional stress
B. Occupational habits
   1. Thread-biting—seamstresses
   2. Holding pins and needles in the teeth—seamstresses
   3. Holding nails in the teeth
      a. Cobblers
      b. Upholsterers
      c. Electricians
      d. Carpenters
      e. Telephone repairmen
      f. Wood-lathers
      g. Furriers who are "nailers" (who spread, stretch and dry skins)
   4. Biting on cigar during manufacture—cigar workers
   5. Playing of reed instruments—musicians
   6. Holding a cork between the teeth—package wrappers
   7. Grinding teeth in rhythm with work
C. Miscellaneous habits
   1. Pipe smoking
   2. Abuse of the teeth with a cigarette holder
   3. Biting on various object, such as safety pins and hairpins
   4. Opening tops of bottles
   5. Cracking nuts with the teeth
   6. Chewing on bones
   7. Abuse of teeth by acrobats during stunts requiring mouth props
   8. Incorrect toothbrushing method
   9. Chewing on cigars
   10. Abnormal reading and sleeping habits—pressure of fingers against the teeth
   11. Mouth breathing—lowered tissue tone caused by drying of the mucous membrane, particularly in the anterior part of the mouth
   12. Pressure on the teeth by the hand supporting the head
   13. Thumb-sucking
   14. Unilateral mastication
   15. Use of tongue depressor or other hardwood implements to influence the position of malposed teeth
   16. Use of rubber appliances to strengthen the gums
   17. Wedging of toothpick between the teeth
   18. Orange-sucking by athletes

3. **Palpation:** Locate the areas which are painful and find which muscles may be overdeveloped or in spasm. Place the little fingers in the ears to determine if any backward thrust of the condyles occurs after the first contact of the teeth are made, and if it causes the patient pain or discomfort. Clicking, crepitation, and rubbing can be felt as well. Auscultation should also be utilized to confirm these findings. (See Figure. 9-20, A-V).

4. **Radiographs:**
   A. Intraoral—Full mouth series/periapical x-rays
   B. Extraoral—Panoramic survey, transcranial films, cephalometric films, computerized axial tomography scanning, magnetic resonance imaging

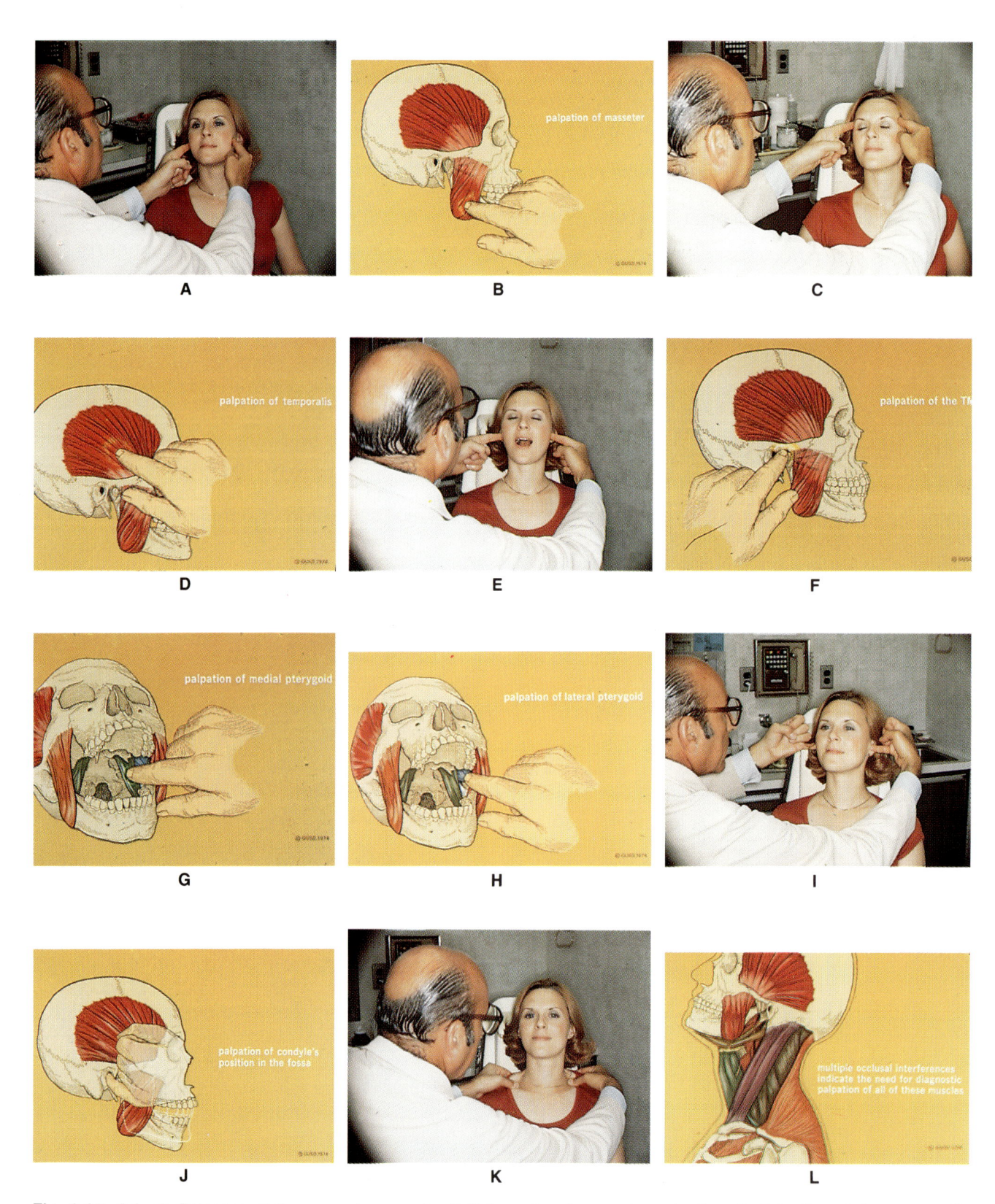

Fig. 9-20, A-L. A, Palpation of the masseter muscle. **B**, Schematic of masseter palpation. **C**, Palpation of the temporalis muscle. **D**, Schematic of temporalis palpation. **E**, Palpation of TMJ. **F**, Schematic of TMJ palpation. **G**, Schematic of medial pterygoid palpation. **H**, Schematic of lateral pterygoid palpation. **I**, Palpation of the condyle's position in the fossa. **J**, Schematic of condyle palpation. **K**, Palpation of the trapezious muscle. **L**, Schematic of cervical musculature. *(continued)*

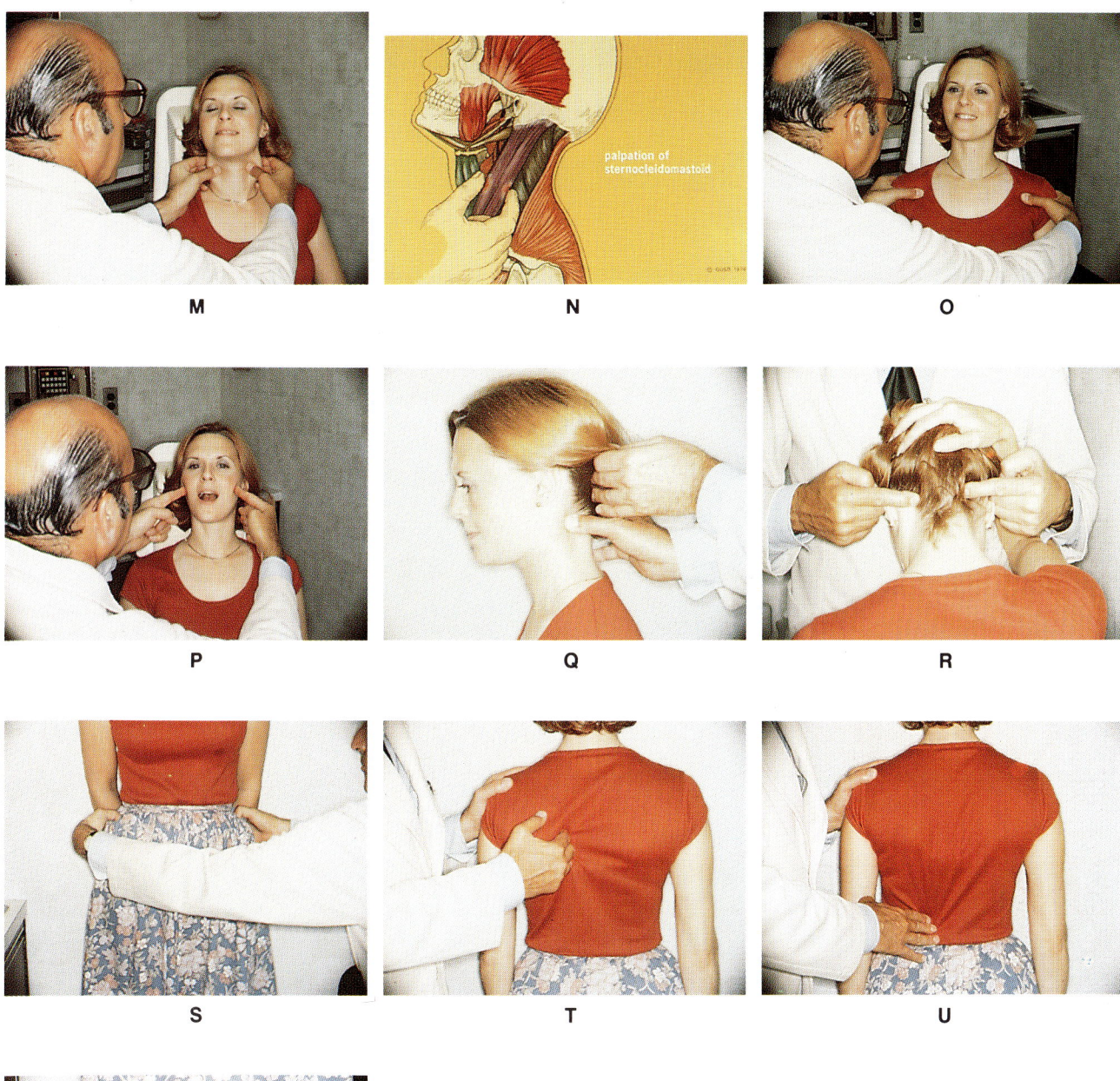

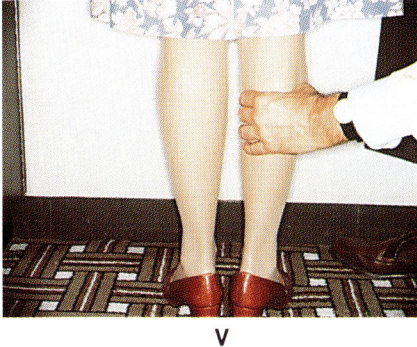

CHAPTER 9   An Orthopedic Approach to Craniocervical Mandibular Disorders   237

Fig. 9-20, M-V. M, Palpation of the sternocleidomastoid muscle. **N**, Schematic of sternocleidomastoid palpation. **O**, Palpation of the deltoid muscle. **P**, Palpation fo the coronoid process. **Q**, Palpation of the posterior cervical muscles. **R**, Palpation of the suboccipital muscles. **S**, Palpation of the iliac crests. **T**, Palpation of the scapular muscles. **U**, Palpation of the sacrospinal muscles. **V**, Palpation of the gastrocnemious muscle.

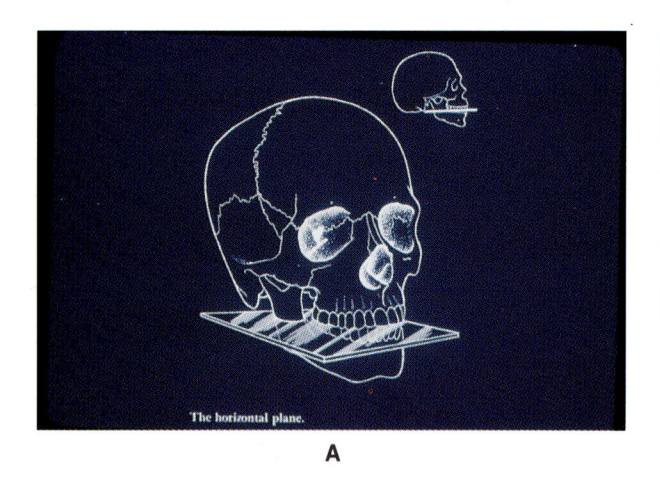

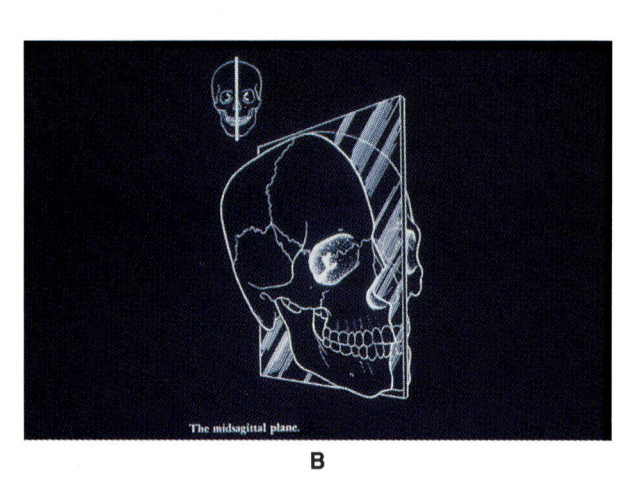

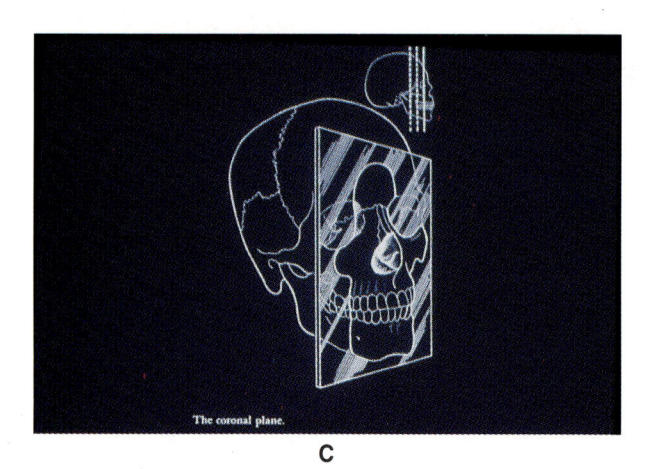

238 New Concepts in Craniomandibular and Chronic Pain Management

Fig. 9-21. A, The Horizontal Plane. **B**, The Midsagittal Plane. **C**, The Coronal or Transverse Plane. *(Reprinted with permission from Grieder, A., Cinotti, W.R. Periodontal Prosthesis, The C.V. Mosby Co., St. Louis, 1968, pp 44-46.)*

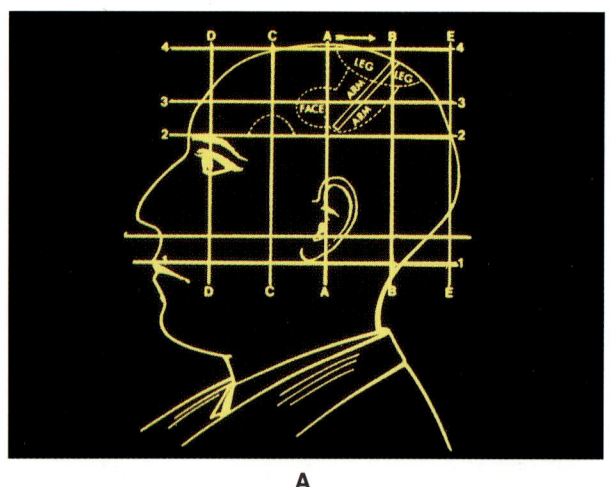

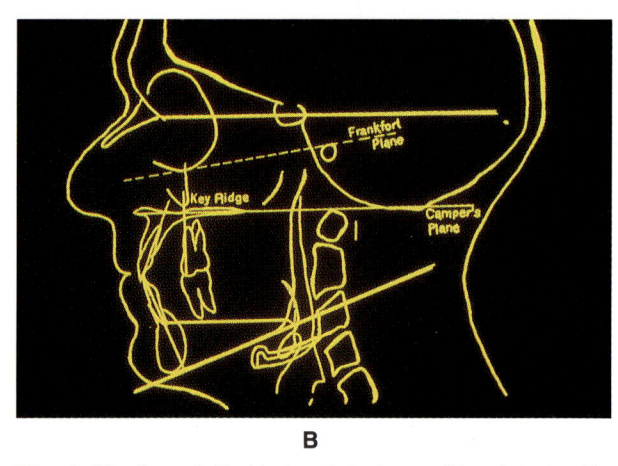

Fig. 9-22. A and **B**. Horizontal plane. *(Reprinted with permission from Lieb, M.M.: Oral Orthopedics in Gelb, H.: Clinical Management of Head, Neck, and TMJ Pain and Dysfunction, 2nd edition, W.B. Saunders Co., 1985, p. 38.)*

5. **Analysis of Aberrations:**
   The attempt is then made to diagnose the patient's given relationship and any or all aberrations from the correct and most natural relationship structurally and functionally. The aberrations are corrected in realignment and retraining of the components previously mentioned.

A. Incorporation of a three-dimensional approach to the overall diagnostic picture supersedes past endeavors which focused their greatest attention on variances in vertical dimension. By utilizing three planes of orientation—the horizontal, midsagittal, and transverse—it is possible to establish reference points (for each patient) from which deviations from normal are much more readily observed (Fig. 9-21, A-C).

   1) Horizontal—this plane may be said to be the MEAN plane of occlusion for the specific patient and

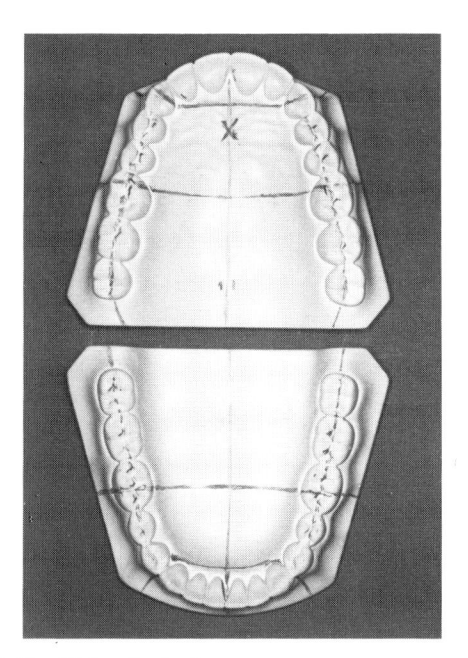

Fig. 9-23. Midsagittal plane.

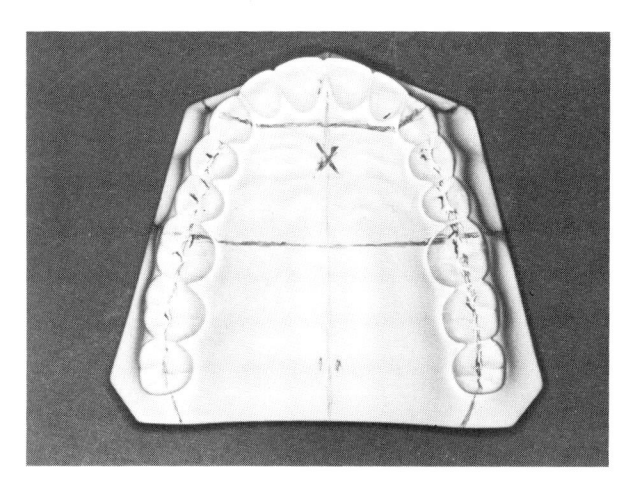

Fig. 9-24. Transverse or coronal plane.

should ideally pass through the mesiolingual cusps of the upper first molars and occipital protuberances. It should be parallel to a plane describing the "flattening" part of the hard palate, and to the level of the eyes. With the head and body in correct posture (patient sitting upright in the dental chair without the backrest, or standing upright in a relaxed condition) this plane should then be parallel to the floor (Fig. 9-22, A and B).

2) Midsagittal—this plane passes through the midline of the head anterioposteriorly. On the upper model it would bisect the fovea palatinae posteriorly and a midpoint between the junction of the second and third set of palatal rugae. If the upper and lower teeth were in proper position, it would bisect the upper and lower central incisors. Posteriorly, it should be midway between the lines bisecting the ridges of properly formed maxillary and mandibular arches (Fig. 9-23).

3) Transverse or coronal—this plane lies at right angles to the midsagittal and horizontal planes. It generally passes through the mesiobuccal cusps of the upper first molars. We utilize this cusp with its root because, with our patient in proper position, a line bisecting this cusp and root also bisects the right and left Key ridges at their lowest points, and is also perpendicular to the other two planes (Fig. 9-24).

By utilizing these three planes we are then able to analyze the dental mass within itself, and to determine its relationship to the cranium.

In relating the two jaws to one another statically (Fig. 9-25, A-D), several points should be confluent:

1. The midline of the upper dentition should be continuous with the midline of the lower dentition, anteriorly as well as posteriorly.
2. A line drawn through the height of contour of the labial aspect of the upper cuspid will fall between the lower cuspid and lower first bicuspid.
3. A line drawn through the height of contour of the labial aspect of the mesiobuccal cusp of the upper first molar will fall into the buccal groove of the lower first molar.
4. The upper and lower ridges will be parallel to one another and to the mean flat part of the hard palate, as well as to the level of the eyes.
5. Posteriorly, the line bisecting the ridges of the upper arch will be equidistant from

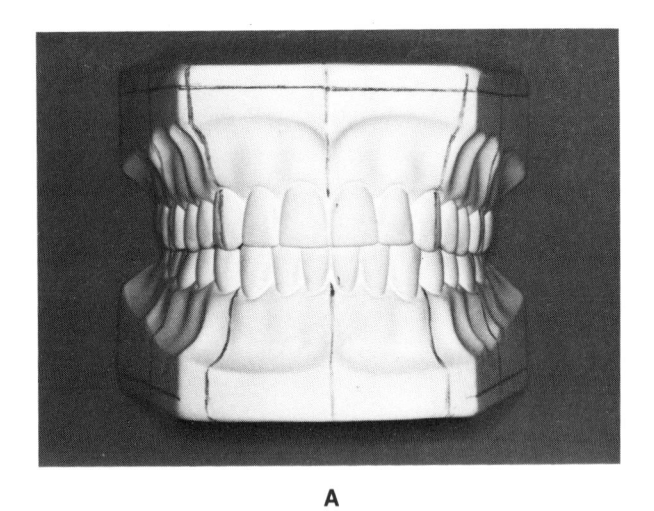

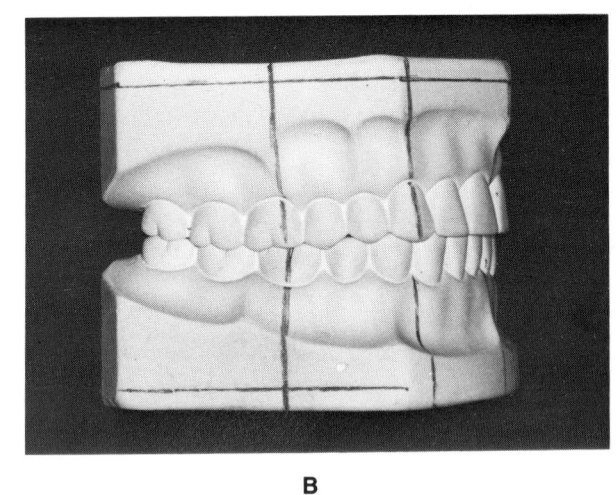

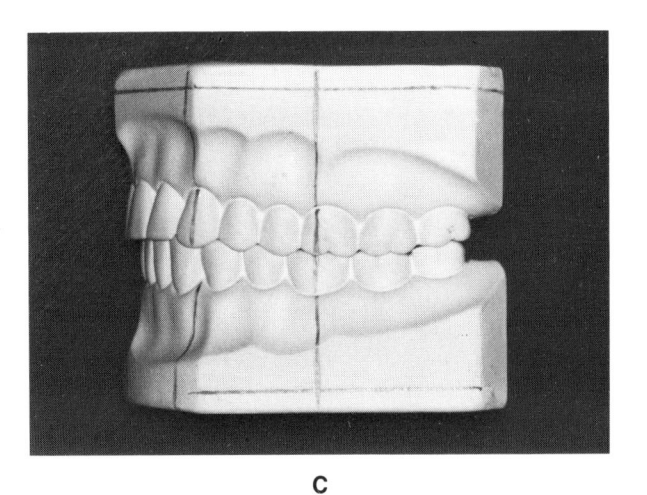

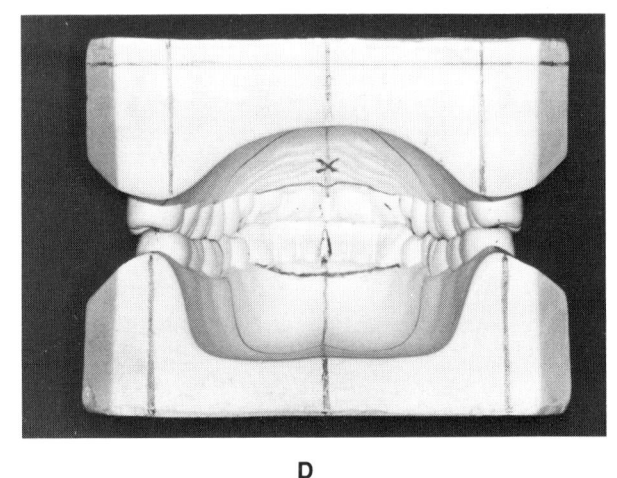

Fig. 9-25. A-D. Statistical relationship of the jaws.

the line bisecting the ridges of the lower arch. These lines as a rule bisect the tuberosities of the upper arch and the retromolar pads of the lower arch.

First, the landmarks on the upper case are established according to the planes above since they are fixed in the skull. The landmarks are then set up on the Galetti articulator, which we have found to be the instrument of choice, although any instrument which will duplicate all the movements of the mandible can be used. The lower cast is mounted to it in the prevailing occlusion of the patient. Deviations from normal can then be more easily discerned (See Fig. 9-26, A and B).

A splint is never constructed until a diagnostic treatment bite is tried in at a consultation visit, when the patient's original symptoms are reevaluated. Serial TMJ x-rays can be taken with the treatment wax bite in position, so that it can be compared to the habitual occlusal position.

The most important problem we are dealing with here is the determination of which mandibular position or range of positions is best for our patient. Once we have established this by using all the diagnostic criteria mentioned above, we can then progress along definite lines of therapy.

6. **Phonetics:**

    Use of closest speaking space—an incisal gap of 1-1.5 mm using surd and sonant forms of the silibant. Words having the following letters: S, SH, CH, J, Z, and ZH. We use the words hiss, house, church, judge, and zebra. Clinical rest position

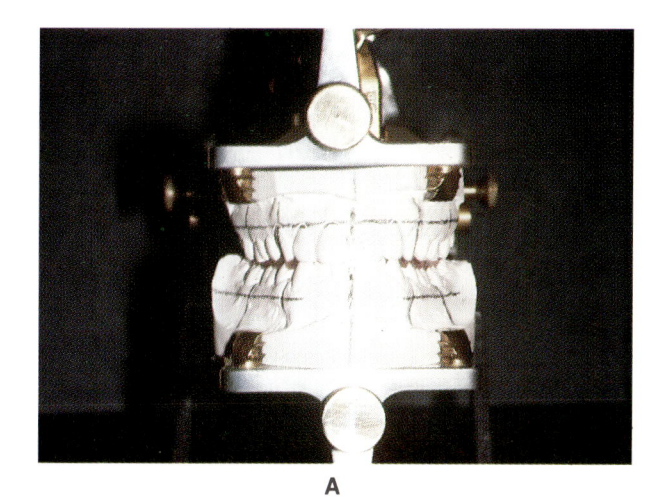

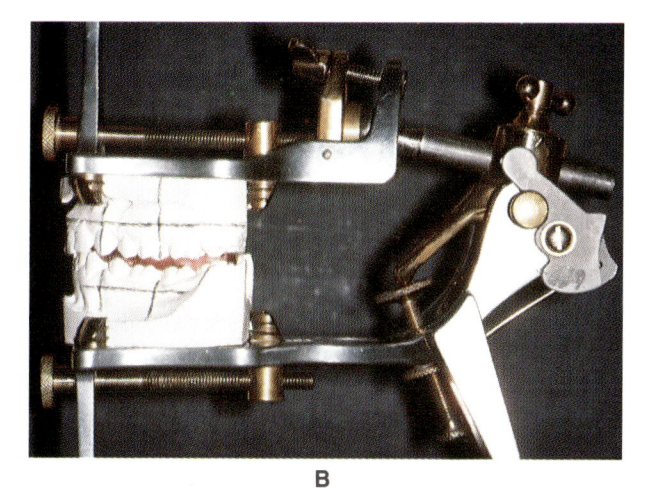

Fig. 9-26, A and B. Mounting of casts.

has been shown to be 2.1 mm for both men and women.[53]

7. **Applied Kinesiologic Testing Procedures:** Applied Kinesiology means the application of muscle testing to aid in the diagnosis and treatment of physiological conditions and anatomic problems. There are six major applications of applied Kinesiology in craniocervical mandibular joint therapy:[54]

   1) To improve muscular function;
   2) To further verify the diagnosis of occlusal dysfunction;
   3) To facilitate efficiency of treatment and effectiveness of mandibular repositioning, appliances, and occlusal therapy;
   4) To verify the impact and appropriateness for temporomandibular joint treatment;
   5) To psychologically motivate patient compliance in following the recommended program of therapy;
   6) To determine the therapeutic needs of temporomandibular joint muscle support services;

Four fundamental concepts must be understood in order to appreciate the dynamics of applied kinesiology:

1. The concept of physiopathology, which assumes that physiologic processes may develop "habits" that create an environment conducive to the development of organic disease and/or structural deterioration.
2. The concept of relative dysfunction, which assumes that physiologic processes may operate at various degrees of efficiency and may react to stress with varying degrees of response and recovery.
3. The concept of muscle reactivity and reciprocity, which assumes that change in the length and tension of any particular muscle group results in a change of length and tension in some associated musculature.
4. The concept of therapy localization, which assumes that digital contact of any area of the body which has an electromagnetic imbalance will cause all muscle groups of that individual to experience a relative "weakness." Although the physiologic mechanisms that account for the dynamics of therapy localization are not completely understood at present, the physiologic consequences of therapy localization may be replicated with remarkable consistency.

It is the author's opinion that applied Kinesiology may prove to be one of the major diagnostic and therapeutic advances of our time. It has revolutionized many practices in the health field, and the coming decade should see related changes in those branches of the healing arts which are open to change and progress.

Those dentists utilizing applied kinesiology

in their practices have discovered their role in improving a patient's general health and well being. When the patient is at the proper centric occlusion and vertical dimension, many muscle groups within the body exhibit greater strength. This has significant implications for improving the performance of athletes.[58,59] It may also help to reinforce and explain the concept of the physiopathology of functional disorders as proposed by Whatmore and Kohli.[57]

Several recent studies have demonstrated the efficacy of the mandibular or maxillary orthopedic repositioning appliance in improving muscular strength as well as performance of athletes and other individuals.

In particular, recent studies[58,59] at well-known teaching institutions showed a positive relationship between changes in jaw relationship and increases in strength and muscle efficiency. One study showed a highly significant increase in muscle efficiency (power), recorded by vertical jump and grip tests, for a group of athletes. In that study, however, there was no significant increase in strength recorded by maximum hip sled and bench press tests.[58] The other study tested 23 athletes, comparing mandibular position with appendage muscle strength. Three different mandibular positions were tested, as were all four appendages. Results indicated that mandibular position affects appendage muscle strength and may be important to all well being. However, considerable variability of optimum muscle strength by muscle groups and mandibular positions was observed.[59]

A controlled double blind field study[60] was conducted to see the effects of the Mandibular Orthopedic Repositioning Appliance (MORA) on football players on the 1982 C.W. Post College football team. Forty players were randomly divided into two groups, one wearing the MORA (21) and the other wearing the Conventional Mouthpiece (CM) (19).

They were tested to see the effects of the MORA on performance; number, type, and severity of injuries; and on three measures of physical fitness which included strength, jumping ability, and balanced with agility.

Overall results were in favor of the MORA. Significant findings favored the MORA in reducing the severity of all injuries, reducing the incidence of knee injuries, in increasing strength, and in overall satisfaction. No significant findings favored the CM. The findings show the importance of the MORA to football players. The author suggests that the study be replicated with planned periodic readjustments to the mouthpiece.

Verban et al. conducted a study to examine the effects of a mandibular orthopedic repositioning appliance (MORA) on human shoulder strength.[61] Twenty volunteer undergraduate college students were randomly selected. Following oral examination by Verban, two appliances were constructed: a MORA splint which repositioned the mandible in three dimensions as described by Gelb (1977), and a placebo splint which did not alter the individual's normal bite. Data was collected, using a Cybex 11 dynamometer, as the subjects were seated in a stabilized chair. Information was obtained for three bite conditions: a normal bite, a normal bite with a placebo splint inserted, and with the MORA splint inserted. Three trials were recorded for each of six shoulder movements: abduction, adduction, flexion, extension, external rotation, and internal rotation. Statistically significant results were determined between the MORA and the normal bite condition for shoulder extension peak torque, shoulder extension average torque, and external rotation average torque. No statistical differences were observed between the placebo and the normal bite condition. Post hoc tests of the interaction effects of a MORA, placebo, and the normal bite condition revealed that the MORA does affect shoulder strength in certain movements. The key to what happened to a patient is what was done with the appliance, and where the condyle was on the posterior slope of the eminence.

It should be noted at this point that how the testing procedure is performed is important, as well as the position which the orthopedic repositioning appliance places the subject's mandible. The key to jaw position is that the approach and correction must be three-dimensional.

The figures below show the author testing a patient in habitual occlusion, rest position, and the three-dimensional repositioned jaw relationship (Figs. 9-27, A-F).

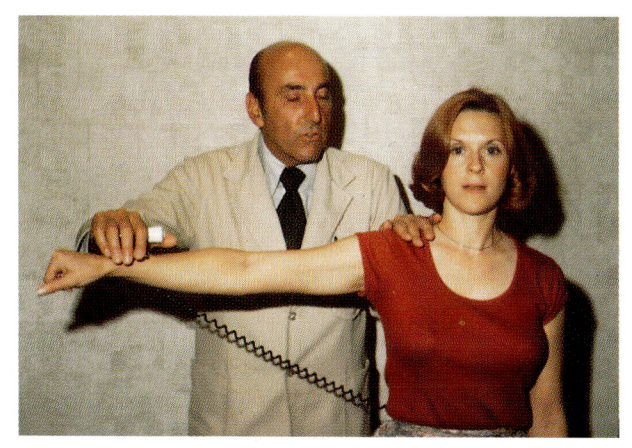

CHAPTER 9 An Orthopedic Approach to Craniocervical Mandibular Disorders

Fig. 9-27 A. Deltoid press kinesiological test. Mouth slightly open to check muscle strength base line.

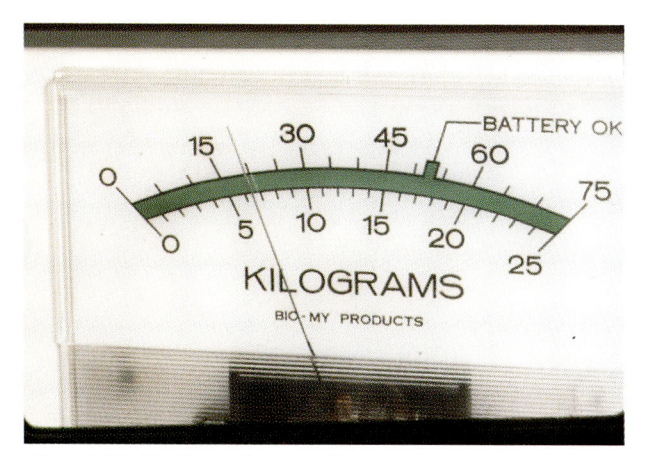

Fig. 9-27 B. Base line reading.

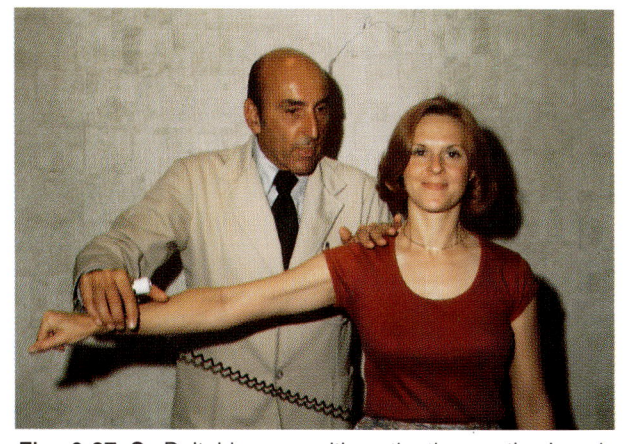

Fig. 9-27 C. Deltoid press with patient's mouth closed in habitual occlusion.

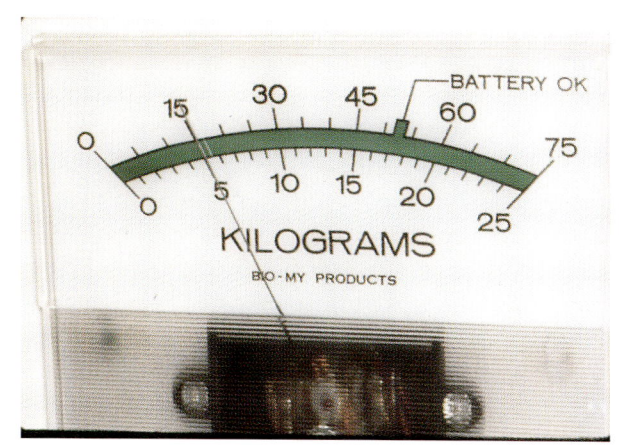

Fig. 9-27 D. Kinesiometer reading is lower.

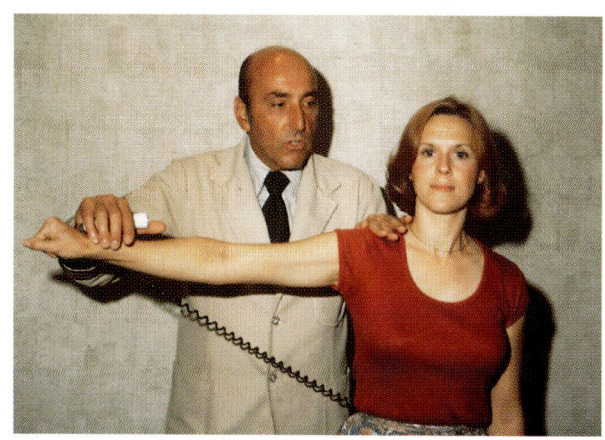

Fig. 9-27 E. Deltoid press. Mouth closed with MORA in place at corrected centric and vertical dimension.

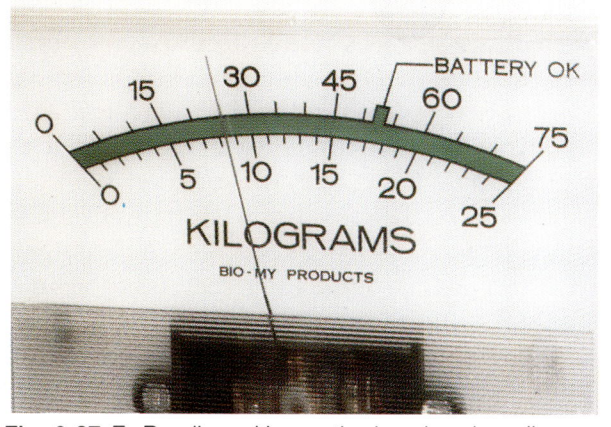

Fig. 9-27 F. Reading with mouth closed and appliance in place.

In another recent article,[62] the "Influence of the Vertical Dimension in the Treatment of Myofascial Pain Dysfunction Syndrome," (*Journal of Prosthetic Dentistry*, 1983), some interesting observations were made. The vertical dimension of least EMG activity was determined for each of 75 randomly selected patients who were then divided into three groups according to the height at which their splints were constructed. Group I occlusal splints were constructed at 1 mm from the occlusal vertical dimension, Group II splints at 4.422 mm, and Group III splints at 8.15 mm. The findings showed a faster and more complete reduction in clinical symptoms for Groups II and III than for Group I.

The authors concluded that temporary use of occlusal splints with a vertical height exceeding the physiologic rest position did not encourage a greater muscular tonus or hyperactivity of jaw muscles. In essence, the elongation of elevator muscles to or near the vertical dimension of least EMG activity by means of occlusal splints is more effective in producing neuromuscular relaxation.

Earlier, Rugh and Drago[53] found that minimal muscle activity in a sampling of men took place at 10.4 mm and in women at 6.8 mm, but the clinical rest position (where there was some EMG activity) for both groups was 2.1 mm. The results of this study show that in an upright position, certain jaw muscles must be in slight contraction to maintain the jaw in clinical rest position. They go on to state that what has been referred to as "clinical rest position" may be more appropriately called an upright postural position.

Treatment

First, the patient is relieved of any pain as soon as possible. Generally, the pain seen in these cases is due to muscle spasm, and definite trigger areas can be palpated. These areas are sprayed with ethylchloride or flourimethane with the muscles under stretch. We can also inject into the affected muscles (after we first digitally locate the trigger points by palpation), using a normal saline solution or lidocaine. Dry needling may also be utilized. The most common trigger points that the dentist is likely to discover, their major causes and effects, as well as their pathways of referred pain are graphically depicted in Figure 9-28, A-L. With many patients who present with a decided malalignment of the mandible of long standing duration, temporary acrylic mandibular occlusal splints in conjunction with myofunctional therapy must also be utilized.

When we reposition the mandible, temporary orthopedic repositioning appliances are utilized because:

1. They can be constructed quickly and are easy to correct and adjust.
2. They provide the patient with functional comfort in the shortest period of time.
3. The operator has an opportunity to familiarize himself with the case and effect any changes that he deems advisable.
4. If not effective, they can be discarded without damaging teeth.
5. They are hygienic, comfortable, inconspicuous, and inexpensive.
6. The dentist has an opportunity to discover if psychogenic factors are more deep-seated, requiring the patient to seek psychiatric consultation and therapy.
7. Phonetically, they can be checked to see that they do not invade the freeway space.
8. If myofunctional therapy has to be instituted, the tongue can contact the palate without a layer of acrylic in its way during deglutition and speech.
9. If the patient should go into a lateral excursion, they can contact the natural cuspids. With an upper appliance, acrylic generally covers the linguals of the upper cuspids, altering the mechanics of the joint structures when the appliance is removed prior to reconstruction of the dentition.
10. The patient can make optimal contact in protrusion, and still disocclude posteriorly where permissible.
11. From the standpoint of conservation, the dentist truly has a functional architectural rendition of the correct jaw relationship in all planes of space. Since the habitual jaw relationship was a factor in the etiology of the symptoms, time is required to decondition the neuromuscular reflexes involved, and to recondition the structures to a more harmonious muscle, jaw, and tooth relationship. At this time, it is important to restate that, in most instances, if properly diagnosed, the optimal interarch relationships must be produced by the guidance and assistance of the dentist, and can not be obtained by the patient alone.

The splints can be made entirely of acrylic, a combination of metal and acrylic, or all metal depending upon the needs of the case. In edentulous cases, the lower denture teeth are overlaid with acrylic of the same shade as the teeth. In partially edentulous cases, fast-curing tooth-shade acrylic is added to the occlusal surfaces of the saddle areas to attain the correct height. These cases are first mounted on the Galetti articulator, and a diagnostic wax bite registration is taken and then tried into the mouth over the denture. This is then replaced with fast-setting acrylic by dividing the wax in half and doing one quadrant at a time.

The final mandibular orthopedic repositioning appliance fabricated by us covers the bicuspids and molars and is placed and balanced according to the following criteria:

1. Head posture: patient feels and looks better, shows a more symmetrical appearance and postural improvement.
2. Balance for Parafunction
   A. Maximum intercuspation at centric occlusion at proper vertical dimension
   B. Right and left lateral excursions - may be group function but generally cuspid protection
   C. No balancing side interferences
   D. Optimum contact in protrusive, disocclude posteriorly
   E. No centric relation prematurities

After the acrylic sets, the occlusal surfaces are trimmed so that only slight depressions for the cusps remain, allowing the patient full freedom in lateral movement. The appliances are then bite corrected so that the forces applied during mastication will be directed within the root portions of the abutment teeth. The appliances are balanced with the patients sitting upright in the dental chair, standing, and in the supine position, the reason being that we have different prematurities in those three positions. The patients are instructed to wear the splints full time. They are not always restricted to a soft diet. Then muscular therapy begins.

Whereas the discrepancies in jaw posture have been ongoing for many years, it can be readily understood that accompanying degenerative changes occur in the neuromusculature and joints. These range from fibrosis to contracture, and there are concomitant changes in habit patterns. In order to restore the patient to a more normal relationship, new habit patterns have to be established. We endeavor to return the patient to what we believe is their normal unstrained mandibular position. However, degenerative changes in the musculature and in the joints will of necessity alter our course. Time is an essential factor in solving the problem.

A recent study comparing the therapeutic effect of three appliance designs (Sved, Gelb, and stabilization) found the the Gelb mandibular orthopedic repositioning appliance was most effective in treating dysfunction of the superior cervical column.

Where there is a cessation or major reduction in symptoms, and the patient is comfortable for several months without exhibiting a reoccurance of symptoms, permanent restorations can be made, or orthodontic therapy can begin.

Discussion

In a recent study,[43] observations made of 200 private practice craniomandibular (TMJ) patients revealed a number of interesting findings.

The patients in this study had undergone numerous medical consultations, complicated and expensive medical tests and hospitalization, unnecessary surgical dental procedures, and had become addicted to various medications, and suffered the destructive effects of long-term chronic pain as well as associated personality changes.

The patients were divided into seven ten-year age groupings (Table 9-1). Almost 70% of the patients were between 21 and 50 years of age. The ratio of women to men was 2.7:1. Another study[64] had a similar proportion of the sexes.

In the five year period preceding their initial examination, 46 patients had had some type of traumatic injury to the skeletal system, such as whiplash, blows to the head or face, or broken bones. Ninety-nine patients reported a history of trauma occurring more than five years prior to their first visit.

The muscles most frequently in spasm and/or tender to digital palpation were the

Table 9-1. Age groupings of symptoms

	Age group							
	10-20	21-30	31-40	41-50	51-60	61-70	71-80	Total
Men	3	20	14	6	8	1	2	54
Women	15	34	37	28	16	12	4	146
Muscles in spasm								
Internal pterygoids	15	41	41	28	16	11	4	156
External pterygoids	17	44	46	31	19	12	5	174
Masseters	16	50	44	28	22	11	5	176
Temporal	15	44	42	25	16	10	5	167
Sternocleidomastoid	16	46	45	29	18	10	4	168
Posterior cervicals	15	45	43	27	17	10	3	160
Mylohyoids	12	34	35	27	16	9	4	137
Trapezius	16	44	45	29	16	10	4	164
Others	17	52	50	33	21	12	6	191
Ear symptoms								
Tinnitus	3	15	24	10	9	6	4	71
Hearing loss	2	9	19	5	5	5	4	49
Temporomandibular joint								
Clicking	6	30	36	23	7	8	3	113
Pain	16	54	51	33	21	13	6	194
Bruxism	9	29	35	19	12	10	2	116
Head pain								
Facial	5	14	19	9	9	6	1	63
Occipital	1	13	9	6	7	2	2	40
Cervical	1	10	9	9	5	5	1	40
Temporal	2	12	29	17	8	5	4	77
Vertigo	3	13	30	12	11	6	4	79
Stuffiness	6	20	28	17	13	6	5	95
Popping or whooshing noise on opening or closing	10	43	43	22	14	5	5	142

masseter 88%, external pterygoid 87%, and sternocleidomastoid muscles 84%. Most of the patients examined (95.5%) had some involvement of nonmasticatory muscles listed under the heading of "others." Included in this group were the deltoid; upper, middle, and lower back muscles; pectoralis major; and the gastrocnemius.

Pain on preauricular lateral palpation of the temporomandibular joints was elicited in 194 patients. Upon palpation of the condyles through the external auditory meatus, pain was elicited in 152 patients. Of this number 114 had unilateral anterior wall tenderness, while 38 had bilateral pain.

One hundred and seven patients exhibited some type of joint click. Forty-nine patients exhibited reciprocal opening and closing clicks on the same side. Twenty-eight patients had single-sided opening clicks only and a similar number had single-sided closing clicks only. Three patients had bilateral opening clicks and seven had bilateral closing clicks.

The patients examined commonly had a right eyebrow higher than the left; the right eye was also higher and larger; the lip line generally turned up to the right side; the right ear was higher than the left; the right nostril tended to be higher and larger than the left and the midline of the teeth and lips also tended to be off to one side or the other. The facial high side often corresponded to a greater deficiency in vertical dimension of occlusion on that side which was further

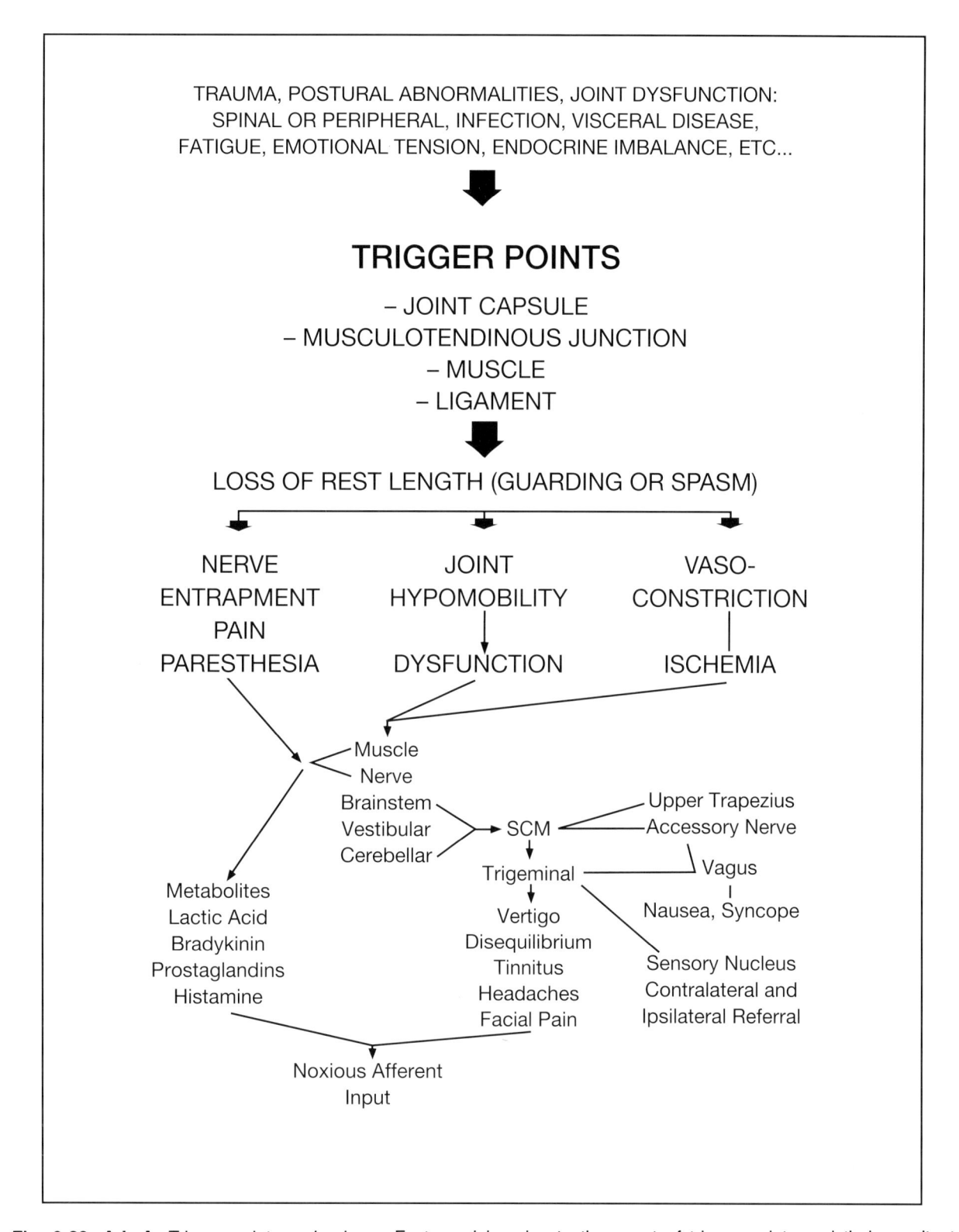

CHAPTER 9 An Orthopedic Approach to Craniocervical Mandibular Disorders

```
TRAUMA, POSTURAL ABNORMALITIES, JOINT DYSFUNCTION:
SPINAL OR PERIPHERAL, INFECTION, VISCERAL DISEASE,
FATIGUE, EMOTIONAL TENSION, ENDOCRINE IMBALANCE, ETC...
                          ⬇
                   TRIGGER POINTS
                   – JOINT CAPSULE
              – MUSCULOTENDINOUS JUNCTION
                      – MUSCLE
                     – LIGAMENT
                          ⬇
           LOSS OF REST LENGTH (GUARDING OR SPASM)
           ⬇              ⬇              ⬇
         NERVE          JOINT           VASO-
       ENTRAPMENT    HYPOMOBILITY    CONSTRICTION
          PAIN            ⬇               ⬇
       PARESTHESIA    DYSFUNCTION       ISCHEMIA
```

- Muscle
- Nerve
- Brainstem
- Vestibular → SCM ← Upper Trapezius / Accessory Nerve
- Cerebellar
- Trigeminal → Vagus
- Vertigo   Nausea, Syncope
- Disequilibrium
- Tinnitus   Sensory Nucleus
- Headaches   Contralateral and
- Facial Pain Ipsilateral Referral

Metabolites
Lactic Acid
Bradykinin
Prostaglandins
Histamine

Noxious Afferent Input

Fig. 9-28, A-L A. Trigger point mechanisms. Factors giving rise to the onset of trigger points and their resultant signs and symptoms. *Reprinted with permission from Mannheimer, J.S. and Lampe, G.N. Clinical Transcultaneous Electrical Nerve Stimulation. Philadelphia, PA, F.A. davis Company, 1984, p. 122.* (continued)

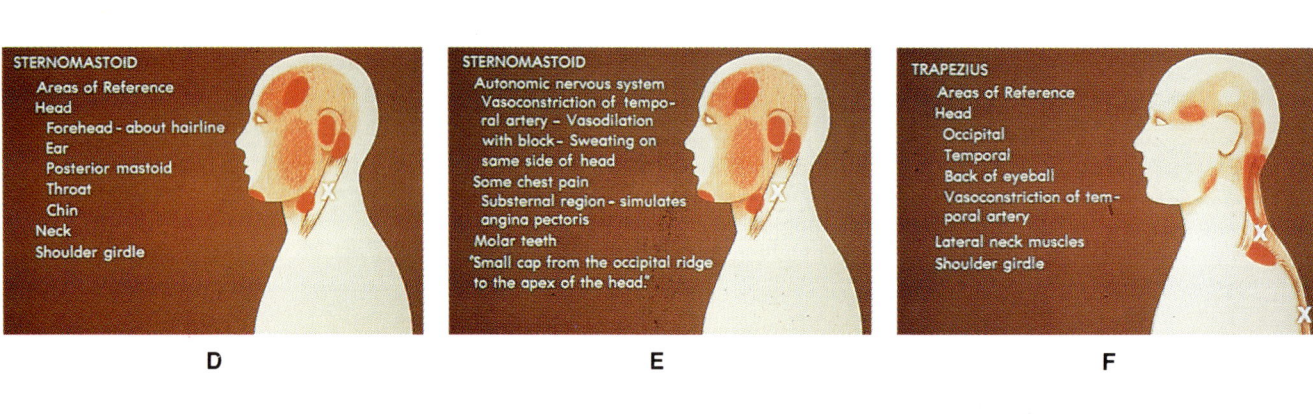

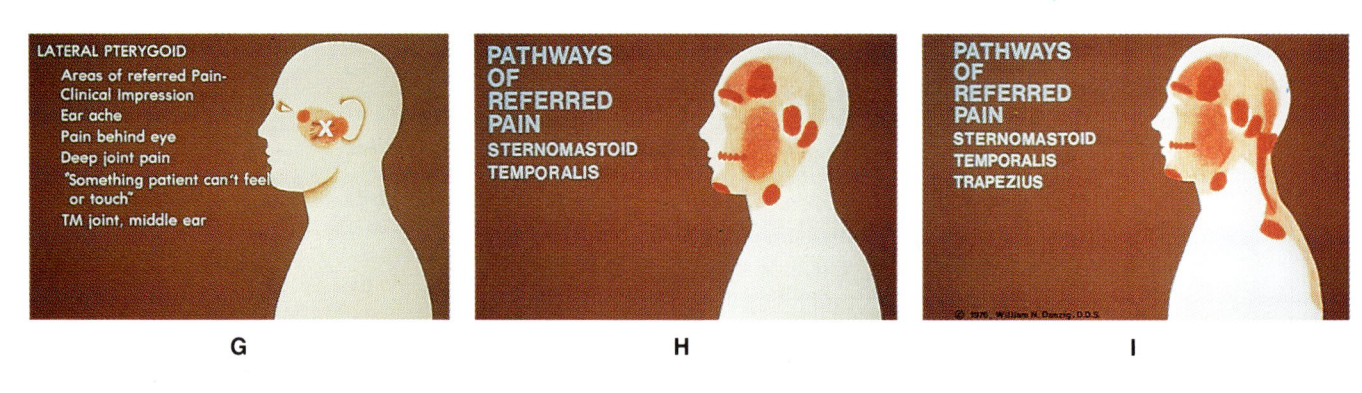

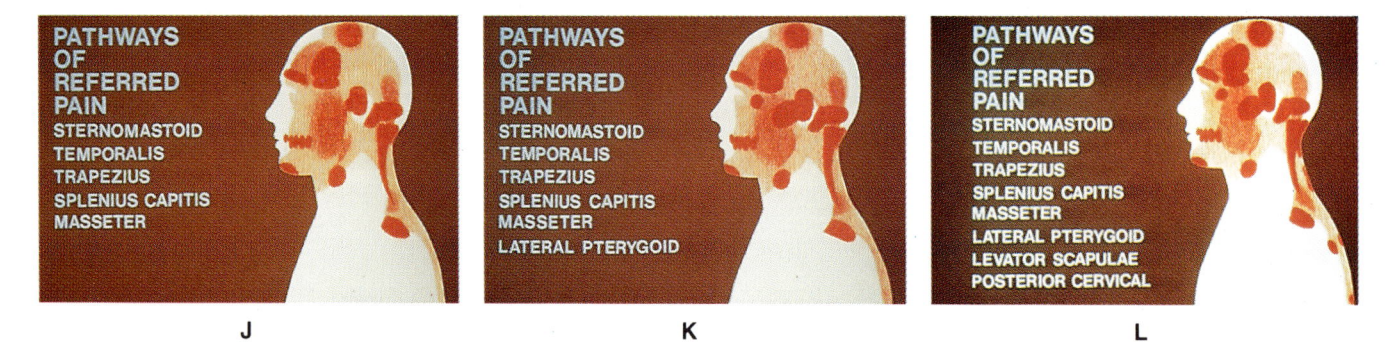

248   New Concepts in Craniomandibular and Chronic Pain Management

Fig. 9-28, B-L. *Reprinted with permission. Danzig, W.N., D.D.S., Walnut Creek, California (as modified from Travell, J. and Bonica, J.J.).*

Fig. 9-29 A.

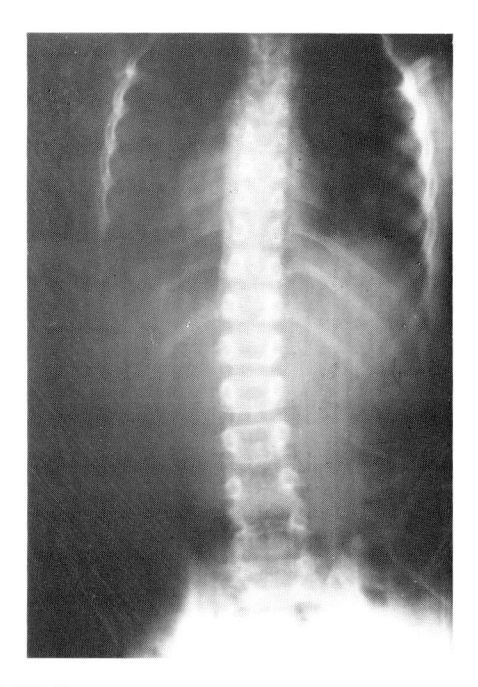

Fig. 9-29 B.

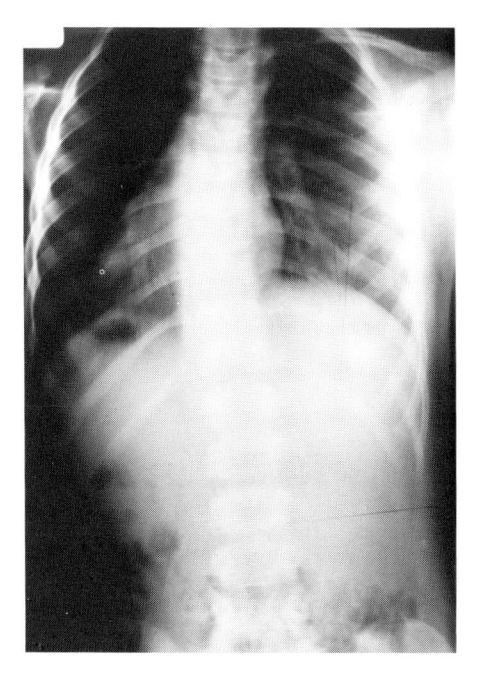

corroborated by palpation of the condyles through the external auditory meatus, transcranial or tomographic x-rays, and phonetics. Interestingly, if one were to stand in front of one of these patients with their mouth open, the plane of occlusion in the mandibular lower left quadrant would frequently be higher than the corresponding plane of occlusion on the right side.

The level of the shoulder was generally lower on the right side than on the left, which was also true for the level of the breasts and hips. This also corresponds to leg length discrepancy, which was discussed in detail in the preface of this book. The iliac crest was generally higher on the left side (123 patients). The gastrocnemius was tender to palpation on the right side in 102 patients, but only 16 were tender on the left side.

In ideal posture, a plumb line should pass (on profile) through the tragus of the ear, the tip of the shoulder, the hip joint, posterior to the patella of the knee joint, and anterior to the ankle bone (Fig. 9-12).[45]

As observed not only in this study, but also in most craniomandibular (TMJ) patients seen, the head is forward of the plumb line. The head is in hyperextension in response to keeping the bipupillary line horizontal with the ground. The body will shift as necessary so that it can maintain the pupil in a horizontal plane.[65] Obviously, the position of the head in space will materially affect the posture of the rest of the body.

As a result of the postural imbalance seen in most craniocervical mandibular patients, we have found certain muscles to be tender to palpation on a fairly routine basis. On the left side of the patient, the muscles most frequently affected would be the suboccipitals, the sternocleidomastoid, the trapezius, the splenius capitus, the pectoralis major, and the upper, middle, and lower back muscles. The left iliac crest is usually tender as well. On the right side, the posterior cervicals, the deltoid, and the gastrocnemius are usually tender. When the muscle tenderness is more diffuse, then we must consider such factors as nutritional deficiencies, endocrine imbalances, chronic infection, allergy, psychological stress, nerve entrapment, congenital skeletal abnormalities, trauma to muscles, and cranial faults.

Whenever mandibular neuromuscular tension is present, the abnormal maxillomandibular relationship affects the normal physiologic posture of the cervical vertebrae, resulting in abnormal strains on the muscles of the upper torso, which affect the posture of the head, neck, and shoulder girdle.[43]

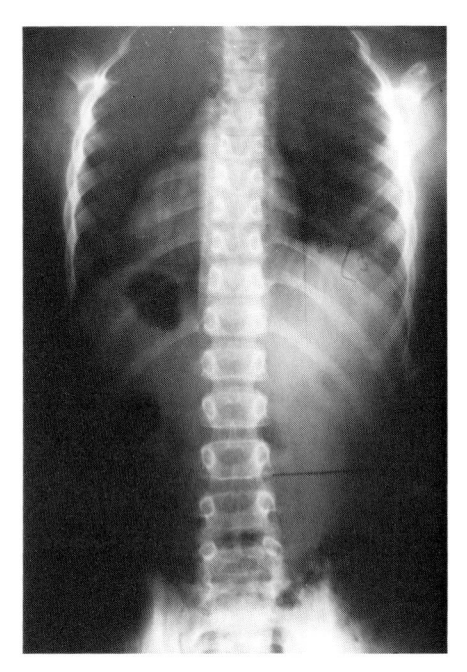

Fig. 9-29 C.

Conclusion

At the present time, the full magnitude of patients' suffering from craniomandibular (TMJ) disorders has not been fully recognized by health professions or by the public. There is sufficient evidence that craniocervical mandibular disorders, to a great extent, create anxiety states and vice versa. They act as potent chronic stressors since they are operant twenty-four hours a day. Logically, the condition will become more common as civilization becomes more advanced and mechanized. Epidemiological studies have placed the number of persons suffering from this disorder at twenty per cent of the population or more.

The dental profession must be prepared to work with and educate allied health professionals, such as the otolaryngologist, neurologist, orthopedist, rheumatologist, phsiarist, endocrinologist, physical therapist, osteopath, and chiropractor who are often unaware that temporomandibular joint pathology and its ramifications play an important role in treating seemingly unrelated nondental complaints. Headaches, neckaches, backaches, eye and ear pain, and other problems previously discussed are not symptoms that have traditionally lent themselves to a consultation by a dentist as part of a differential diagnosis.

Treating patients with craniomandibular disorders is not necessarily an obligation for every dental practitioner. However, the dental profession has an obligation to visualize, listen attentively, and palpate muscles in order to identify those patients who can benefit from treatment for craniomandibular disorders. These individuals do exist in unbelievable numbers and are present in every dental practice.

Case Study #1

A ten-year-old boy presented for orthodontic consultation in January 1978. After assembling the base line records (clinical exam, palpation, history, radiographs, and study models), the probability of a craniomandibular disorder was ascertained. The patient had a Class II molar relationship, decreased vertical dimension, an overbite, and flat cusps on the maxillary and mandibular deciduous cusps. The patient was under the care of a local orthopedist for scoliosis, and the orthopedist had prescribed exercises for him.

During March 1978, a Gelb mandibular orthopedic repositioning appliance was inserted to correct the maxillomandibular imbalance in order to begin treatment of his craniomandibular (TMJ) disorder. From January to November 1978, while he was being treated for his TMJ disorder, he did not see the orthopedist. He also did not perform any of the prescribed exercises for the scoliosis. On December 19, 1978, the child was informed by the orthopedist that his scoliosis had been cured. Figure 9-29A shows an x-ray of the spine with a 10° curve taken September 30, 1975. Figure 9-29B, taken on November 30, 1977, exhibits an increase in the curvature of the spine to 25°. Figure 9-29C, taken on December 19, 1978, shows a decrease in the curvature to 3°. It should be noted that treatment for a TMJ problem, not scoliosis, was originally planned.

Case Study #2

A thirty-year-old woman originally reported on referral with a complaint of left-sided facial

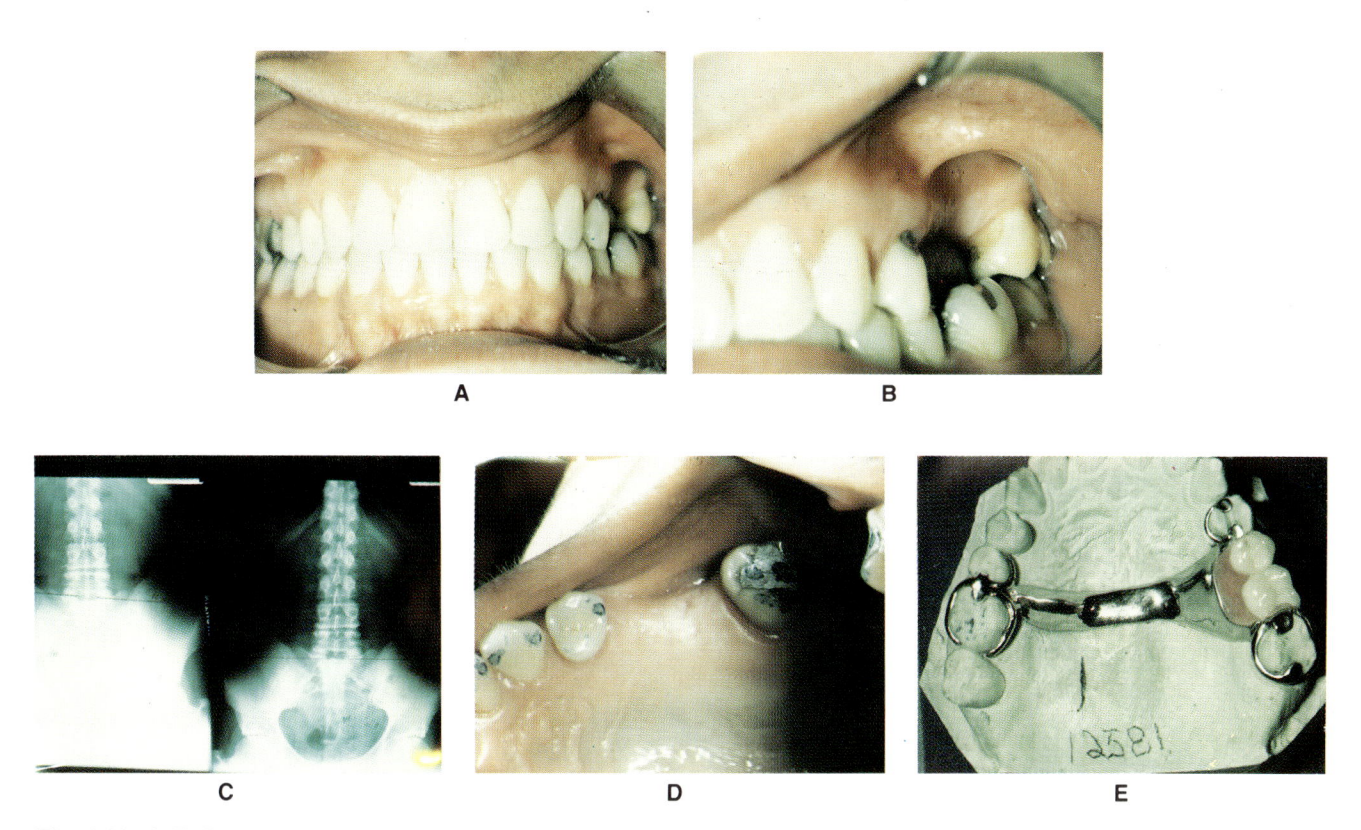

Fig. 9-30, A-E. *Reprinted with permission of Stephen D. Smith, D.M.D., Director Temporomandibular Center, Osteopathic Medical Center of Philadelphia.*

pain and earache with pain radiating to the left temple and left ear/mastoid process region.

The patient's occlusion was Class I, with excellent midline alignment and excellent overjet/overbite relationship. The functional excursions, on protrusion and lateral movements, were also within normal limits. However, the left side "vertical dimension" had collapsed slightly with the missing second bicuspid and first molar. When the patient closed, she could touch the incisors and the entire right quadrant, but posterior support in the left quadrant was slightly shortened, requiring extra muscular pressure and causing pressure on the temporomandibular joint. The patient could not hold a strip of cellophane in the left posterior area without excessive pressure. Palpation of the left temporomandibular joint revealed tenderness, particularly of the lateral capsule and the lateral pterygoid muscle which was markedly tender as well (Fig. 9-30A). A close-up of this area revealed that when the incisor and cuspid areas touched, approximately one-fourth of a millimeter of space occurred between the second upper molar and the lower first and second molar (Figs. 9-30, B and C).

A postural standing x-ray of the lumbar and sacral/pelvic area was taken. The x-ray on the left shows a sacral based declination toward the left with a shortening or apparent rotation of the right pelvis. The right femur (hip) is higher than the left. The radiologist drew the sacral base, which was not level, and the lumbar had a tilt toward the right. The same photograph was taken thirty days later, after occlusal treatment (which was the only modality used in this case) without spinal manipulation. The radiologist again took the postural standing x-ray (stocking feet) and noted the leveling of the sacral base, the apparent pelvic rotation into a normal position with the hip/femoral head height being level, and the elimination of the lumbar tilt. Again, it should be noted that no manipulation or osteopathic or chiropractic treatment had been done.

The main therapy was occlusal therapy, with the addition of support in the fossa of the upper left 2nd molar and the addition of an amalgam overlay in the one-half millimeter to one-fourth millimeter range (Fig. 9-30D). At this point, the incisal contacts and the posterior occlusal contacts matched without any additional muscular pull or compression within the temporomandibular joint. It was this occlusal stabilization that was the primary treatment. Again, thirty days after the treatment, the postural standing x-ray was taken, showing the apparent spinal corrections which had occurred. The final treatment, after occlusal stabilization, was the insertion of a removable, (cast) partial prosthesis replacing the bicuspid and molar which had been missing (Fig. 9-30E). Simultaneous with this therapy was the elimination of the patient's complaint of pain in the joint and ear, and a radiating temporal headache.

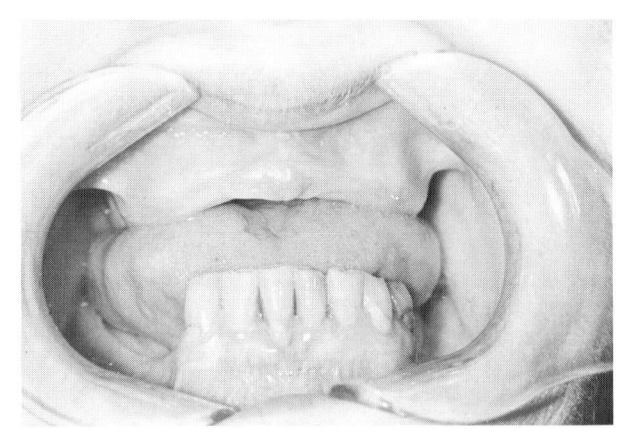

Fig. 9-31 A. This view shows the patient's mouth as it would be during sleep, with the complete upper denture out, few remaining lower anterior teeth, and bilateral missing posterior bite support.

Case Study #3

A white woman, age 58 years, presented with the chief complaint of discomfort in the left ear. She described a sense of ear fullness, Eustachian tube blockage, and mild tinnitus. She experienced frequent loss of balance, with attacks of vertigo, dizziness, and nausea. The patient had continual shortness of breath and extreme tiredness. She noted tingling and numbness of the left arm and hand, which was most pronounced on her awakening in the morning. She stated that she had difficulty in swallowing, with an apparent susceptibility to choking. Her voice tone was fluctuant as she continually had to clear her throat. As a child, the patient exhibited incoordination, stooped posture, and structural imbalance. The patient's eustachian tube had always been closed, particularly on the left side, with specific hearing involvement since the age of 14. She visited her physician for suspected otitis media, but findings were essentially negative. She was also a mouth breather. She had even experienced bouts of pneumonia. The patient had delivered five children and had had ovarian surgery between 1935 and 1945.

In 1948, she took a fall while skating, traumatizing the coccyx and sacral area. Although there was no apparent fracture, severe back pain became recurrent. In 1952, the patient was diagnosed as having a "pinched nerve" in the metatarsal areas and was on crutches for 6 weeks. Both an orthopedic surgeon and a chiropractor discovered a tilt of the right hip and a short right leg.

In January 1969, after several years of menstrual disorders, a benign tumor was found at total hysterectomy. Two weeks postoperatively, one embolism occurred in the right lung and then another clot moved first into the left lung and then apparently to the heart area. Congestive heart failure occurred. A major myocardial infarction developed.

She experienced subsequent heart attacks in years 1971, 1972 (two), 1973, and 1975. Bypass surgery was not considered an option, so she was placed on a low-fat diet. During this same period, a hiatal hernia was discovered which put unnecessary pressure on the heart muscles, causing additional chest pain, especially on chewing and swallowing. She was prescribed belladonna before meals and nitroglycerin for any chest pain attacks. She also experienced pain in her teeth. Her cardiologist restricted her stair climbing and recommended that she move to a one-story residence. Since 1975, her sleeping pattern had not been normal.

In January 1975, the patient experienced a seventh myocardial infarction. After this heart attack, she noticed definite changes in her voice, with weakness and strained vocal patterns—stress on speech exertion. She had

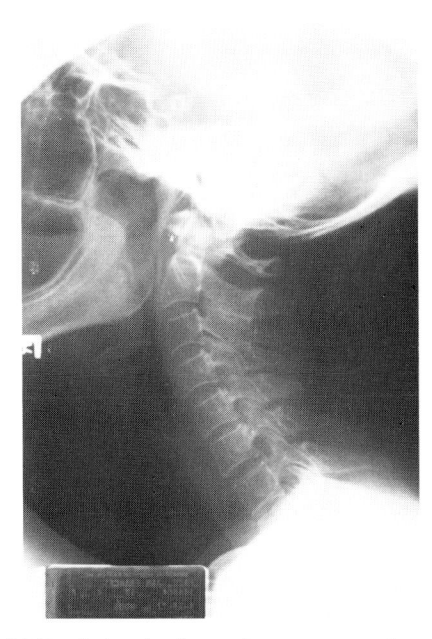

Fig. 9-31 B. Lateral view shows excessive forward extension of the head, cervical muscular contractions, and excessive cervical lordosis.

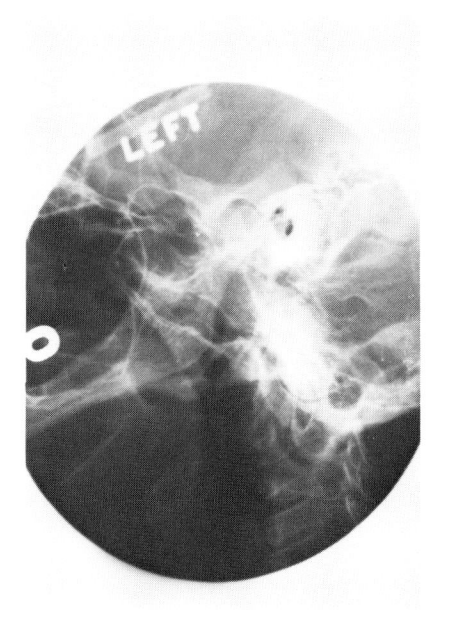

Fig. 9-31 C. Transcranial view of the symptomatic left temporomandibular joint, shows distal or posterior retrusion of the mandible with a narrowed joint space compressed toward the ear canal. View is without the lower prosthesis in.

to walk very slowly and experienced a feeling of tightness in the chest if she proceeded with any mild activity.

In April 1975, the patient developed pancreatitis and liver involvement with pain in the liver, pancreas, and bladder. At that time, temporary paralysis of the arms and legs and a loss of voice control ensued. In May, cytoscopic examination revealed multiple cysts of the bladder. In March 1976, she experienced cystitis with excessive bladder pain. Since that time, she had been susceptible to fatigue, with constant shortness of breath and limitations in mobility.

Her past dental history revealed that the patient had had all the lower posterior teeth extracted 23 years before, and had never had prosthetic replacements. She had been wearing a complete upper denture for that entire time, but reported that she usually left it out at night (Fig. 9-31A).

Muscle examination revealed tenderness on palpation of the right and left shoulder musculature. The temporalis muscle was sore, primarily on the left. Palpation of the left masseter elicited severe pain radiating up to the temple. Both external and internal pterygoids on the left were sensitive to intraoral palpation. The right sternocleidomastoid muscle and both trapezius muscles were sore, as were the right and left posterior cervical muscles. Palpation of the left mylohyoide muscle created pain in the throat.

Very obvious spinal lesions were found on palpation. The most obvious were on the left side in the T2, T3, and T4 areas, as well as T7-9. On the right side, sensitivity was present at T2-3 and T9-12. These findings of somatic dysfunction are most common and significant in the heart patient as well as in the chronically ill.

Palpation of the condyle through the external auditory meatus with the little finger showed tenderness in the left ear canal. An opening click on the left, as well as crepitation in the temporomandibular joint, were evident. Opening and closing patterns showed no significant deviation, and the widest interincisal opening was within normal limits (40 mm).

The insertion of a wax bite to test vertical dimension and jaw posture showed immediate improvement in facial muscle tone. Palpation of the tender left masseter muscle revealed significant reduction of sensitivity. The insertion of the wax bite also relieved the pain evident on palpation in the thoracic paravertebral areas where the osteopathic lesions

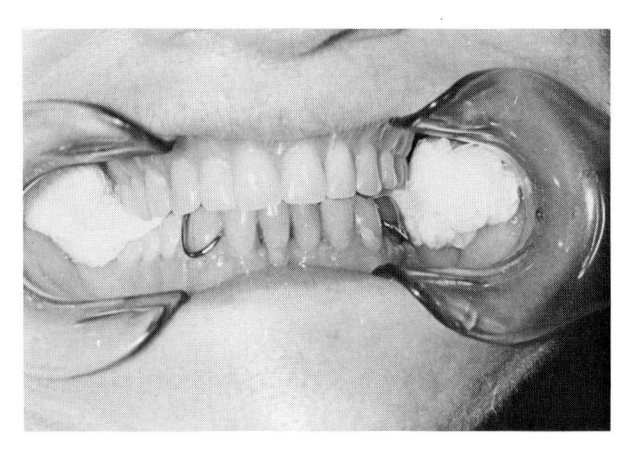

Fig. 9-31 D. Upper denture with newly made lower prosthesis. Additional molar support was still needed. Gauze square supports were used temporarily and diagnostically to build up the needed additional height.

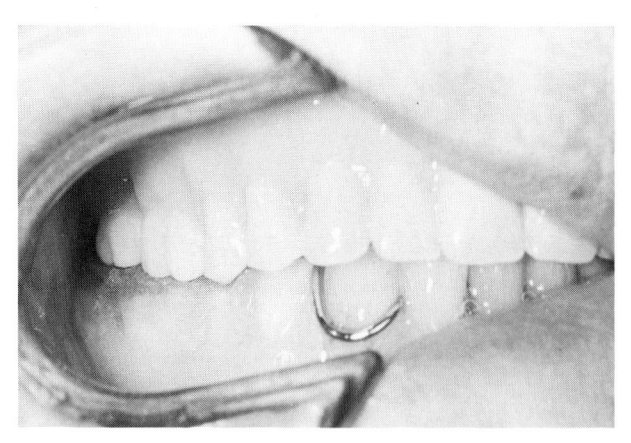

Fig. 9-31 E. Acrylic overlay material was added to the posterior teeth as a transitional measure to get ideal jaw support-height, prior to long-term prosthetic stabilization.

were located, particularly the left T3-4 area. Once the jaw was correctly repositioned with the wax support, palpation of these points showed no anterior chest pain (which was present beforehand). Additionally, the patient's ability to show increased muscular strength was determined subjectively, using an isometric deltoid press. Objective measurements also can be ascertained with the use of either the Cybex dynamometer, or more practically for the patient, with the Kinesiometer, which measures muscle resistance in kilograms over time duration in seconds.

X-ray films taken of the patient's posture in the cervicocranial region confirmed the visual impression of increased cervical lordosis with the head in extension and forward posture (Figs. 9-31, B and C). A slight narrowing of the intervertebral disk space between C5 and C6 was evident on lateral radiographic examination (Fig. 9-31B). The patient was also tested for a pelvic tilt and a short right leg. When a 3/8-inch lift was placed under the short right leg in the heel area, muscle testing of the arm showed improved arm muscle strength. The radiologist's evaluation indicated that the L5-sacral space was closed, with some evidence of osteoarthritis. A comparatively normal Ferguson's angle was evident. Scoliosis was seen on the right side, with a convexity to the left with a 1/2-inch differential at the femoral head acetabular area. The joint spaces of the sacrum-iliac were acceptable. It was observed that with the lift in the heel, the splint-bite molar area on the same side was high; without the heel lift, the bite pattern changed. This was determined by occlusal articulating paper and muscle kinesiology testing, and can be better understood by the findings presented in Chapter 5.

Treatment was undertaken by first taking impressions of the upper denture and lower arch, along with a reregistered occlusion with increased vertical dimension of the jaws. The lower jaw was brought slightly downward and forward, and was tested kinesiologically (isometric deltoid press). A lower partial removable prosthesis was fabricated, and then adjusted to provide sufficient molar support (Fig. 9-31D). Without this type of support, the patient was not able to walk up a flight of stairs without chest pain. The prosthesis was further adjusted for ideal head-neck balance (Fig. 9-31E). The patient was instructed to leave the maxillary denture in place at night, but to remove it for approximately two hours for a daily rest period to stimulate the oral mucosa and palate.

No osteopathic manipulation or heel lifting procedures were carried out. The clinical course of this case involved initial improvement in overall health, followed by a reappearance of symptoms in reverse order, and finally by eventual recovery. The case finally demonstrated a correlation between dental and TMJ stress and the involvement of the cardiac plexus, as well as the importance of a multidisciplinary approach.

By the tenth month of treatment, the patient was free of chest pain. She was now able to

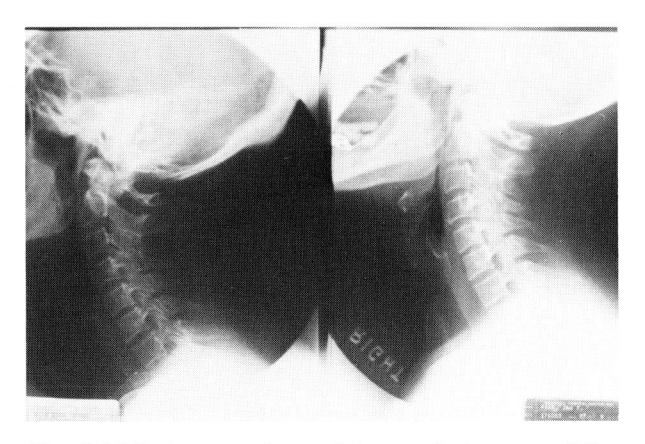

Fig. 9-31 F. A comparison of the cervical x-rays of the patient one year apart. There are less cervical lordosis and less head flexion-extension problems. The head is positioned one inch farther backward.

chew food much better. There was no recurrence of hiatal hernia pain. The belladonna and nitroglycerin were no longer needed. The patient was able to climb stairs approximately 15 times per day without fatigue. Her balance problem was considerably improved. Palpation of the thoracic and paravertebrral areas no longere elicited pain. The ringing or buzzing in the ear that she had experienced were gone, and her sleep pattern seemed stabilized. Since 1972, she was taking one half tablet of Inderal four times per day on the advice of her cardiologist.

X-ray films of the patient one year after fabrication of the lower partial denture showed improvement of the cervical curvature (Fig. 31F). The position of the head, which had been in excessive extension, had normalized itself, and the nuchal crest area was one inch less prominent than originally.

By 1980, a comparison of her eye levels to photographs taken in 1973 showed head posture and eyes to be much more level compared to the prior tilt. She was quite comfortable with the upper and lower prostheses and had not suffered any recurrent chest pains or significant shortness of breath. She felt that she had been healed from her multiple physical disabilities. The patient, then age 60, had experienced no "replays," or relapses, since the period of January through March 1979. As of February 1980, her voice was strong and clear. The patient stated that she hadn;t felt so well for 20 years. She said that she actually felt 10 years younger. The buzzing in her ear had been gone for two years. She was able to move up and down stairs easily. Her cardiologist said that the electrocardiogram was normal and her condition had stabilized enough so that he did not need to see her again for six months. Her physician also gave her permission to enroll in an aerobics class. The patient's dosage of Inderal was down to one tablet per day. Her hand coordination had improved to the point where she could do fine hand drawings. An open palate denture was made for night time wear, and as a result, her sleeping pattern became stable. She had no chest pain, overall body pain, or sickness that entire winter. She began to notice a slight sensation in her left ear, but it was not acute. Since it was time for her annual oral-TMJ check-up, she might have required a thin layer of rebasing material. As with most TMJ patients, whether they are prosthodontic or splint patients, long-term annual follow-up should be considered. With denture patients especially, hard and soft tissues can change and shift, so the follow-up is important to guard against the possible return of the symptomatology which was treated in the transitional temporomandibular orthopedic treatment period.

The clinical progress of this particular patient gives some indication of the major interrelationships that exist between jaw posture, occlusal stability, and TMJ function and the entire body. The possible consequences in terms of fiscerosomatic or somatovisceral disease are certainly obvious.

Case Study #4

A 16-year-old boy with scoliosis and other defects of posture. His occlusion and maxillomandibular relationships were diagnosed as being unphysiologic. The jaw relationship was corrected by the insertion of occlusal restorations in several posterior mandibular teeth to provide dominant molar support. The results of the therapy can be seen in Figures 9-32, A and B.

Case Study #5

These skeletal x-rays represent a 21-year-old male patient with very bad posture. He

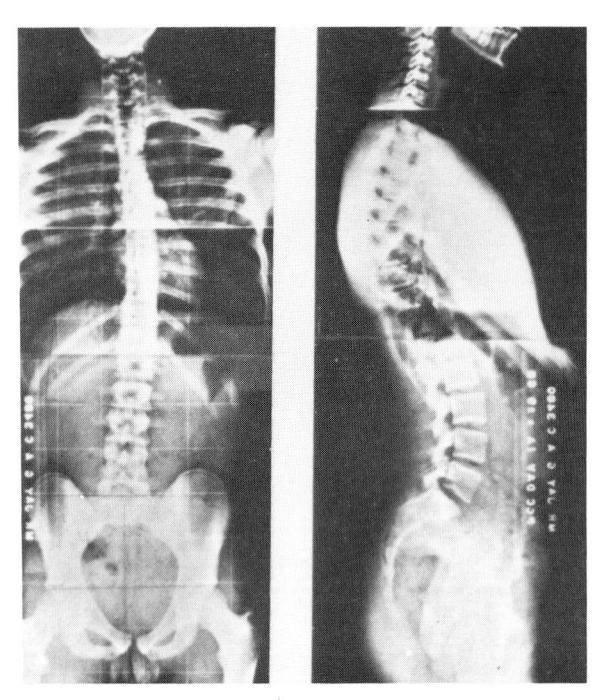

Fig. 9-32 A. Anteroposterior and lateral views before treatment.

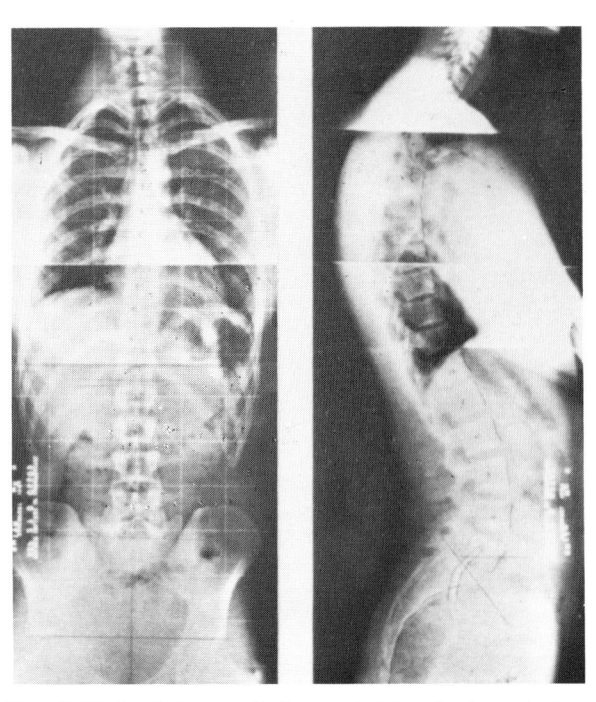

Fig. 9-33 A. Anteroposterior and lateral views before treatment.

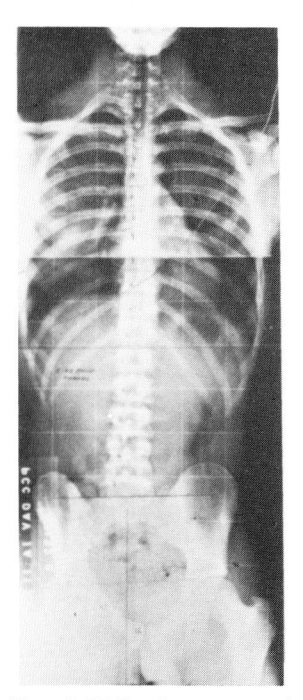

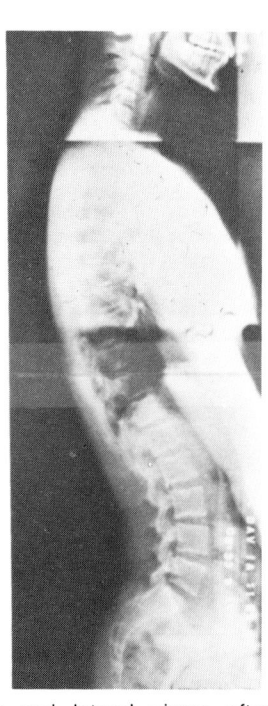

Fig. 9-32 B. Anteroposterior and lateral views after treatment. *(Reprinted with permission of the Academy of Physiological Dentistry, the American Academy for Functional Prosthodontics, and Dr. A.C. Fonder, Rock Falls, Illinois.)*

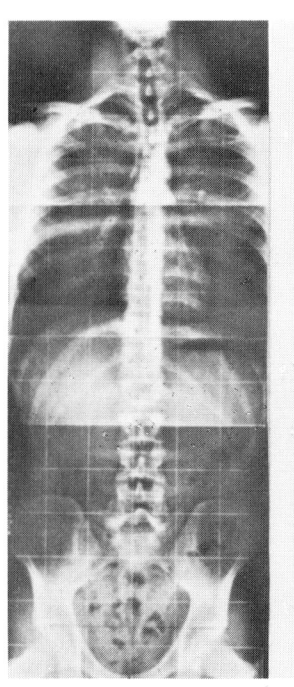

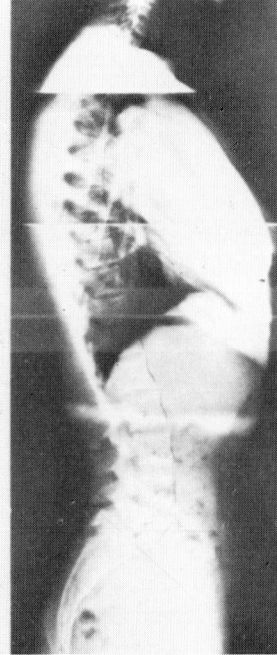

Fig. 9-33 B. Anteroposterior and lateral views after treatment. *(Reprinted with permission of the Academy of Physiological Dentistry, the American Academy for Functional Prosthodontics, and Dr. A.C. Fonder, Rock Falls, Illinois.)*

presented with a deep overbite, primarily caused by all his lower posterior teeth being in linguoversion. In this particular case, therapy involved the use of upper and lower removable expansion appliances to upright all the posterior teeth. The improvement in posture can be viewed in Figures 9-33, A and B.

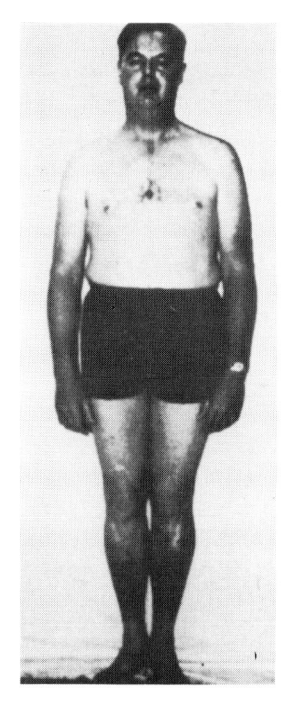

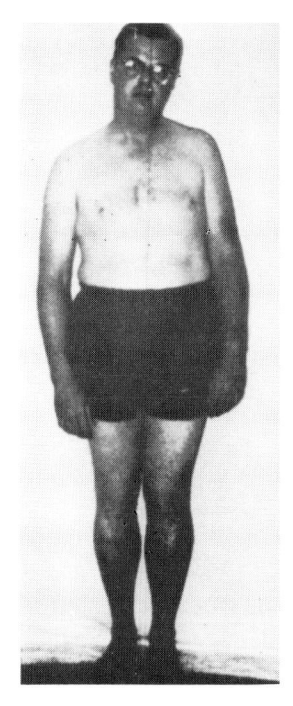

Fig. 9-34 A. Frontal views. *Left:* before treatment. *Right:* after treatment.

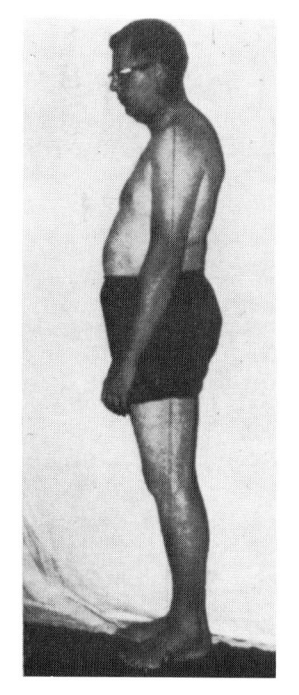

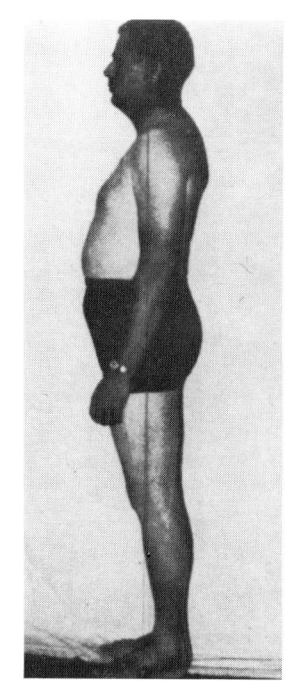

Fig. 9-34 B. Lateral views. *Right:* after treatment. *Left:* before treatment. *(Reprinted with permission of the Academy of Physiological Dentistry, the American Academy for Functional Prosthodontics, and Dr. A.C. Fonder, Rock Falls, Illinois.)*

Case Study #6

A 39-year-old clergyman was referred by a specialist who suspected that a relationship might exist between the patient's malocclusion and his respiratory and allergy problems. In addition, he suffered from psoriasis and scoliosis. He stood flat footed on one foot, but only the toes of the other foot were able to touch the floor. The psoriasis was of twenty years duration, and he had sought treatment from every major medical center in the U.S., but to no avail. He had been placed on allergy pills around the clock, and was usually hospitalized every spring and fall with pneumonia or near pneumonia.

Molar support was provided by self-curing acrylic inlay-overlay fillings on all mandibular and maxillary first and second molars to increase vertical dimension. The itching of his legs stopped the first day afterward. Two days following this build-up, he stood normally. He was able to discontinue the allergy pills and went five years without a cold. After six weeks, the skin of the legs began to appear more normal.

Gold inlay-onlays were finally placed on all posterior teeth. Numerous chronic problems he had experienced disappeared, along with his sinusitis, rhinitis, psoriasis, kyphosis, lordosis, and scoliosis.

Nine years after treatment, the patient still reported being asymptomatic.

The postural changes that took place during therapy can be viewed in Figures 34 A and B.

REFERENCES

1. Gelb H. An orthopedic approach to occlusal imbalance and temporomandibular joint dysfunction. *Dent Clin North Amer.* 1979;23:181-197.
2. Dixon D. Can you see the mouth for the teeth? *Bul Acad Gen Dent.* March 1968.
3. Eighth International Conference on Human Functioning. Biomedical Synergistic Institute, Wichita, Kansas. September 1984.
4. McNeill C, et al. Craniomandibular (TMJ) disorders: the state of the art. *J Pros Dent.* 1980;44(4):434.
5. Travell JG, Simons DG. *Myofascial Pain and Dysfunction: The Trigger Point Manual.* Baltimore, Md: Williams and Wilkins; 1983:104-164.
6. Fricton JR, et al. Myofascial pain syndrome of the head and neck: a review of clinical characteristics of 164 patients. *J Oral Surg.* 1985;60:615-623.
7. Kraus S, ed. *Growth and Development Influences on the Craniomandibular Region in TMJ Disorders:*

Management of the Craniomandibular Complex. New York, NY: Churchill Livingston; 1987.

8. Howard J. Clinical diagnosis of temporomandibular joint disorders. In: Moffett B, Westesson PL, ed. *Diagnosis of Internal Derangements of the TMJ*. Univ of Washington Cont Dent Ed.

9. Williamson EH. The role of craniomandibular dysfunction in orthodontic diagnosis and treatment planning. *Dental Clin North Amer*. July 1983:541-560.

10. Vig PS, Showfety BS, Phillips C. Experimental manipulation of head posture. *Am J Orthod*. 1980;77:258-268.

11. Solow B, Tallgren A. Head posture and craniofacial morphology. *Am J Phys Anthropol*. 1976;44:417-436.

12. Solow B, Tallgren A. Dentoalveolar morphology in relation to craniocervical posture. *Angle Orthod*. 1977;47:157-163.

13. Linder-Aronson S. Effects of adeniodectomy on dentition and facial skeleton over a period of five years. *Trans Eur Orthod Soc*. 1983:177-186.

14. Solow B, et al. Airway adequacy, head posture, and craniofacial morphology. *Am J Orthod*. 1984;86:214-223.

15. Solow B, Greve E. Craniocervical angulation and nasal respiratory resistance. In: McNamara J. Jr ed. *Naso-Respiratory Function and Craniofacial Growth*. Ann Arbor, MI: University of Michigan; 1979:87-119.

16. Marcotte M. Head posture and dentofacial proportions, *Angle Ortho*. 51:208.

17. Schwartz AH. Kopfhaltung and Kiefer. *A Stomathol*. 1926;24:669-744.

18. Bezuur JN, et al. The recognition of craniomandibular disorders IV: condylar asymmetry in relation to myogenous and arthrogenous origin of pain. *J Oral Rehab*. 1988:61-67.

19. Habets LLMH, Bezuur JN, Naeije M, Hansson TL. (1)The OPG, an aid in TMJ diagnostics, (2) The vertical Symmetry. *J Oral Rehab*. 14 (in Press).

20. Ayub E, et al. Head posture: a case study of the effects of the rest position of the mandible. *JOSPT*. 1984;5:179-183.

21. Mohl ND. Head posture and its role in occlusion. *NY State Dent J*. 1976;42:17-23.

22. Pullinger AG, et al. A tomographic study of mandibular condyle position in an asymptomatic population. *J Pros Dent*. 1985;53:711.

23. Goldstein DF, et al. Influence of cervical posture on mandibular movement. *J Prosth Dent*. 52:421-426.

24. De Bont LGM, et al. Osteoarthritis of the temporomandibular joint: a light microscope and scanning electron microscopic study of the articular cartilage of the mandible condyle. *J Oral Maxillofac Surg*. 1985;43:481-488.

25. Lagaida M, White GE. Unilateral mastication and facial formation. *J Pedod*. 1983:127-134

26. Solow B, Kreiborg S. Soft-tissue stretching: a possible control factor in craniofacial morphogenesis. *Scand J Dent*. 1977;85:505-507.

27. Dibbets J, et al. Symptoms of TMJ dysfunction: indicators of growth pattern. *J Pedod*. 1985;9:265-284.

28. Rocabado M. Biomedical relationship of the cranial, cervical and hyoid regions. *J Craniomand Pract*. June 1983;1:61.

29. Darnell M. A proposed chronology of events for forward head posture. *J Craniomand Pract*. September 1983;1:50.

30. Bjork A. Cranial base development. *Am J Orhod*. 1955;41:198-255.

31. Harvfold EP, Vargerik K, Chierici KG. Primate experiments on oral sensation and dental malocclusions. *Am J Orthod*. 1973;63:494-508.

32. Moss ML, Rankow RM. The role of the functional matrix in mandibular growth, *Angle Orth*. 1965;38:95-103.

33. Moss ML. The functional matrix concept and its relationship to temporomandibular joint dysfunction and treatment. *Dental Clin N Am*. July 1983:445-455.

34. Sicher H, DuBrul EL. *Oral Anatomy*. 6th ed. St. Louis, MO: The C.V. Mosby Co; 1975.

35. Thurow RC. *Atlas of Orthodontic Principles*. 2nd ed. St. Louis, MO: The C.V. Mosby Co;1977:131.

36. Price W. *Nutrition and Physical Degeneration* San Diego, Calif: Price-Pottenger Nutritional Foundation Inc;1970.

37. Hashi H. Comparative morphology of the mammalian mandible in relation to food habit. *Okajimas Folia Anat*. Japan: 1971;48:333-345.

38. Muhl ZF, Newton JH. Change in digastric muscle length in feeding rabbits. *J Morph*. 1982;171:151-157.

39. Corruccini RS, Hander JS. Temporomandibular joint size decreases in American blacks: Evidence from Barbados. *J Dent Res*. 1980;59:1528

40. Bouvier M, Hylander WL. Effect of bone strain on cortical bone structure in macaques (Macaca Mulatta). *J Morphol*. 1981;167:1-12.

41. Herring SW. Functional design of cranial muscles: comparative and physiological studies in pigs. *Am Zool*. 1980;20:283-293.

42. Rocabado M. Arthrokinematics of the temporomandibular joint. *Dental Clin N Am*. July 1983:573-594.

43. Gelb H, Berenstein IM. Clinical evaluation of 200 private patients with TMJ syndrome. *J Prosth Dent*. 1983;49:234-243m.

44. Fonder AC. *The Dental Physician*. Blackbury, Va: University Publications; 1977:51.

45. Lieb M. Oral orthopedics. In: Gelb H ed. *Clinical Management of Head, Neck and TMJ Pain and Dysfunction*. 2nd ed. St. Louis, Mo: Ishiyaku EuroAmerica; 1991:37.

46. Rocabado M, et al. Physical therapy and dentistry: an overview. *J Craniomandibular Pract*. June-August 1983;1:61-66.
47. Sorrin S. Habit: an etiologic factor in periodontal disease. *Dent Digest*. 1935;41:291.
48. *Dorland's Illustrated Medical Dictionary, 25th Edition*. W.B. Saunders Co; 1974.
49. Posselt U. *Physiology of Occlusion and Rehabilitation*. Philadelphia, Pa: F.A. Davis Co;1962:186.
50. *Course in Clinical Oral Orthopedics*. Institute for Graduate Dentists. 1953.
51. Posselt U. *Physiology of Occlusion and Rehabilitation*. Philadelphia, Pa: F.A. Davis Co;1962:37,66,73,88.
52. Mongini F. Influence of function on temporomandibular joint remodeling and degenerative disease. *Dent Clin N Am*. 1983;27:479-494.
53. Rugh JD, Drago CJ. Vertical dimension: a study of clinical rest position and jaw muscle activity. *J Prosth Dent*. 1981;45:670-675.
54. Eversaul GA. Biofeedback and Kinesiology: *Dental Applications*. Las Vegas, Nev; Private Publications; 1977.
55. Linn JB. Lecture—Kinesiology testing of a sample group of basketball and football players. *New Orleans Dental Conference*. 1979.
56. Smith SS. Muscular strength correlated to jaw posture and the temporomandibular joint. *NY State Dental J*. 1978;44:278.
57. Whatmore GB, Kohli DR. *The Physiopathology and Treatment of Functional Disorders*. New York, NY: Grune and Stratton; 1974.
58. Bates RF, Atkinson WB. The effects of maxillary MORA's on strength and muscles efficiency tests. *J Craniomandib Pract*. 1983;1:37.
59. Williams MO, Chaconas SJ, Bader JP. The effects of mandibular position on appendage muscle strength. *J Prosth Dent*. 1983;49:560.
60. Kaufman A, Kaufman RS. Effects of the MORA on members of a football team. *Quintessence International*. June 1983;6:671-681.
61. Verban EM Jr, et al. A biochemical analysis of the effects of a mandibular orthopedic repositioning appliance on shoulder strength. *J Craniomand Pract*. 2(3):232-237.
62. Manns A, Miralles R, Santander H, Valdivia J. Influence of the vertical dimension in the treatment of myofascial pain-dysfunction syndrome. *J Prosthet Dent*. 1983;50:700-709.
63. Valdivia J, Manns A, Miralles R. Myofascial pain dysfunction syndrome: comparative clinical evaluation of the therapeutic basis of three appliance designs. *Chilian Orthodontic Review*. 1985;2:108-116.
64. Rocabado M. Lecture—Physical therapy in the treatment of TMJ Dysfunction. *Institute of Graduate Dentists*. New York, NY: April 1979.
65. Weinberg LA, Lager L. Clinical report on the etiology and diagnosis of TMJ dysfunction-pain syndrome. *J Prosthet Dent*. 1980;44:642.

Chapter 10

The Effect of Macroposture and Body Mechanics on Dental Occlusion

Noshir Mehta, DMD, MDS, MS
Albert G. Forgione, PhD

The field of dental occlusion is filled with references to occlusal interferences and their effects on masticatory function,[1-4] techniques of occlusal equilibration,[5-8] prosthetic reconstruction,[5-9] orthodontic correction,[9] and other methods used to "stabilize" the occlusion.[10] All such references assume that interferences are damaging to the masticatory system.[11] However, occlusal interferences are actually part of normal occlusion, occurring when opposing teeth meet. During intercuspation, the cusp fossa arrangement relies mainly on the integrity of the the teeth and proper movement of the mandible to prevent occlusal interference.

Mandibular movements are affected by a wide variety of influences. The most recognized include muscle contraction patterns of the masticatory muscles, mechanoreceptors of the temporomandibular joints, and proprioceptors of the periodontal ligaments of teeth and mucosa.[12] These are further affected by proper nerve impulses and function.[13]

Less known is the effect of head and body posture[14] on occlusal contacts and mandibular position. In some patients with apparent unequal leg lengths, it has been suggested that occlusion differs when the patient is standing as opposed to sitting.[15]

As early as 1965, Strachan and Robinson[15] demonstrated that a hip rotation associated with one leg appearing longer than the other was associated with abnormal electromyographic (EMG) patterns during mastication. The EMG pattern returned to that of normal occlusion when a lift was inserted in the shoe. Emphasizing that occlusion was not an isolated function, Gelb[16] was a forerunner in underlining the importance of posture in craniomandibular syndrome. Our own clinical observations have reinforced our belief in this general principle, that the attainment of jaw stability requires examination and treatment of more than just the occlusal contacts.

The purpose of this chapter is to provide documentation which supports our conclusion that the macroposture of the body indeed affects the microposture of occlusion. Of the many factors which can affect occlusal contact and muscle activity patterns, three which are often overlooked have been selected for further discussion here. These are:

1) Body posture at the time of evaluation and treatment (standing versus sitting).
2) Relationship of hip balance and leg length to masticatory muscle activity and occlusal pattern.
3) Relationship of the atlas/axis complex to occlusal pattern and masticatory activity.

RECORDING INSTRUMENTATION

Recent advances in electronics have allowed information on occlusal contacts and muscle function to be collected simultaneously in a clinical setting. All the recordings cited in this chapter were made with a Davicon's bilateral surface electromyograph[17] in conjunction with the T-Scan occlusal analysis system.[18]

Dry, active EMG electrodes were applied to alcohol-wiped skin over each masseter mus-

Fig. 10-1 A

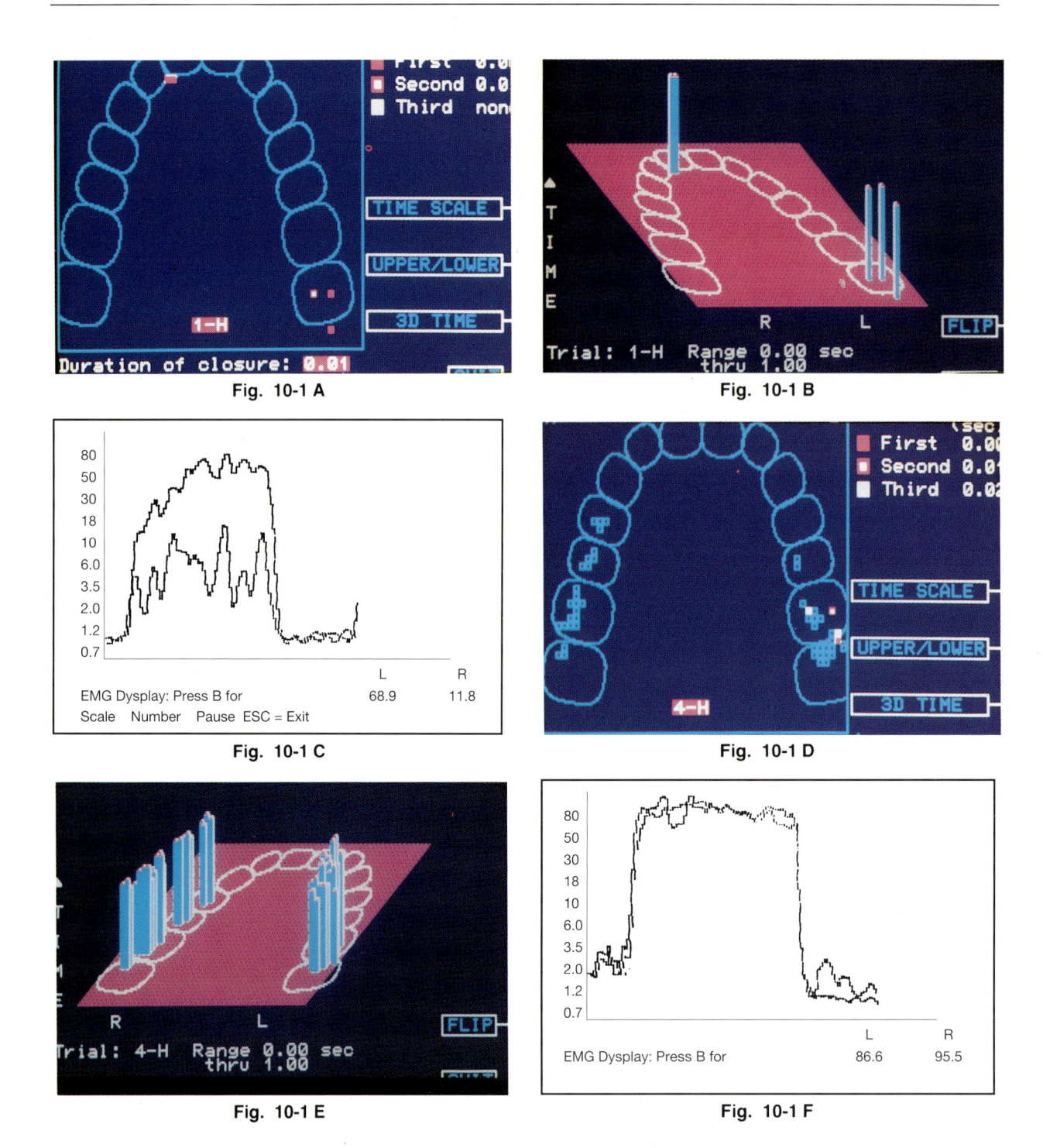

Fig. 10-1 B

Fig. 10-1 C

Fig. 10-1 D

Fig. 10-1 E

Fig. 10-1 F

cle with double sticky discs. Active electrodes were aligned with the direction of the muscle fibers. The Davicon system employs a linearized power detector circuit configuration. It combines the advantages of RMS measurement and full wave averaging to more closely represent changes in muscle force over time.

The T-Scan system utilizes a thin, disposable occlusal sensor held in place by a plastic holder. When placed between the patient's teeth, a pointer on the holder is positioned between the central upper incisors. This ensures a constant position for the sensor from trial to trial. This computerized device records sequence, duration, and location of occlusal contacts, and also analyzes contacts in the form of a balance plot, time display, and comparison screen. These modes allow easy visualization of different occlusal patterns, and also facilitate comparisons.

Figure 10-1 is an example of the form of the recordings. This figure presents the case

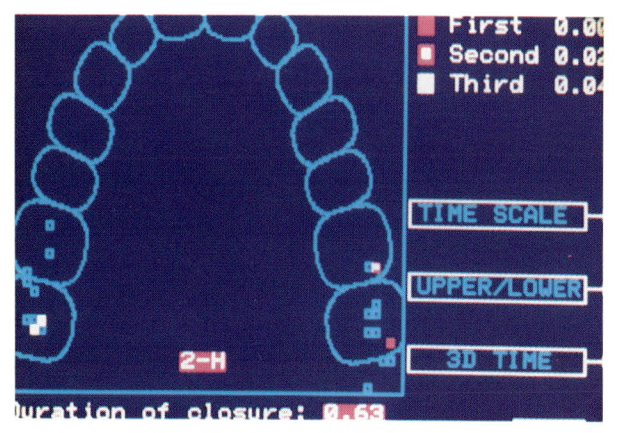

CHAPTER 10 The Effect of Macroposture and Body Mechanics on Dental Occlusion

Fig. 10-2 A

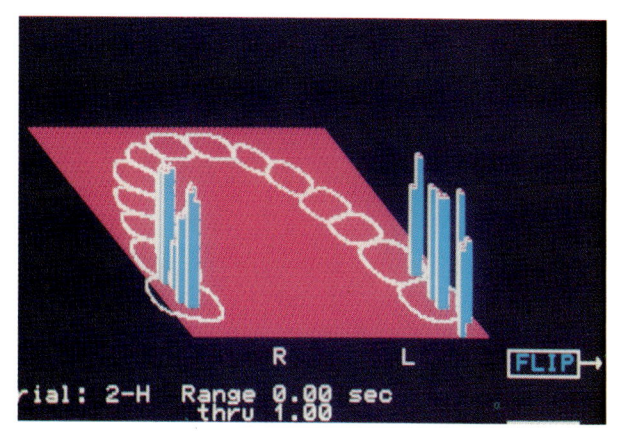

Fig. 10-2 B

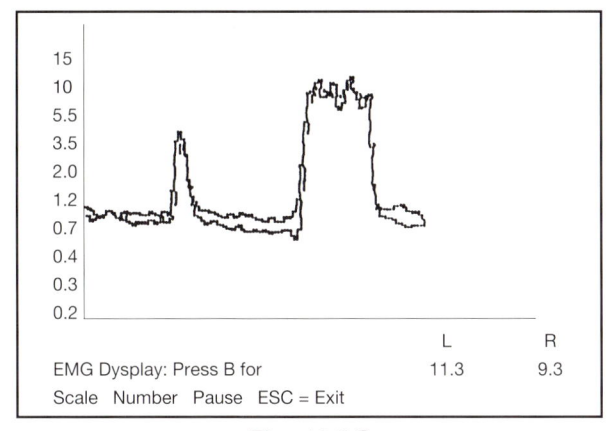

Fig. 10-2 C

of a patient with no postural imbalances and with contacts on two teeth only (left incisor and right second molar). Sequence analysis reveals that both contacts occured within 0.01 second (Fig. 10-1A). The duration histogram plots are essentially equal (Fig. 10-1B). The somewhat steady EMG trace of the left masseter shows an average peak value of 68.9 uV during a sustained bite, while the right masseter shows an irregular and faltering trace with an average peak value of only 11.8 uV

(Fig. 10-1C). With the same patient biting on a balanced occlusal splint of 0.5 mm thickness, there is initial contact on the right first molar within 0.2 second; all other contacts occur almost simultaneously (Fig. 10-1D). The duration histogram plot represents the more distributed and balanced occlusal pattern (Fig. 10-1E). The EMG traces are in perfect harmony in the brisk acceleration, maintenance and deceleration of the bite force. The average peak values are greater, show less variability, and differ by less than ten percent at 86.6 uV left and 95.5 uV right (Fig. 10-1F).

The three areas of discussion are represented in case form. These cases are not unique, but rather true representations of the occlusal instability frequently seen in individuals with head, neck, and hip problems.

THE EFFECTS OF BODY POSTURE ON OCCLUSION

The first case demonstrates the complexity of the interaction of various postural variables and their influence on mandibular function. It will become clear that a postural imbalance in the hip-leg relationship will produce different bites when standing or sitting, while balance in the hip-leg relationship will result in a more consistent bite regardless of position.

Figure 10-2 shows that in the seated position the T-Scan occlusal time analysis (Fig. 10-2A), duration histogram plot (Fig. 10-2B), and the EMG (Fig. 10-2C) are those of a closely balanced bite. In the standing position, however, there is a dramatic shift in the bite.

The initial contact shifts from the right second molar to the left second molar (Fig. 10-3A), while the distributed contacts on the left disappear and the entire contact pattern on the right shifts forward to two contacts on the canine and first bicuspid. This reversal is also manifested in the EMG (Fig. 10-3B). For clarity, dots are superimposed on the right masseter trace (the first peak is a swallow). As the bite force is increased, the right trace, initially lower, crosses over to become the one with higher tension, as the trace of the left masseter falters to approximately one third of the level of the right. The duration histogram plot is shown in Figure 10-3C.

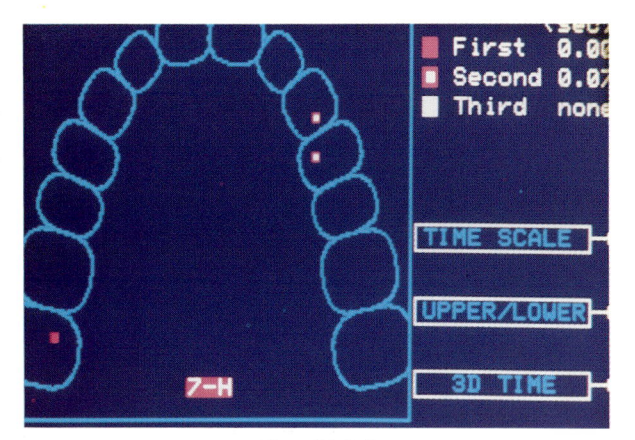

264 New Concepts in Craniomandibular and Chronic Pain Management

Fig. 10-3 A

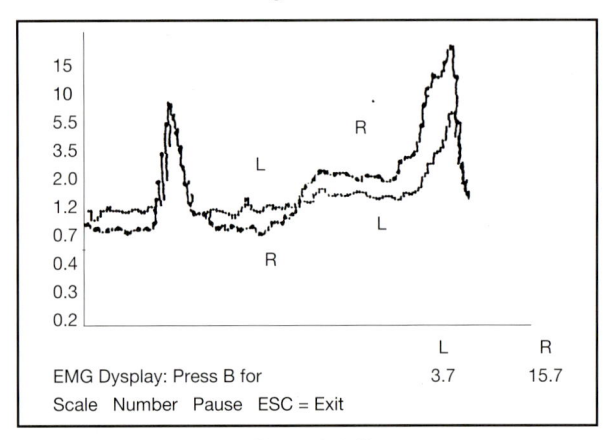

Fig. 10-3 B

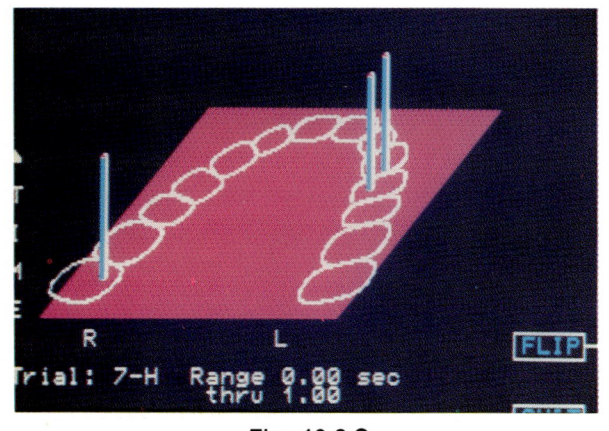

Fig. 10-3 C

Dramatic shifts such as these between the standing and sitting positions constitute a valuable diagnostic aid in identifying a hip rotation and associated leg-length discrepancy. The presence of this phenomenon can be substantiated by palpation of the ischial prominences of the pelvis and determining whether they are level. The diagnosis can be further verified by remonitoring the bite in both positions after a lift of approximate height has been inserted under the foot of the appropriate leg (it is not always the apparently shorter leg).

In this case, the lift (a 1.5 mm cork heel) was inserted under the apparently longer leg to produce the results shown in Figures 10-4 and 10-5. Notice that while standing 10-4A, the contacts upon the second molars are almost simultaneous and the duration histogram plots are similar (Fig. 10-4B). The EMG traces are also more harmonious and do not shift in value as the bite force increases (Fig. 10-4C). Upon sitting (from the standing, lift-inserted position), the bite remains consistently balanced, with only a slight retrusion (Fig. 10-5, A and B). The EMG trace (Fig. 10-5C), although not identical to that of the standing position, shows harmony during the bite and has similar average peak values (49.7 uV left and 42.2 uV right).

Even with the sophisticated monitoring devices used for this report, a dentist examing this case only in the erect, seated position might well conclude that the bite was within the acceptable range of balance. However, upon recording the standing bite, the dramatic shift in occlusion immediately identifies the influence of macropopostural imbalance upon the occlusion. It has been our frequent observation that such dramatic shifts in occlusion do not occur when an atlas/axis derangement is the patient's only problem. However, in a case such as that above, if the occlusion does not approach balance after lift insertion, this indicates an atlas/axis derangement in addition to the hip imbalance. This will be discussed further below.

THE EFFECT OF PURE HIP ROTATION IN OCCLUSION

A second case example reinforces the first finding. This patient reported discomfort in the right trapezius, right zygomatic arch, and right masseter.

The data presented in Figures 10-6 and 10-7 show the instantaneous occlusal equilibration which results from the insertion of a 1.5 mm cork lift. Although it is not the purpose of this chapter to present the therapeutic course of lift therapy, it is worthy of mention here that in most cases such as this one, the lift

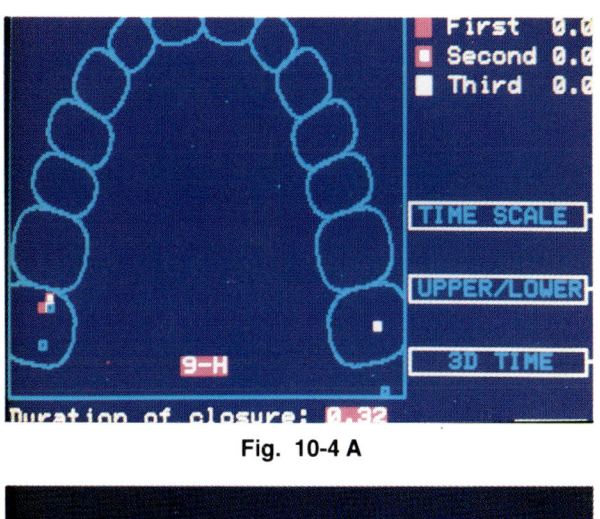

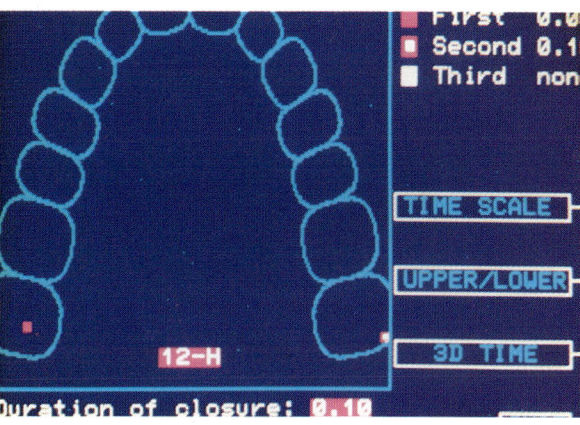

CHAPTER 10   The Effect of Macroposture and Body Mechanics on Dental Occlusion   265

Fig. 10-4 A

Fig. 10-5 A

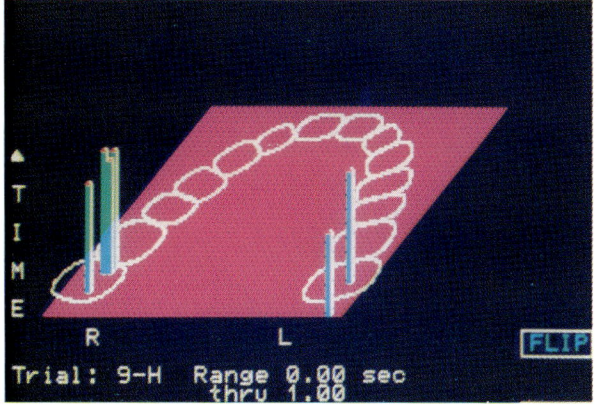

Fig. 10-4 B

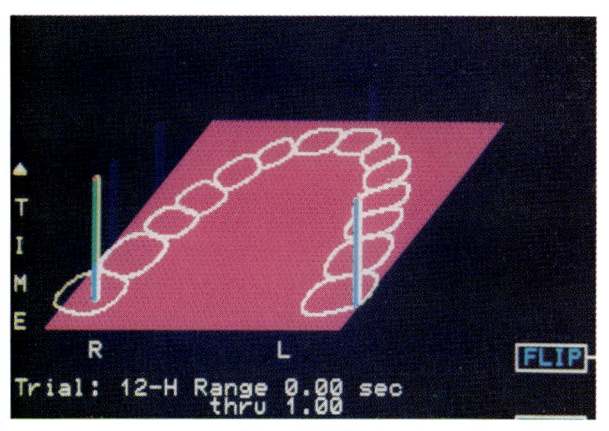

Fig. 10-5 B

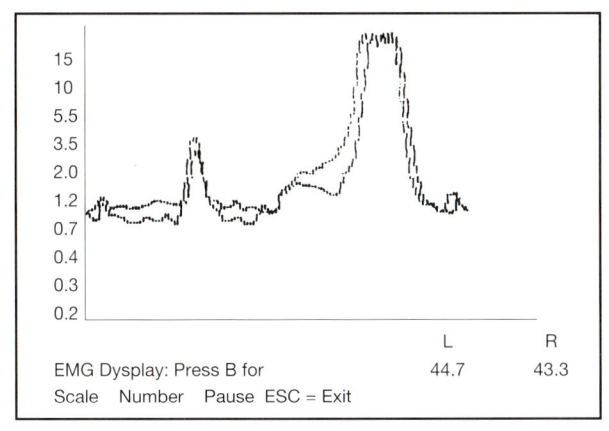

Fig. 10-4 C

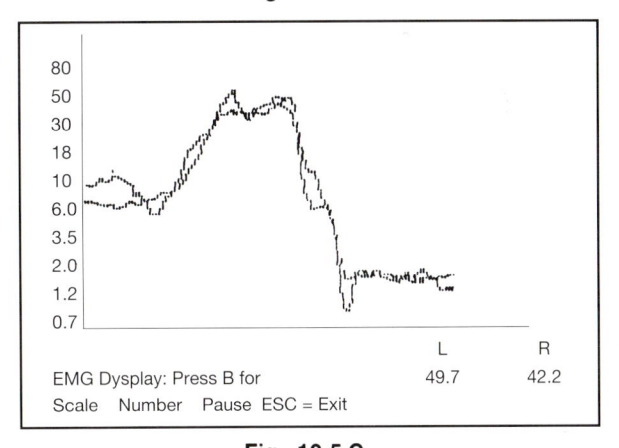

Fig. 10-5 C

is gradually reduced in height over the course of two to three weeks until it is no longer necessary.

THE EFFECT OF ATLAS IMBALANCE ON OCCLUSION

One of the first areas to examine when dealing with suspected head and neck dysfunction is the position of the atlas or C1 vertebra. The position and configuration of the atlas makes it of primary importance in the carriage of the skull. Travell[19(p 323)] shows that the arrangement of the associated muscles predicts that excessive tension in the posterior neck muscles will tend to displace or rotate the vertebra. It has been our experience that unilateral and bilateral subluxation of the atlas is found in many chronic craniomandibular syndrome patients who do not respond to conservative splint therapy.

The most common chiropractic method of

Fig. 10-6 A

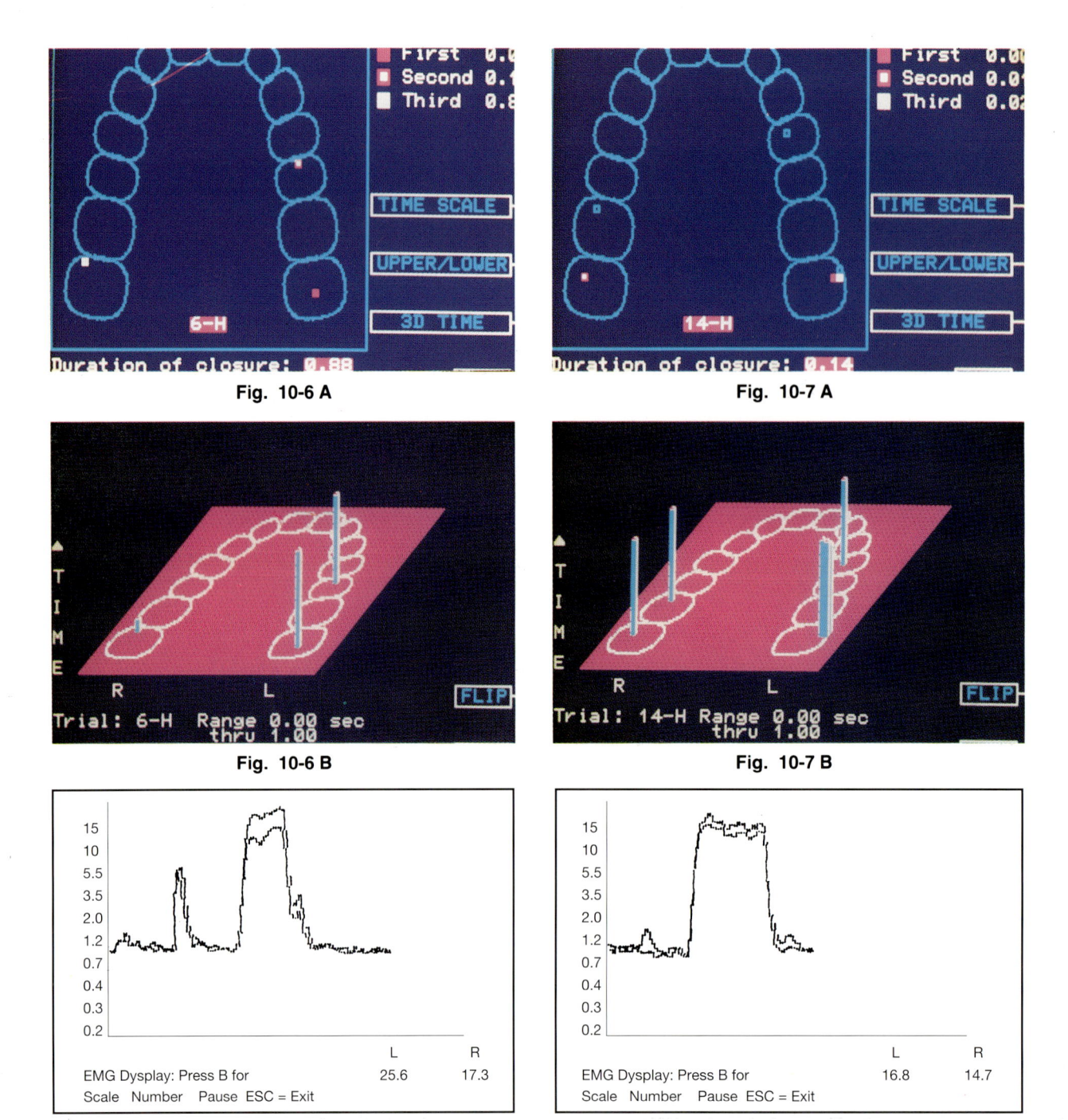

Fig. 10-7 A

Fig. 10-6 B

Fig. 10-7 B

Fig. 10-6 C

Fig. 10-7 C

cervical alignment, head rotation and rapid hyperextension (aside from being violent and frightening to a patient in pain) may not always position the atlas correctly. The more conservative method of gentle distraction along with slight, posteriorly directed pressure applied at the level of the transverse processes (at the point between the ramus of the mandible and mastoid process) is sufficient to relieve tension in the muscles maintaining the atlas in the forward position. This maneuver is usually followed by a slight light headedness and a spread of warmth in the neck area below the earlobe. Often the patient will remark that their *teeth fit together differently*, along with reporting a marked reduction of pain in the zygomatic area, masseter, and trapezius. The common report that "the bite feels different" following posteriorly directed direct pressure on the transverse processes of C-1 is substantiated in Figures 10-8 and 10-9.

CHAPTER 10 The Effect of Macroposture and Body Mechanics on Dental Occlusion 267

Fig. 10-8 A

Fig. 10-9 A

Fig. 10-8 B

Fig. 10-9 B

Fig. 10-8 C

Fig. 10-9 C

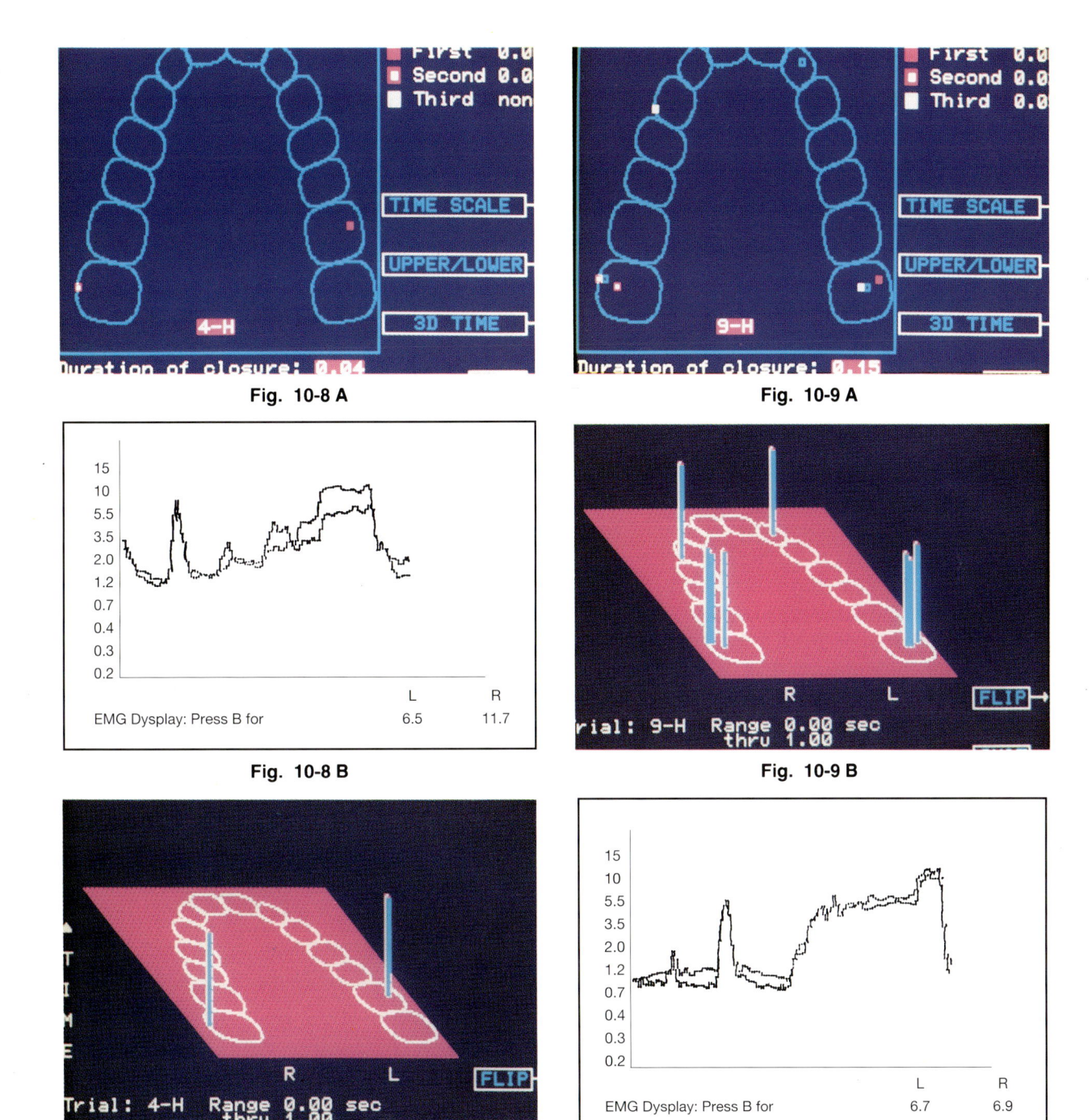

The T-Scan initially records two contacts: a primary contact on the right first molar and the next contact on the labial surface of the left second molar 0.04 seconds later (Fig. 10-8A). Masseter EMG activity (the initial peak records a swallow) during increasing bite force before C-1 release shows greater tension in the right masseter throughout, indicating an imbalanced bite (Fig. 10-8B). Following the atlas release (Fig. 10-9), masseter tension is essentially equal during swallow and gradual bite (note also the more vigorous and coordinated acceleration of tension of the bite in this second condition). The T-Scan reveals a dramatic shift in the bite (Fig. 10-9A). First contact now occurs on the right second molar; second contact occurs more lingual on the left second molar 0.02 seconds later; third contact occurs both more lingually on the right second molar and the left canine 0.03 seconds thereafter, with sequential contacts occurring on the left second molar, right second molar, and right second incisor. Although not ideal, the bite following the atlas release is significantly more balanced (Fig. 10-9B and C). This evidence indicates that one must proceed with caution when contemplating adjustment of the obvious premature contacts or the simple adjustment of a bite appliance to balance contacts when a deranged atlas is suspected. Such actions may lock in the imbalanced vertebra or promote further migration of C-1 forward.

DISCUSSION

It is evident from the information presented that occlusal contacts are affected by imbalances of the cervico/pelvic system.

In a study of 325 patients at the Gelb Craniomandibular Center at Tufts Dental School,[20] 60% were found to have cervical problems related to the atlas/axis complex. In these patients, the final occlusal position could not be achieved until the cervical area was stabilized. The concept of craniosacral technique[21] now used for patients with chronic head, neck, and back problems also suggests that there is a relationship between the pelvis and the cervical area. In these cases where there is cervical dysfunction, it is also common for patients to complain about low back pain and sciatica.

Treatment of these problems should be instituted before finalizing the occlusion through any definitive irreversible technique involving shaping, building, or moving teeth.

In such instances, it is important that the occlusion be maintained through the use of reversible techniques until the patient has had treatment for the cervical and pelvic problems. The best method is by the use of occlusal bite appliances which can be made to conform to the occlusion of the teeth. Where the occlusion is unstable but no other jaw problems exist, the operator can adjust the appliance instead of the teeth to balance the occlusion. This would need to be repeated as ongoing therapy for the neck and hip continues. When the new body posture has been stabilized, the appliance is removed and an occlusal adjustment is performed if necessary. If the occlusion can not be stabilized by selective grinding alone, then restorative or orthodontic means must be employed to achieve occlusal stability.

SUMMARY

The purpose of this chapter has been to make the reader aware of the dramatic shifts in occlusion brought about by the macroposture of the body. This is an area which has not previously been the focus of attention in dentistry. The advent of more sophisticated technology has now allowed us to evaluate clearly these effects on occlusion. Our treatment techniques will need to reflect this new information if true, enduring occlusal stability is to be achieved.

REFERENCES

1. Haddad AW, Mehta NR, Glickman I, Roeber F. Effects of occlusal adjustment on tooth contacts. *J Periodon*. October 1974;45(No.10):714.
2. Munlemann HP. Tooth mobility—its causes and significance. *J Periodon*. 1965;36:148.
3. Carranza F. The pole of morphofunctional occlusal factors in periodontal disease and temporomandibular diseases. In: *Glickman's Clinical Periodontology*, 6th ed. Philadelphia, Pa: WB Saunders; 1984:427.
4. Mehta NR, Roeber F, Haddad AW, Glickman I, Godman J. Stresses created by occlusal prematurities in a new photoelastic model system. August 1976;93:334.
5. Dawson PE. *Evaluation, Diagnosis, and Treatment of Occlusal Problems*. St. Louis, Mo: CV Mosby Co; 1975:56.
6. Schuyler CH. Fundamental principles in the correction of occlusal disharmony, natural and artificial. *J Am Dent Assoc*. 1935;22:1193.
7. Jankelson BA. A technique for obtaining optimal functional relationship for the natural dentition. *Dent Clin North Am*. 1980:4131.
8. Glickman I, Pameijer JHN, Roeber FW, Brion MAM. Functional occlusion as revealed by miniaturized radio transmitters. *Dent Clin North Am*. 1967;13:667.
9. Zarb G, Fenton A. Prosthodontic operative and orthodontic therapy. In: *A Textbook of Occlusion*. Chicago, Ill: Quintessence Publishing Company; 1988:Ch. 22.
10. Hudis MM. Occlusion in removable partial dentures. *Dent Clin North Am*. 1981;25(No.3):533.
11. Wank GS, Kroll YJ. Occlusal trauma: an evaluation of its relationship to periodontal prostheses. *Dent Clin North Am*. 1981;25(No.3):511.

12. Kawamura Y Jr. Neurogenesis of mastication. *Frontiers of Oral Physiology.* 1974;1:24.
13. McCall W Jr. The musculature. In: *A Textbook of Occlusion.* Chicago, Ill: Quintessence Publishing Company; 1988:Ch. 7.
14. Funakoshi M, Fujita N, Takenama S. Between occlusal interferences and jaw muscle activities in response to changes in head positioning. *J Dent Res.* 1976;55:684.
15. Strachen F, Robinson MJ. Short leg linked to malocclusion. *Osteopath News.* April 1965.
16. Gelb H. Effective management and treatment of the craniomandibular syndrome. In: *Clinical Management of Head, Neck and TMJ Pain and Dysfunction.* Philadelphia, Pa: Ishiyaku EuroAmerica; 1991.
17. Davicon. 79 Second Avenue, Burlington, Mass: 01803 (The MyoDental System/3).
18. TEKSCAN, Inc., 451 D Street, Boston, Mass: 02210 (The T-Scan).
19. Travell JG, Simons DG. *Myofascial Pain and Dysfunction: The Trigger Point Manual.* Baltimore, Md: Williams & Wilkins; 1983.
20. Mehta NR, Forgione A. Incidence of TM. joint, myofascial pain and cervical/spinal dysfunctions in craniomandibular dysfunctional patients. (In preparation)
21. Upledger JE, Vredevoogd JD. *Craniosacral Therapy,* 5th ed. Eastland Press; 1986:Ch. 2.

Chapter 11

Craniomandibular Dysfunction in The Growing Child

Murad N. Padamsee, BDS
George E. White, DDS, PhD, FAGD

INTRODUCTION

Disorders of the craniomandibular system, though well established in adults, are thought to occur rarely in children. The only consistent symptoms that children usually present with are headaches and earaches (commonly regarded as allergic manifestations), sinusitis, and otalgia. Thus, pediatricians are frequently the first diagnosticians to observe the symptoms. The disorders then often go misdiagnosed, allowing the condition to mature into the characteristic picture of temporomandibular and myofascial pain dysfunction syndromes. This vicious cycle is further perpetuated by nasal allergies and mouth breathing patterns.

Several investigators[1-5] have demonstrated that mouth breathing predisposes towards a lowered mandibular posture, in addition to downward and forward tongue posture, all of which in turn may lead to forward head posture, causing excessive strain in the cervical area. These changes are reflected down along the spine and influence the posturing of the body. Since we are dealing with rapid periods of growth and development as the child matures, it is of immense importance that the dentist be aware not only of headaches, earaches, and clicking or popping within the temporomandibular joints (TMJ), but also of compromised breathing patterns, parafunctional habits, forward head position, and possible loss of the physiological curvatures of the spine at an early age. This vigilance on the dentist's part will increase the success of treatment for craniomandibular dysfunction, and more importantly, allow development to be facilitated to its fullest potential.

It is unfortunate that skeletal muscles are often ignored as a source of pain to the head, neck, and face. Active trigger points in the muscles of the masticatory system, head, and neck may refer pain and tenderness to distal areas, which often mimic symptoms of internal derangement of the TMJ's, thus masking underlying pain syndromes that may exist as myofascial pain dysfunction and/or cervical strain.

In the course of this chapter, attention will be drawn to three principal areas: 1) TMJ dysfunction and guidance of the dentition to optimal interarch relationships, 2) myofascial dysfunction, and 3) cervical and spinal dysfunction.

LITERATURE REVIEW

Little has been written about TMJ dysfunction in children as compared to the epidemiological studies done on the adult population. But with the growing attention to functional disorders and their role in TMJ dysfunction, there has also been a growing interest in undertaking studies of children and adolescents.

In 1971, Geering-Gaerny and Rakosi[6] studied 241 children aged 8-14 years, and assessed 41% of these children as displaying one or more of the following: joint sounds such as clicking or grating, pain on palpation of the joints and masticatory muscles, and deviation of the mandible on maximal opening. However, not even one child complained of any pain.

Lindquist[7], in 1974, found muscle tenderness in 27% of the twelve-year-old children studied. Siebert[8], in 1975, studied children of 12-16 years of age in pre- and post-orthodontic groups, reporting TMJ-muscle tenderness in 80% and 60% respectively.

In a 1977 longitudinal study on 112 children with Class II Division 2 malocclusion, Dibbets[9] assessed signs and symptoms of functional disturbances. Twelve percent of the subjects were reported to have had pain, clicking, or limitation of mandibular opening.

Williamson[10] in 1977 studied 304 pretreatment adolescent patients between 6-16 years, and reported a strong tendency for TMJ dysfunction in patients exhibiting Class II Division 2 or Class I deep bite malocclusions. Thirty-five percent of the children were found to have pain on palpation of the TMJ muscles, and 19% exhibited clicking. The lateral pterygoid muscle most frequently exhibited palpatory tenderness, followed by the medial pterygoid and the masseter. Of interest was that 24% of the group showed radiographic deformation of the condyles.

In the same year, Wigdorowicz[11] examined 2,100 children aged 10-15 years and reported TMJ dysfunction associated with bruxism in 40.4%, as compared to only 26.9% in children without a history of bruxism.

Four years later, Egermark-Eriksson, Carlson, and Ingervall[12], in an epidemiological study of 402 children in three age groups of 7, 11, and 15 years, demonstrated that the prevalence of subjective symptoms was 39%, 67%, and 74%, respectively. The signs of dysfunction were shown to have increased with age, from about 30% in the youngest to 60% in the oldest group.

The same year, Nilner and Lassing[13], examined 440 children aged 7-14 years, of which 36% were symptomatic, with 15% exhibiting recurrent headaches and 13% reporting clicking of TM joints. Seventy-five percent of the children reported at least one of the following parafunctional habits: grinding, clenching, lip and cheek biting, nail biting, or thumbsucking. Sixty-five percent experienced pain on palpation of muscles, and 39% claimed pain on palpation of the TMJ.

In a 1985 epidemiological study of 800 adolescents, Grosfield, Jackowska, and Czarnecka[14] reported 67% as having TMJ dysfunction, and found that the condition was significantly more prevalent in girls than boys. Magnusson, Egermark-Eriksson and Carlsson[15], reported in 1986 on a five-year longitudinal study in 119 adolescents, 15 years old at the first examination and 20 years old at the follow-up. Sixty-two percent had mild signs of mandibular dysfunction, whereas moderate to severe signs were found in 17%.

An interesting though disturbing finding was that almost half of those who clicked at 15 years had no clicking at 20 years, and half of those with clicking recorded at 20 years had no clicking at 15 years. In a 1986 study on children only 3-5 years old, Bernal and Tsamtsouris[16] reported clicking in 5% of the sample. Though this percentage is lower than those reported by the other studies, the relatively low age of the subjects may explain the low incidence. The incidence of clicking has been shown to increase with age.

Thus, TMJ dysfunction is shown to be commonly found in both children and adolescents. These patients exhibit increasing signs and symptoms with age, including joint sounds and deviation on opening and closing. Muscle tenderness is also often related to jaw position, e.g., Class II Division 2, and parafunctional habits, e.g., clenching, grinding, lip and cheek biting, nail biting, or thumbsucking.

DEVELOPMENT OF THE TMJ

The TMJ is one of the last joints in the body to develop, and unlike other joints that develop from a single blastema, the TMJ develops from two blastemmata that grow towards each other. The articulating surfaces of the TMJ are covered by fibrous tissue, unlike the hyaline cartilage which covers other joint surfaces.

TMJ development is initiated during the 8th week of intrauterine life and occurs as a condensation of mesenchymal cells, derived from the neural crest on the dorsal end of the mandible.[17] At birth, the mandibular condyle is also relatively flat, covered by a thick layer of cartilage. The mandible is displaced downward and forwards as the condyle grows in a posterior-superior direction, attaining its mature contour during the late-mixed dentition. At birth, the disc too is flat, and develops its accentuated S-shaped profile as the articulator tubercle develops.[18] Early development is characterized by vascularization of all components, which are replaced by fibrous tissue. Growth and maturation of the TMJ is not completed till the end of the second and third decades of life.

Due to their anatomic locations, the condyles are vulnerable to trauma. Any fall or blow to the chin may affect their growth and development. This type of macrotrauma may be common in children as they learn to walk and play, sustaining many falls during the developing years.[19] Poor posture in the classroom, cradling the chin against the palm of the hand, or tilting the head to one side, and resting against the heel of the palm in such a manner that excessive pressures are sustained by the lateral aspect of the TMJ may all adversely affect its development. Microtrauma, such as bruxing, clenching, unilateral mastication, and occlusal and/or functional interferences may also have long-term effects.

Dibbits[20], in a study of 175 children over a 15-year period, reported that TMJ dysfunction occurred during periods of active growth. This group was more retrognathic, with a shorter ramus, decreased mandibular length, reduced posterior facial height, and steeper mandibular plane angle caused by a backward rotation of the mandible. Lagaida and White[21] reported that unilateral chewing affects the dentition, facial development, and possibly TMJ development. In their study of 7-11 year olds, they found that the side with the higher eye and greater vertical development is associated with the unilateral chewing.

Ricketts[22] reports that both macro- and microtrauma may affect the condrogenic area of the condyle, which may lead to degenerative changes and growth deformities. This is often expressed as a flattening of the eminence, or as a small condyle in a large fossa.[19]

A TRIAD OF DYSFUNCTION

Mehta et al.[23] described the "TMJ-triad of dysfunction" as being three distinct and separate dysfunctions, interposed upon each other. The three dysfunctions were: a) TMJ dysfunction or internal derangement, b) myofascial pain dysfunction (MPD), and c) cervical and spinal dysfunction (CSD).

TMJ dysfunction is specific to the TM joint and consists of pain in and around the joint, popping and clicking joint sounds, and even locking and degenerative changes within the joint itself.

MPD refers to muscle tension and hypertonicity within the muscles of the head, neck, and face, leading to pain and dysfunction. Trigger points arise within these muscles as a loci of hyperirritability within the muscles or fascia and refer pain in a characteristic pattern often distant to the site of the trigger point. These pain patterns often mimic those that arise from internal derangement within the TMJ.

CSD is related to the spine, the cervical region in particular, and to the vertebrae, ligaments, and muscles. A forward head position, uneven shoulder height, loss of cervical lordosis, cervical nerve entrapments, trigger points in the suboccipital and posterior cervical muscles may affect the harmony of the craniocervical system. This may also translate down into the upper thoracic spine, and a compensatory effect upon the lumbar spine and pelvic girdle may further influence the craniocervical region. Pain and dysfunction arising from this area often mimic and are frequently superimposed upon internal derangement of the TMJ and MPD syndromes. The key to treatment is precise diagnosis of the symptom complex affecting the craniomandibular region. Categorizing these symptoms and signs into the appropriate dysfunctional syndrome will itself dictate the modalities of treatment. As the etiology is multifactorial, the treatment must be interdisciplinary.

TMJ DYSFUNCTION

TMJ dysfunction has been defined as a set of symptoms rather than by the etiology or an exact diagnosis.[24] Most of the symptoms include: 1) pain in the TMJ region, and tenderness, soreness or fatigue in the muscles associated with the joint; 2) sounds during condylar movement, such as popping or clicking;

and 3) limitation of mandibular movement and eventually locking (closed) of the TMJ. Preteens usually manifest only headaches and earaches. Unless they are specifically questioned about them, they usually do not complain about either. As they move into the teens, the presenting complaints include popping, clicking, headaches, earaches, and tinnitus. As early as the second or third decade, crepitus within the joint may be evidenced.

Since children present with different signs of dysfunction, it is important to correlate these with condylar position to obtain an integrated viewpoint and arrive at an accurate diagnosis and treatment plan.

Condylar Position

The diagnosis of internal derangement may be aided with radiographs of the TMJ. The panoramic view gives the least reliable view of the TMJ's. Only the head of the condyle is seen in a lateral projection, and its position in the fossa is distorted. Changes in the shape of the condylar head from a smooth rounded surface can be detected. The transcranial projection if the most commonly used technique. It is useful for viewing the lateral aspect of the joint, and six views are taken on one film, in the intercuspal position, postural rest position, and on maximal opening. Beaking, lipping, and arthritic changes can be observed, as well as the position of the condylar head. If changes are suspected in the middle and medial pole, tomograms and CT scans offer more accurate information. The recent advent of magnetic resonance imaging holds great promise in viewing hard and soft tissues of the joints with no associated radiation. Due to the practicality and radiation involved, the transcranial projection is a very useful preliminary screening radiograph.

Although the disc cannot be seen on the radiograph, its position can be inferred by the relative position of the condyle in the fossa. On the normal radiograph, the condyle in the closed jaw position is seated concentrically or slightly forward in the fossa, and there is at least 2 mm of surrounding joint space. Internal derangement is defined as an anterior displacement of the disc associated with a posterior-superior displacement of the condyle in the intercuspal position. When diagnosing from the radiograph alone, the disc cannot be seen. Therefore, if the relative position of the condyle to the fossa changes in the intercuspal position, then the position of the disc must also be changed.

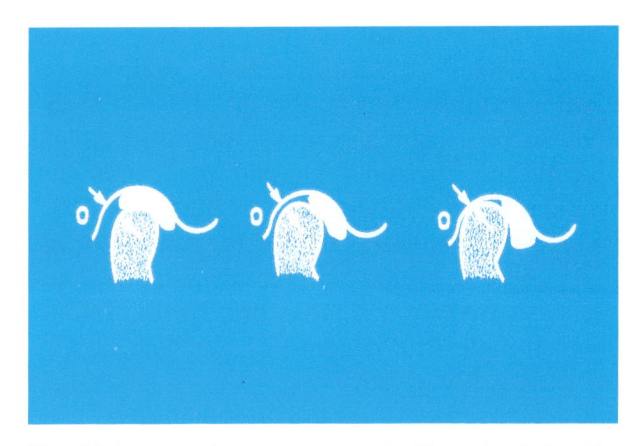

Fig. 11-1. Internal Derangement. **A.** Normal relationship of the condylar head to the disc. **B.** Decrease in posterior joint space with anterior disc displacement. **C.** Advanced disc displacement.

When the condyle is centered in the fossa, the disc is in a 12 o'clock position with respect to the head of the condyle (Fig. 11-1A). If the condyle is driven posterosuperiorly, the posterior attachment will stretch and the disc will migrate anteriorly (Fig. 11-1B). Radiographically, there will be a decrease in joint space. If the condition worsens, the posterior attachment will become even more stretched, thinner and weaker, and the disc will migrate even further anteriorly. Radiographically, the posterosuperior displacement of the condyle is seen in Fig. 11-1C. With such a narrow posterior joint space, the disc must be situated anterior to the condyle.

There have been many attempts to define the normal position of the condyle in the fossa. Ricketts[25] found that the space between the glenoid fossa and condyle was 1.55 mm anteriorly, 2.5 mm superiorly and 7.5 mm posteriorly to the center of the auditory meatus. Stack and Funt[26] describe normal joints with condylar heads located somewhat mesial and inferior to the center of the fossa.

Gelb[27] describes the normal position of the condyle by drawing lines tangent to the roof of the fossa and eminentia, and drawing a third line halfway between these two lines. Next, two vertical lines are drawn, one from

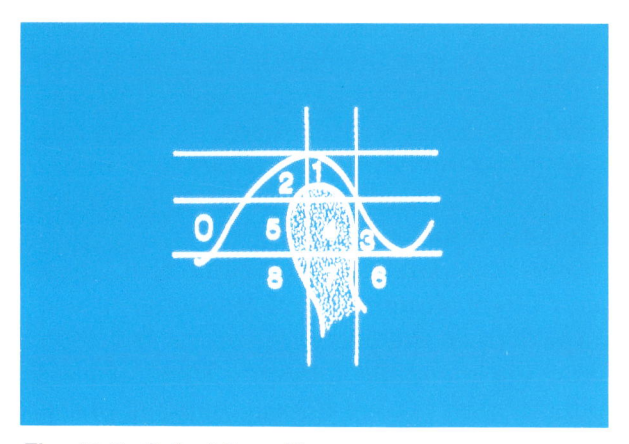

Fig. 11-2. Gelb 4-7 position.

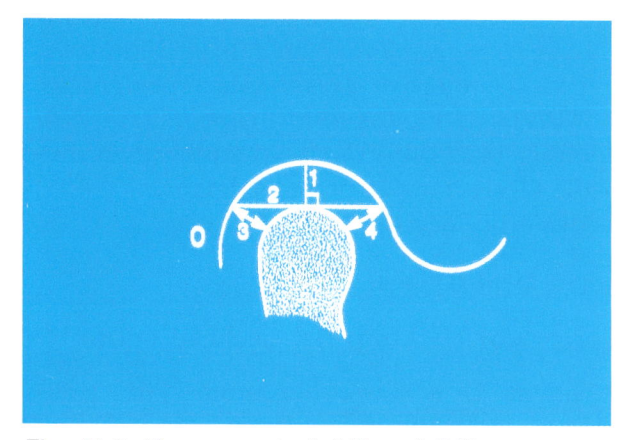

Fig. 11-3. Measurement of AJS and PJS.

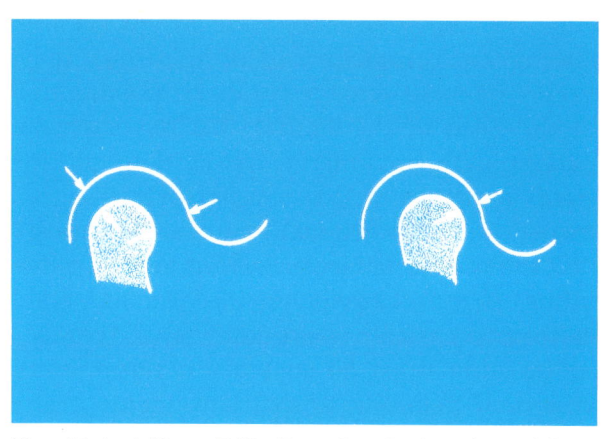

Fig. 11-4. AJS > PJS: Posterior displaced condyle.

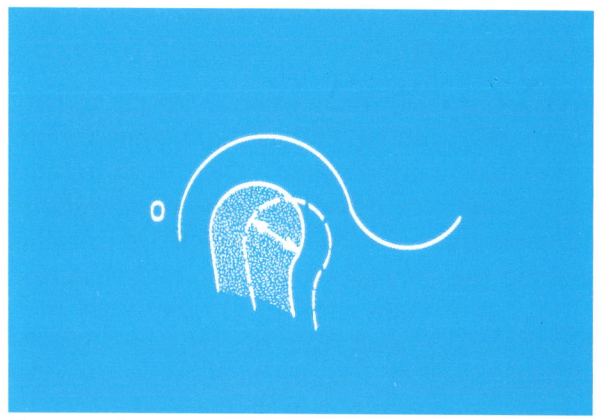

Fig. 11-5. Owens' therapeutic range. Solid line represents concentric position. Broken line represents 4-7 position.

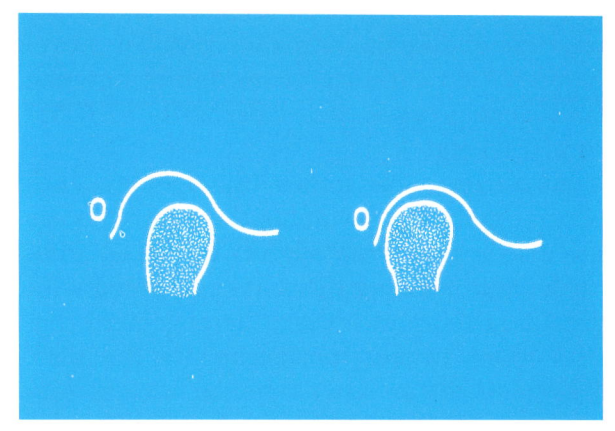

Fig. 11-6. Pre- and Post-treatment condylar position.

the highest point of the roof of the fossa and the other from the point where the middle horizontal line intersects the descending slope of the eminence. The normal position of the condyle is in areas 4 and 7 (Fig. 11-2:4-7 position).

Owens[28] regards the concentric positioning of the condyle to be the most ideal. It is calculated as follows: a) a vertical line (line 1 is drawn from the fossa center to the top of the condyle; b) a horizontal line is drawn perpendicular to line 1; c) line 3 is the shortest distance to the condyle from the intersection of line 2 with the posterior joint space (PJS); d) line 4 is the shortest distance to the condyle from the intersection of line 2 with the eminence and represents the anterior joint space (AJS) (Fig. 11-3). In a concentric position, the AJS equals the PJS. A posteriorly displaced condyle has an AJS greater than the PJS. An anteriorly displaced condyle has a PJS greater than the AJS (Fig. 11-4).

Owens[28] has also defined a therapeutic range in which the posterior limit is the concentric or 12 o'clock position, and the anterior limit is the Gelb 4-7 position (Fig. 11-5).

Pre- and post-treatment condylar positions offer a prognostic value. Consider the following example (Fig. 11-6):

In the above situation, the prognosis following the completion of orthodontics may be unfavorable due to the distal positioning of the head of the condyle[29]. Conversely, a patient with an anterior positioning of the condyle with a slight mandibular retrusion, treated with a functional appliance to reposition the mandible forwards, may result in the riding of the condyles on the articular eminence and possible resorption[30]. Thus, condylar position must be considered throughout treatment planning so that iatrongenic problems may be avoided.

Anterior Disc Displacement with Reduction

Anterior disc displacement with reduction, commonly known as clicking, refers to the condyle (usually posteriorly displaced), reducing the anteriorly displaced disc on mandibular opening. An opening click occurs the instant the condyle slips past the posterior border and snaps into the thinner avascular portion of the disc. This may be classified as an early click if it occurs within the first 22 mm of opening, or late if it occurs towards the end of the opening cycle. A closing click occurs when the condyle slips upwards and backwards, the disc being displaced anteriorly near the end of the retrusive condylar movement. When clicking occurs during opening and closing cycles, it is referred to as reciprocal clicking.

In general, the earlier the opening click occurs, the more favorable the prognosis, as the disc is being only slightly displaced anteriorly. Late opening clicks are associated with greater severity of internal derangement due to a more anterior positioning of the disc. Treatment for an early opening click is easily accomplished by an acrylic flat occlusal full coverage splint, which opens the vertical dimension to reduce the click. A late opening click, however, will be reduced only if the mandible is repositioned anteriorly with an increase in posterior vertical dimension. This is frequently accomplished with a pull-forward mandibular repositioning splint and/or with functional appliances. The anterior repositioning splint is made by modifying the flat occlusal splint. Cold-curing acrylic is added to the functional surface and the mandible is repositioned to the "non-click" position, the bite being registered in the cold-curing acrylic. After it hardens, excess acrylic is trimmed off and grooves are left in the custom-made functional surface to guide the mandible into full closure.

Once the patient is symptom free, these cases often require "splint finishing" procedures to open the posterior vertical and reposition the mandible forward. Thus, Phase I splint therapy is used to treat the acute phase, after which Phase II splint finishing techniques involve orthopedic-orthodontic procedures to stabilize the dentition and TMJ's.

As we are dealing with mixed dentitions, the same objective of anterior repositioning would be achieved with concomitant bite opening using the Occlus-o-guide or Orthopedic Corrector (described later).

Case History #1

Reciprocal clicking, flat occlusal splint

Patient 1, a 9-year-old white girl, complained of ear pain, stuffiness, and loss of hearing for the past six years. She experienced frontal headaches and severe tinnitus in the right ear, accompanied by stuffiness and pain. Secondary complaints included dryness of her throat and difficulty in swallowing. Palpation of her TMJs revealed early reciprocal clicking of both jaws, pain on lateral palpation of the right joint, and a 1 mm deviation of the mandible to the left on opening. Her maximal opening was 46 mm.

Palpation of her musculature revealed tender masseters, temporalis, medial and lateral pterygoids, sternomastoids, and trapezzi muscles. Her right iliac crest and gastrocnemius were tender.

She had multiple allergies to dust, mold, and certain antibiotics. She had had tubes placed in her ears and multiple ear operations to her right ear.

A diagnosis of TMJ dysfunction and MPD were made. An acrylic full-coverage mandibular flat occlusal splint was placed, and the occlusion balanced kinesiologically (Figs. 11-7, E and F). The flat occlusal splint reduced the early clicking in both joints.

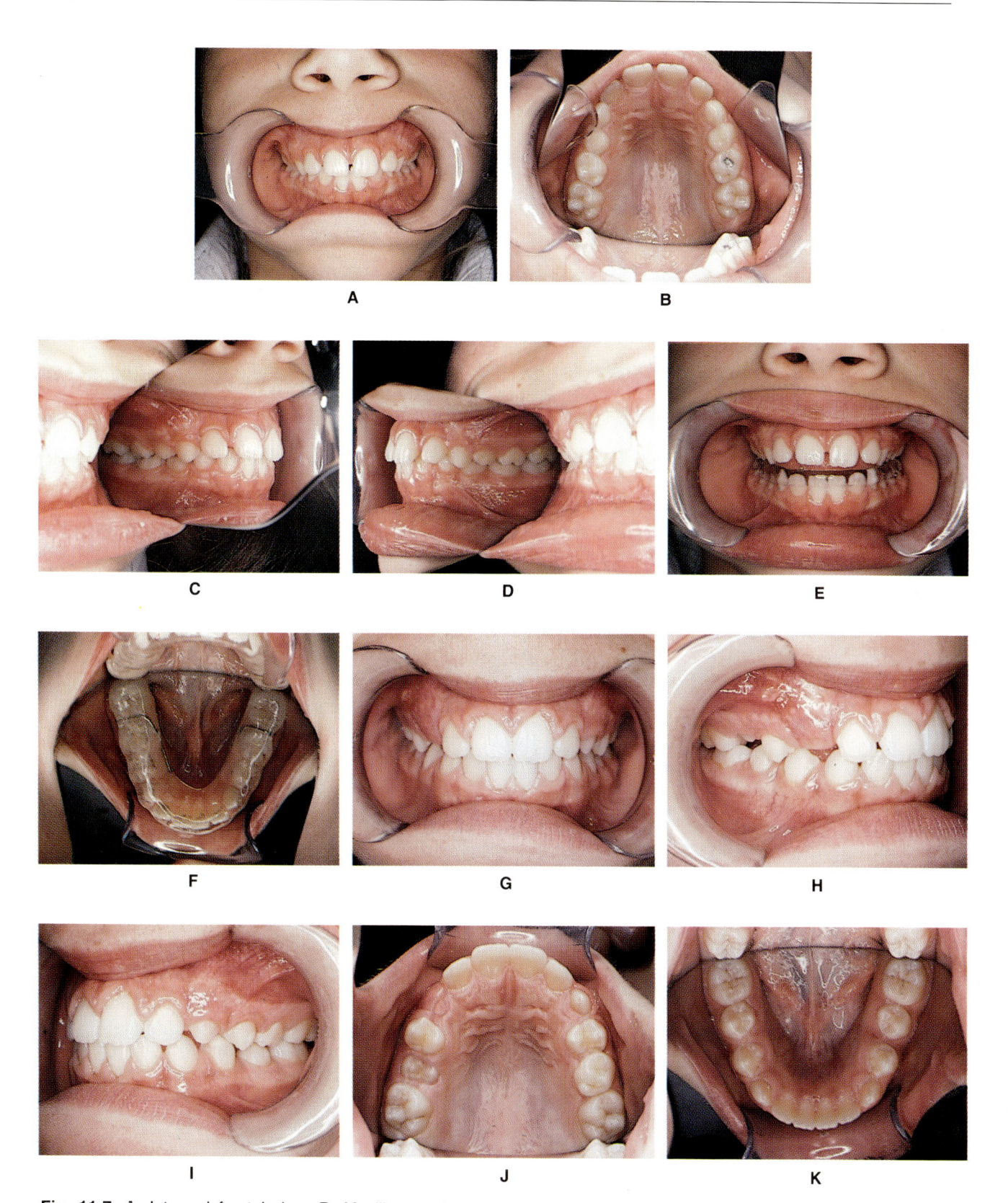

CHAPTER 11 Craniomandibular Dysfunction in the Growing Child   277

Fig. 11-7. A, Intraoral frontal view. **B,** Maxillary occlusal view. **C,** Left lateral view. **D,** Right lateral view. **E,** Mandibular flat occlusal splint. **F,** Mandibular flat occlusal splint. **G,** Splint finishing Occlus-o-guide appliance, frontal view of dentition. **H,** Right lateral views of dentition being guided into full occlusion. **I,** Left lateral views of dentition being guided into full occlusion. **J,** Occlusal view of maxillary and mandibular arches. **K,** Occlusal view of maxillary and mandibular arches.

One month later, the patient was symptom-free: no frontal headaches, tinnitus, or stuffiness in her right ear. She experienced no difficulty in swallowing, and her joints were free of clicking. After three months of symptom-free wear, splint finishing procedures were instituted, using an Occlus-o-guide (eruption guidance) appliance (Fig. 11-22). Now the case is one of simple guidance of the erupting teeth into the full permanent dentition (Figs. 11-7, G-K). The patient remains symptom-free to this date.

Comment: Children and adolescents respond very quickly and dramatically to appropriate treatment, often in 1-3 months. With adults the time span is considerably lengthened due to the chronicity of the case and other complicating factors.

The Occlus-o-guide appliance offers excellent posterior vertical development while maintaining the anterior-posterior correction in the anterior region, ensuring a favorable condylar position. (The Occlus-o-guide will be dealt with fully later in this chapter.)

Anterior Disc Displacement Without Reduction (Closed Lock)

Disc displacement with reduction is often a precursor to a complete anterior displacement that will not reduce. When a displaced disc forms a physical barrier to anterior translation of the condyle, the result is a closed lock. Incompetency of the bilaminar zone is the pathophysiologic mechanism, and this may be associated with damage to the elastic tissue and fibrosis. The pressure of the condyle upon the richly innervated posterior menisca attachment may well be a major cause of pain in this condition.[31] Mandibular opening is limited to 22 mm or less and is often deviated to the affected side.

Case History #2

Closed lock reduction

Patient 2, a 16-year-old white girl, presented on an emergency basis with excruciating pain over the left side of her face and inability to open her mouth. She had had third molar extractions done two weeks prior, and on first impression, the pain and trismus were attributed to the wisdom teeth extractions. But on examination, the sockets of the extracted teeth showed little inflammation. On further questioning, then, it was elicited that the patient's jaw had been locking on and off for over a year, and the left-sided jaw and face pain was exacerbated after the extractions, which may have contributed to her closed lock.

She described her symptoms as follows: "My jaw feels stuck on the left side. There is a constant pain in the jaw near the ear, and I have had locking of my jaw for over a year now." She experienced left temporal headaches; pain in the forehead, cheeks, and around the eyes, accompanied by a sensation of pressure in the left eye; tinnitus and excruciating pain in the left ear; excruciating pain also in the TMJs, and a closed lock of the left joint. Maximum opening was 22 mm, and lateral excursions were very painful. The patient's history of a fractured nose a few years before was also elicited.

Muscles tender to palpation were the medial and lateral pterygoids, left masseter, and left temporalis.

Of immediate concern was the closed lock, and the following closed lock reduction technique is presented.

1. As the mandibular opening was 22 mm, an alginate mandibular impression was taken, and an acrylic flat occlusal splint was fabricated on a vacupress machine.
2. The outline of the condyle, coronoid process, and sigmoid notch in the open mouth position was drawn on the skin over the left TMJ.
3. Asking the patient to open as far as possible, with the index finger of one hand palpating the condyle, a few drops of Xylocaine (without epinephrine) was infiltrated posterior to the condyle into the lower joint space, to anesthetize the innervation of the joint by the auriculotemporal nerve fibers (Fig. 11-8B).
4. As the lateral pterygoid is most often in spasm on the same side, it was injected by an extraoral approach. The overlying skin was swabbed with betadine, which was then cleaned off with an alcohol

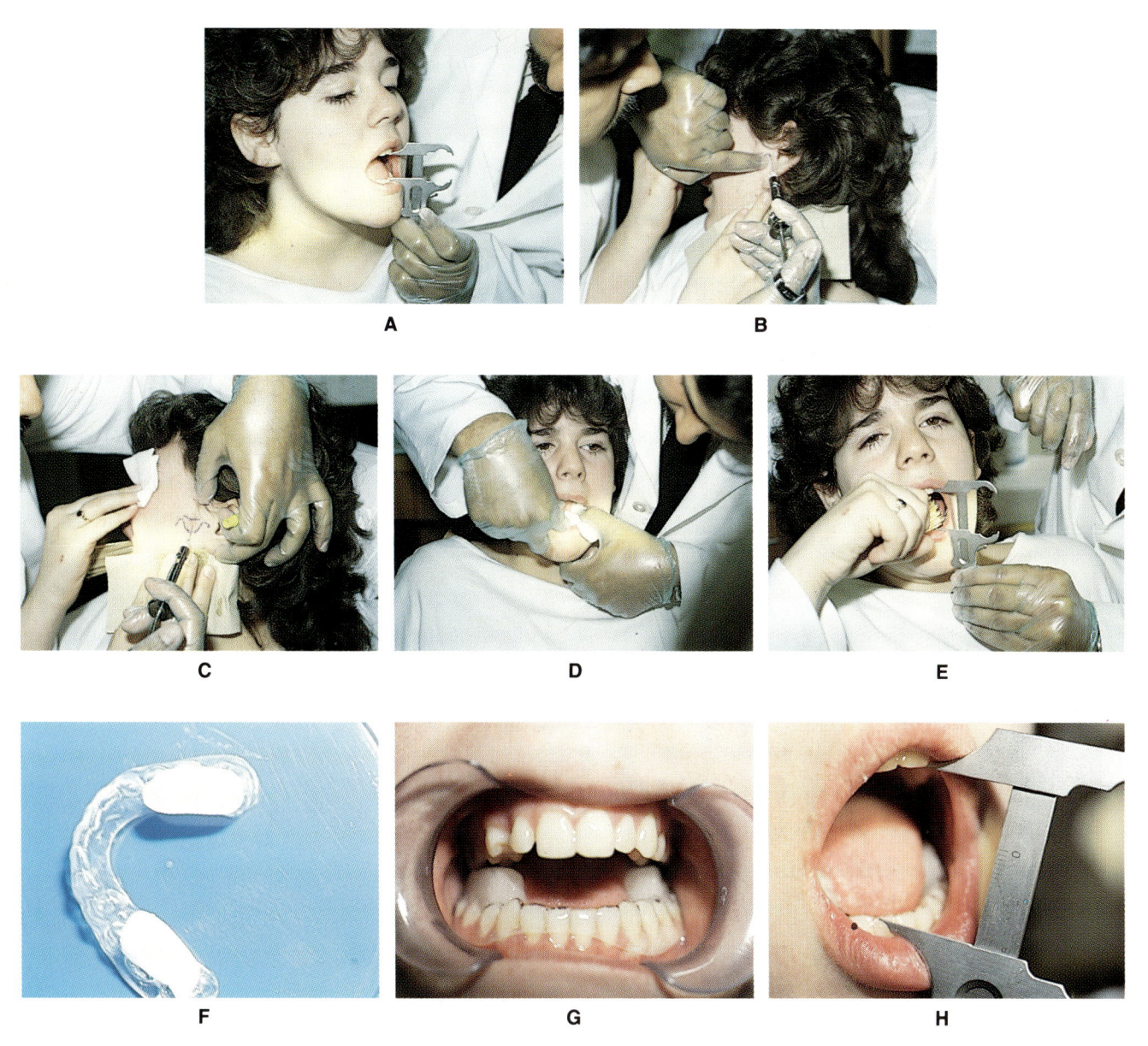

Fig. 11-8. Patient 2, closed lock reduction. **A**, Acute closed lock. 22 mm maximum opening. **B**, Lower joint space being infiltrated to anesthetize auriculotemporal nerve fibre innervation. **C**, Lateral pterygoid trigger point injection through an extraoral approach. **D**, Reduction of closed lock. **E**, Closed lock reduced, mouth propped open with throat sticks. Maximum opening 34 mm. **F**, Self-curing resin placed on flat occlusal splint. **G**, Interincisal opening temporarily increased to prevent left recurrence of locking. **H**, Maximum opening 38 mm.

wipe. Using a Fluori-Methane vapocoolant spray, the area was sprayed to make the insertion as painless as possible, and the lateral pterygoid trigger point injection was performed (Fig. 11-8C).

5. Standing behind the patient, the clinician held the mandible between the thumb and index fingers, and the patient was instructed to relax the jaw as much as possible. An inferior distracting force was applied, guiding the mandible forward to reduce the disc. The patient was instructed to protrude the jaw, and upon reduction to open as wide as possible, thus reducing the closed lock. Note that at this point care must be taken to ensure that the mandible be kept open until the splint is inserted. Failure to do so may cause the locking to recur (Fig. 11-8D).

6. Self-curing acrylic was added to the posterior quadrants of the flat occlusal splint, which was inserted into the mouth. The

patient was instructed to close into the acrylic slowly in a forward position (usually edge-to-edge), with an interincisal opening of 2-4 mm. The patient was then asked to open to ensure that the disc was still reduced. If the closed lock were to recur, the vertical opening would have to be increased, and/or the mandible repositioned to a more anterior position.

7. The patient was instructed to wear the splint at all times, only removing it for purposes of oral hygiene, at which time two fingers were to be placed in one side of the mouth while the other side was being brushed.

8. As children recover rapidly, in 2-3 weeks the vertical dimension may be lowered to the non-click position, provided the joint does not lock again.

9. Patients must continue to wear the splints until they are symptom-free, after which splint-finishing procedures are instituted.

MYOFASCIAL PAIN DYSFUNCTION (MPD)

Myofascial pain dysfunction should not be mistaken for myofacial pain, which refers to the face. Myofascial pain dysfunction arises from the muscles of the face, head, and neck.

Myofascial pain is referred from trigger points within the muscles in a specific pattern characteristic of each muscle. This pain pattern is rarely felt at the trigger point zone, but rather at a distant reference zone. The pain is often dull and aching, varying in intensity from mild discomfort and tightness to severe incapacitating pain. The referred pain can usually be elicited or increased in intensity by digital pressure on the trigger point[32].

A myofascial trigger point (TP), is a hyperirritable locus within a taut band of skeletal muscle or associated fascia. This area is exquisitely tender and refers a characteristic pain pattern to a distant zone. Normal muscles do not contain TPs. They have no taut bands of muscle fibers, are not tender to palpation and do not refer pain in response to palpation[32]. Muscles that are strained by trauma or stress are the most likely to develop TPs, and are shortened because of tense myofascial bands. Tenderness to palpation may arise from the sensitivity of the muscle's own TPs or it may be referred pain from the sternomastoid or trapezius TPs.

To exemplify the nature of pain referral, TPs of the upper trapezius are most commonly the source of tension neckache. The referred pain may extend along the side of the neck to the mastoid process, or the side of the head centering in the temples and back of the orbit (retro-orbital). Its zone of reference may also include the angle of the mandible, the occiput, postauricular region and the mandibular molars.

Retro- and supraorbital pain may be referred from the TPs in the sternomastoid, temporalis, spenius cervicis, masseter, trapezius, and occipital muscles.

Vertex pain in the top of the head is characteristically referred from TPs in the sternomastoid (sternal head), and splenius capitis.

Pain within the joint is often referred from TPs within the deep fibers of the masseter, medial, and lateral pterygoids, but can also come from TPs in the clavicular head of the sternomastoid. These pain patterns often mimic pain of the internal derangement within the joint; therefore, TP examination and treatment greatly facilitates splint therapy in treating TMJ syndromes.

Recommended is Travell and Simon's excellent text, *Myofascial Pain and Dysfunction: The Trigger Point Manual*[32] for an indepth study of the subject.

Case History #3

MPD, TMJ dysfunction, trigger point injection

Patient 3, a 15-year-old female, was referred to the department of pediatric dentistry, Tufts University School of Dental Medicine, for evaluation of considerable pain in the face while eating, and limited jaw opening.[33]

Since 10 years of age, the patient had experienced frontal and bilateral temporal headaches. These had gotten progressively worse, and on eating she now had consider-

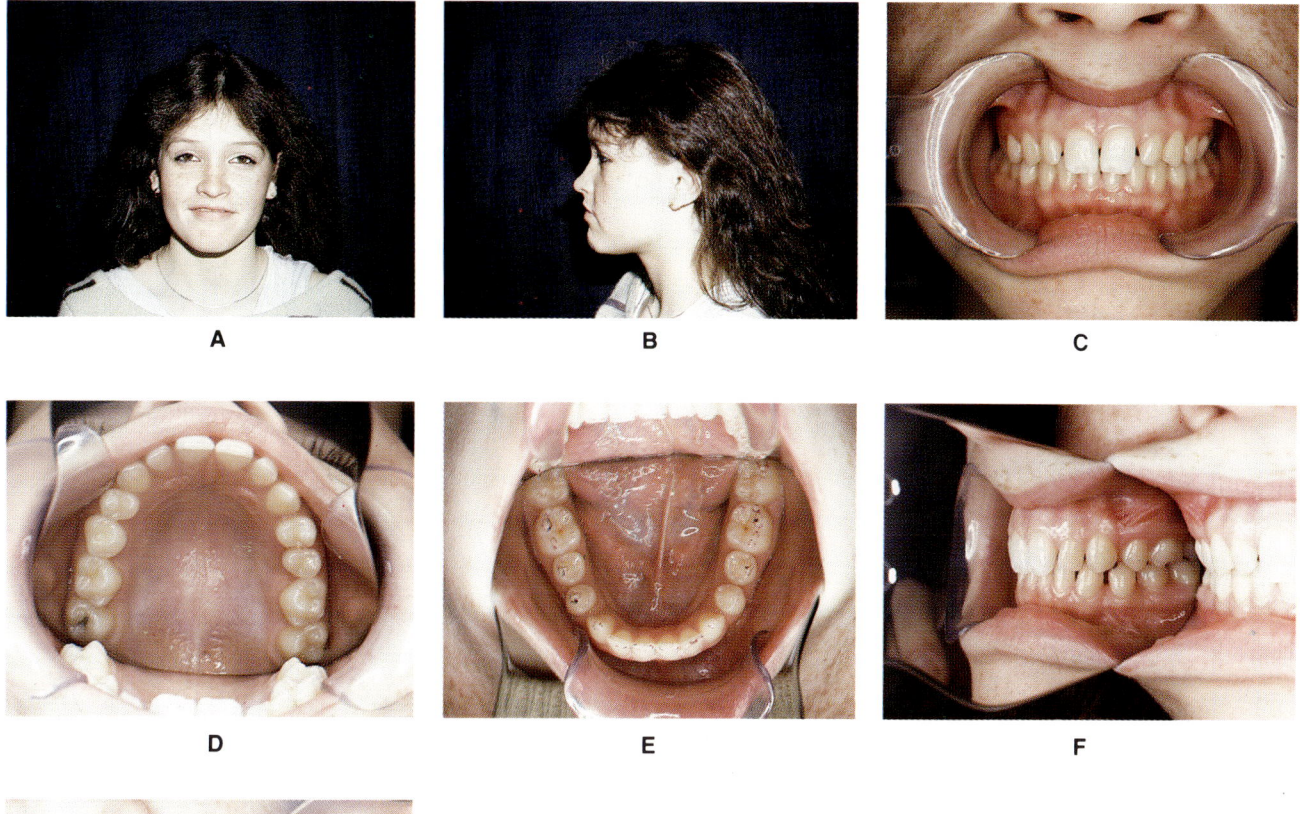

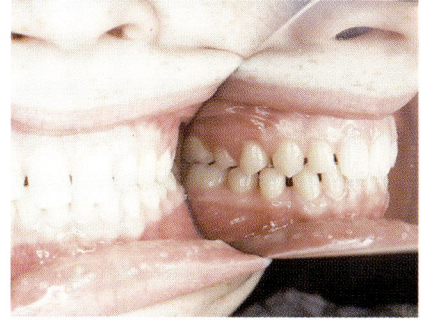

Fig. 11-9. A, Facial view of patient 3. **B,** Profile view of patient 3. **C,** Intraoral view of incisor region. **D,** Mirror view of maxillary arch. **E,** Mirror view of mandibular arch. **F,** Mirror view of right side. **G,** Mirror view of left side. (continued)

able pain in her cheeks, TM joints, and around the eyes. She felt the worst on awakening, with headaches, pain, stuffiness, and ringing in both ears. She felt pressure behind her eyes and occasionally had sharp twinges of piercing pain behind her right eye. Throughout the day, she experienced tightness in her neck with upper back pain, clicking of both TM joints and limited jaw opening.

Her medical history revealed no serious illness or known drug allergies. She took 3 to 4 aspirins a day for her headaches, and Dramamine at night to sleep.

The only history of trauma elicited was a fall at the age of 3 to 4 years, in which she sustained a severe blow to her chin. Positive history of clenching during the day and bruxism at night was obtained. The psychological evaluation showed a very depressed and anxious young individual.

Clinical examination revealed pain on lateral palpation over both TM joints, and posteriorly displaced condyles with early reciprocal clicking of both joints. She had pain on opening and closing, with maximal opening being limited to only 26 mm. She had good lateral excursions and protrusive excursions of her mandible and was not closed locked. Orthodontic evaluation revealed a Class I cuspid and molar relationship, with a 50% deep bite (Figs. 11-9, A-G).

A panoramic radiograph revealed no bony pathology. The transcranial radiograph (Fig. 11-9H), revealed a steep articular eminence,

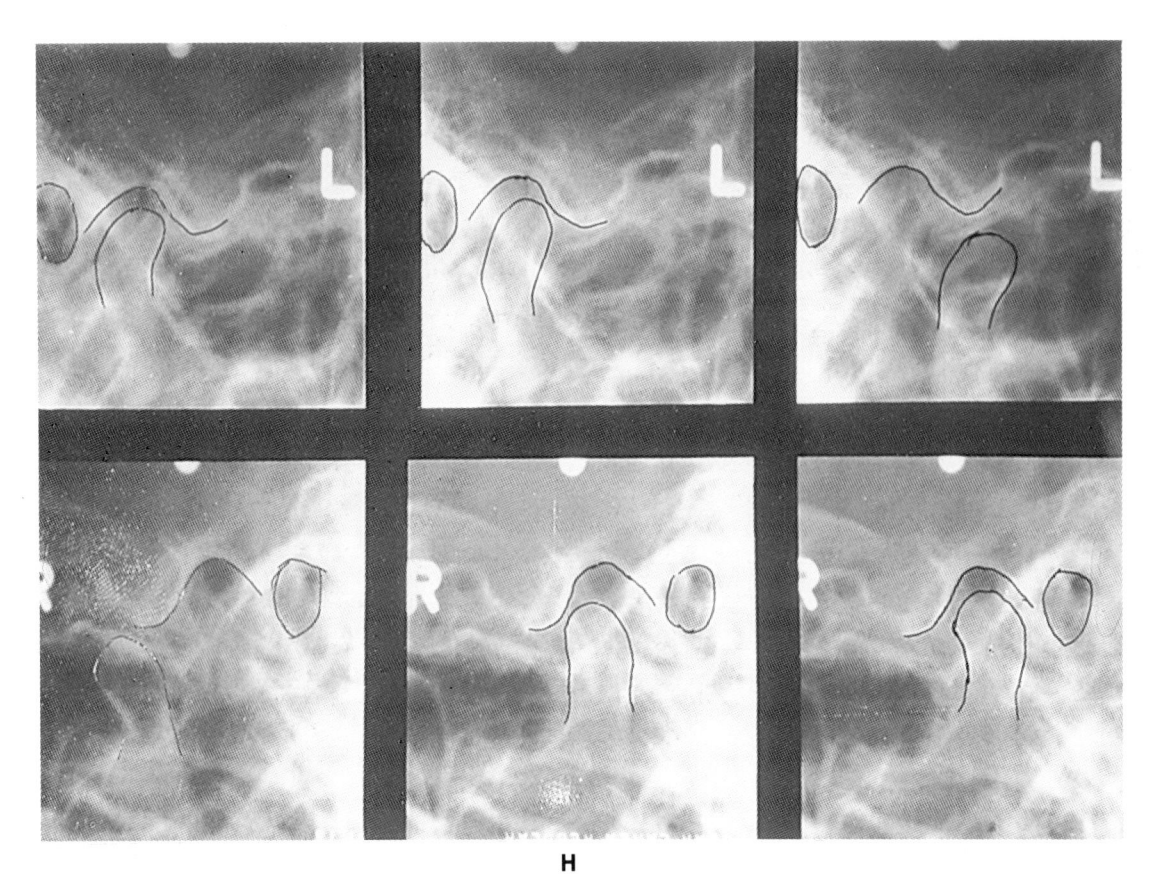

Fig. 11-9. H, Transcranial radiograph showing reduction of posterior joint space from rest position to centric occlusion. Left to right: left condyle position in centric occlusion, rest, and maximal opening; right condyle on maximum opening, rest, and centric occlusion. (continued)

and a reduction of the posterior joint space as the mandible moved from the rest position to the centric occlusion position. On anteriorly repositioning the mandible to the position in Fig. 11-9I, the early reciprocal clicking was reduced.

On palpation of the musculature, tenderness was elicited in the following muscles: R-L masseters, R-L temporalis, R-L medial and lateral pterygoids, R-L sternomastoids, and L-trapezius.

The diagnosis of TMJ and MPD syndrome was made. A maxillary soft mouthguard (nighttime wear) and a mandibular acrylic flat occlusal splint (daytime wear) to reposition the mandible anteriorly and increase the vertical dimension were inserted on 1-16-86 (Figs. 11-9, J and K). Notice that the position of the mandible resembles the non-click position determined during the initial evaluation (Fig. 11-9I). The following description shows the progress of the patient's treatment.

2-6-86   Less pain in the face. Headaches are 50% better, less pressure behind the eyes, ringing in the ears less frequent. Appliance equilibrated.

3-7-86   Pain in the joints and cheeks are 50% better. Headaches almost gone. Infrequent attacks of sharp retro-orbital pain (right). Pressure in the eyes almost gone. "When the splint is in, the joint doesn't crack any more." She is sleeping very well at night and has stopped Dramamine and aspirin tablets. Appliance checked and equilibrated.

4-29-86 No headaches at all, very infrequent joint pain. No ringing, stuffiness, or pain in the ears. Experiences a tired feeling in the masseters and attacks off and on of retro-orbital pain (right). Neck and upper back stiffness are still present, no improvement noted. Re-

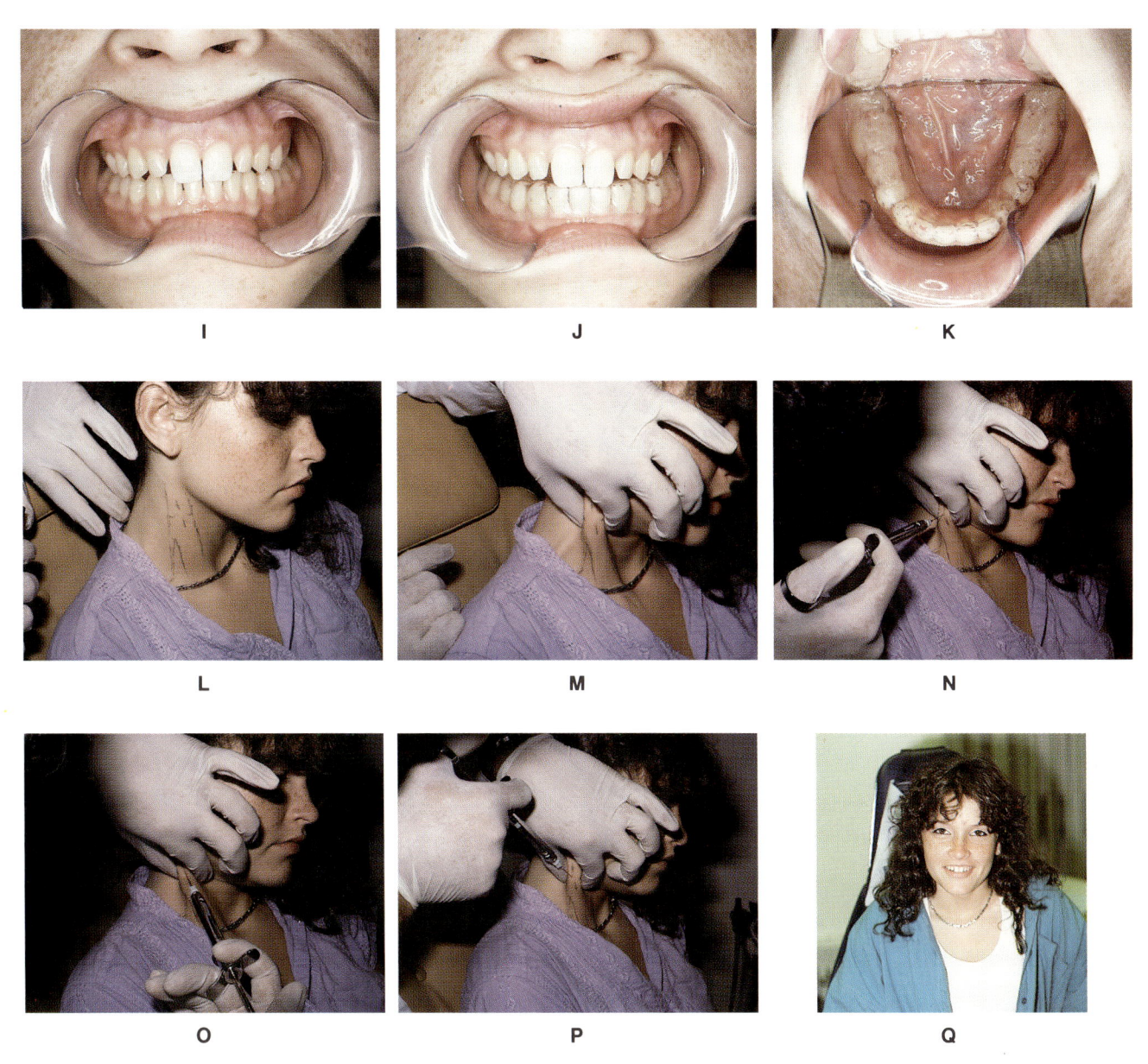

Fig. 11-9. (continued) **I**, Anterior repositioning of the mandible reduces reciprocal clicking if opening is initiated from this position. **J**, Mandibular flat occlusal splint, facial view. **K**, Mandibular flat occlusal splint, occlusal view. **L**, Right sternomastoid TP located between interrupted horizontal and vertical lines. **M**, Sternomastoid muscle lifted off underlying neurovascular vessels. **N**, TP injected—notice startle response when the exact TP is encountered. **O**, The muscle is fanned to intercept satellite TPs. **P**, The muscle is fanned to intercept satellite TPs. **Q**, Frontal view of patient 3 after therapy.

ciprocal clicking eliminated and tenderness to palpation only elicited in masseters, sternomastoids, and trapezius muscles. Appliance equilibrated.

6-23-86 Patient is asymptomatic, except that stiffness in the neck and upper back remains unchanged, and she experiences some attacks of retro-orbital pain (right). Palpation of the sternomastoid and the trapezius reveal presence of TPs. Digital palpation of the TP in Fig 11-9L of right sternomastoid referred pain to behind the right eye. Palpation of the left trapezius TP referred pain up along the side of the neck to the nuchal line. As this was the most tender TP in the trapezius, this along with the TP in the right sternomastoid were scheduled to be treated at the next appointment.

7-25-86 TP injections done into TPs of

right sternomastoid and left trapezius, using xylocaine without epinephrine (epinephrine is a muscle irritant), with a 24 needle. Within a few minutes, she was feeling better, describing a feeling of a great weight being lifted from her shoulders.

Technique

1) The TP in the right sternomastoid muscle is located by palpation as the most tender spot in the taut band of muscle that refers pain to a distant zone upon palpation. The overlying skin is marked to recall the precise position of the TP (Fig. 11-9L).

2) The area is then swabbed with betadine.

3) The betadine is then cleaned off with an alcohol wipe.

4) Using ethyl chloride or fluoromethane vapocoolant, the area is sprayed to make the needle insertion as painless as possible.

5) The course of the external jugular vein is outlined by blocking the vein with a finger just above the clavicle. The muscle is then supported by the thumb and forefinger and lifted off the underlying blood vessels. The TP is injected with a few drops of Xylocaine (without epinephrine); the needle is then withdrawn partially and redirected in a fan-shaped direction to intercept satellite TPs (Figs. 11-9M-P). Penetration of the needle into the TP at the precise point is confirmed by the experience of exquisite tenderness and referral of pain to distant sites.

6) The needle is then withdrawn and an alcohol wipe is held with pressure for 1 to 2 minutes till hemostasis is achieved.

7) A similar procedure is carried out for TP injection into the left trapezius muscle.

8) After the trigger point injection, the trapezius and sternomastoid are placed under a gentle stretch. Vapocoolant is applied in slow, even, uninterrupted sweeps in one direction only, "from the trigger point, to the zone of referred pain."

CERVICAL AND SPINAL DYSFUNCTION (CSD)

Even though the connection between craniocervical findings and TMJ dysfunction is not always clear, the clinician should be able to recognize the presence of significant craniocervical symptoms.[34]

In the screening examination, attention to a cervical spine dysfunction may be directed by an affirmative answer to the following questions (adapted from Clarke, G.T.):[34]

1. Have you ever had an injury to your neck (whiplash)?
2. Do you suffer from frequent or severe headaches or neck pain?
3. Does your neck every make clicking, grating, or popping noises on movement?
4. Does your head or neck ever get stuck momentarily in one position so you cannot move it?
5. Is your neck pain worse on awakening?
6. Do you have pain or numbness in your arms, fingers, or hands?

Forward head position

A forward head position is one which causes the head to be anterior to the center or gravity. If the weight of the head is 10 pounds, and it is 3-4 inches forward of the center of gravity, the cervical spine bears the equivalent of 30-40 pounds of excess load. To maintain direct vision, the head must rotate upwards and backwards, thus increasing cervical lordosis. By virtue of the increased cervical lordosis, the intervertebral foramina are compressed and the posterior articulations become more weight bearing. The erector spinae (cervical) muscles must go into a constant state of isometric shortened contraction to support the cantilevered head. Thus the foraminal closures and increased weight bearing of the facets cause local and radiating pain. Persistence of increased cervical lordotic posture can become an aggravating cause of degenerative spondylosis.[35] With the upper cervical segments bending backwards onto each other, space is at a minimum. Due to this compression, the greater and lesser occipital nerves may also become involved.[36] Children displaying poor postural habits, such as sitting hunched over a table, supporting the head by resting the chin in the palms, and displaying a forward head position merit immediate attention.

Airway obstructions

The forward head position may also be secondary to airway obstructions. These include frequent allergies, congested nasal mucosa, enlarged tonsils and adenoids, deviated nasal septum, and nasal polyps, to name a few. These may lead to reduced nasal breathing in favor of an oral breathing pattern in which the tongue is held in a lowered position, leading to a lowered mandibular posture, in turn predisposing to a Class II malocclusion and posterior condylar displacement. Mouth breathing may also cause increased activity of the anterior and lateral cervicals, which causes the middle and upper cervical vertebrae to be pulled forward and down as the thorax is more fixed. With the occiput placed anterior to the center of gravity, the strong posterior cervical muscles contract and exert a backward bending force on the occiput. To orient the visual gaze to the horizontal, the lower cervical and upper thoracic portions of the spine bend forward, producing a cervicothoracic kyphosis.[36]

Parents must be asked if the child suffers from allergies, repeated attacks of sore throats, inability to breathe through the nose, and snoring episodes at night.

The loss of the physiological curvature of the spine at an early age is a fundamental process, the interception of which all dental specialists must know about in order to prevent early degeneration of the cervical spine.[37]

Posterior condylar position

In the forward position, the occiput is rotated backwards and upwards, which causes a lowered mandibular position and retraction of the mandible. When the mandible closes with the occiput rotated backwards, the suprahyoid and infrahyoid muscles come under increased tension. As the position of the mandible and hyoid are changed, the tongue may assume a lowered position and abnormal swallowing patterns may result. The retroposition of the mandible causes posterior condyle displacement, and this sets up a vicious cycle of altered occlusal contact patterns and TMJ mechanics.[36]

Scoliosis

Scoliosis is one of the leading causes of postural problems in children, and may present as lateral deviation, or as bending, rotation, and anatomic changes of the spinal vertebrae. These children may eventually have chest deformities that compromise lung function by restricting lung capacity. This may lead to compensations in breathing patterns and to abnormal craniocervical posturing.[39]

As symptoms in early scoliosis are often diagnosed accidentally, it behoves the dental practitioner to screen for this deformity, especially if differences in shoulder height or iliac crest are noticed. Since symptoms are minimal or even absent in the early stages, the diagnosis of scoliosis is often not made until deforming changes have taken place. The three significant residual effects of scoliosis that justify early treatment are: a) cosmetics, b) pain, and c) cardiopulmonary symptoms.[37]

Cailliet[37] has described evaluation for scoliosis as follows. First, the child is examined in an upright posture with the upper body well exposed. Both feet are parallel and knees fully extended. The balance of the spine can be easily detected by a surveyor's plumb line with the string held at the base of the occiput and the plumb weight below the gluteal crease. The lateral deviation of the string from the midline can be accurately measured and recorded.

Frequently, scoliosis does not appear in the erect, standing child, but upon examination with the spine flexed forward, an incipient or functional scoliosis becomes apparent. Forward flexion of the thoracic spine accentuates or reveals a thoracic scoliosis often not recognized in the erect position. This fact demands that all children whose spine is examined must be viewed from behind, with the body bent forward. Any adverse findings must be communicated to the child's pediatrician and/or to therapists in manipulative medicine.

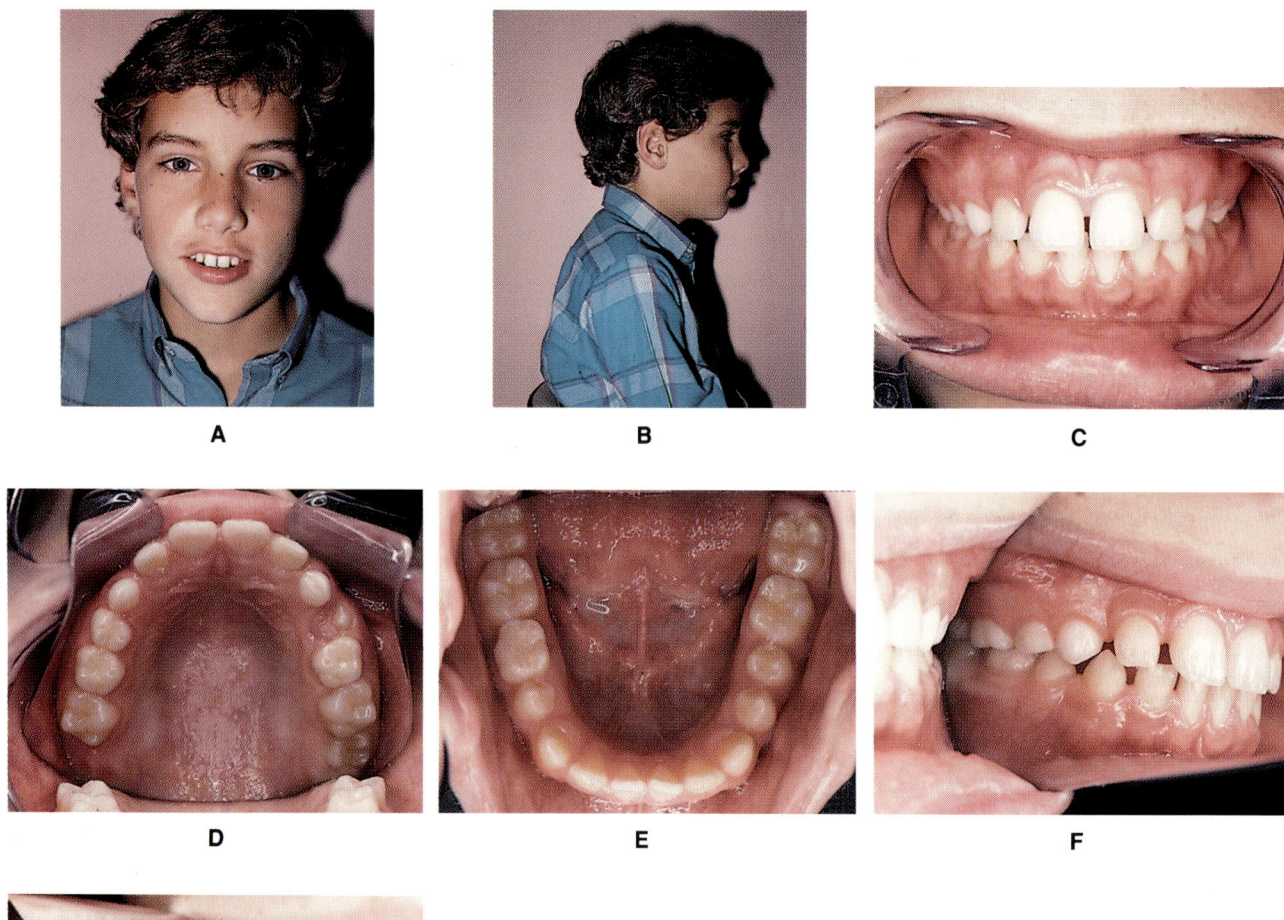

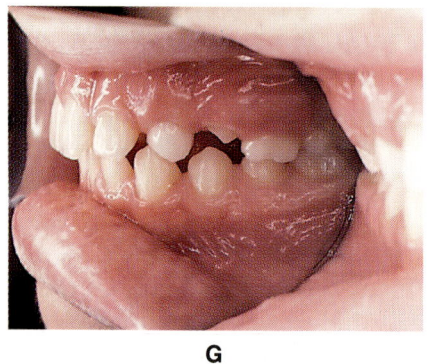

286 New Concepts in Craniomandibular and Chronic Pain Management

Fig. 11-10. A, Patient 4, frontal view. **B,** Patient 4, profile view. Note forward head position and rounded shoulders. **C-G,** Intraoral views of the dentition. (continued)

Case History #4
Cervico-spinal dysfunction, MPD, TMJ dysfunction

Patient 4, an 11-year-old white boy, complained of headaches over the past two months. He had first experienced them one year previously for a brief interval, after which they went away. The headaches occurred in the temporal and parietal regions, toward the afternoons and evenings. He experienced stuffiness and ringing in both ears and stiffness in the lumbar region.

On palpation of the TMJs via the external auditory meatus, the right condyle was found to be posteriorly displaced and early bilateral opening clicks in both joints were elicited. Only the medial and lateral pterygoids were bilaterally tender to palpation. A pattern of clenching during school hours and periods of active study, as well as bruxism at night, was elicited.

The patient had had a lower thoracic vertebra fracture four years before, and the right clavicle had been fractured at childbirth. The postural examination revealed an apparent asymmetry. The head was tilted to the right; the right shoulder was lower; an unequal pelvic base was evident, and the left foot was pronated. Thus, the patient was referred to a physical therapist for an evaluation, which was as follows:

Physical Therapy Report (Figs. 11-10, H-L) "The patient presents with postural asym-

H I J

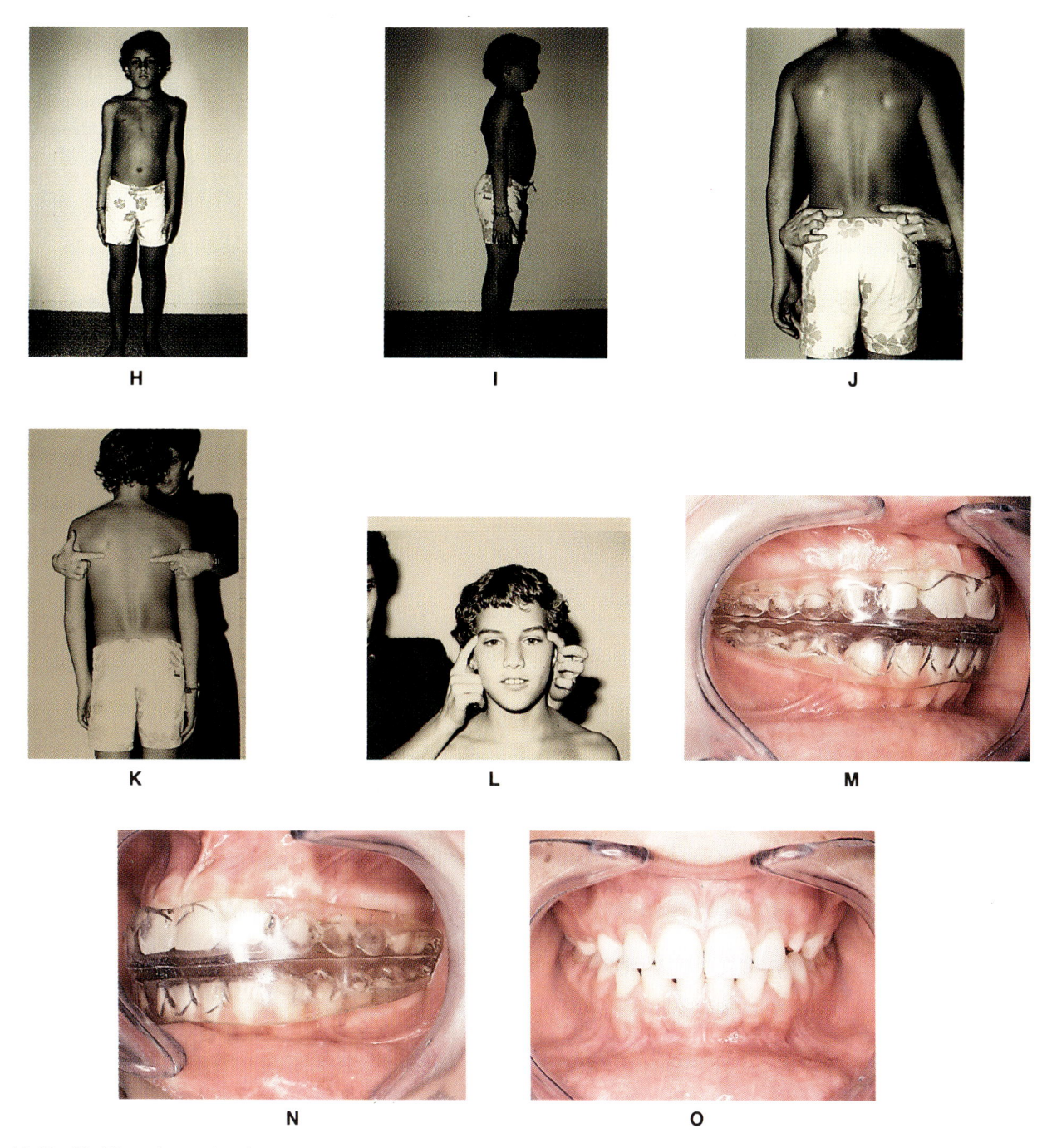

K L M

N O

Fig. 11-10. **H**, View from the feet upwards. Left foot pronation. Left hip external rotation (toe out). **I**, Right side of body shows hyperextension of knees, increased lumbar lordosis, winging of the shoulders, rounded shoulders, and increased thoracic kyphosis. **J**, Posterior aspect shows left PSIS lower. **K**, Posterior aspect shows right scapula lower. **L**, Right eye and earlobe lower, right lateral tilt of sphenoid. **M** and **N**, Patient 4 wearing the Occlus-o-guide appliance. **O**, Closure of diastemata with Occlus-o-guide wear.

metries and deviations which may be contributing to his headaches and may become a potential problem as he grows older. He has a history of two significant traumas. The first occurred during childbirth, resulting in a fixed clavicle. The second occurred four years ago, resulting in a lower thoracic vertebral fracture. These traumas and possibly other minor falls may have created the functional asymmetries that he presents with at the early age of 11 years.

Postural evaluation revealed left foot pronation, left hip external rotation, hyperextension of both knees, right lumbar lateral shift, increased thoracic kyphosis, rounded shoulders, increased forward head position, right lower scapula and shoulder, right cervical lateral tilt, left splenius muscle spasm, and a lower right eye. His spinal motion was pain free, and within normal limits except for cervical forward flexion producing a left upper thoracic pull. Both hamstrings were tight.

Myofascial restrictions in his pelvic transverse plane were moderate, whereas those in his thoracic transverse plane were moderate to severe. His sphenoid was found to be compressed and sidebent to the right. Craniosacral rhythms in the sacrum were limited and sluggish in flexion and in right torsion during extension.

The patient's young age made it easier for his soft tissue to respond to the therapy to help correct his postural asymmetries and deviations, and to bring his body into a well-balanced state for optimal, pain-free function."

The patient was given the Occlus-o-guide appliance (Figs. 11-10, M and N) to wear all night and at least 4 hours a day, in school during periods when he was not required to speak actively, and at home especially during study hours.

Within two weeks, he was free of symptoms. This was attributed to the appliance acting as a cushion during periods of clenching during the day and of grinding at night. The appliance also had his dentition in a super Class I position, thus facilitating an anterior repositioning of the mandible. An added benefit of the appliance was that it closed the diastemata anteriorly (Fig. 11-10 O) and guided the dentition into optimal interarch relationships. The patient also continued with the physical therapist's recommendations for correcting postural and spinal disharmony.

CLINICAL EVALUATION OF THE PEDIATRIC PATIENT

History taking

A brief screening examination and history pertinent to temporomandibular disorders is taken to determine the need for a more extensive evaluation. Careful efforts to ascertain the child's emotional status often reveal excessive anxiety and stress, particularly with respect to the school environment and relationships at home. Every effort to ascertain a positive history of clenching and bruxism should be made, as this parafunctional activity may cause excessive loading of the joint and trigger points in associated muscles of mastication. Any history of trauma to the head and neck is of paramount importance: incidents involving whiplash injuries, falling downstairs, a blow to the head with a baseball bat, and so on must be carefully elicited.

Palpation of the TMJ

Digital palpation of the TMJ may be carried out bilaterally over the joint to determine the character of joint activity. A posterior positioning of the condyle may be felt, by palpating via the external auditory meatus, as a backward push of the condyles against the pulp of the palpating fingers. At times, one condyle is felt posteriorly first on one side and then the other, suggesting that the mandible may be torqued or is closing asymmetrically.

Another excellent method of ascertaining clicking within the joint is to palpate the inferior border of the mandible at the gonial angle, as the ramus is an excellent conductor of joint sounds. Joint sounds may also be assessed by auscultating with an amplifying stethoscope or with a Doppler (3 Brothers) and recording the clicking sounds on graph paper via a Dopplergram.[40]

Palpation of the musculature

The smaller size of the child makes palpation difficult, as often the child may react positively regardless of the muscle being tender or normal. Palpation of the muscles of the hand may be done first, explaining the difference between normal palpatory tenderness and trigger points. The referral of pain to a distant zone in palpating trigger points must be explained. Each muscle is examined with a soft but firm thrust, across the direction of muscle fibers, the fingers compressing the adjacent tissue in a gentle back-and-forth motion. Pain and tenderness on palpation and the presence of trigger points are noted.[41]

The reader is referred to the Travell and

Simons text, *Myofascial Pain and Dysfunction: The Trigger Point Manual*,[32] for an in-depth study of the subject.

Mandibular movements — Let's play baseball!

Determination of the range of movement of the mandible is a simple and objective method of assessing function. Reduced range of movement may be a sign of disorder of the musculature and/or of the TMJ. The interincisal opening may be measured by a ruler or Boley gauge, assessing the maximal opening. Ingervall[42] found the mean maximal opening to be 46 mm in a 7-year-old child, and 51 mm in a 10-year-old. An incisal opening of less than 40 mm may indicate dysfunction.

Asymmetries of mandibular opening or midline deviation can be seen by marking a vertical line across the labial surfaces of the maxillary and mandibular incisors and observing mandibular opening and closing. If the disc is displaced on one side, say anteromedially, then movement is limited on that side and the mandible deviates to the affected side.

Lateral excursions and protrusive movements may be likened to playing baseball. The intercuspal position is home base, with the right lateral excursion being first base. The left lateral excursion is third base, with the protrusive motion being second base. Normal lateral movements range from 8-10 mm. Decreased movements on one side may often reflect disharmonies of the contralateral joint.

Occlusal considerations

An examination of the occlusion should include molar and canine relationships, along with any abnormalities of the overbite, overjet, anterior, and posterior crossbites. In the evaluation, posterior crossbites, deviation, and shifts of the midline are noted. Spacing or crowding is also taken into account, with factors such as interproximal decay, missing teeth, loss of arch length, rotations, incisal interferences, and axial inclination of the teeth carefully noted. Lateral and anterior shifts of more than 1 mm are also noted. Bruxofacets indicate improper tooth contacts, and parafunctional habits such as bruxism and clenching may be manifestations of anxiety, stress, and emotional tensions.

In most cases, the problem is not a loss of vertical dimension, but rather that the optimum vertical has never developed. Often a retruded mandible, deep bites and large overjets, or a Class II tendency prevents the vertical from developing. Repositioning the mandible to an optimal overjet and overbite causes a separation in the molar region, indicating the amount of vertical dimension that needs to be developed.

Parafunctional habits

Parafunctional habits place abnormal and excessive functional demands on the TMJ and associated muscles. Of these, bruxism and clenching abuse the masticatory muscles and cause excessive loading of the TMJ. Bruxism is one of the prime causes of trigger points in the lateral pterygoid muscles. These can also be precipitated by excessive gum chewing, by playing a wind instrument, or holding the mandible in a protruded position. In some instances, cradling a violin may also exacerbate these dysfunctions. Careful history-taking of both parents and children is essential in revealing all possible contributing etiologic factors.

Children often thrust their mandible forward and in side-to-side bruxing motions, imitating their peers. Children with clicking TMJs often exacerbate the condition by demonstrating the click at every opportunity to their friends. History of these parafunctional habits must be carefully elicited and strongly discouraged.

The presence of abnormal swallowing and tongue thrusting may contribute to an increased tension in the suprahyoid and infrahyoid muscles, thereby contributing to a forward head position. Squirting water into the mouth and parting the lips as the patient swallows frequently reveals abnormal swallowing and tongue thrusting patterns.

Airway evaluation

This is a simple chairside evaluation that is completed within a few minutes. The par-

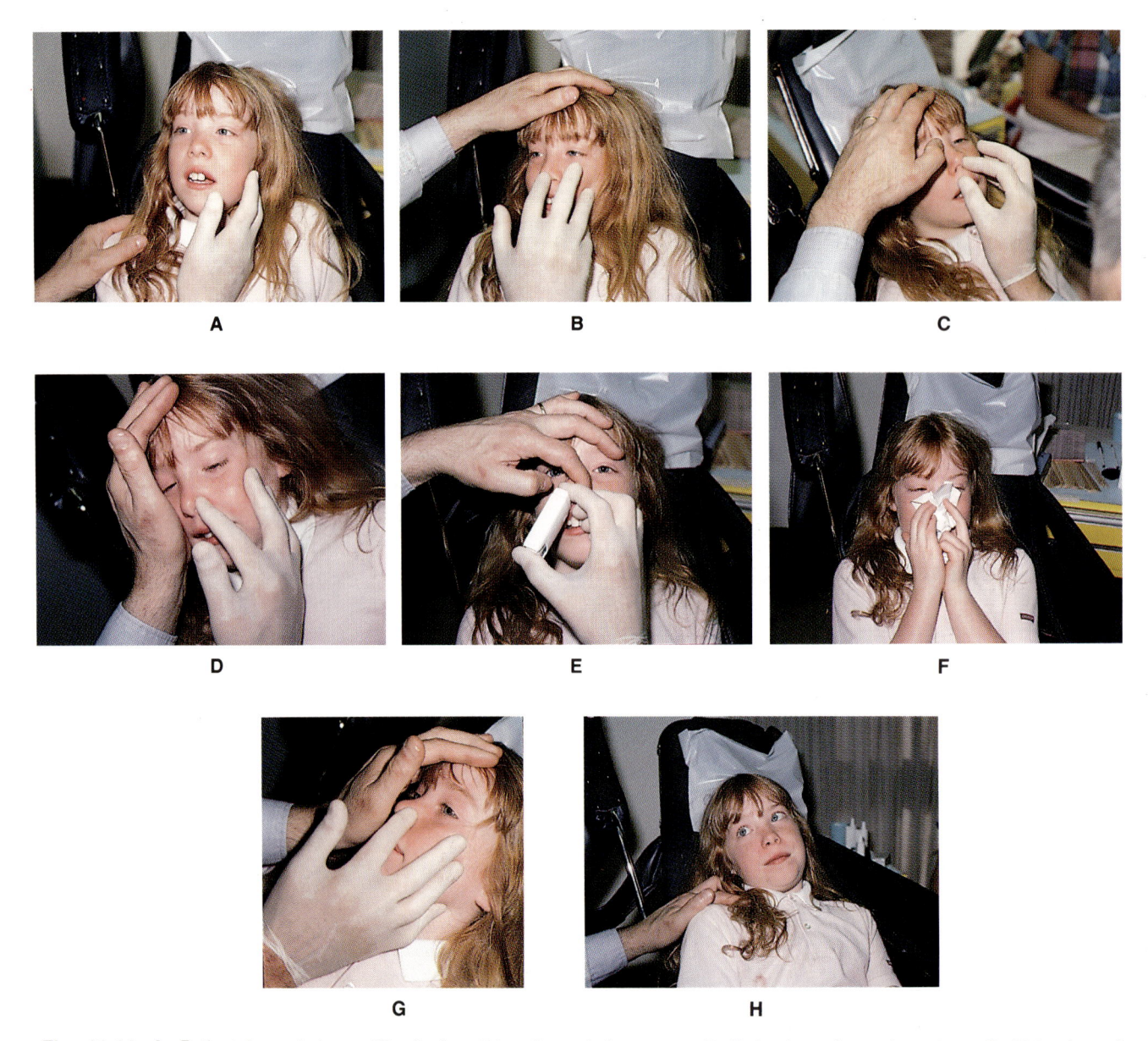

Fig. 11-11. A, Patient has obvious difficulty breathing through her nose. **B**, Palpation of nasal septum. **C**, Palpation of the external nares, to assess differences in size. **D**, Patency of right nostril being assessed. **E**, Neo-Synephrine spray being administered. **F**, Excess spray cleared by blowing into a tissue. **G**, Airflow through right nostril being assessed after the use of Neo-Synephrine. **H**, Patient breathing comfortably through her nose.

ents are asked during history-taking if the patient suffers from frequent colds or tonsillitis attacks, and if he/she snores at night. The sequelae of mouthbreathing and its relationship with lowered mandibular posture and forward head posture has been discussed earlier.

The clinician palpates the external nares bilaterally for discrepancies in size, and palpates the nasal septum, checking for deviations between the two sides (Figs. 11-11, A-C). A deviated nasal septum causes an obstruction to nasal airflow on the deviated side during the nasal cycle.[5]

To check the patency of the right and left nasopharynx, the following procedures are performed:

1. To test the right side of the nose, the patient is instructed to take a deep breath. With the lips together, the operator's index finger seals off the left nostril. The patient is then asked to exhale against the operator's left palm (Fig. 11-11D).

2. This is repeated on the left side and the difference in nasal airflow is ascertained.
3. Congested nasal mucosa is a common factor in decreased nasal airflow. To ascertain this, the operator sprays a small dose of *Neo-Synephrine* (Winthrop), a rapid acting nasal decongestant, into the compromised side, and the patient is asked to take a deep breath through that nostril and subsequently clear the excess by blowing into a tissue (Figs. 11-11, E and F).
4. After a few minutes, the airflow on the compromised side is checked as in step 1. If an improvement occurs, the etiology may very well be congested nasal mucosa.
5. The patient is referred to an allergist or ENT surgeon for a thorough evaluation. Long term use of *Neo-Synephrine* is contraindicated, as it causes a rebound congestion of the nose. Considerable success has been obtained in treating nasal allergies with a *Beconase* (Glaxo) nasal inhaler which delivers a metered dose of beclomethasone dipropionate.

Cervical examination

Movements of the craniocervical complex can be divided into 3 planes:

1. Flexion and Extension: Ask the child to nod his/her head forward in a "yes" movement. He/she should be able to touch the chin to the chest (flexion), and look up at the ceiling (extension). Whiplash injuries often cause a limitation in the range of this motion and disruption of a smooth movement.
2. Rotation: Ask the patient to turn his/her head from side to side. Normal range of movement allows the chin to approximate the shoulder on each side. Torticollis frequently limits this motion.
3. Lateral Bending: Have the patient try to touch his/her ear to the shoulder, making sure the shoulder is not raised to compensate for limited motion. The head in lateral bending tilts approximately 45 degrees towards each shoulder. However, it is more important to observe the quality of this motion. The movement should be accomplished in a smooth arc, rather than in a halting fashion. Discrepancies from one side to another are noted.

Craniocervical muscles are palpated in conjunction with the myofascial examination of the neck.

Bony process palpation

The lateral processes of the first cervical vertebra may be palpated behind the posterior aspect of the ramus and anteroinferior to the mastoid process. These should be symmetrically positioned. Palpation of one side significantly more than the other may suggest a displacement of C1 to that side. This is often very tender in a dysfunctional state.

The spinous processes of all seven cervical vertebrae may be palpated and evaluated for symmetry, paravertebral muscle tenderness and normal cervical lordosis.[36]

Postural examination

The postural examination is done with the child in a standing position. The evaluation should include an assessment of the symmetry of the iliac crests, shoulder evaluation, shoulder girdle position, waist creases, and arm-to-body spaces. Leg lengths should also be assessed if possible. The alignment of the head over the shoulders and the gluteal cleft is an important assessment for problems of forward head position, hyperextension of the neck and spinal curvature.

Forward bending should be observed in each child for the existence of thoracic and lumbar prominences that may indicate scoliosis.[38]

By the age of 10-11 years, the child's posture resembles that of an adult. Kendall and Kendall[43] describe the ideal body alignment in a child as follows:

FRONT VIEW
 Head erect, not turned or tilted to one side
 Level shoulders
 Hips level, with weight equally distributed
 Patella facing straight forward
 Feet pointing straight ahead, or slightly toed-out

BACK VIEW
- Head erect
- Shoulders level
- Straight cervical, thoracic, and lumbar spine
- Neutral positioning of scapulae with medial borders parallel
- Legs and heelcords straight

SIDE VIEW
- Head erect and back, chin above notch between clavicle, with a slight forward curve in the neck
- Shoulders in line with the ear
- Upper back erect
- Abdominal wall flat
- Slight lordosis in the lower back
- Pelvis in a neutral position
- Knees slightly flexed
- Feet pointed straight or slightly toed-out

The clinician need not be proficient in diagnosing and treating cervical and spinal disharmonies. However, if the clinician is alert that such a disharmony may exist, then an appropriate referral may be made to specialists in physical therapy and manipulative medicine, for evaluation and treatment.

The clinician then departs from just treating interarch relationships, and enters a team of health professionals delivering whole-body care to the growing child.

FIVE CLINICAL FINDINGS IN EXAMINING THE PEDIATRIC PATIENT

Deep bites

Deep bites are often associated with Class I deep bite or Class II Division 2 malocclusions. As the overbite increases, the lower teeth and mandible proprioceptively retreat posteriorly to avoid anterior interferences. This predisposes to posterior condylar displacements and anterior disc displacements (Fig. 11-12). When the overbite is corrected, the mandible is free to reposition itself anteriorly.

When the lower incisors are not seen due to excessive overbite, the face is sending a message that the clinician must not ignore: increase the vertical dimension—open up the bite.

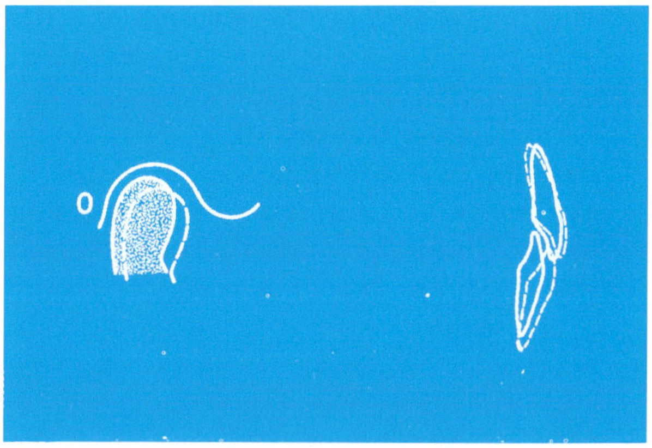

Fig. 11-12. Deep overbite. The solid line represents deep overbite and postcondylar displacement. The broken line represents optimal position.

Overbite correction may be effected by intruding the anteriors, erupting the posterior teeth, or both. In TMJ dysfunction, with posterior condylar displacement, eruption of the posterior vertical is preferred as it favors condylar repositioning to the therapeutic zone. This may be accomplished with the Occlus-o-guide or Orthopedic Corrector appliances, which anteriorly reposition the mandible and simultaneously enhance vertical development. In the permanent dentition, if brackets are already present, the Biofinisher appliance,[44] developed by Jack Lynn, may be used at night for rapid eruption of the posterior vertical dimension.

In a Class II Division 2 malocclusion, the lingoversion of maxillary anteriors may first be corrected with a sagittal appliance with occlusal coverage (to act as a TMJ splint), or a maxillary utility arch to labialize the retroclined anteriors. When the maxillary anteriors are aligned, a mandibular repositioning appliance such as an Occlus-o-guide or the Orthopedic Corrector may be used to correct the Class II retrusion and stimulate posterior vertical development. This allows the posteriorly displaced condyles to reposition to a more favorable anterior position.

Large overjets

Large overjets are frequently accompanied by flared maxillary anteriors presenting with the characteristic picture of a Class II Division 1 malocclusion. The retrusive mandibular position predisposes to posterior condylar

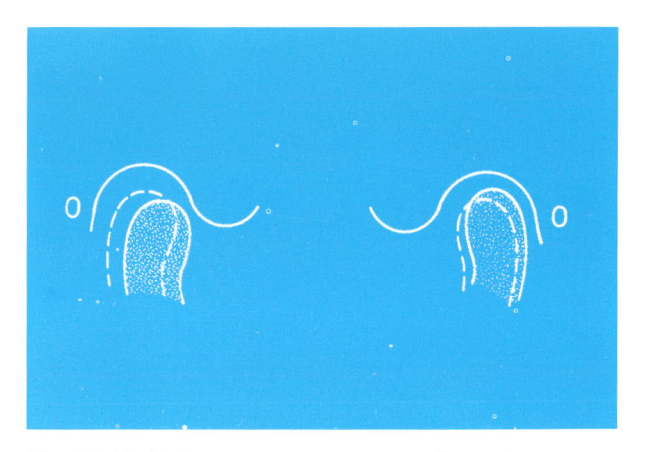

Fig. 11-13. Unilateral left crossbite. **A**, Contralateral side shows anterior displacement. **B**, Ipsilateral side shows distal displacement.

displacement. It is difficult to treat Class II Division 1 cases with only fixed orthodontics. Treatment goals are geared towards repositioning the mandible forward, correcting the Class II tendency, and positioning the condyles anteriorly into the therapeutic range. This may be accomplished by functional and/or fixed orthodontics. If the maxillary anteriors are procumbent, they can be lingualized with a maxillary utility arch first, followed by anterior repositioning of the mandible.

A note of caution. When using mandibular repositioning appliances, vertical growth tendencies must be taken into account, since most of these appliances open the bite by lengthening the face. Thus, for a patient with a Class II tendency, with a short and lower face height, deep bite, and retrusive chin, anterior repositioning will dramatically improve the profile. Conversely, a patient with a dolichocephalic tendency, or long face, Class II malocclusion with an open bite, would look worse on mandibular repositioning as the face would be lengthened even further. Thus patients with vertical excesses have to be carefully evaluated.

Crossbites
Posterior crossbites

The posterior crossbite is usually the result of a constricted maxillary arch. Upon closure, the mandible makes a lateral shift in order to accommodate the occlusal discrepancy, resulting in an unilateral crossbite. The condyle on the ipsilateral side is frequently posteriorly displaced, whereas the contralateral condyle is displaced anteromedially (Fig. 11-13).

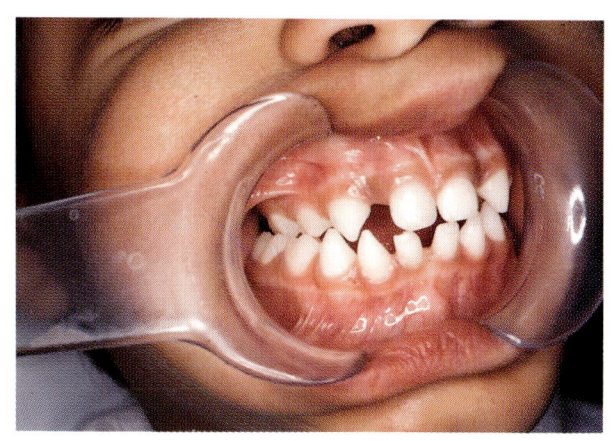

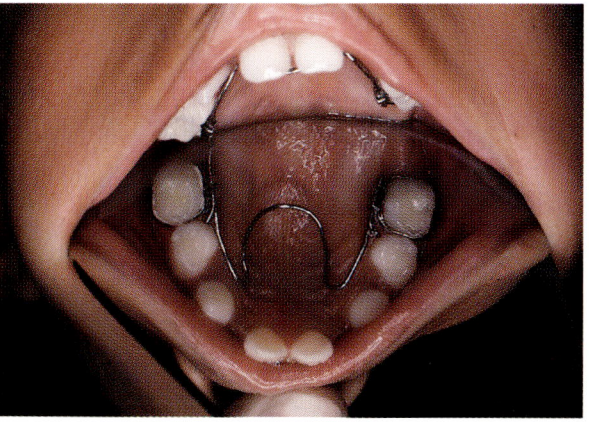

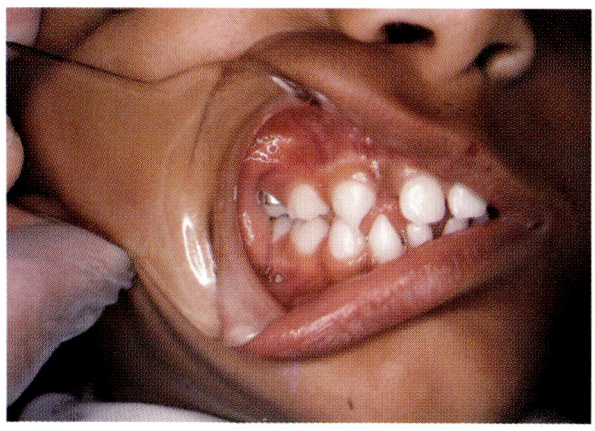

Fig. 11-14. Porter arch. **A**, Pre-treatment posterior crossbite. **B**, Cemented Porter arch. **C**, Posterior crossbite corrected.

Crossbites are best corrected as early as possible for two reasons: 1) the earlier the correction, the more stable the result, and 2) the growing TM joint assumes an adult

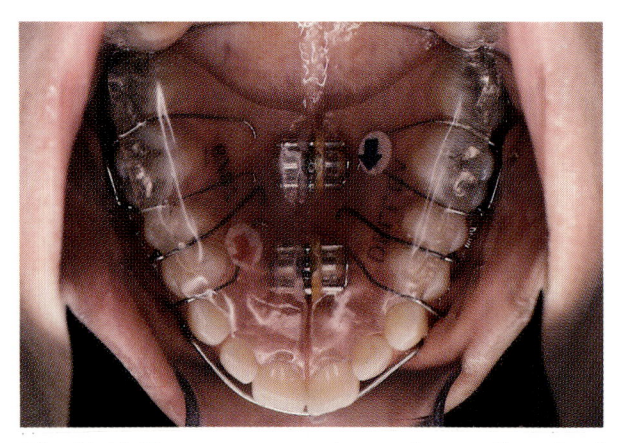

Fig. 11-15. Transverse expansion appliance with occlusal coverage.

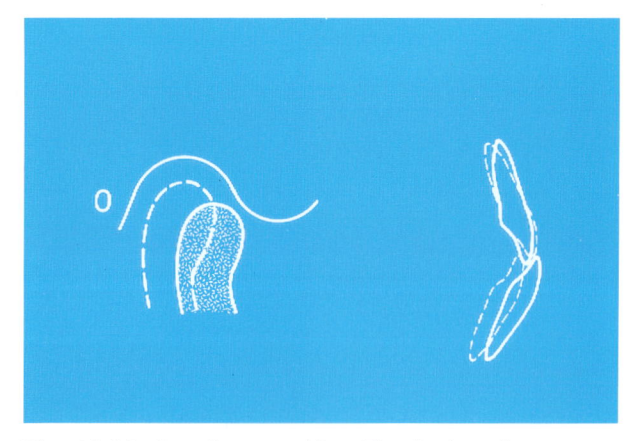

Fig. 11-16. Anterior crossbite. The broken line represents optimal position; the solid line represents anterior displacement.

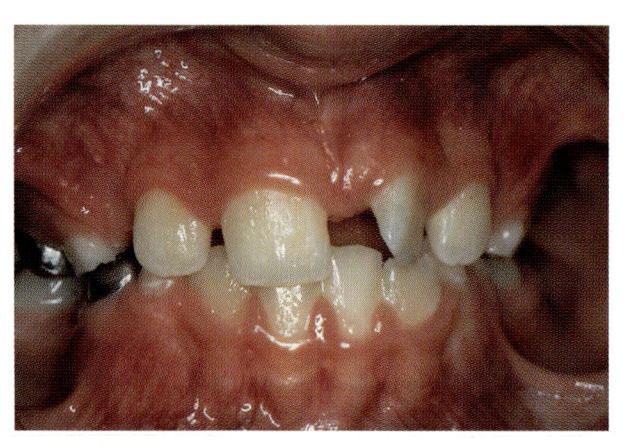

Fig. 11-17. Incisal interference

shape at approximately 8-9 years of age, thus allowing the joint to develop in a favorable environment.

Treatment of posterior crossbites in the primary dentition is accomplished with cemented Porter arches (Fig. 11-14) and Quad helix appliances. In mixed dentition, they may be corrected using a transverse expansion appliance (Fig. 11-15) with occlusal coverage (to act as a TMJ splint if needed), or with rapid palatal expansion if severe maxillary construction exists.

Anterior crossbites

Anterior crossbites or pseudo-Class III malocclusions occur when the mandibular anteriors overlap anteriorly with the maxillary anteriors. Early treatment is advisable because of potentially unfavorable growth patterns leading to possible Class III malocclusions. The condyle may be positioned downward and forward and may lead to anterior resorption of the condyle and/or articular eminence. This may be corrected by a removable appliance with finger springs or a maxillary sagittal appliance to procline the anteriors.

Incisal interferences

Incisal interferences can cause posterior condylar displacement by a proprioceptive shift distally of the mandible on closure. Consider the following example (Fig. 11-17):

The maxillary incisor is rotated so that the distal marginal ridge faces posteriorly. The mandible can come no further forward than the most palatally inclined maxillary anterior tooth.

This incisal interference is often very deceptive. A maxillary canine may be deflected palatally, contacting the labial aspect of a labially positioned mandibular cuspid. Proprioceptively, the mandible would be deflected posteriorly, predisposing to a posterior condylar displacement.

It is good practice to view study models from the posterior aspect to check for incisal interferences.

Such interferences may also exist naturally in the classic Class II Division 2 deep bite malocclusions. Here the maxillary anteriors are palatally inclined. Upon full closure, the lower anteriors contact the palatal aspect of the maxillary anteriors and are guided posteriorly into a retruded position. This can lock the mandible permanently into a pretreatment Class II retruded position.

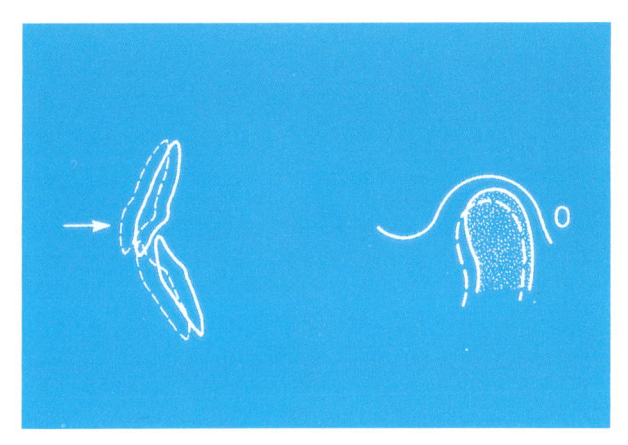

Fig. 11-18. Over-retraction of maxillary teeth.

Treatment may be easily accomplished with either the sagittal appliance or a utility arch. In doing so, if a splint is desired to alleviate joint symptoms, the sagittal with occlusal coverage is an excellent choice. The utility arch may be used to align the anteriors and advance them to the correct antero-posterior position in the dental arch. This treatment is indispensable when used in an interceptive manner to eliminate the predisposition to an incisal interference or a Class II Division 2.

Over-retraction of anterior teeth

When using headgear therapy or intermaxillary elastics, care must be taken not to over-retract maxillary anterior teeth. A distal force vector may cause a deflection posteriorly of the condylar head (Fig. 11-18). Properly torqued teeth, with an interincisal angle of 125—130 degrees, are ideal aesthetically, and provide for good anterior guidance. If the maxillary anteriors are too upright, the overbite gradually deepens and the mandible may be deflected posteriorly to avoid anterior interferences.

TREATMENT CONSIDERATIONS

Splint therapy, functional jaw orthopedics, or fixed orthodontics?

In the past, too much emphasis has been placed on correcting dental malocclusions by treating the teeth alone and allowing the TMJ to adapt to a new position. Correct condylar position and muscular harmony of the craniomandibular system is of primary concern.

To summarize, the goals of early treatment are:

1. Functional considerations
   -joint integrity
   -airways
   -myofascial and cervico-spinal harmony
2. Orthopedic (skeletal) considerations
3. Orthodontic (dental) considerations
4. Optimal esthetics

Treatment planning should fulfill all of these objectives. To ignore the airways or myofascial triggerpoints may result in a relapse of the dysfunction and dentofacial correction. Correct positioning of the condylar head in order to prevent arthritic changes or disorders in later years is also of prime importance. Orthopedic corrections are best achieved with the use of orthopedic appliance therapy to provide the best possible skeletal base for the dental units. Orthodontic correction is most commonly achieved with the use of multi-bracketed appliances. All three considerations must complement each other if an integrated treatment objective is to be achieved. Correction of a malocclusion cannot be contemplated without consideration of TMJ function.

Treatment may be broken down into 2 phases:

Phase I — Acute phase
Phase II — Splint finishing phase

PHASE I THERAPY usually consists of treating the acute symptomatology of the dysfunction. The internal derangement component may be managed by the use of splint therapy, either flat occlusal or anterior repositioning splints. Myofascial and cervico-spinal dysfunctions, if present, are referred to appropriate specialists who use manipulation, massage, ultrasound, electric galvanic stimulation, myofascial release, craniosacral techniques, and traditional physical therapy modalities. Trigger points respond well to injections of a few drops of 0.5% procaine anesthetic solution. Airway obstructions, if present, are referred to allergists and ENT specialists. Emotional tensions, stress, clenching, and bruxing respond well to biofeedback, relaxation modalities, and a soft maxillary mouthguard. Tongue thrusting, tense peri-

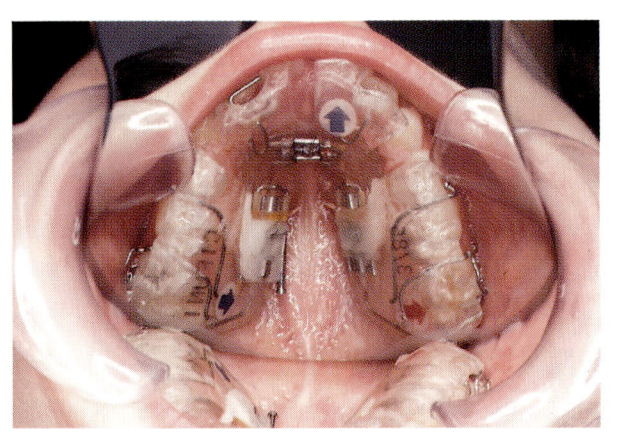

Fig. 11-19. 3-way Sagittal appliance. Sagittal screws filled with acrylic to stabilize appliance and convert it into a retainer.

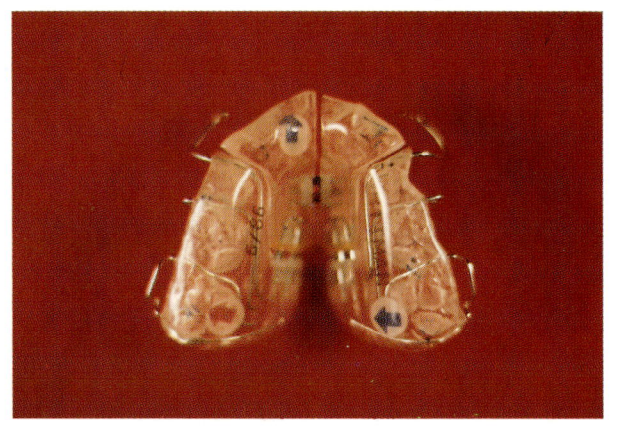

Fig. 11-20. Occlusal coverage acts as TMJ splint.

oral musculature, and abnormal swallowing patterns are referred to myofunctional therapists.

Phase I therapy ends when the patient is free of pain and presenting symptomatology, and remains pain free for 3-6 months.

PHASE II THERAPY consists of splint finishing techniques. Most patients need posterior vertical eruption and/or mandibular anterior repositioning, which is then instituted with functional jaw orthopedics (FJO), using appliances such as the Sagittal, Orthopedic Corrector, Biofinisher, and Occlus-o-guide. Splint finishing may also begin with fixed orthodontics (utility arch), and/or a combination of fixed and functional orthodontics.

A unique factor with respect to pediatric patients is that Phase I and Phase II (splint therapies and splint finishing) may often be combined into a single mode of treatment. Even as the acute phase is being treated, the dentition is being guided into a new relationship.

In addition to splint therapy, a simple system of four appliances will be presented to guide the developing dentition if early treatment is instituted. This system consists of the following:

Development of Anterior Guidance:
1. Sagittal appliance.
2. Utility arch.

Development of Posterior vertical:
3. Occlus-o-guide appliance.
4. Orthopedic Corrector

Sagittal appliance

The sagittal is an arch-lengthening appliance (Fig. 11-19), moving teeth in an anteroposterior direction along the crest of the alveolar ridges. It may be used to develop immature premaxillae, relieve anterior crowding, unlock retroclined maxillary anteriors (as in Class II Division 2) and distalize the molars. The acrylic over the occlusal surfaces acts as a splint, while the sagittal screws simultaneously affect dental and skeletal changes (Fig. 11-20). With the first (and second) permanent molars present, 80% of the expansion occurs anteriorly, which is desired in a Class II Division 2 malocclusion with posteriorly displaced condyles. By adjusting the acrylic lingual to the anterior teeth, different tooth movements may be accomplished as desired. For example, if the maxillary anteriors need to be torqued labially and no movement of the premaxilla is desired, acrylic is relieved on the tissue side of the palatal rugae, creating a differential pushing effect on the maxillary anterior teeth instead of the premaxilla.[46]

The appliance is worn 24 hours a day, especially while eating. The patient is instructed to turn the screws twice per week, on Wednesdays and Sundays, recording this in their progress report books. Once the anterior crowding or lingualization is corrected, the appliance is converted into a retainer or splint by filling in the screws with self-curing resin. The occlusal coverage (which acts as a splint) is adjusted at each visit to ensure balanced intercuspal contacts. The sagittal is worn till the acute TMJ symptomatology subsides and desired tooth movement is achieved, followed by the Orthopedic Corrector or Occlus-o-guide appliances to guide the developing dentition.

The utility arch

The utility arch utilizes straight wire fixed mechanics in the mixed dentition.[47] It is termed the utility arch because it performs a number of roles and functions due to the uniqueness of the basic design and the many modifications that will allow it to achieve the following treatment objectives:[48]

1. Proper overbite
2. Proper overjet
3. Proper molar relationship
4. Proper jaw relationship and
5. Proper lip seal

The utility archwire is formed by banding the molars, bracketing the incisors, and bending the straight wire arch form into the utility arch shape to bypass the posterior primary teeth of the maxillary or mandibular arches.[48] These arch wires not only level, align, and rotate the two permanent molars and four anterior teeth, but may also be used to retract or advance, intrude, or torque the four anteriors (creating optimal anterior guidance), open the bite, maintain or regain space, develop the dental arches, and assist in the correction of Class II to Class I.[48] After optimal anterior guidance is achieved, the dentition is easily guided in with straight wire mechanics, or preferably with an Occlus-o-guide appliance.

Case History #5

Utility arch in a developing Class II Division 2.

Patient 5, a 9-year-old white girl, presented to the clinic with a chief complaint of an ectopically erupting right mandibular incisor (Fig. 11-21D). Her medical history was contributory only for "tubes in ears," as a child.

On examination, a developing Class II Division 2 and a bilateral posterior crossbite was observed (Fig. 11-21F). The permanent right mandibular right lateral incisor was erupting ectopically, necessitating the premature loss of the right primary cuspid. She complained of occasional headaches and ringing in both ears. Digital palpation revealed bilateral posterior condylar displacement. No other TMJ symptomatology was elicited. Palpation of her musculature revealed tender medial and lateral pterygoids.

This case presents with the early developing picture of a TMJ dysfunction often associated with a Class II Division 2 malocclusion. Treatment objectives were to expand the upper arch, correcting the bilateral posterior crossbite; labialize the retroclined maxillary centrals; correct the ectopically erupting lateral; effect mandibular incisor rotations; and achieve good anterior guidance, allowing the mandible to reposition itself into a Class I relationship and optimal condylar position.

Treatment was initiated with a maxillary expansion appliance to correct the posterior crossbite (Figs. 11-21, G and H). The occlusal coverage on the appliance served to open the bite and allowed the condyles to move downward and forwards. (Treatment time, 5 months). At the same time, a mandibular 016 sentinol archwire was inserted after banding the molars and bracketing the lower incisors (Fig. 11-21 I). With the help of a chain elastic, the mandibular lateral was moved mesially, and the four anteriors were leveled, aligned, and had rotations corrected (2 months). Thereafter, a lower utility arch, 016 round steel, was inserted for 2 months followed by an 016x016 square utility arch (Figs. 11-21, J-M). (Notice that the "E" space is being maintained.)

Following the expansion of the maxillary arch, a similar sequence of maxillary utility arches accomplished leveling, aligning, and rotating of the maxillary anteriors (Figs. 11-21, J,R). Time elapsed from initiation of treatment to the end of this phase was 10 months. The utility arches were debanded and an Occlus-o-guide (size 4 1/2 G) was inserted, as the case became one of simple guidance (Figs. 11-21, S and T). The Occlus-o-guide acted as an excellent retainer for the corrections thus accomplished, allowing posterior eruption to open the bite and correct the increased overjet. With good wear and excellent cooperation the bite opened at the rate of about 1 mm per month.

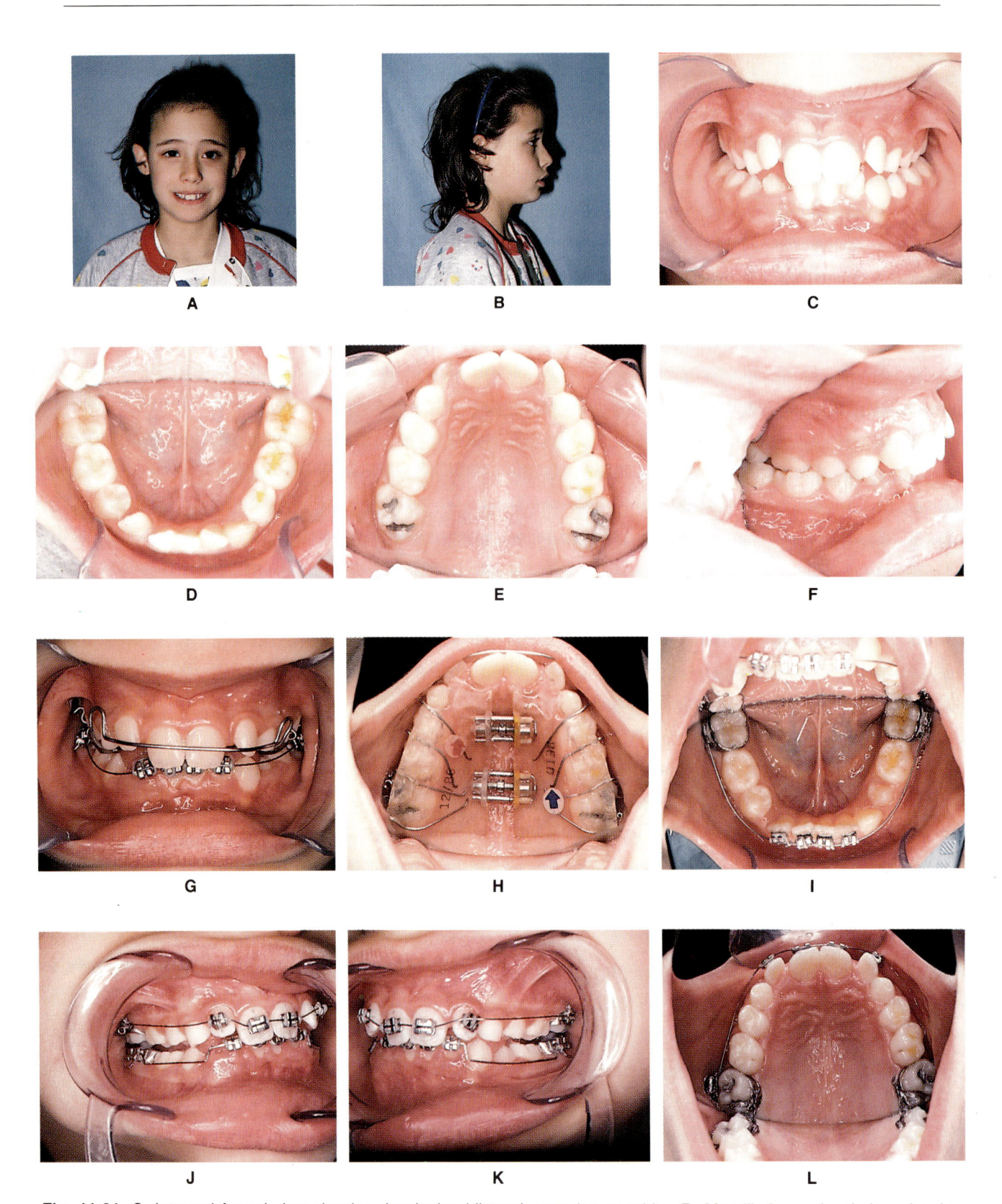

Fig. 11-21. C, Intraoral frontal view showing developing bilateral posterior crossbite. **D,** Mandibular occlusal view showing ectopically erupting right lateral incisor. **E,** Maxillary occlusal view showing incisor rotations and arch construction. **F,** Lateral view showing posterior crossbite and developing Class II Division 2. **G,** Maxillary expansion plate and 016 sentinol archwire inserted. **H,** Expansion screws activated to correct posterior crossbite. **I,** Right mandibular lateral being aligned, with 016 sentinol. **J,** Right lateral view show maxillary 016 sentinol and mandibular utility arch. **K,** Left lateral view show maxillary 016 sentinol and mandibular utility arch. **L,** Maxillary occlusal view showing anterior rotations being corrected. (continued)

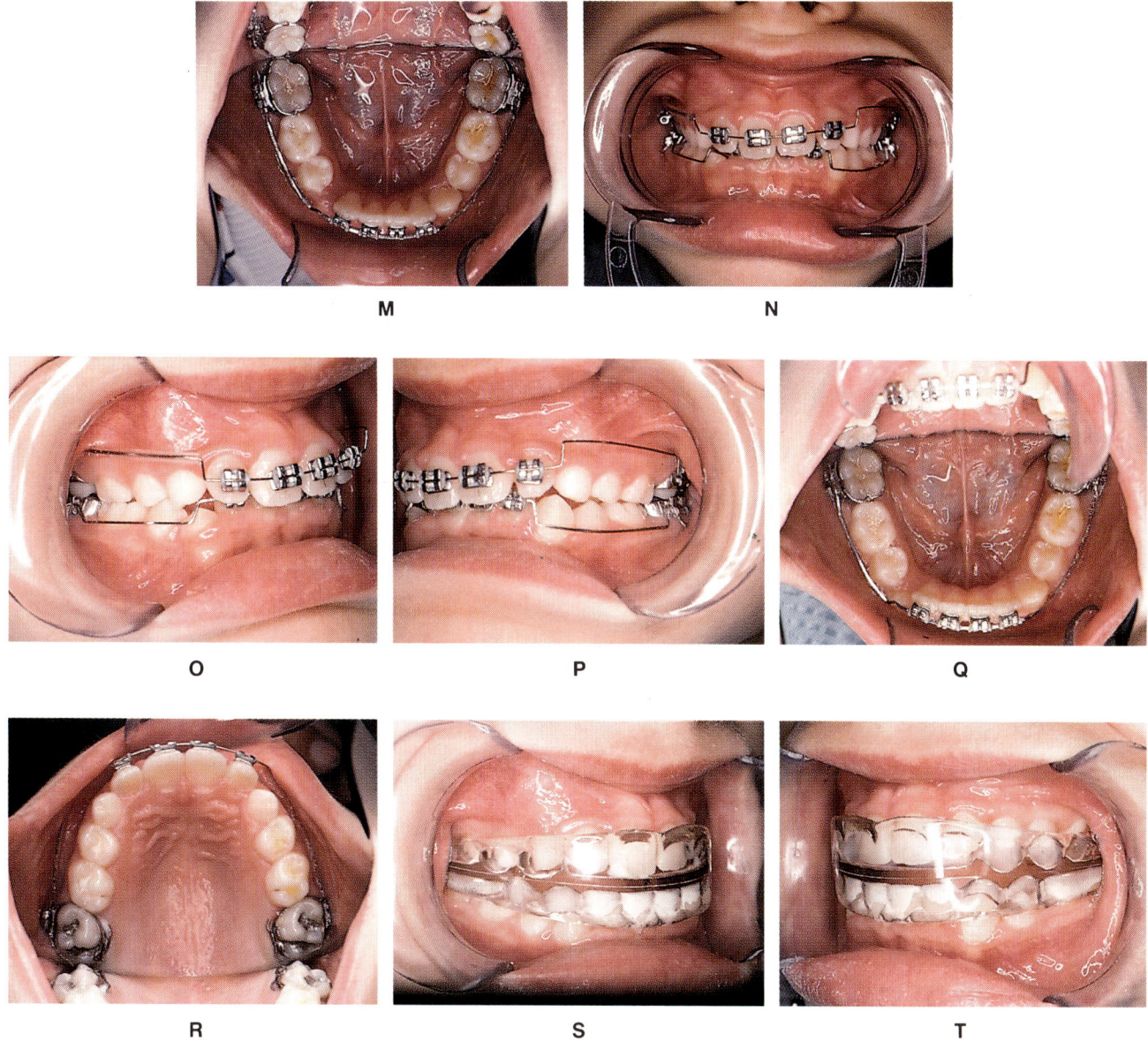

CHAPTER 11 Craniomandibular Dysfunction in the Growing Child

Fig. 11-21. **M**, Mandibular 016x016 utility arch inserted. **N**, Maxillary 016 utility arch inserted. **O**, Maxillary anteriors aligned. **P**, Maxillary anteriors aligned. **Q**, Mandibular cuspids erupting, note preservation of "E" space. **R**, Occlusal view of maxillary arch with anteriors aligned. **S**, Occlus-o-guide inserted after debanding utility arches. **T**, Occlus-o-guide inserted after debanding utility arches.

Comment:
The utility arch was the treatment of choice in this case, as it required correction of individual tooth rotations, retroclinations, and so on. The posterior crossbite correction could easily have been accomplished with the utility arches alone. However, the expansion plate was used, as its occlusal coverage served as a splint, opening the bite, and allowing the early symptoms of headaches and ringing to subside.

After leveling, aligning, and rotating the anteriors, the utility arches were debanded and an Occlus-o-guide inserted. An alternative approach could have been to continue with fixed mechanics, opening the bite and guiding in the permanent dentition. However, if cooperation is not an issue, the Occlus-o-guide is an excellent choice for finishing such a case. If worn all night and 4 hours per day, deep bite correction is achieved at approximately 1 mm/month.

Occlus-o-guide appliance

The Occlus-o-guide appliance or the Eruption Guidance appliance developed by Bergersen,[49] is a combination of a functional appliance and a positioner. This appliance corrects overbites and overjets like a functional appliance while simultaneously rotating anterior teeth, aligning the arches, and intercuspating teeth like a positioner. It is premanufactured in several graduated standard sizes. A single measurement of maxillary or mandibular incisors is made, and the measured size is selected out of stock and inserted into the mouth.[50]

The Occlus-o-guide resembles a standard positioner, but unlike the positioner, it makes contact vertically only in the anterior region, allowing the posterior teeth to develop excellent vertical as they are guided into position within the slots of the appliance. This vertical correction requires 3-4 hours of biting force in increments of 20 minutes at a time during the day, in addition to passive nighttime wear. Overjet correction is caused by the muscles adapting to the mandible held in a protrusive position within the appliance. Severe overjet corrections are most successfully treated during active periods of facial growth, while minor overjet problems (5 mm or less), may be treated at any time.[49] The perfect bite is built into the appliance and "orthodontic finishing," in most cases, is not required. This appliance performs well in correcting overbites and overjets, which are often the most significant causes of posterior condylar displacements. If crowding is not present to an extent of 3 mm or more, this may be the only appliance used to correct the dysfunction. In crowded cases, space must be created before this appliance can be used. Rotations of 2 mm or more or procumbent anteriors may first be corrected with a utility arch, followed by the Occlus-o-guide. In a Class II Division 2 malocclusion, either a sagittal or a utility arch can correct the retroclination of maxillary anteriors, following which the Occlus-o-guide may be used to finish the case.

In addition to splint finishing techniques with the Occlus-o-guide, we have found that myofascial dysfunction patients respond very favorably to this appliance. During daytime wear, the patient is asked NOT to clench into the appliance, but rather to wear it passively. At night, the appliance maintains the mandible in an end-to-end incisor position and doubles as a soft nightguard.

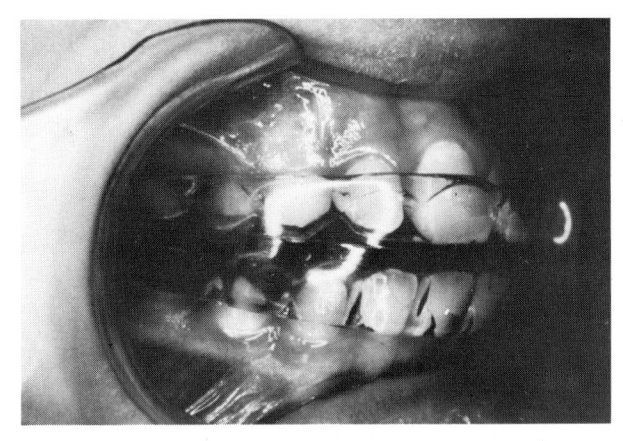

Fig. 11-22. Occlus-o-guide appliance.

Case History #6

Overbite, overjet correction in the primary dentition

Patient 6, a 5-year-old white girl, presented with primary dentition displaying a deep bite and Class II tendency (Figs. 11-23, A-C). Her medical history was non-contributory. On examination, her overbite was 3.15 mm and overjet 3.5 mm. The primary cuspids displayed a Class II relationship, and the flush terminal relationship was distal step. The first permanent molars were erupting into the oral cavity. No TMJ symptomatology was elicited at this age.

As this case displayed all signs of developing into a full Class II Division 2 malocclusion and a possible TMJ problem in later years, treatment with an Occlus-o-guide appliance was instituted to correct the Class II tendency, achieve optimal anterior guidance, and promote development of the TMJs in the best possible environment.

She was instructed to wear the appliance only at night, passively, while sleeping (no day wear). The following is the progress of correction of the overbite and overjet over a 16-month period.

The patient, now 6 1/2 years of age, has a Class I relationship and good anterior guid-

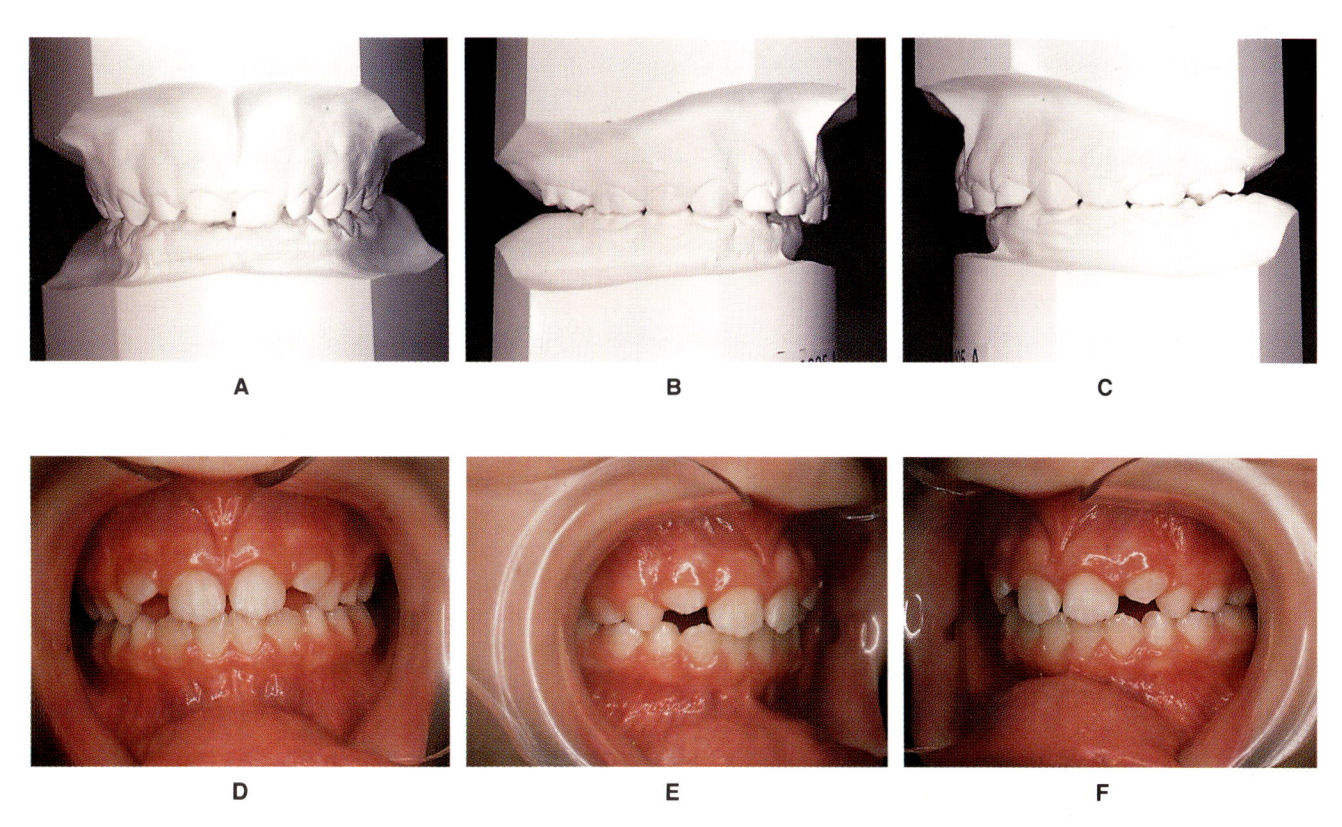

Fig. 11-23. **A-C**, Pre-treatment models (patient 6) showing an impinging deep bite, large overjet, and developing Class II in the primary dentition at 5 years of age. **D-F.** Post-treatment intraorals, 16 months later show development of good anterior guidance, correction of deepbite, Class I relationship, with only nighttime wear of the Occluso-guide appliance.

		Overbite (mm)	Overjet (mm)
19 July 86		3.2	3.5
11 Aug 86		1.7	2.9
4 Oct 86	Mand. centrals erupting	1.7	2.3
22 Nov 86	Mand. centrals erupt fully Mand. laterals erupting	1.7	2.2
13 Dec 86		2.1	2.7
31 Jan 87	Max. central erupting	—	—
28 Mar 87	Max. central erupted fully	0.9	1.7
18 Apr 87		1.3	2.2
16 May 87	Mand. laterals fully erupted	1.6	2.5
20 Jun 87		1.6	2.0
11 Jul 87		1.8	2.4
8 Aug 87		1.7	2.0
26 Sept 87		1.3	2.0
14 Nov 87	Max. laterals erupting	1.6	2.2

ance (Figs. 11-23, D-F). The case now becomes one of guidance only. This same case, if allowed to develop into a full Class II Division 2, would have taken approximately 2-2 1/2 years at age 12 to correct, with the possibility of developing TMJ symptomatology.

Comment: The previous examples have illustrated the use of the Occlus-o-guide in the treatment of mixed dentitions as a finishing appliance. This case illustrates its use in the primary dentition in treating deep bites and/or large overjets. This is accomplished easily with only nighttime wear, as changes are very rapid. The usual treatment time is between 6-9 months for the correction of impinging deep bites and large overjets. Care must be taken not to open the vertical to an edge-to-edge position, as that may lead to a Class III malocclusion. Critical in succeeding with a child aged 3-5 years is correct motivation and constant reinforcement of both the child and the parents.

Orthopedic Corrector 1 (to open the bite)

The Orthopedic Corrector is a functional appliance, a modification of the Bionator, its main function being to reposition the mandible downward and forwards, correcting a Class II malocclusion to a Class I. This increases vertical dimension, thus developing the entire face. It is not a "tooth" appliance, but an arch-developing appliance.[52] Its big advantage is that it moves the mandible as a whole and unlocks posteriorly displaced condyles, allowing a more favorable (anterior) condylar repositioning.

The appliance has an upper portion that fits against the palate and the lingual surfaces of the upper teeth, while the lower portion has grooves into which the lower lingual surfaces fit and rest. The labial shelf of acrylic receives the incisal edges of the mandibular anterior teeth, and the tongue occupies the area beneath its palatal portion and lateral flanges. The Orthopedic Corrector has three expansion screws. The midline screw, in conjunction with the palatally located coffin spring, may be used for lateral expansion and unravellng crowded mandibular anteriors. Two additional screws are located lingually to the premolar areas, and slow the mandibular anterior portion to be advanced independently from the rest of the appliance. This is particularly valuable in large overjet cases of 10-13 mm.[53]

As the construction bite is taken, with the mandible advanced anteriorly to an edge-to-edge position, or to the non-click position, a posterior open bite develops. The lingual flanges of the appliance are grooved to allow the eruption of the posterior quadrants, thus allowing click correction and splint finishing to be achieved with the same appliance. For an in-depth study, the reader is recommended Witzig and Spahl's text, *The Clinical Management of Basic Maxillofacial Orthopedic Appliances*.[51]

Case History #7

Class II, splint finishing, Orthopedic Corrector I

Patient 7, a 17-year-old Chinese girl, presented to the clinic to have a crown made for the mandibular left first permanent molar. Her medical history was non-contributory. On examination, she elicited a left early opening click and right mid-opening click. Palpation of the condyles revealed posteriorly displaced condyles. She exhibited a Class II cuspid and molar relationship with slight lower incisor crowding (Figs. 11-24, A-E). Her overbite was 40% and overjet 4 mm. She did not present with any obvious TMJ symptomatology.

To ascertain if the clicks were easily reduced, the mandible was repositioned to an edge-to-edge position, and she was asked to open as far as possible. Opening clicks were felt bilaterally. She was now asked to close forward to the edge-to-edge incisor position. Opening and closing a few times from this position did not elicit any clicks, indicating that the disc was easily reducible.

To simultaneously treat the Class II malocclusion, the opening clicks, and encourage posterior vertical development to finish the case, the Orthopedic Corrector was selected as the appliance of choice (Figs. 11-24, F-I).

An Orthopedic Corrector I (to open the bite) was inserted, and instructions were given to wear it all day and all night (or at least 18 hours/day), except for purposes of oral hygiene. The midline expansion screw and coffin spring were activated twice to unravel slight lower anterior crowding. By the second month, the opening clicks were reduced. In six months, the bite had opened up to an edge-to-edge position, and the cuspid and molar relationships were Class I (Figs. 11-24, J-L).

The appliance was discontinued, and the case was allowed to "settle." Final finishing with fixed orthodontics was recommended, which was declined as she liked the result. Both joints are free of clicking and a solid Class I relationship has been established.

Comment: This example is one of splint finishing with an Orthopedic Corrector I. This appliance was chosen over the Occlus-o-guide appliance due to the age of the patient. It would be very unlikely to obtain a Class II correction to Class I, with only 4 hours/day and nighttime wear, at the age of 16. This could only have been achieved with 18-20 hours/day wear. Remarkable bite opening was achieved in only 6 months, to an edge-to-edge position. This was attributed to excellent wear by the patient. The case was overtreated and

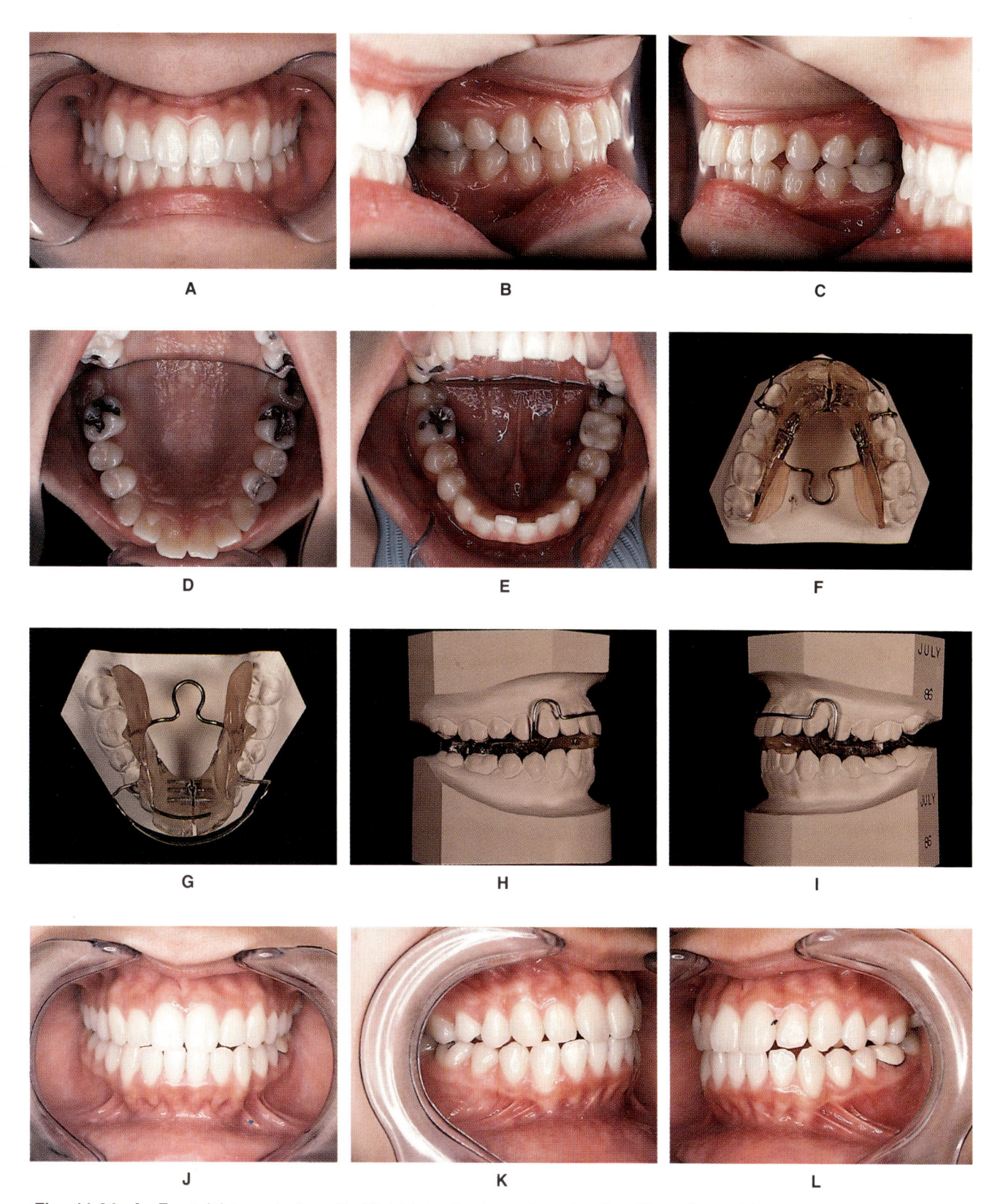

Fig. 11-24. **A**, Frontal intraoral view. **B**, Right lateral mirror view showing Class II cuspid and molar relationship. **C**, Left lateral mirror view showing Class II cuspid and molar relationship. **D** and **E**, Maxillary and mandibular occlusal view. **F** and **G**, Maxillary and mandibular occlusal view of Orthopedic Corrector I on study models. **H**, Right lateral view of Orthopedic Corrector I on study models. **I**, Left lateral view of Orthopedic Corrector I on study models. **J**, Intraoral facial view after 6 months of treatment. Overbite reduced to an edge-to-edge position. **K**, 6 months post-treatment, right lateral view showing Class I cuspid and cmolar relationships. **L**, 6 months post-treatment, left lateral view showing Class I cuspid and molar relationships.

was then allowed to relapse. Final finishing is often required, after skeletal bases and disc displacements have been corrected.

Case History #8

Splint finishing, Orthopedic Corrector I

Patient 8, a 19-year-old white girl, presented with a chief complaint of "popping and clicking joints" over the preceding one year. Her medical history was non-contributory. Past history of trauma included trauma to side of head in a skiing accident 10 years ago, and numerous car accidents, the most recent in the past year.

She complained of pain and stuffiness in both ears; pain, redness and aching sensation in her right eye; pain in both TMJs; and cracking of her neck and upper back. She had locked open once, and gave a positive history of clenching and bruxing. On examination, late opening clicks of both TMJs were felt, masseters and temporalis were very tender to palpation, and a forward head position was observed.

She was treated with a mandibular flat occlusal splint (day wear), and soft maxillary nightguard, and was recommended physical therapy and biofeedback. She responded very well to the above treatment and was asymptomatic with the lower splint in four months (Fig. 11-25E). However, without the mandibular splint, she still experienced the opening clicks in both joints. Any reduction of the posterior vertical on the splint resulted in pain. Thus, it was decided to institute splint finishing, with the Orthopedic Corrector I appliance, to erupt the posterior vertical.

The appliance was fabricated to the non-click position, as determined by the splint, and she was asked to wear it all day and all night (at least 18 hours/day) (Figs. 11-25, F-H). The patient had had a convex profile, which dramatically improved with the appliance (Figs. 11-25, I and J). In 6 months significant bite opening had been achieved (Figs. 11-25, O and P), and the late clicks were reduced. At this juncture, an Occlus-o-guide appliance was inserted to complete the bite opening (Fig. 11-25Q), as she was tired of the all-day wear with the Orthopedic Corrector I. Six months later with the Occlus-o-guide, the bite opening was complete (Figs. 11-25, R-V). In this instance, the Occlus-o-guide was used as a positioner for final finishing of the case.

CONCLUSION

TMJ dysfunction in children presents challenging problems and unique opportunities. Unlike adults, the dentist is faced not only with treating the presenting symptomatology, but also guiding the developing dentition into a state of normalcy. It is with this view in mind that certain treatment modalities have been presented, comprising a simple system to treat most of the dysfunctions, which involve internal derangement of the TMJs, and myofascial and cervico-spinal dysfunctions. Often, the only presenting signs are deep bites, retroclined maxillary anteriors, or posteriorly displaced condyles, which predispose the child to the unfolding sequence of TMJ dysfunction.

The alert clinician recognizes these signs early and has the unique opportunity with younger patients to intervene with interceptive techniques, guiding the developing dentition and influencing indirectly the whole body. The establishment of optimal anterior guidance, encouraging posterior vertical development, serves to provide the developing TMJs a favorable environment. With this in mind the use of the sagittal and utility arch have been presented.

Children with history of trauma to the head or neck, whiplash injuries, postural problems, or multiple trigger points are best treated in conjunction with physical therapists, and/or chiropractors. Compromised airways, allergies, and parafunctional habits are easily screened at the chairside examination and referred to appropriate specialists. It is always amazing how dramatically and easily children and adolescents respond to this multifactorial problem when dealt with through an interdisciplinary approach. The reward for the clinician is to see his clientele develop into young, dynamic individuals with healthy TMJs, full faces, and broad smiles.

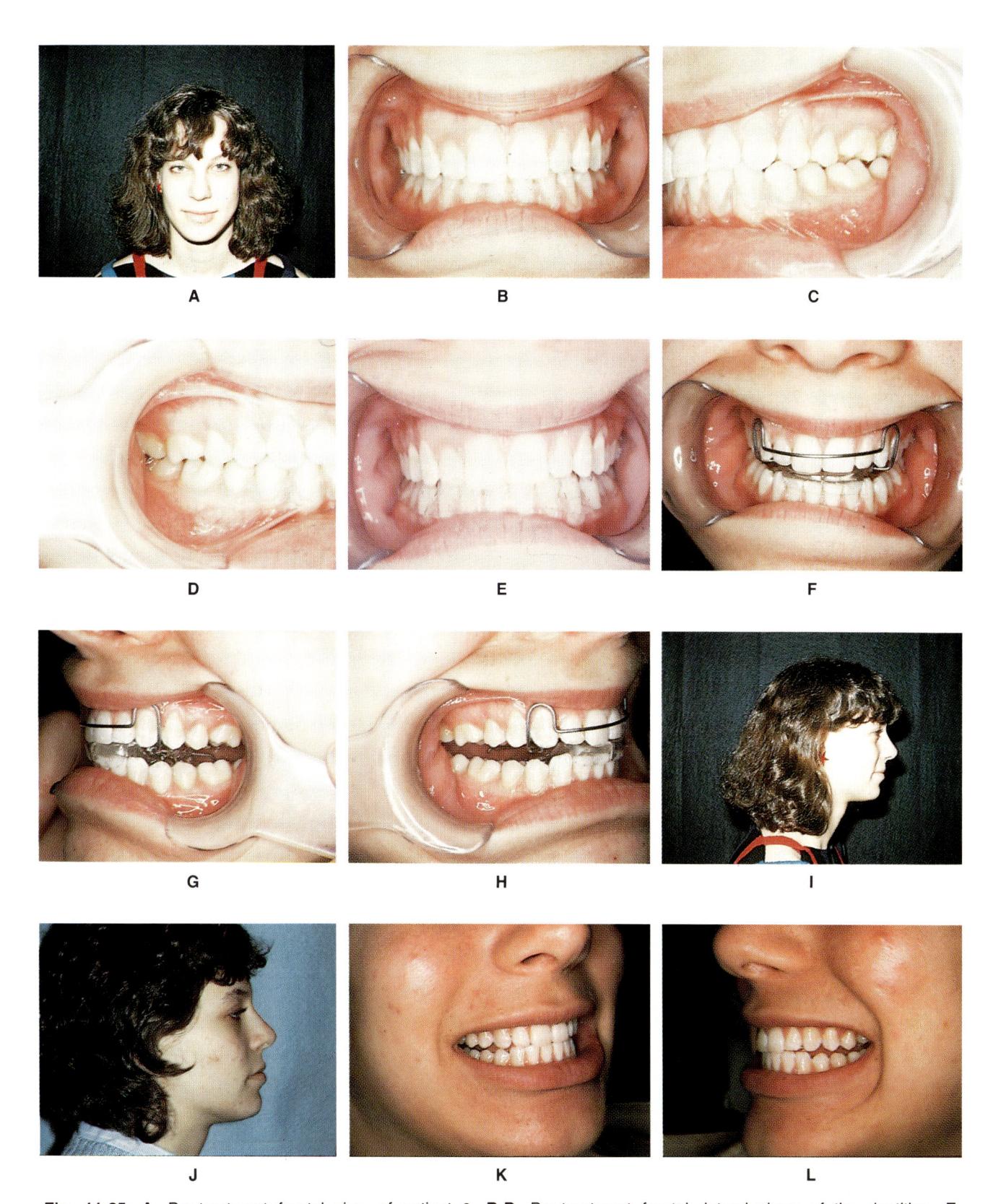

CHAPTER 11 Craniomandibular Dysfunction in the Growing Child 305

Fig. 11-25. **A**, Pre-treatment frontal view of patient 8. **B-D**, Pre-treatment frontal, lateral views of the dentition. **E**, Patient 8, asymptomatic with flat occlusal splint. **F-H**, Orthopedic Corrector I inserted to open the bite. **I**, Pre-treatment convex profile. **J**, Profile full and straight, on insertion of Orthopedic Corrector I. **K** and **L**, Mandibular repositioning after one week of wearing Orthopedic Corrector I. (continued)

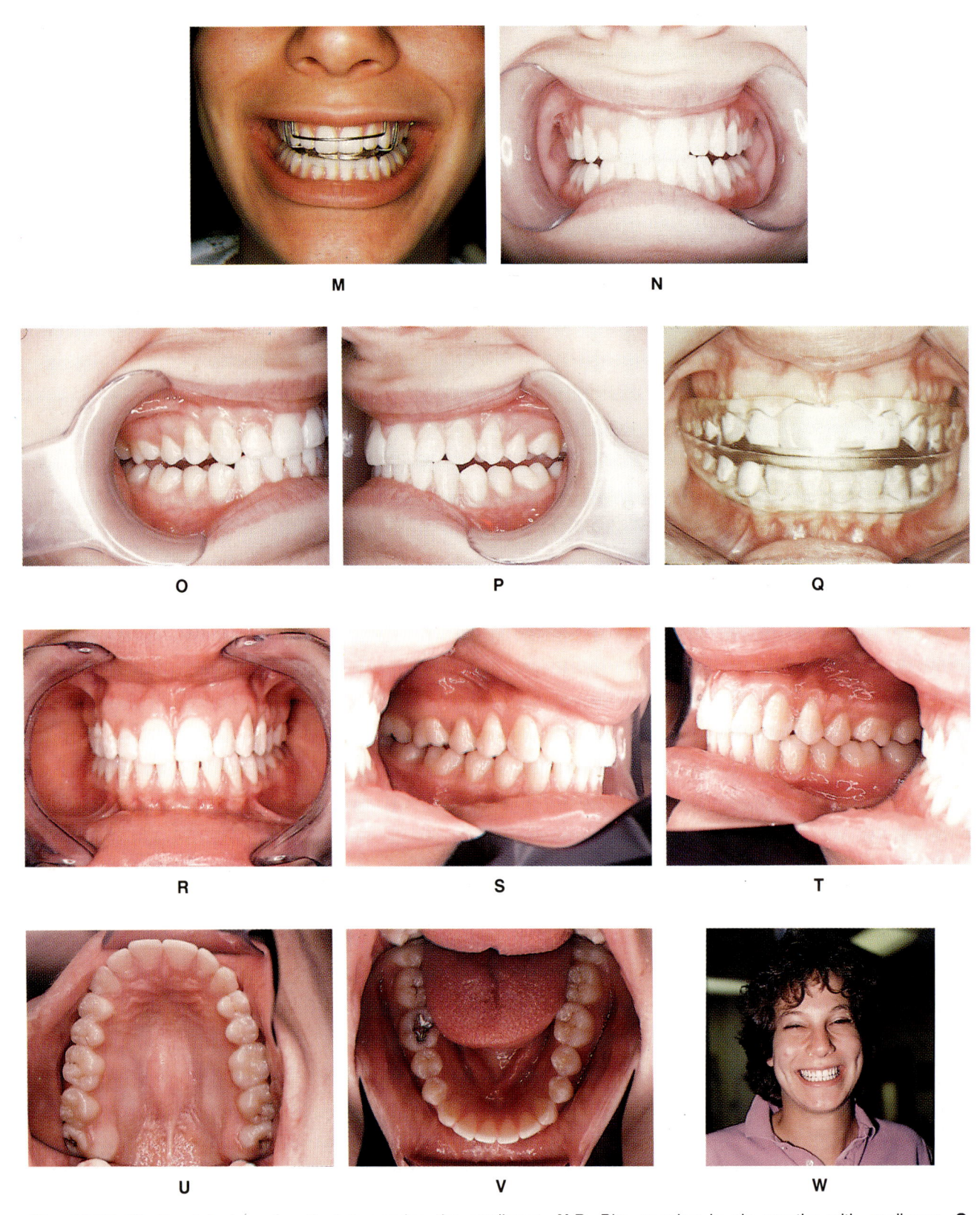

306 New Concepts in Craniomandibular and Chronic Pain Management

Fig. 11-25. M, Frontal view of patient 8 wearing the appliance. **N-P**, Bite opening in six months with appliance. **Q**, With Occlus-o-guide appliance. **R-W**, Bite opening is complete.

ACKNOWLEDGEMENT

Our sincere appreciation and gratitude are extended to Dr. Noshir Mehta for his invaluable suggestions, critique, and thought-provoking questions; to Dr. Earl Bergersen for his contribution of the Occlus-o-guide correction in the primary dentition; and to Cynthia Rowe for her physical therapy evaluation of the child in case history #4.

REFERENCES

1. McNamara J Jr. Influence of respiratory pattern on craniofacial growth. *Angle Orthod.* 1981;51;4:269-299.
2. Linder-Aronson S. Effects of andenoidectomy on the dentition and facial skeleton over a period of five years. Trans Third Int Orthodont Congress. 1973; 85.
3. Linder-Aronson S. Effects of adenoidectomy on the dentition and nasopharynx. *Am J Orthod.* 1974;65;1:1-15.
4. Solow B, Siersback-Nielson s, and Greve E. Airway adequacy, head posture and craniofacial morphology. *Am J Orthod.* 1984;86;3:214-222.
5. Weimert T. Airway obstruction in orthodontic practice. *JCO.* 1986;20;2:96-104.
6. Geering-Gaerny M and Rakosi T. Initialsymptome von kiefergelenk-storungen bei kindern im alter von 8-14 jahren. Schweiz Monatsschir Zahnheilkd. 1971;81:691-712.
7. Lindquist B. Bruxism in twins. *Acta Odontol Scand.* 1974;31:177-187.
8. Siebert G. Zur frage okklusaler interferenzer bei jugendlischen. *Dtsch Zahnastzl.* 1975;30:539-543.
9. Dibbets J. Juvenile TMJ dysfunction and craniofacial growth. Thesis. Rijkuniversiteit te Groningen. 1977; 96-98.
10. Williamson E H. Temporomandibular dysfunction in pretreatment adolescent patients. *Am J Orthod.* 1977;72:429-433.
11. Wigdorowicz, Makowerowa N, et al. Epidemiological studies on prevalence and etiology of functional disturbances of the masticatory system. *J Prosthet Dent.* 1979;41:76-82.
12. Egermark-Eriksson I, Carlsson GE, and Ingervall B. Prevalence of mandibular dysfunction and orofacial parafunction in 7, 11, and 15-year-old Swedish children. *Eur J Orthod.* 1981;3:163-172.
13. Nilner M and Lassing S. Prevalence of functional disturbances and diseases of the stomatognathic system in 7-14 year olds. *Swed Dent J.* 1981;5:173-187.
14. Grosfield O, Jackowska M, and Czarnecka B. Results of epidemiological examinations of the TMJ in adolescents and young adults. *J Oral Rehab.* 1985;12:95-105.
15. Egermark-Eriksson I and Carlsson G E. Five-year longitudinal study of signs and symptoms of mandibular dysfunction in adolescents. *J Craniomand Prac.* 1986;4;4:339-343.
16. Bernal M and Tsamtsouris A. Signs and symptoms of TMJ dysfunction in 3-5 year old children. *J Pedod.* 1986;10;2:127-140.
17. Keith D. Development of the human temporomandibular joint. *Br J Oral Maxillofac Surg.* 1982;20:217-224.
18. Wright D and Moffett B Jr. The postnatal development of the human temporomandibular joint. *Am J Anat.* 1974;141:235-250.
19. Lawrence E S and Samson G S. "Growth and development influences on the craniomandibular region." In: *TMJ Disorders; Management of the Craniomandibular Complex.* Kraus S L, ed. Edinburgh, United Kingsom: Churchill Livingstone; 1988:258-262.
20. Dibbets J, Vander-Weele L, and Boering G. Craniofacial morphology and temporomandibular joint dysfunction in children. In: Development aspects of TMJ disorders: Craniofacial growth series, monograph #16; Carlson D S, ed. Center for Human Growth and Development, Univ of Mich (Ann Arbor); 1985.
21. Lagaida M and White G. Unilateral mastication and facial formation. *J Pedod.* 1983;7:127-134.
22. Ricketts R. Clinical implications of the temporomandibular joint. *Am J Orthod.* 1966;52:416.
23. Mehta N R, et al. TMJ triad of dysfunctions: a biologic basis of diagnosis and treatment. *J Mass Dent Soc.* 1984;33;4:173-213.
24. Morawa A P, et al. *TMJ Dysfunction in Children and Adolescents: Incidence, Diagnosis and Treatment.* Chicago, Ill: Quintessence Pub Co; 1985;11:771-777.
25. Ricketts R M. Laminography in the diagnosis of TMJ disorders. *J Am Dent Assoc.* 1953;46:620.
26. Stack B C and Funt L A. TMJ problems in children. *J Pedod.* 1977;1:240-247.
27. Gelb H, ed. Clinical management of head, neck and TMJ pain and dysfunction. Philadelphia, Penn: W. B. Saunders Co; 1977:109.
28. Owen A H. Orthodontic-orthopedic treatment of craniomandibular pain and dysfunction. *J Craniomand Prac.* 1984;2:238-249.
29. Padamsee M, et al. Functional disorders of the stomatognathic system: Part II - a review. *J Pedod.* 1985;10;1:1-21.
30. Owen A H. Orthodontic-orthopedic treatment of craniomandibular pain and dysfunction. *J Craniomand Prac.* 1984;2:334-349.
31. Katzberg R W, Messing S G, and Helms C A. "Arthrography of the TMJ." In: *Clinical Management*

of Head, Neck, and TMJ Pain and Dysfunction. Philadelphia, Penn: W. B. Saunders Co; 1977:557.

32. Travell J and Simons D. *Myofascial Pain and Dysfunction: The Trigger Point Manual*. Baltimore, Md: Williams and Wilkins; 1983.

33. Padamsee M, Mehta N R, and White G E. Trigger point injection: a neglected modality in the treatment of TMJ dysfunction. *J Pedod*. 1987;12:72-92.

34. Clark G T. Examining TM-disorder patients for cranio-cervical dysfunction. *J Craniomand Prac*. 1983;2;1:56-63.

35. Cailliet R. *Soft Tissue Pain and Disability*. Philadelphia, Penn: F. A. Davis Co; 1986:132.

36. Darnell M W. A proposed chronology of events for forward head posture. *J Craniomand Prac*. 1983;1;4:50-54.

37. Cailliet R. *Scoliosis, Diagnosis and Management*. Philadelphia, Penn: F. A. Davis Co; 1986:49-52.

38. Rocabado M and Tapia V. Radiographic study of the cranio-cervical relation in patients under orthodontic treatment, and the incidence of related symptoms. *J Craniomand Prac*. 1987;5;1:37-41.

39. Connolly B. "Postural applications in the child and adult." In: *TMJ Disorders: Management of the Craniomandibular Complex*. Kraus, SL, ed. Edinburgh, United Kingdom: Churchill Livingstone; 1988.

40. Doppler, Dopplergram. 3 Brothers Enterprises. P O Box 1001, East Hampstead, NH 03826.

41. Ahlin J H, et al. *Maxillofacial Orthopedics: A Clinical Approach for the Growing Child*. Chicago, Ill: Quintessence Pub Co; 1984: Chapter 10.

42. Ingervall B. Range of movement of mandible in children. *Scand J Dent Res*. 1970;78:311-322.

43. Kendall H O and Kendall F P. Developing and maintaining good posture. *Phys Therapy*. 1968;48;4:319-336.

44. Lynn J W. The Biofinisher. *Funct Orthod*. 1985;2;2:36-41.

45. Witzig J W and Spahl T J. "The sagittal appliance." In: *The Clinical Management of Basic Maxillofacial Orthopedic Appliances*. Littleton, Mass: PSG Pub Co; 1984:217-275.

46. Stack B C. Orthodontic treatment methods, part I. *J Funct Orthod*. 1984;1;3:11-22.

47. Witzig J W and Spahl T J. "The straight wire appliance." In: *The Clinical Management of Basic Maxillofacial Orthopedic Appliances*. Littleton, Mass: PSG Pub Co; 1987:501-519.

48. Brehm W and Carapezza L J. Space age pedodontics: The use of the utility arch wire appliance. *J Pedod*. 1987;11:201-229.

49. Bergersen E O. The eruption guidance myofunctional appliance: how it works, how to use it. *J Funct Orthod*. 1984;1;3:28-35.

50. Bergersen E O. The eruption guidance myofunctional appliance: case selection, timing, motivation, indications, and contraindications in its use. *J Funct Orthod*. 1985;2;1:17-33.

51. Witzig J W and Spahl T J. "The Bionator." In: *The Clinical Management of Basic Maxillofacial Orthopedic Appliances*. Littleton, Mass: PSG Pub Co; 1987:501-519.

52. Stack B S. Orthodontic treatment methods. *J Function Orthodont*. 1984;1;4:22-33.

Chapter 12

Skeletal Facial Types — "The Missing Link"

Richard A. Pertes, DDS

It is generally accepted that the concept of an all-inclusive craniomandibular syndrome with like signs and symptoms and a single method of treatment is no longer valid. This is due primarily to the recognition that the etiology of craniomandibular disorders is often multifactorial and may not always be clearly discernible.[1]

Clark and Solberg have broken down the most likely etiologies into four major events: 1) trauma, 2) repetitive loading, 3) arthritic disease, and 4) stress-induced muscle tension.[2]

While the role of occlusal factors remains unclear, their importance as "the" primary etiological factor has diminished as awareness of the adaptive capacity of the individual to occlusal disharmony has increased. Nevertheless, some occlusal discrepancies are important in masticatory muscle complaints while others may play a role in disorders involving the joint structures.

In recent years, the role of the cervical spine and of head posture as both an etiological and a perpetuating factor in craniomandibular disorders has been recognized. Poor posture is endemic to our society, and the influence of head posture upon the postural rest position of the mandible, masticatory muscle activity, and dentoalveolar development is well documented.[3,4]

Perhaps Rugh and Solberg's classic statement that "the central question is not which factor is involved, but how much of each is involved" is the key to understanding etiology.[5]

A knowledge of craniofacial morphology involving skeletal facial types may well provide the "missing link" in our understanding of the complex relationship between occlusion, head posture, and craniomandibular disorders, thus affecting craniomandibular therapy.

FACIAL TYPES AND MALOCCLUSION

Malocclusion has been defined by Ricketts as "improper fitting of the teeth which is, therefore, aberrant from the normal and is characterized by irregularity of or deviation from the normal in anatomic relationships".[6] Although emphasis is now placed on functional aspects of occlusion more than on the anatomic, the classification of dental malocclusion developed by Angle in 1907 is still commonly accepted. He noted that "... all teeth are essential, yet in function and influence some are of greater importance than others, the most important of all being first permanent molars... They are by far the most constant in taking their normal positions... especially the upper first molars... which we call the keys to occlusion."[7] On this basis, Angle defined the following classifications of malocclusion:

Class I (neutroclusion). The anteroposterior relationship of the maxillary and mandibular first molars is correct. Crowding and spacing of teeth may be present with one or more anterior teeth in malposition.

Class II (disotoclusion). The lower first molars are distal to the maxillary first molars. This class has two divisions, based on the position of the maxillary incisors.

    Division 1. The maxillary incisors are protruding, creating an overjet.

Division 2. The maxillary central incisors are inclined lingually, and the maxillary incisors overlap the central incisors. A deep incisal overbite is usually present.

Class III (mesioclusion). The lower first molars are mesial to their maxillary counterparts, and the mandibular arch is usually forward of the maxillary teeth.

Attempts to relate craniomandibular disorders to a specific malocclusion have not been successful. However, Pullinger et al. found that TMJ tenderness was more frequent in Class II Division 2 malocclusions than in Class I Malocclusions.[8]

While serving a useful purpose in identifying dental malocclusion, Angle's classifications were inadequate for describing the accompanying craniofacial skeletal relationship. Accordingly, many cephalometric analyses have been developed over the years to overcome this shortcoming.

One of the first analyses to deal primarily with craniofacial morphology and relationships was published by Sassouni in 1969; it was based on geometric proportions. On the basis of similar characteristics, he defined four abnormal basic facial types: two with vertical disproportions which he referred to as skeletal deep bite and skeletal open bite, and two types with anteroposterior disproportions, skeletal Class II and skeletal Class III.[9]

Currently, a great deal of emphasis is placed on the vertical dysplasias of craniofacial morphology. Indeed, they are often associated with anteroposterior dysplasias and may even be at the origin of the dysplasias. Thus multidimensional combinations are possible: e.g., Class II deep bite, Class II open bite, Class III deep bite, and Class III open bite. In addition, while a Class I skeletal facial type is considered to be normal in an anteroposterior direction, it can be associated with a skeletal deep bite or an open bite. If a malocclusion is present, it frequently reflects the skeletal type, but variation is possible because of dentoveolar adaptation.[9,10]

Facial characteristics are determined by both genetic and environmental factors. In an anteroposterior direction, genetic factors appear to be primary. In the vertical plane, growth is more susceptible to changes induced by environmental factors, especially those involving breathing. Any skeletal combination may be involved in a craniomandibular disorder. From the viewpoint of understanding the relationship between craniomandibular disorders and craniofacial morphology, however, the vertical discrepancies have more significance and will be discussed in detail. A brief description of the vertical discrepancies is in order.

SKELETAL CLASS II

In a skeletal Class II, there is a maxillary protrusion or a mandibular retrusion or a combination of both. The skeletal Class II can be viewed either as a dimensional problem or as a positional deviation. For example, the maxilla and mandible may be in correct position with respect to the cranium, but a discrepancy in size may be responsible for the Class II facial relationship.

Usually, the most frequent cause of a dimensional Class II is a small mandible. On the other hand, both the maxilla and the mandible may be in proportion but a Class II is present because of a positional discrepancy. A prime representative of this situation would be a normally positioned maxilla accompanied by a mandibular retrusion. Since postional and dimensional deviations are not mutually exclusive, combinations of the two may be found in an individual. An Angle Class II dental malocclusion is usually associated with a Class II skeletal facial pattern.[9,10]

SKELETAL CLASS III

A skeletal Class III can be a dimensional problem with a small maxilla and/or a large mandible. But it may also represent a postional deviation resulting from a maxillary retrusion, a mandibular protrusion, or both. Often dimensional and positional deviations may be associated, creating a variety of composite Class III types, most of which are accompanied by an Angle Class III malocclusion.[9,10]

In general, a Class II skeletal type, characterized by a mandibular retrusion, is more

CHAPTER 12 Skeletal Facial Types — "The Missing Link" 311

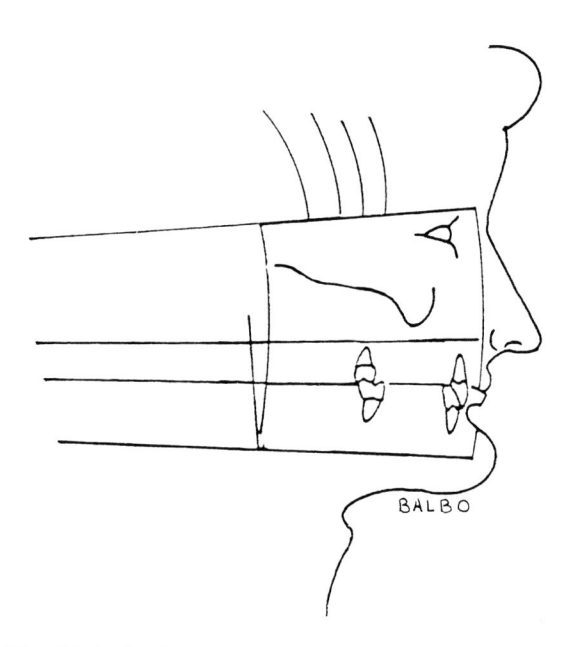

Fig. 12-1. Skeletal deep bite facial type. Facial planes are horizontal and nearly parallel to each other. Anterior facial height is short and gonial angle is small. (Modified after Sassouni)

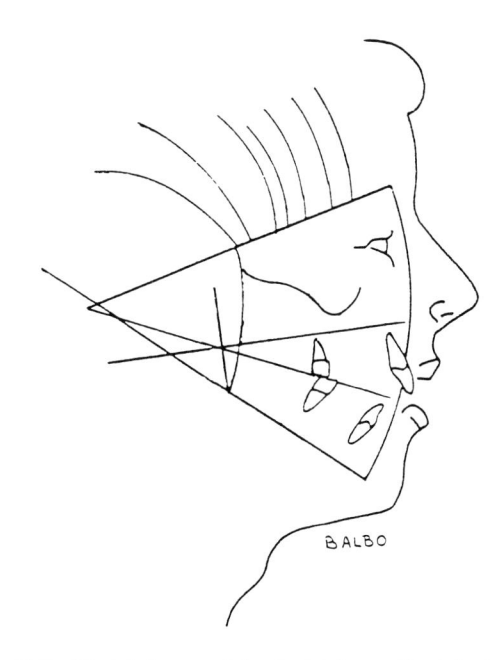

Fig. 12-2. Skeletal open bite facial type. Facial planes are steep to each other. Anterior facial height is long and gonial angle is large. (Modified after Sassouni)

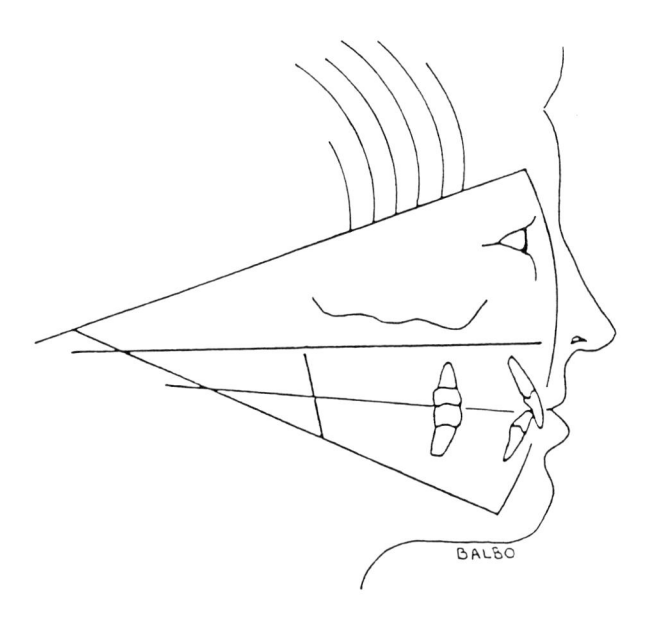

Fig. 12-3. Normal Facial type.

SKELETAL DEEP VERSUS SKELETAL OPEN BITE

Both extreme vertical facial types have in common an alteration in the lower anterior facial height. Because each facial type shares similar cephalometric, occlusal, and esthetic features, the term "syndrome" is often used to describe the facial type. Since Sassouni, a great deal of research has been devoted to comparisons of individuals with vertical facial dysplasias. Therefore, different terms have been introduced to describe the clinical esthetic impression created by the disharmony in facial proportion. The term skeletal deep bite has been used interchangeably with "short-face syndrome," "low angle type," and "hypodivergent face." "Long-face syndrome," "high angle type," and "hyperdivergent" are often used instead of skeletal open bite. Because no single parameter is sufficiently accurate to describe each facial type, for the purposes of this chapter, Sassouni's original terms of skeletal deep and open bite will be employed. In the author's opinion, they still remain the most comprehensive. However, the characteristic features of each facial type described in the following sections reflect the work of many researchers.[9,10,12-14]

likely to have posterior condylar displacement, creating a predisposition to a possible internal derangement of the TMJ. Paradoxically, it is not unusual to find a posterior condylar position in a Class III facial type. Therefore, each TMJ patient must be evaluated on an individual basis without any preconceived concepts.

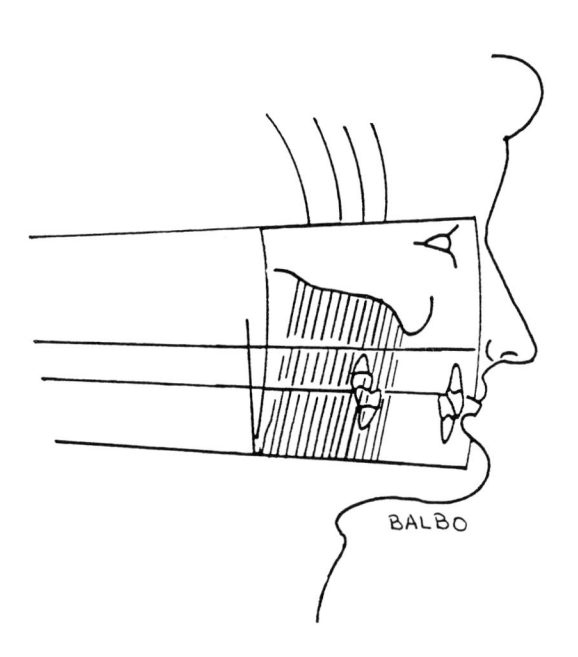

Fig. 12-4. Skeletal deep bite facial type. Large, well-developed masticatory elevator muscles attach to mandible directly over molars. Verical development of alveolar processes is inhibited, permitting mandible to be rotated in a counterclockwise direction. (Modified after Sassouni).

Fig. 12-5. Skeletal open bite facial type. Elevator muscles are small and weak and attach to mandible behind molars. Vertical development of alveolar processes is excessive and the mandible is rotated in a downward and backward direction. (Modified after Sassouni).

FACIAL PLANES

In a deep bite, the four planes of the face (supraorbital, palatal, occlusal, mandibular) are horizontal and nearly parallel to each other. This is in contrast to an open bite, where the same planes are steep to each other, giving the face a hyperdivergent appearance (Figs. 12-1 through 12-3).

FACIAL HEIGHT

A deep bite is characterized by a short anterior facial height (decreased chin-nose distance) and usually has a long posterior facial height due to a long mandibular ramus length. The posterior border of the ramus is nearly vertical and the gonial angle (ramus to corpus) is small. Another subgroup has been described by Opdebeeck and Bell which also has a decreased lower anterior facial height but has a short ramus and a more normal gonial angle.[12]

Conversely, in an open bite face, the anterior facial height is long and the posterior facial height is frequently shortened because of a short mandibular ramus. The posterior border of the ramus is tilted posteriorly, the gonial angle is steep and an antegonial notch may be present. Another subtype has been delineated by Opdebeeck, Bell, et al., which has long ramus contributing to the large lower facial height.[13]

MASTICATORY MUSCLES

In a deep bite, the elevator muscles are large and well-developed and stretch in nearly a straight line vertically, thus placing the molars directly under the impact of masticatory forces. Occlusal forces are strong, and there is decreased vertical development of the alveolar processes, resulting in a flat mandibular plane angle and short face seen in skeletal deep bites. This lack of vertical alveolar development also permits the mandible to rotate in a counterclockwise direction (Fig. 12-4).

Elevator muscle mass in an open bite face is considerably smaller than in the deep bite face. These muscles are inclined posteriorly and are attached to the mandible behind the first molars, reducing their mechanical advantage.

Proffitt and Fields have shown that, as a result, only about half as much biting force is present in an open bite compared to that of a normal facial type.[15] Sassouni has demon-

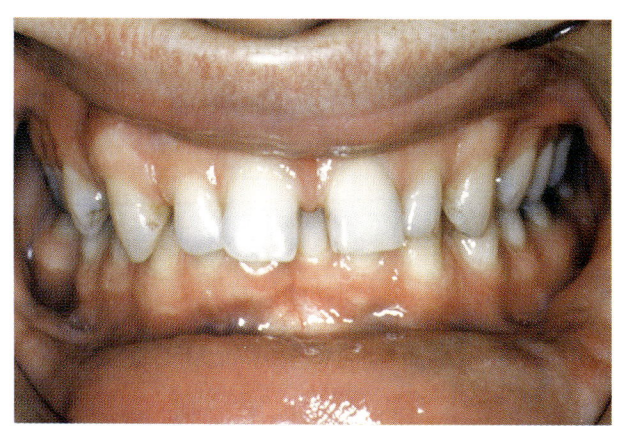

Fig. 12-6. Skeletal deep bite occlusion. A deep overbite is present as a result of lack of occluded vertical dimension. Note the broad maxillary arch, small teeth, and spacing.

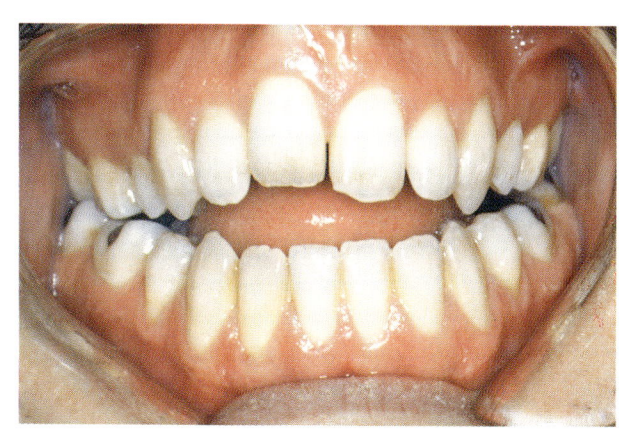

Fig. 12-7. Skeletal open bite occlusion. Excessive maxillary vertical alveolar development has resulted in a dental open bite which is maintained by a tongue thrust. The maxillary arch is constricted, teeth are large, and crowding is present even after bicuspid extractions and orthodontics.

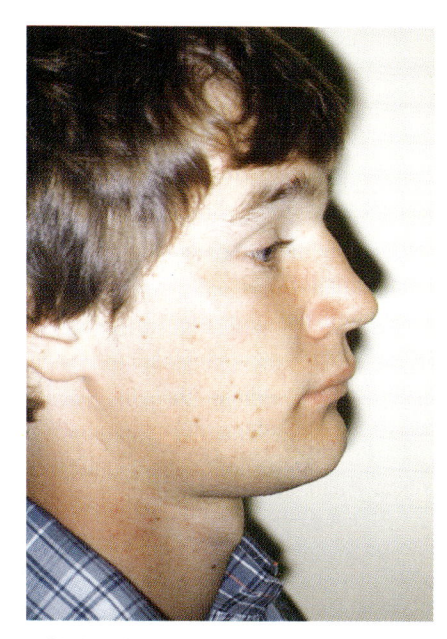

Fig. 12-8. Skeletal deep bite facial type. Facial form is rectangular, the mandible is prominent, and bidental retrusion is present, giving face a concave appearance. Mouth breathing is uncommon.

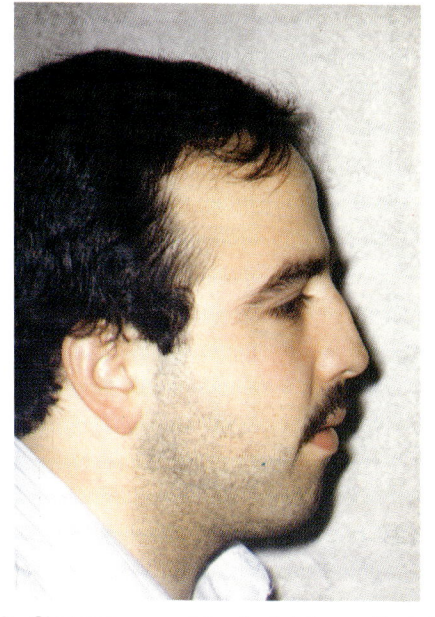

Fig. 12-9. Skeletal open bite facial type. Facial form is triangular and the mandible is rotated down and posteriorly, giving the face a convex appearance. Mouth breathing and tongue thrusting is common.

strated that in open bite faces, a biting force of 50-60 pounds is present at the molar level, compared to a biting force of 150-200 pounds in the deep bite[10] (Fig. 12-5).

A clear correlation between muscle activity, which is a measure of muscle strength, and craniofacial morphology was also found by Ingervall and Thilander. They noted a high degree of temporalis and masseter activity during chewing, and maximal bite in deep bite faces which substantiated previous studies.[16-19]

OCCLUSION

A relationship exists between tooth eruption, vertical growth of the alveolar processes, and rotation of the mandible during growth.

In a deep bite, strong occlusal forces prevent vertical development of the alveolar processes leading to a vertical maxillary insufficiency. A large interocclusal space is present between the molars, and the vertical dimension of occlusion is small.

On a dental level, the teeth are small and prone to abrasion, and there is a high percentage of congenitally missing teeth. The flat palatal vault contributes to a wide, broad maxillary dental arch. Spacing is common, but there may be crowding in the lower incisor area. Due to a lack of occluded vertical dimension and the upright position of both upper and lower incisors which allow these teeth to extrude past each other, a deep overbite is present. The dental arches are in bidental retrusion relative to their bony bases, giving the face a "dished-in" or concave appearance (Fig. 12-6).[9,10]

In an open bite, lower occlusal forces allow greater eruption of posterior alveolar processes, creating a vertical maxillary excess. This vertical growth encourages a downward and backward rotation of the mandible. A small interocclusal space is present and there is a large occluded vertical dimension.[13]

Large teeth contribute to frequent crowding in the dental arches and irregularities along with impacted third molars. A dental open bite is usually present and the lips are often apart at rest. The dental arches are protruded, giving the face a full and convex appearance (Fig. 12-7).[10]

FACIAL SHAPE

Deep bite faces are wide, have broad nasal apertures, a palatal vault which is flat and wide, and a large pharyngeal space. These features are consistant with an absence of mouth breathing. In profile, the facial form may be characterized as rectangular, with considerable depth of the face and prognathism (Fig. 12-8).

On the other hand, open bite faces tend to be narrow, with diminished nasal apertures, a high palatal vault, and a constricted pharyngeal space. These individuals are frequently mouth breathers and tongue thrusters. Whether the facial features are a result of mouth breathing and nasal obstruction or a predisposing factor to these noxious habits is a subject open to considerable debate. In profile, the facial form is triangular and exhibits retrognathism (Fig. 12-9).

CRANIAL SHAPE

In a deep bite, the skull is usually round or brachyfacial with a bulging forehead. A dolichofacial or oval-shaped head is associated with an open bite facial type.

In summary, the skeletal deep bite is a clinically recognizable facial type with a reduced lower anterior facial height and may be divided into two subgroups. The first group is characterized by a long ramus and a sharply reduced gonial angle. The second group has a shorter ramus, a slightly reduced gonial angle, and a sharply reduced posterior maxillary height of the alveolar processes. Both groups can be designated as having, to a varying degree, a vertical maxillary deficiency, which accounts for the short facial height; also, the mandible is rotated in a counter-clockwise direction.

An increase in lower anterior facial height is the characteristic feature of the skeletal open bite. Two subtypes have been described, both of which show a vertical maxillary excess. This encourages a clockwise rotation of the mandible along with the hyoid, tongue, and pharynx. This may be in response to the necessity of maintaining a patent airway at the level of the base of the tongue.

SKELETAL DEEP BITE AND CRANIOMANDIBULAR DISORDERS

Skeletal deep bite is characterized by excessive incisor overbite, excessive freeway space, and a diminished occluded vertical dimension. This can lead to an abnormal functional pattern and the likelihood of posterior condylar displacement, which has been implicated as a prime predisposing factor in internal derangements of the TMJ. In order to understand the possible relationship between deep overbite and posterior condylar displacement, it is necessary to explore vertical dimension in some detail.

There are essentially two vertical dimensions:

Postural Vertical Dimension (PVD). The vertical dimension of the face when the mandible is in its physiologic rest position. At this position, the patient is upright and looking straight forward and the mandibular musculature is in a state of minimal tonic contraction to maintain posture and to overcome the force of gravity. Recent studies have indicated that the mandible is capable of continuously adjusting to body posture and respiratory changes and that a single resting position of the mandible does not exist.

Occluded Vertical Dimension (OVD). The vertical dimension of the face when the teeth are occluded in their habitual position of maximum intercuspation.

Normally, when the mandible is in its postural rest position, a space is present between the occlusal surfaces of the maxillary and mandibular teeth, known as the interocclusal or freeway space. According to Ramfjord and Ash,[21] this space usually measures 1-3 mm in the anterior part of the mouth, but Rugh and Johnson[22] caution that because rest position of the mandible is not constant, any optimum interocclusal space measurement may not be valid.

As the teeth and supporting alveolar bone erupt into the oral cavity, they are subject to the influence of various muscular and occlusal forces. As previously stated, in a skeletal deep bite, the alveolar processes are prevented from erupting to their full genetic potential by strong elevator muscle activity, creating a reduced occluded vertical dimension and an excessive freeway space. Should the tongue rest between the dental arches, or if it is thrust bilaterally between the posterior teeth during swallowing, it too can inhibit eruption of teeth and alveolar processes.

In individuals with a reduced occluded vertical dimension as indicated by an excessive freeway space, the posterior fibers of the temporalis and the deep masseter become dominant in closing from rest position to centric occlusion, thus moving the condyle posteriorly and superiorly, predisposing the patient to a possible internal derangement.[23]

Deep bite faces may also be more susceptible to joint problems because of joint anatomy. Ingervall found a marked height of the articular eminence to be associated with a deep bite type of face and a small height of the eminence in open bite faces.[24]

Extreme height and inclination of the articular eminence may constitute another predisposing factor in disc-interference problems of the joint. As the disc-condyle complex moves forward in translation, full surface contact between the condyle and the eminence is accomplished by rotation of the disc posteriorly on the condyle. Therefore, as Bell has written, the greater the inclination and height of the aricular eminence, the greater the demand for rotation of the disc to accomplish smooth, silent, unobstructed translatory movements.[25]

In the same vein, skeletal deep bite patients are more likely to experience subluxation or joint hypermobility as a result of their steep eminences and deep overbite. Subluxation has been defined by Bell as partial or incomplete dislocation of the articulating surfaces of a joint.[25] It is primarily due to excessive mouth opening in response to the functional requirement of separating the jaws to traverse the steep eminence and overcome the vertical overlapping of the incisors.

While abnormal joint function may be an important etiologic factor in the development of symptoms in skeletal deep bite patients, the role of muscles as a source of symptoms cannot be ignored. A common muscle disorder affecting the masticatory apparatus is the myofascial pain dysfunction (MPD) syndrome. Laskin, in defining the MPD syndrome, stated that masticatory muscle spasm, resulting from muscle fatigue produced by chronic parafunctional habits such as bruxism, was the primary factor responsible for symptoms.[26] Since deep bite patients have strong muscles of mastication and have more activity in chewing and closing in centric occlusion than patients with normal or open bite faces, it is possible that they may show an exaggerated response to bruxing by developing muscle spasm and/or trigger areas. Graber brings in another factor when he writes, "Clinical experience has shown that there is a high incidence of bruxism associated with overbite."[23]

The effect of a reduced occluded vertical dimension on the muscles of mastication must also be considered. In these patients, the possibility is strong that in an effort to reach occlusal contact between opposing teeth, the muscles may overcontract, leading to muscle spasm.

Muscles can also be involved secondarily to any posterior condylar displacement, which is often seen in an overclosed condition. Mongini has written, "if the condyles are displaced in intercuspal position, the whole mandible must be displaced."[27] This can cause additional tension in the muscles and lead to spasm.

SKELETAL OPEN BITE AND CRANIOMANDIBULAR DISORDERS

If a reduced occluded vertical dimension and heavy musculature are the main predisposing factors in patients with a skeletal deep bite, what factors would allow the open bite patient to develop symptoms? Obviously, the same factors are not operative. Perhaps the answer lies in exploring the relationship between mouth breathing, which is very common in open bite patients, and its possible adverse effect upon occlusion and head posture.

The characteristic facial dimensions of open bite faces, such as narrow nasal apertures and constricted pharyngeal space, create a potential for mouth breathing. Any chronic obstruction to the flow of incoming air can cause mouth breathing and advancement of the tongue to clear the airway.

This can be due to blockage of the nasal airway resulting from an anatomic deviation within the nasal cavity or allergies or enlarged tonsils and/or adenoids. A major alteration in craniofacial and cervical muscle function, occlusion, head posture, and subsequent growth is likely to occur.[28,29]

Abnormal tongue posture frequently causes a narrow maxillary arch, which may result in an end-to-end occlusion. Many patients will shift their mandible laterally to avoid cuspal interferences, thus creating a unilateral posterior crossbite in centric occlusion. Studies have shown that the resulting jaw shift can cause a disturbed muscular pattern and/or condylar displacement with the possible development of craniomandibular signs and symptoms.[30]

Frequently, skeletal open bite patients exhibit an anterior open bite due to abnormal tongue activity superimposed on a genetic tendency. Mohlin and Kopp were able to relate a lack of incisal guidance to nonworking side and protrusive interferences which also have been implicated in the development of muscle spasm. In addition, a frontal open bite can create an unstable occlusion by decreasing the number of tooth contacts.[31]

Indeed, researchers have studied functional disturbances of the masticatory system and were able to correlate occlusal disturbances with skeletal open bite characteristics.[32] However, it should be remembered that occlusal dysfunction is only one factor in a greater etiologic complex and that individual adaptation is high and therefore symptoms may not develop.

ROLE OF HEAD POSTURE

Abnormal head posture can be an important factor in the etiology of craniomandibular pain and dysfunction as well as craniocervical disorder. To understand this relationship, it is necessary to realize that when the head is in an ideal or orthostatic position, the center of gravity of the head lies slightly anterior to the vertebral column. Constant tension is needed in the strong posterior cervical muscles to counteract gravity and prevent the head from tilting forward. Ideal head posture is also determined by three horizontal parallel lines of reference: the bipupilar, otic, and the transverse occlusal plane. Maintenance of these planes with the ground permits the face and visual gaze to be horizontally oriented. Any change in the normal horizontal and parallel relationship of these planes to each other and to the ground will stimulate mechanoreceptors in the upper cervical spine and the mandible to react to keep those relationships intact. Thus, the head taken as a whole may be considered a lever system with ideal posture being achieved by a balance of all the muscle systems acting on the head. Excess tension in one set of muscles will result in a compensatory tension in other muscle groups to preserve proper head posture.[3,33]

Although head posture is related primarily to resisting the forces of gravity, it is also influenced by various physiologic functions, particularly that of respiration. Several investigators have correlated extension of the head in relation to the cervical spine with nasal obstruction. Ricketts hypothesized that this represented an effort to increase the airway to compensate for nasal obstruction. Other changes were noted in both skeletal and dental variables, including a long lower facial height, a high narrow palatal vault, a tendency toward crossbite and an anterior open bite: all skeletal open facial type characteristics.[29]

Solow and Tallgren were able to clearly define a relationship between craniofacial morphology and craniocervical posture by analyzing cephalometric radiographs on 120 male students. Open bite skeletal facial types were characterized by extension of the head, forward inclination of the cervical column, and a tendency to a reduced cervical lordosis. Conversely, flexion of the head in relation to the cervical column was, on the average, associated with a skeletal deep bite facial type.[34]

Thus, forward head posture appears to be the result of an interplay between genetic factors and external environmental influences. Certainly mouth breathing plays an important role. But any prolonged activity with the head and upper extremities in a more forward position than normal can result in changes in the cervical musculature, which both create and perpetuate forward head posture.[35]

In relating forward head posture to craniomandibular dysfunction, Darnell and Rocabado describe a series of events starting with hyperactivity of anterior and lateral cervical musculature, leading to a forward and downward movement of the middle and upper cervical vertebrae and the shoulder girdle complex. To compensate for this forward movement, the posterior cervical muscles act to bend backward the upper cervical spine and occiput. Mandibular closure with the occiput in an extended position places the suprahyoid and infrahyoid muscles under increased tension, with tightness in the throat and difficulty in swallowing. According to Rocabado, the combined forward head, neck, and shoulder girdle posture, along with increased hyoid muscle tenderness, can cause the mandible to become postured down and back relative to the maxilla. In these situations, the occlusal contact pattern will be altered, with heavier contacts in the last molar region.[33,35] An increase in neuromuscular activity of the masticatory and associated muscles may result. Should the condition persist, then changes in the habitual closing pattern of the mandible may be expected, with altered temporomandibular joint mechanics.

CLINICAL IMPLICATIONS

Craniomandibular therapy is usually divided into two phases: a palliative, reversible Phase I to allow repair and regeneration to occur, and an irreversible Phase II to achieve stabilization of the joint structures.

In most cases, Phase I is accomplished through the temporary use of intraoral occlusal appliances or splints in combination with adjunctive treatment such as physical therapy, biofeedback, medication, and injections. There is currently a great deal of controversy over the design of these appliances, particularly in the area of vertical dimension.

Skeletal deep bite patients usually require an increase in occluded vertical dimension. Care must be taken, however, to preserve some freeway space in order to avoid invoking the myotatic (stretch) reflex. Since posterior condylar displacement is common, mandibular anterior repositioning may also be indicated as part of Phase I therapy. Because of heavy occlusal forces and strong musculature, prolonged wearing of appliances as part of Phase I therapy should be discouraged for fear of intruding posterior teeth. At the University of Medicine and Dentistry of New Jersey TMJ and Facial Pain Center, an upper night appliance is alternated with a lower day appliance to avoid this potential pitfall.

Conversely, in skeletal open bite patients, any increases in occluded vertical dimension are poorly tolerated due to the lack of freeway space. The need for mandibular repositioning is not as great and its direction would depend upon the location of the condylar displacement. Some clinicians use anterior resistance appliances or bite plates without any posterior tooth contact, as either a full-time or night appliance, as part of their appliance protocol. In the author's experience, this type of appliance, when used in open bite cases, has allowed eruption of posterior teeth, resulting in a permanent change in the occlusion and additional rotation of the mandible in a clockwise direction.

After symptoms have been significantly reduced, an attempt is usually made to wean the patient from appliances. In those cases where symptoms return, it may be necessary to proceed to Phase II therapy to achieve stabilization of the joint structures. Since the relationship of the condyle, disc, and eminence is dependent upon the way the upper and lower teeth meet, traditional dental therapies are usually employed to achieve this objective. This can take the form of occlusal equilibration, overlay partials, crowns, and orthodontics, either individually or in combination.

In skeletal deep bite patients, the splint position achieved in Phase I may serve as the occlusal blueprint for any Phase II therapy. Permanent increases both in the occluded vertical dimension and mandibular position are usually well tolerated. These changes should be considered to be orthopedic in nature.

Research has shown a high degree of occlusal interference present in the open bite patient as opposed to the deep bite patient. Therefore, occlusal equilibration to eliminate these interferences may be a necessary part of any Phase II therapy in the open bite patient. This does not infer that equilibration may not be indicated in a deep bite patient, but that orthopedic considerations are more important in the presence of a deep bite. The vertical maxillary excess present in most open bite patients indicates that some reduction in the occluded vertical dimension should be accomplished. In severe cases, maxillary surgery consisting of reduction of the vertical maxillary height in combination with orthodontics may be necessary to allow rotation of the mandible in a counterclockwise direction. In addition, if a forward head posture is present in either a deep bite or open bite pattern, then correction is indicated prior to instituting any Phase II therapy.

CONCLUSION

There are many variations in the size, position, form, and proportion of the structures composing the human face. Although this paper has dealt primarily with two basic facial types with vertical disproportions, the skeletal deep bite and open bite, the majority of craniomandibular patients probably fall somewhere in the range between these two extreme facial types. Nevertheless, even these average facial types may have characteristics of either a deep bite or open bite which may be a contributing factor to the overall symptom complex.

REFERENCES

1. Kopp S. Pain and functional disturbances of the masticatory system—a review of etiology and principles of treatment. *Swed Dent J* 1982;6:49-60.
2. Clark GT, Solberg WK, Monteiro AA. Temporomandibular disorders: new challenges in clinical management, research, and teaching. In: Clark GT, Solberg WK, ed. *Perspectives in Temporomandibular Disorders*. Chicago, Ill: Quintessence Publishing Co, Inc; 1987:14-15.
3. Mohl N. The role of head posture in mandibular function. In: Solberg WK, Clark GT, ed. *Abnormal Jaw Mechanics*. Chicago, Ill: Quintessence Publishing Co, Inc; 1984:97-111.
4. Lawrence ES, Samson, GS. Growth and development influences on the craniomandibular region. In: Kraus SL. ed. *TMJ Disorders, Management of the Craniomandibular Complex*. New York, NY: Churchill Livingstone; 1988;241-273.
5. Rugh JD, Solberg WK. Psychological implications in temporomandibular joint pain and dysfunction. In: Zarb GA, Carlsson GE. ed, *Temporomandibular Pain and Dysfunction*. St. Louis, Mo: CV Mosby Co; 1979:239.
6. Ricketts RM. Occlusion — the medium of dentistry. *J Prosthet Dent*. 1969;21:39-60.
7. Angle EH. *Malocclusion of the Teeth*. 7th ed. Philadelphia, Pa: White Dental Manufacturing Co; 1907.
8. Pullinger AG, Seligman DA, Solberg WK. Temoromandibular disorders, Part II: occlusal factors associated with temporomandibular joint tenderness and dysfunction. *J Prosthet Dent*. 1988;59:363-367.
9. Sassouni V. A classification of skeletal facial types. *Am J Orthod*. 1969;55:109-123.
10. Sassouni V, Forrest EJ. *Orthodontics in General Practice*. St. Louis, Mo: CV Mosby Co; 1971:121-144.
11. Trask GM, Shapiro GG, Shapiro PA. The effects of perennial allergic rhinitis on dental and skeletal development: a comparison of sibling pairs. *Am J Orthod*. 1987;92:286-293.
12. Opdebeeck H, Bell WH. The short face syndrome. *Am J Orthod*. 1978;73:499-511.
13. Opdebeeck H, Bell WH, Eisenfeld J, Mishelvich

D. Comparative study between the SFS and LFS rotation as a possible morphogenic mechanism. *Am J Orthod.* 1978;74:509-521.

14. Schendel SA, Eisenfeld J, Bell WH, Mishelevich DJ. The long face syndrome: vertical maxillary excess. *Am J Othod.* 1976;70:398-408.

15. Proffit WR, Fields HW, Nixon WL. Occlusal forces in normal and long-face adults. *J Dent Res.* 1983;62:566-570.

16. Ingervall B, Thilander B. Relation between facial morphology and activity of the masticatory muscles. *J Oral Rehab.* 1974;1:131-147.

17. Moller E. The chewing apparatus. *Acta Physiol Scand.* 1966;69(Suppl):280.

18. Ahlgren J. Mechanism of mastication. *Acta Odont Scand.* 1966;24(Suppl):44.

19. Ringvist M. Isometric bite force and its relation to dimensions of the facial skeleton. *Acta Odont Scand.* 1973;31:35-42.

20. Grieder A, Cinotti WR. *Periodontal Prosthesis.* St Louis, Mo: CV Mosby Co; 1969.

21. Ramfjord SP, Ash MM. *Occlusion.* 3rd ed. Philadelphia, Pa: WB Saunders Co; 1983.

22. Rugh JD, Johnson RW. Vertical dimension discrepancies and masticatory pain/dysfunction. In: Solberg WK, Clark GT, ed. *Abnormal Jaw Mechanics.* Chicago, Ill: Quintessence Publishing Co; 1984:117-133.

23. Graber TM. Overbite—the dentist's challenge. *JADA* 1969;79:1135-1145.

24. Ingervall B. Relation between height of the articular tubercle of the temporomandibular joint and facial morphology. *Angle Orthod.* 1974;44:15-24.

25. Bell WE. *Temporomandibular Disorders: Classification, Diagnosis, Management.* 2nd ed. St. Louis, Mo: Year Book Medical Publishers, Inc; 107-110, 194-195.

26. Laskin DM. Etiology of the pain dysfunction syndrome. *JADA.* 1969;79:147-153.

27. Mongini F. Abnormalities in condyle and occlusal positions. In: Solberg WK, Clark GT, ed. *Abnormal Joint Mechanics.* Chicago, Ill: Quintessence Publishing Co, Inc; 1984:23-42.

28. Thurow RD. *Atlas of Orthodontic Principles.* 2nd ed. St. Louis, Mo: CV Mosby Co; 1975:43-49.

29. Ricketts RM, Steele CH, Fairchild RC. Forum on the tonsil and adenoid problem in orthodontics—respiratory obstruction syndrome. *Am J Orthod.* 1968;54:485-514.

30. Ingervall B, Thilander B. Activity of temporal and masseter muscles in children with a lateral forced bite. *Angle Orthod.* 1975;45:249-258.

31. Mohlin B, Kopp SA. A clinical study on the relationship between malocclusions, occlusal interferences, and mandibular pain and dysfunction. *Swed Dent J.* 1978;2:105-112.

32. Carlsson GE, et al. Relation between functional disturbances of the masticatory system and some anthropometric physiological variables in young Swedish men. *J Oral Rehab.* 1976;3:305-310.

33. Rocabado M. Diagnosis and treatment of abnormal craniocervical and craniomandibular mechanics. In: Solberg WK, Clark GT, ed. *Abnormal Jaw Mechanics.* Chicago, Ill: Quintessence Publishing Co, Inc; 1984:141-157.

34. Solow B, Tallgren A, Head posture and craniofacial morphology. *Am J Phys Anthrop.* 44:417-436.

35. Darnell MW. A proposed chronology of events for forward head posture. *J. Craniomand Pract.* 1983;1:49-54.

36. Pertes RA, Attanasio R, Cinotti WR, Balbo M. The use of occlusal splint therapy in the treatment of MPD and internal derangements of the TMJ. *J Clin Prevent Dent.* July/August 1989;11:26-32.

37. Pertes RA. Updating the mandibular orthopedic appliance (MORA). *J Craniomand Pract.* 1987;5:351-356.

Chapter 13

Postural Consideration for the Orthodontic Patient

Ira Yerkes, DMD
Grant Bowbeer, DDS, MS

The facial pain patient has often had to undergo a long and tortuous series of visits to any number of professionals, only with varying degrees of success. Recently, the orthodontist has been called upon to help in the management of acute and chronic pain patients. It has become apparent to orthodontists involved with these patients that a multi-disciplinary approach is necessary. A particularly useful collaboration has been that between the physical therapist and the dentist treating patients with craniocervical pain.

HISTORICAL BACKGROUND

Almost half a century ago, on April 22, 1948, a very astute dentist, Victor Stoll, in a lecture delivered before the New Organization of Alumni Associates, related dental occlusion to the head and neck, to spinal posture, and to respiratory, neurological and general health problems. He stated: "Mechanically, the solution to the problem is obvious. When necessary, especially in cases of deep overbite, the mandible should be established in a more forward position to meet the upper teeth correctly and permit proper use of the adjacent soft tissues in addition to other benefits."

In 1971, in the New York Journal of Dentistry, Dr. Harold Gelb, in a classic article, correlated the medical-dental relationship in the craniomandibular syndrome.

In 1973, Dr. Al Fonder received the Nobel Prize in dentistry for his description of the dental distress syndrome.

In 1976, Dr. Norman Mohl authored a landmark article in the New York State Dental Journal, "Head Posture and Its Role in Occlusion." He concluded that studies of head posture were not merely of academic importance, and suggested that head posture be accounted for in occlusal therapy.

In 1980, Dr. Peter Vig, in a study of thirty dental students with no history of allergies, found that total nasal obstruction using a nasal plug **in all cases** resulted in an extended head position. When the plugs were removed, it took an average of 1.5 hours for the head to assume normal posture. In terms of head posture, it seems, therefore, that respiratory requirements dominate as a determinant of the neuromuscular control which regulates cranial orientation.

In the early 1980's, a physical therapist and teacher, Mariano Rocabado, from Santiago, Chile, began a remarkable teaching journey that would eventually affect our profession of dentistry and the specialty of orthodontics. From him, we have learned the need for coordinated treatment between dentists and physical therapists. In an article entitled: "The Biomechanical Relationship for the Cranial, Cervical, and Hyoid Regions," Mariano Rocabado, R.P.T., defined the physical parameters of the physical therapy/orthopedic tracing used in determining the radiographic extent of forward posture. It is with this background in mind that we begin this chapter.

DEFINING THE PROBLEM: DIAGNOSIS

Nasal Insufficiency and Mouth Breathing

Nasal insufficiency as a consequence of early episodes of allergy, increased tonsil and

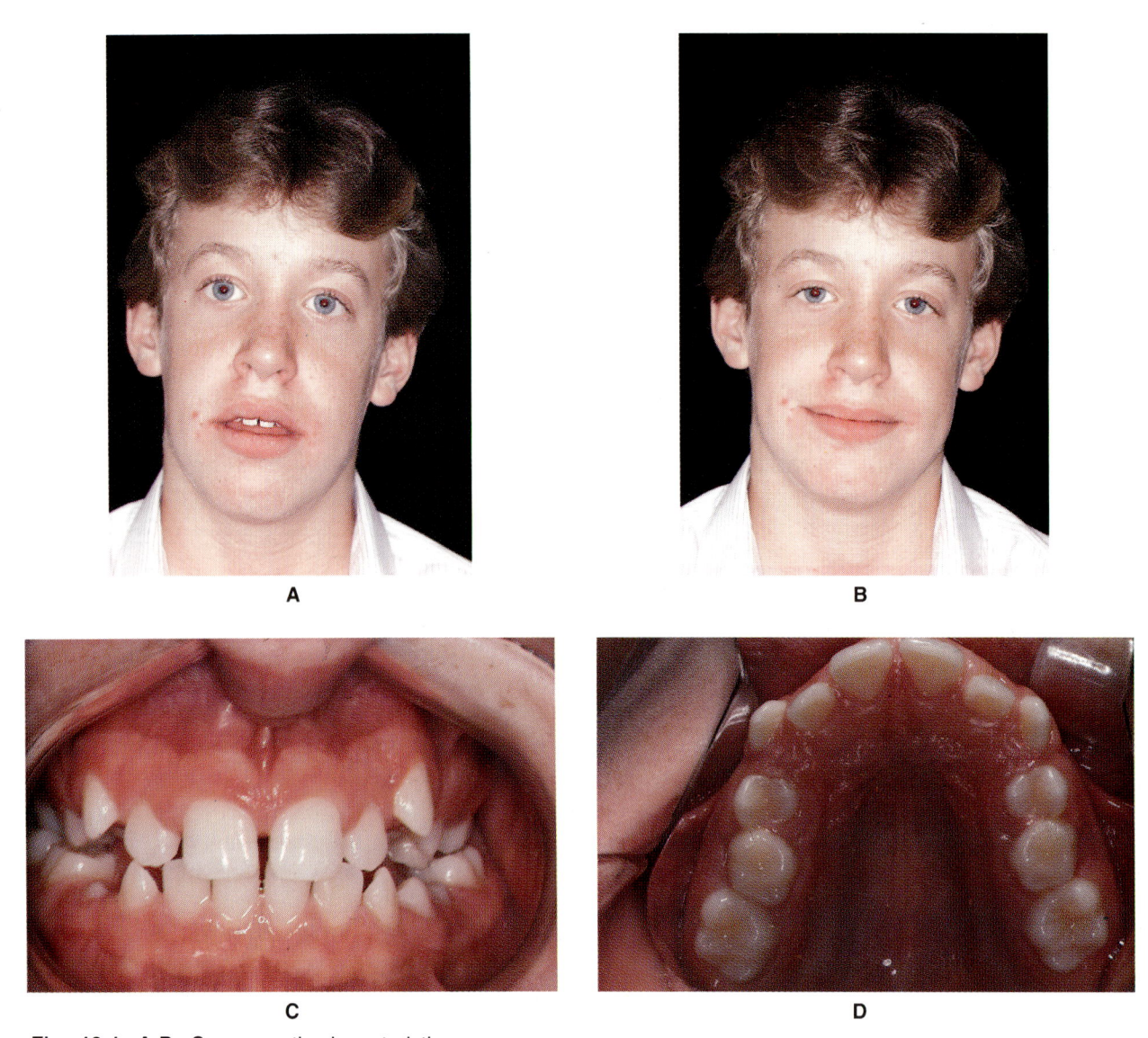

Fig. 13-1, A-D. Open mouth characteristics.

adenoid size, nasal septum blockage, or any other upper airway problem affecting nasal breathing, creates the need for mouth breathing. In order to facilitate mouth breathing, the cranium begins to rotate posteriorly. The head then comes forward to allow for horizontal vision, bringing itself into what is known in the language of physical therapist and chiropractor as "forward head posture."

This tendency toward mouth breathing and the accompanying forward head posture frequently starts early in life. When the causative factors are eliminated, the patient often remains with the head forward in space and the lips remaining open.

Patients who have retained open mouth characteristics as a result of early problems still have the capacity to lip seal (Figs. 13-1, A and B). Excessive parafunctional activity by the lower lip increases the tension of the hyoid muscles. This depressive and retrusive force to the mandible is accompanied by a lowered position of the tongue (Fig. 13-1A). The maxillary constriction that occurs leads to the illusion of maxillary dental crowding (Figs. 13-1, C and D). Maxillary arch constriction also leads to a concomitant mandibular arch constriction, which in turn brings about posterior crossbite (Fig. 13-1C) and/or mandibular dental crowding and possible loss of vertical dimension. Training the patient to breath through the nose with lip seal exercises is essential for the successful treatment of the dysfunctional head, neck, and shoul-

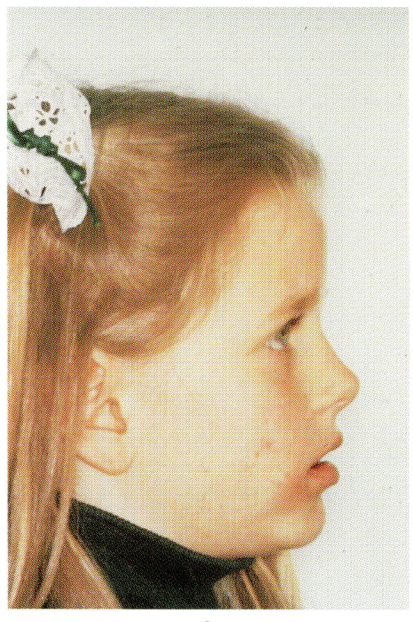

Fig. 13-2, A and **B**. Patient with open lip posture.

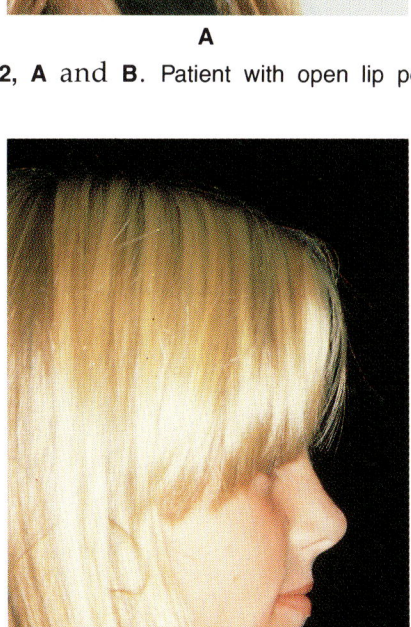

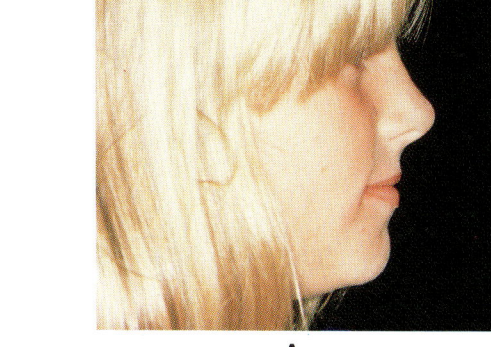

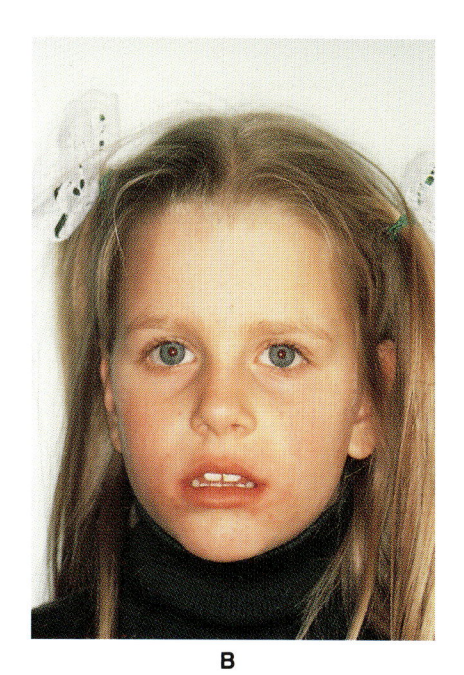

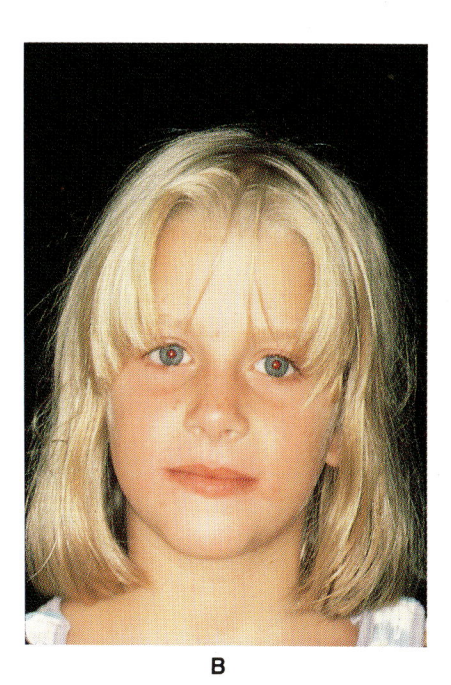

Fig. 13-3, A and **B**. Improved facial esthetics after correction of open lip posture.

der patient. Note the open lip posture on another patient (Figs. 13-2, A and B) and the improvement in facial esthetics when this is accomplished (Figs. 13-3, A and B).

Forward Head Posture

In a patient with normal head posture, the muscles supporting the head are in balance (Fig. 13-4A). The digastric muscles will be in balance and the hyoid bone will lie below the level of the border of the mandible (Figs. 13-4, B and C). The position of the hyoid bone can be confirmed on a cephalogram. When it lies below a line drawn from the most posterior inferior point of the symphysis to the most inferior anterior point of the body of the third cervical vertebra, this is considered a normal

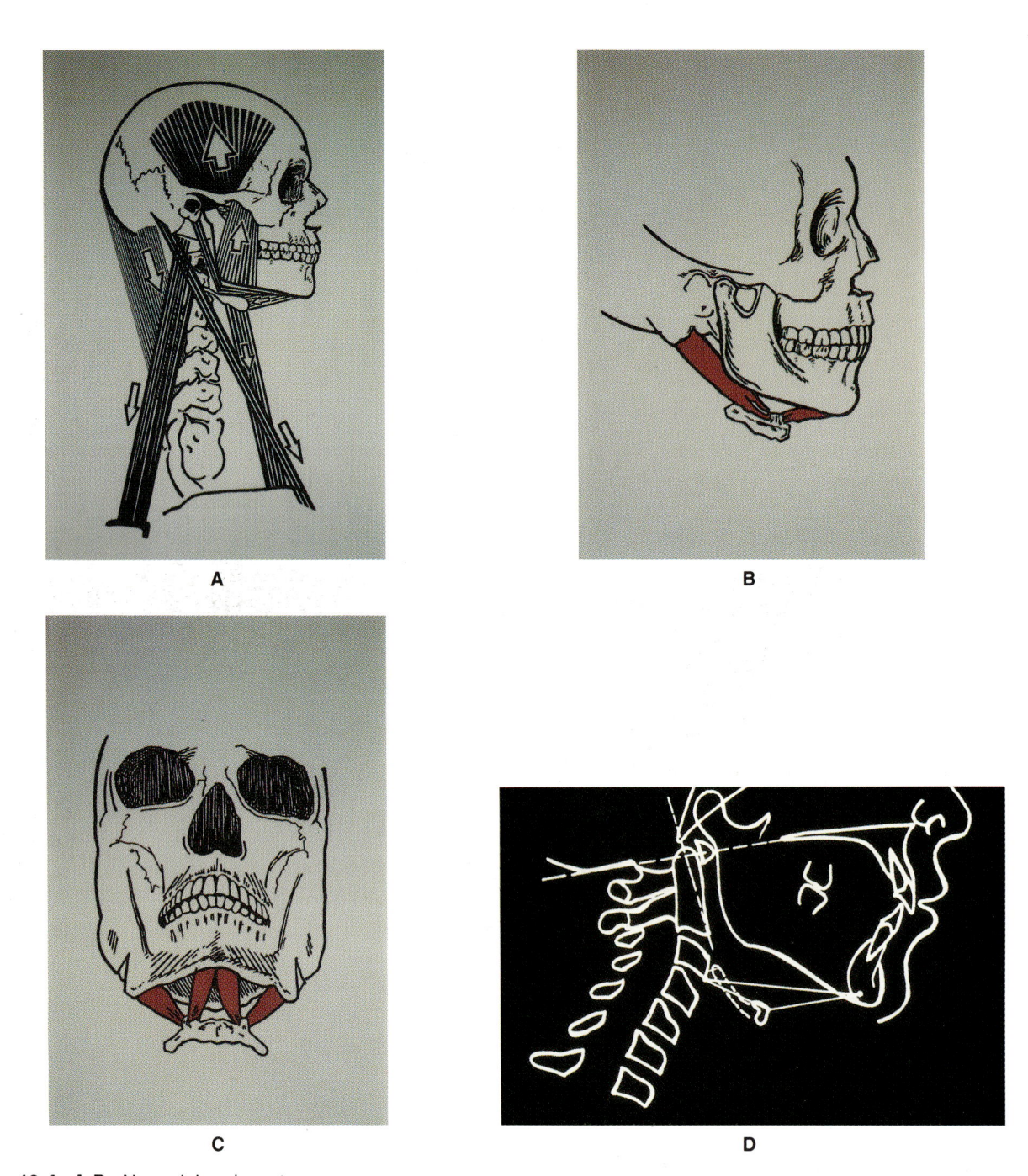

324 New Concepts in Craniomandibular and Chronic Pain Management

Fig. 13-4, A-D. Normal head posture.

hyoid position (Fig. 13-4D). The cephalogram will also demonstrate a normal cervical lordosis. There is also a balance in the pressure between the perioral muscles and the properly positioned tongue during rest and swallowing, maintaining normal maxillary dental arch width.

When the head is forward, there is a depressive, downward, and posterior force exerted on the mandible by the muscles attached to the sternum, leading to mandibular retrusion (Fig. 13-5A). This downward force causes the elevator muscles to constrict (Fig. 13-5, B and C). Compare the difference in head posture of the models in Fig. 13-5D. Also compare the head position of a patient with normal head posture Fig. 13-5E to that of a patient with forward head posture and reduced vertical dimension (Fig. 13-5F), in need of maxillary and mandibular arch expansion, mandibular forward repositioning, and restoration of vertical dimension.

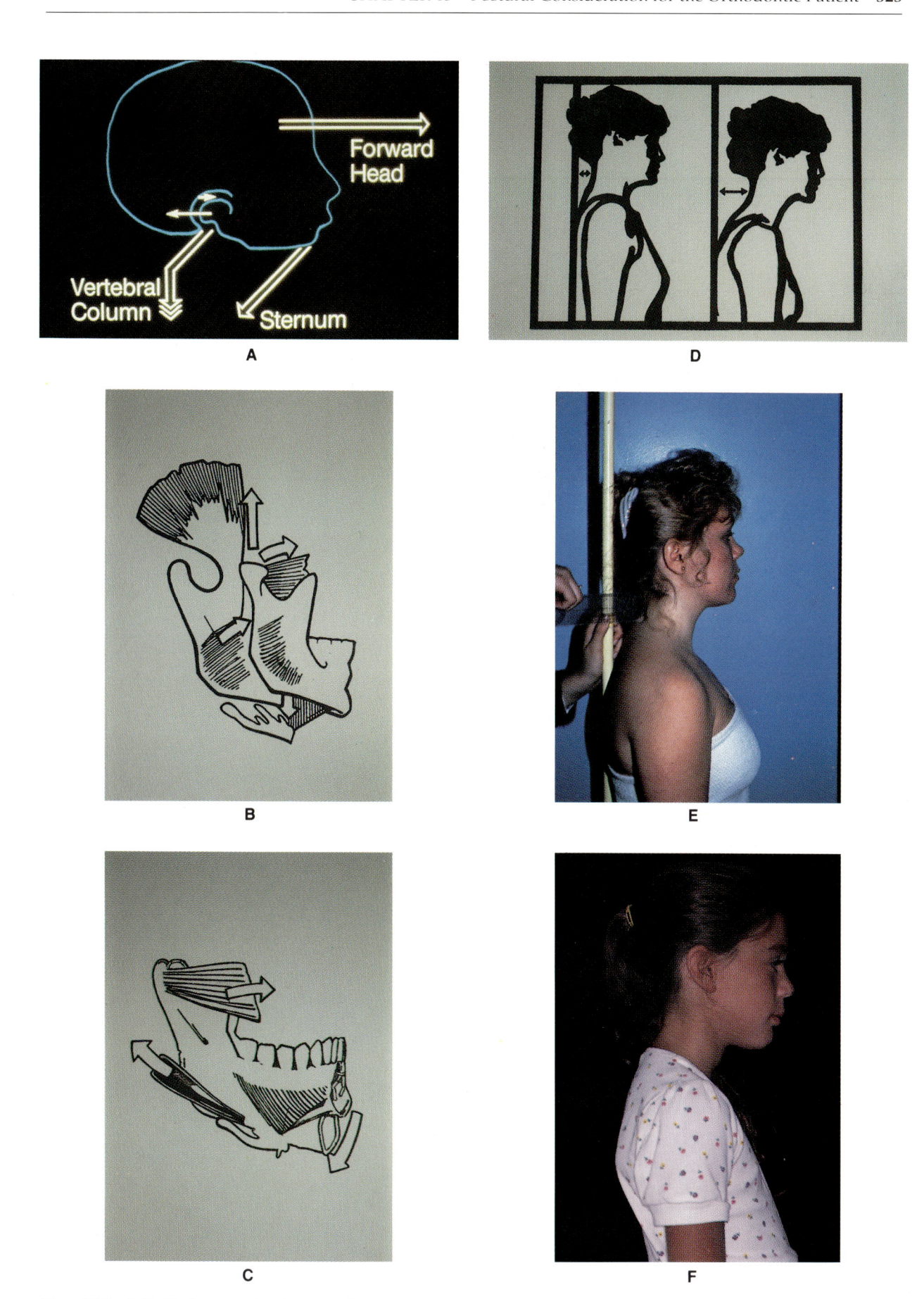

Fig. 13-5, A-F. Various postural comparisons.

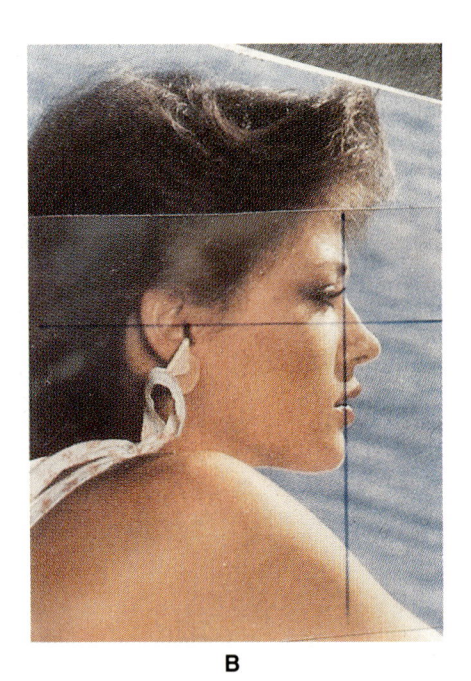

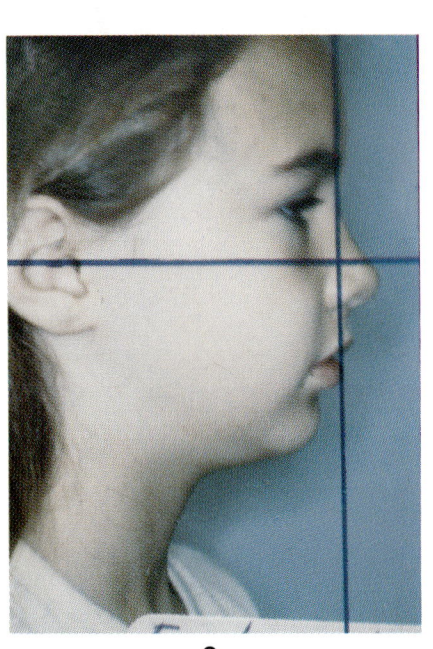

326 New Concepts in Craniomandibular and Chronic Pain Management

Fig. 13-6. The Bowbeer facial analysis.

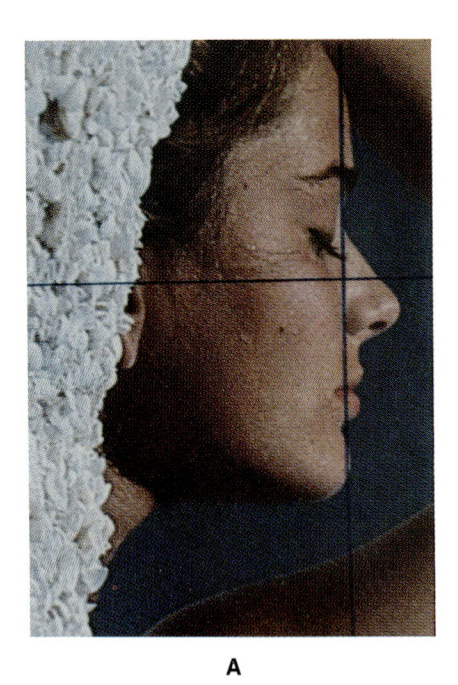

The Myth of the Protruded Maxilla

In the 1400's, scholars thought the world was flat: it certainly looked flat, maps were drawn flat, and there was no reason to think otherwise. When Columbus sailed west in 1492, many were sure he would fall off the face of the earth. As intelligent as these men were, they were wrong. Their concept of the earth being flat was not based on sufficient information.

Looking at an individual with a Class II Division 1 malocclusion, most people, including dental professionals, would once have said the the teeth "stuck out." They certainly looked like the "stuck out." It was believed that this skeletal pattern was inherited and could rarely be altered without surgery. Diagnostic and treatment methods were devised to move the teeth so as to compensate for or "camouflage" the skeletal pattern.

But recent research has demonstrated:

- The maxilla is in a normal position in almost all patients, no matter how far the teeth seem to "stick out" (protrude).
- Almost all (at least 95%) of Class II-1 skeletal malocclusions are due to a retrognathic mandible, and will have a normal or sometimes a retrognathic maxilla.
- Standard orthodontic diagnostic methods will frequently lead to misdiagnosis and incorrect treatment of patients with Class II-1 malocclusions, including constriction and over-retraction of the maxilla with many TMJ implications.

CONFIRMING THE DIAGNOSIS: THE BOWBEER FACIAL ANALYSIS

Bowbeer has developed a facial analysis that matches the profiles of movie stars, fashion models, and beauty contest winners. It is usually done on a facial photograph, using a grid of two lines—the FH (Frankfort Horizontal) and the BNV (Bowbeer Nasion Vertical or Bridge of the Nose Vertical.)*

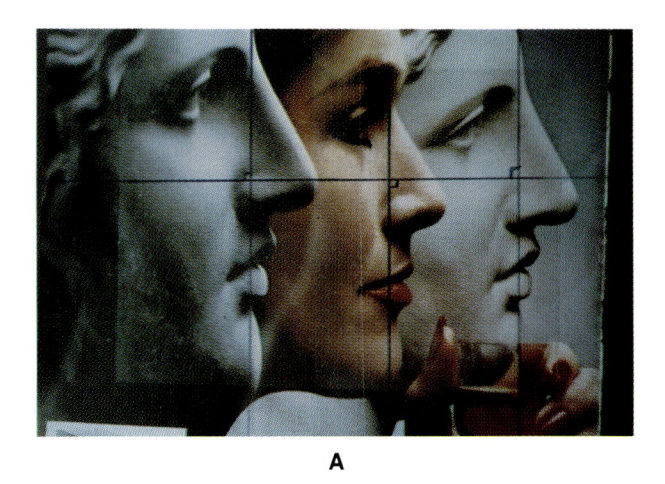

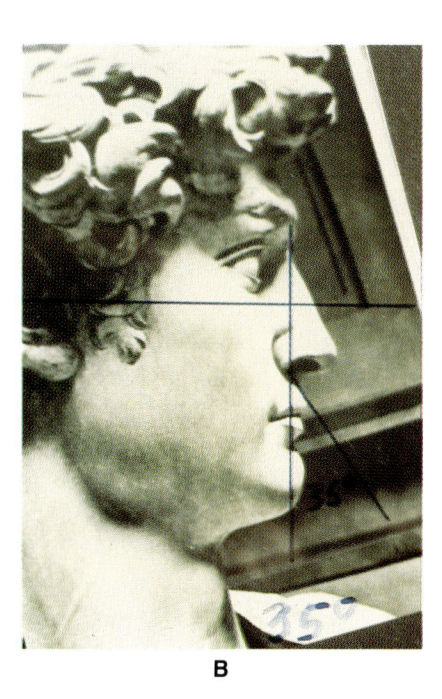

In this analysis, the position of the upper lip and the mentalis crease are related to the BNV (Figs. 13-6, A and B). A beautiful face with a balanced Class I profile will reveal the following:

*The Frankfort Horizontal is a line drawn from the top of the external auditory meatus (top of the tragus of the ear) to the bottom of the orbit. This line will almost always cross 1/2 way down the nose, or slightly lower. The BNV is a vertical line dropped from the bridge of the nose perpendicular to the Frankfort Horizontal.

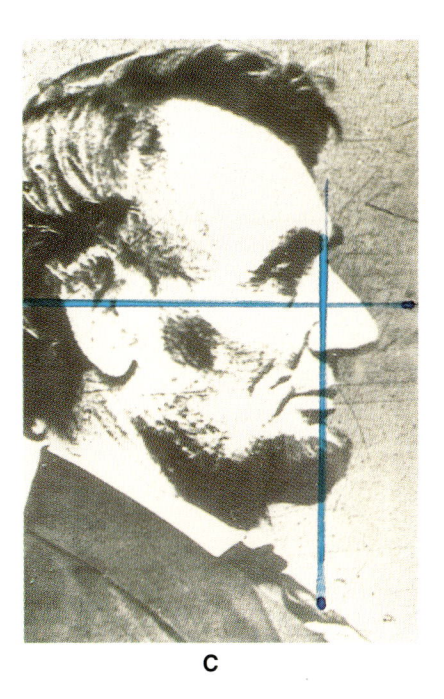

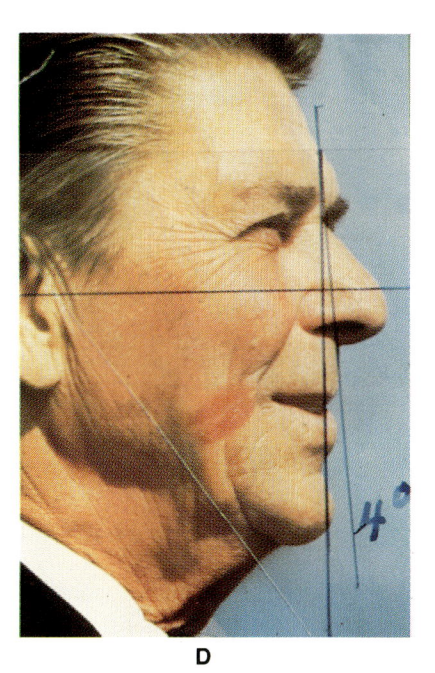

Fig. 13-7, A-D. "Classic" profiles.

MAXILLA
- The upper lip will usually lie at least 1/3-1/2 in front of the BNV.

MANDIBLE
- The mentalis crease will lie on the BNV +/−2mm.

In almost all Class II Division 1 malocclusions (90-95% +):

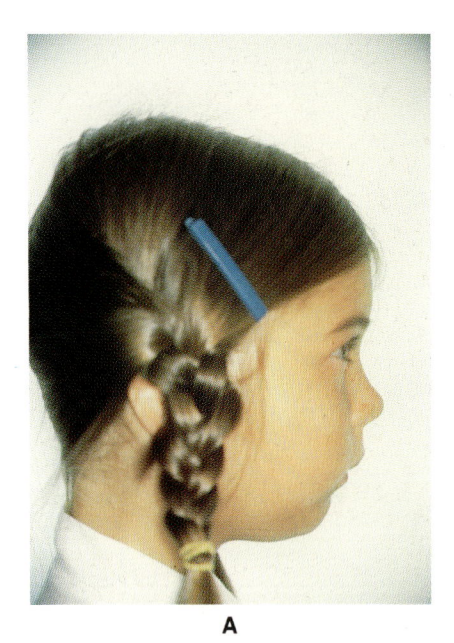

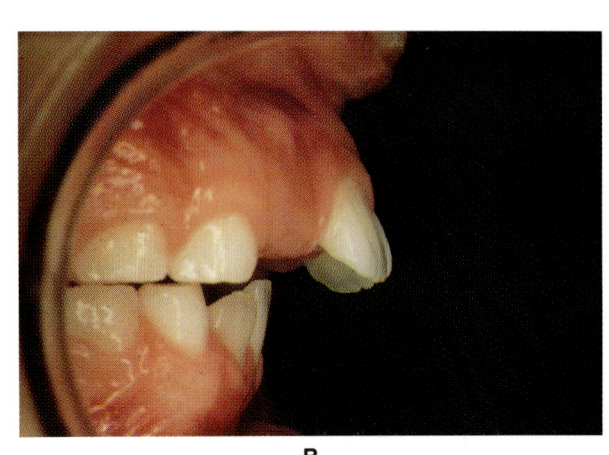

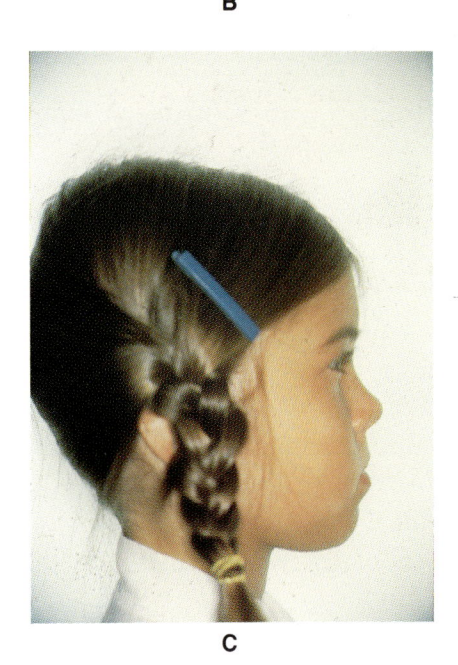

Fig. 13-8, A-C. Patient with a retruded mandible and a severe overjet.

MAXILLA
- The upper lip is usually more retrusive to the BNV (Fig. 13-6C).

MANDIBLE
- The mentalis crease will lie more than 2mm behind the BNV (Fig. 13-6C).
- The more severe the Class II, the farther the mentalis crease will be behind the BNV. (If the mentalis crease is ahead of the BNV more than 2mm, the patient has a Class III skeletal pattern).

Even the Greek artists knew facial balance when they carved their statues (Fig. 13-7A). So did Michelangelo when he carved the statue of David (Fig. 13-7B). Most successful businessmen and world leaders tend to have this straight facial profile and "strong" chin (Figs. 13-7, C and D).

The need to develop the mandible and frequently the maxilla becomes very evident in most patients when these guidelines are used. The patient in Figs. 13-8, A and B has a retruded mandible and a severe overjet. Note how the profile is improved when the lower jaw is brought forward (Fig. 13-8C). Also compare the change in head posture between Figs. 13-8, A and C.

Another Class II-1 patient has retruded mandible and a severe overjet (Figs. 13-9, A through C). Notice how the facial profile is improved when the lower jaw is brought forward to bring the anterior teeth into a proper overjet relationship (Figs. 13-9, D and E). This confirms previous research that maxillas are usually neutral or retruded in Class II-1 malocclusions.

Forward Head Posture and Its Effect on Vertical Dimension

Frequently, vertical dimension is adversely influenced by forward head posture. The reason is not completely understood, but the vertical dimension may be affected in two different ways in patients with a forward head posture:

- An increased vertical dimension, a high mandibular plane angle, and frequently a tongue-thrust open bite.

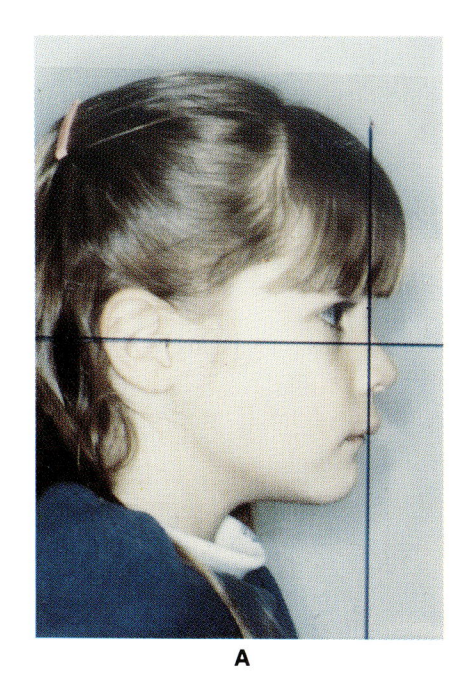

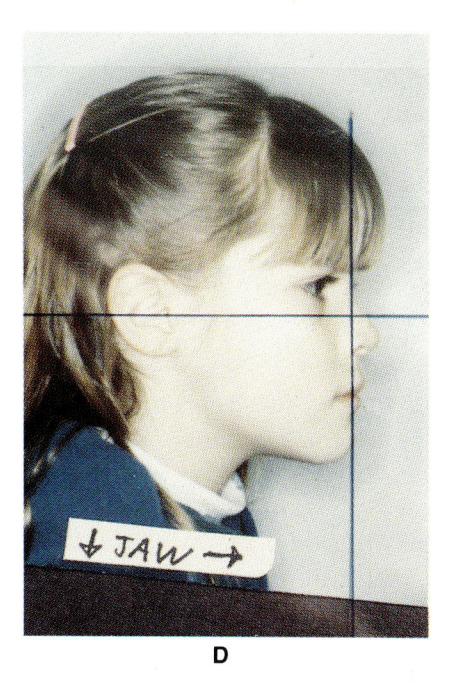

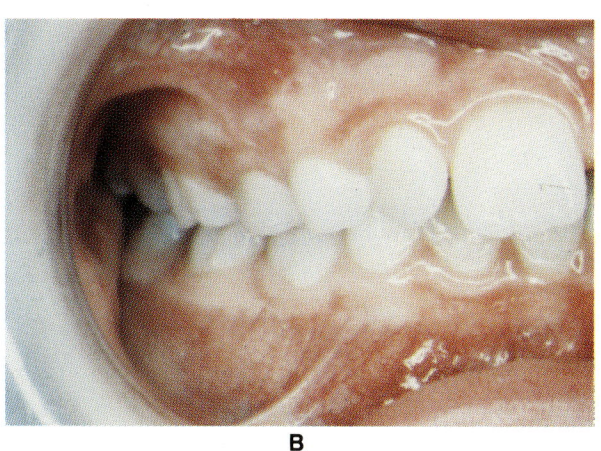

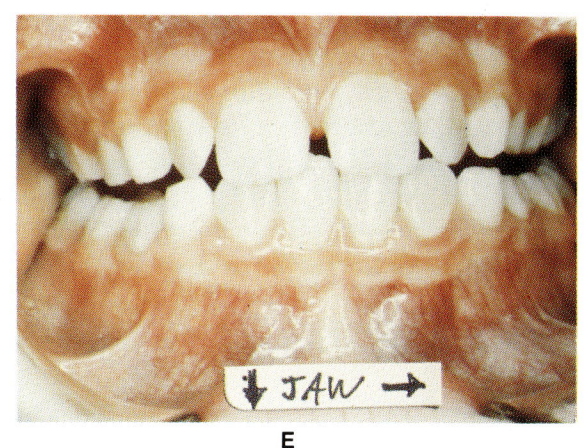

CHAPTER 13 Postural Consideration for the Orthodontic Patient 329

Fig. 13-9, A-E. Another example of improved facial profile in a Class II-1 patient.

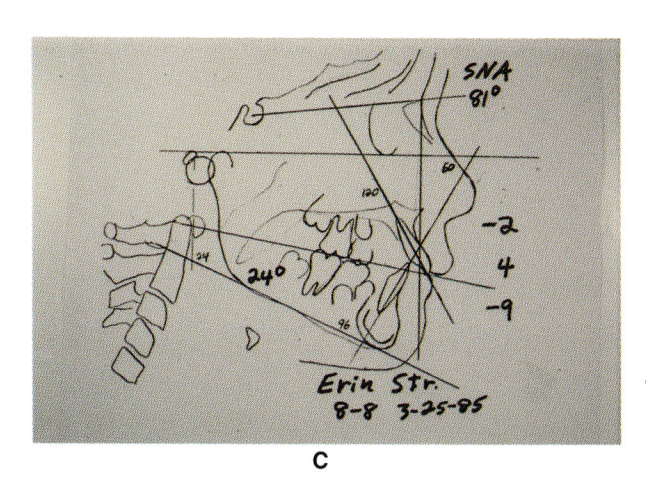

Forward Head Posture/Mandibular Retrusion and Increased Vertical Dimension (Long Face Syndrome)

In this pattern, the patient will usually have a convex facial profile (Figs. 13-10, A and B) and the cephalogram will reveal a high mandibular plane angle (Fig. 13-10C). There may also be a large antigonial notch—as if the body of the mandible had been "bent down" by unfavorable muscle forces.

Most patients who have been diagnosed with forward head posture and an increased vertical dimension have narrow arches, high palatal vaults, and may also have an open bite (Fig. 13-10B). Maxillary and mandibular

- An overclosed vertical dimension and a low mandibular plane angle.

arch expansion and mandibular forward repositioning are needed. If the problem is severe, surgical reduction of the vertical dimension may be necessary.

Forward Head Posture/Mandibular Retrusion and Decreased Vertical Dimension

In this pattern, the patient will usually have a straight facial profile (Figs. 13-11A and B) and the cephalogram will reveal a low mandibular plane angle (Fig. 13-11C). The effect of long term muscle contraction of the elevator muscles is insufficient vertical eruption of the posterior teeth, adding to the vertical dimension loss caused by the mandibular arch constriction (Table 13-1).

Most patients diagnosed as having forward head posture and a decreased vertical dimension have narrow arches, lower palatal vaults, and an impinging overbite. Maxillary and mandibular arch expansion, increased development of the vertical dimension, and mandibular forward repositioning with a functional appliance are needed. If the problem is severe, mandibular advancement surgery may be necessary.

Forward Head Posture, Mandibular Retrusion, Bruxism, Occlusal Wear, and the TMJ

Mandibular retrusion occurs as a result of the combined effect of forward head posture and the depressive force that the hyoid muscles exert. In response to the downward and backward force exerted on the mandible, there is a corresponding constriction of all the elevator muscles, as an antagonist response frequently leading to elevator muscle contraction pain (headache or facial pain) along with clenching, bracing, or grinding (bruxing). This will eventually result in occlusal wear and additional loss of vertical dimension.

Temporomandibular Joint Dysfunction

The combined effect of the depressive and retrusive forces on the mandible, the accompanying constriction of the antagonist elevator

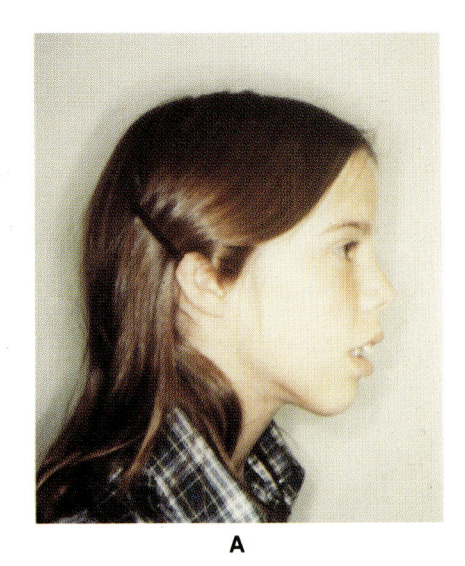

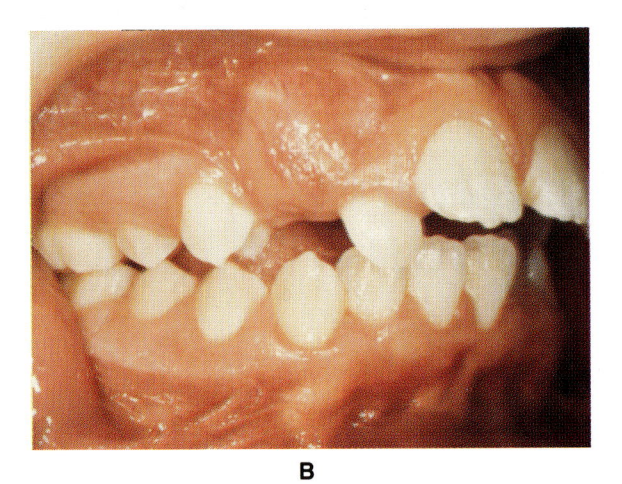

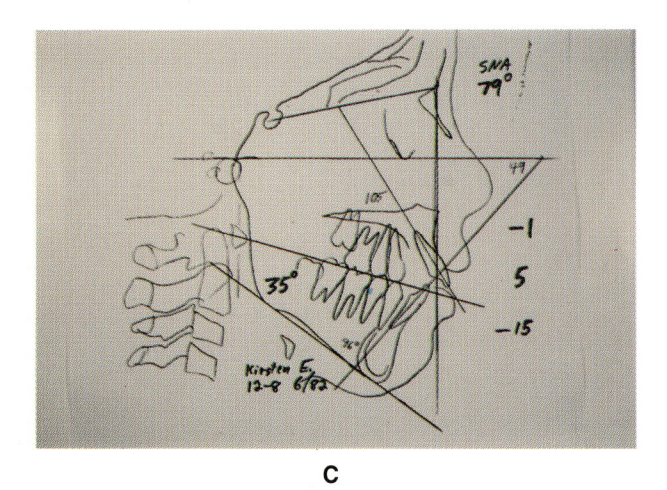

Fig. 13-10, A–C. Long face syndrome.

CHAPTER 13 Postural Consideration for the Orthodontic Patient 331

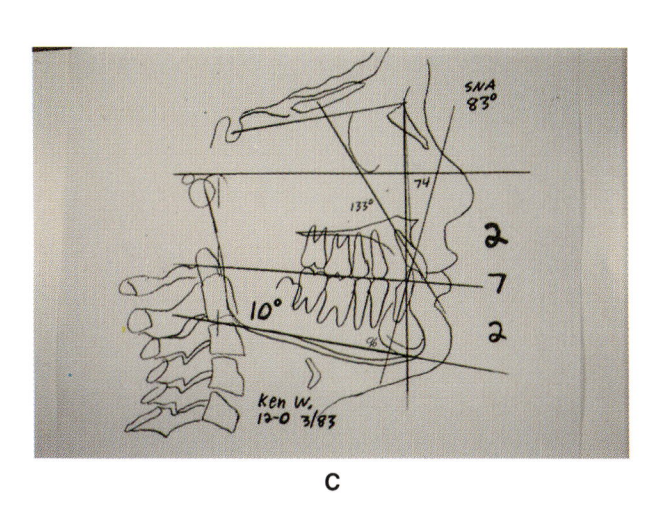

Fig. 13-11, A-C. Forward head posture/mandibular retrusion and decreased vertical dimension.

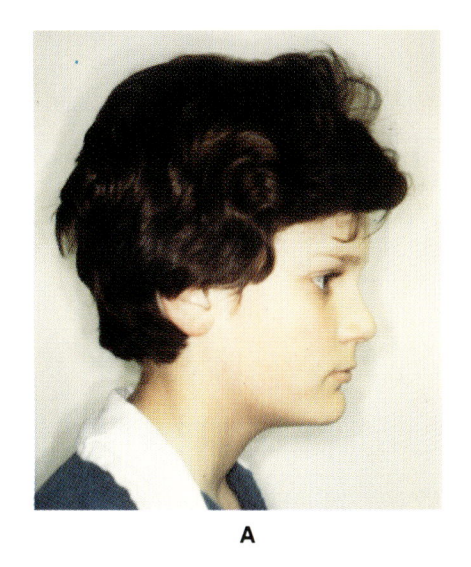

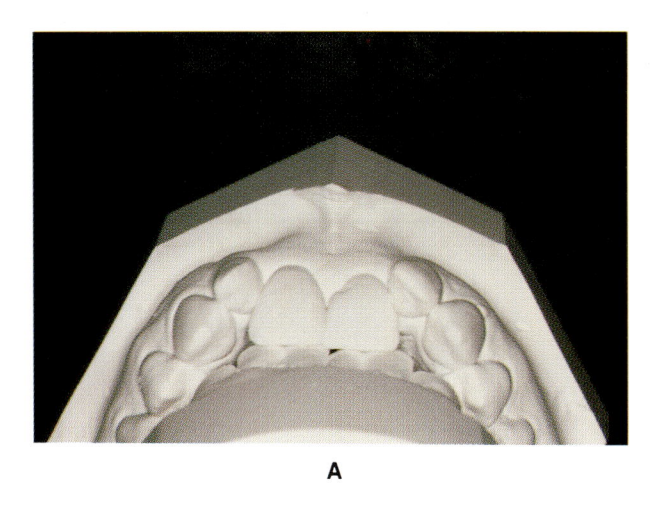

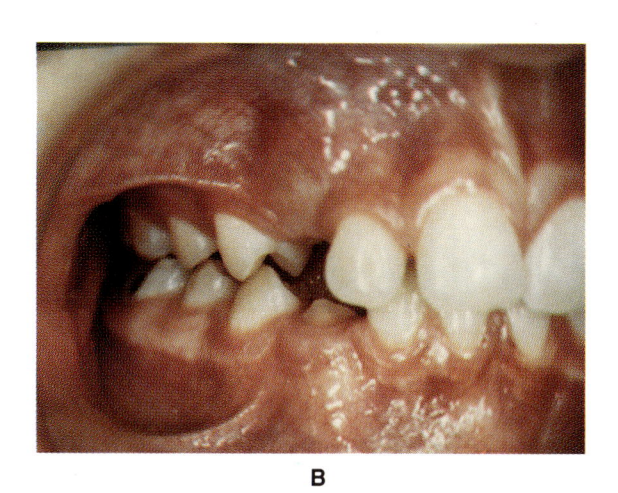

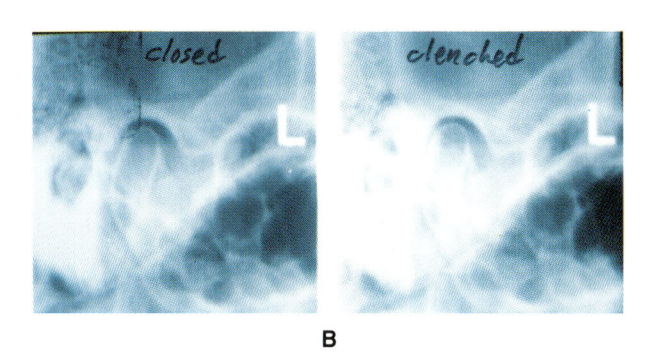

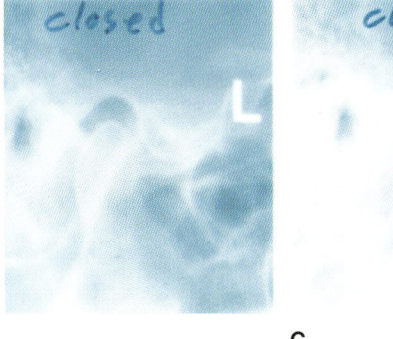

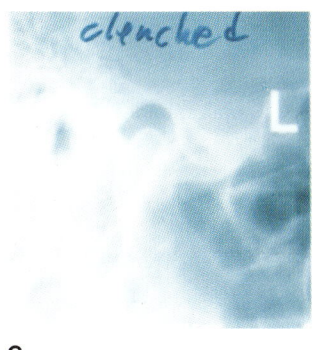

Fig. 13-12, A-C. Temporomandibular joint dysfunction.

muscles, and the resulting clenching, grinding, and bracing—all these lead to posteriorly and superiorly placed condyles within the glenoid fossa. This leads to lack of joint space and an anterior and/or medial displacement of the meniscus, resulting in abnormal joint mechanics. Note the retruded position of the maxillary central incisors (Fig. 13-12A) and the position of the condyle in the transcranial (Fig. 13-12B) compared with a normally positioned condyle (Fig. 13-12C).

332 New Concepts in Craniomandibular and Chronic Pain Management

```
                    ┌─────────────────────┐
                    │  Nasal Insufficiency │
                    │  (Diminished Airway) │
                    └──────────┬──────────┘
                               ▼
                    ┌─────────────────────┐
                    │    Mouthbreathing    │
                    └──────────┬──────────┘
                               ▼
                    ┌─────────────────────┐
          ┌─────────│ Forward Head Posture │─────────┐
          │         └──────────┬──────────┘         │
          ▼                    ▼                    ▼
┌──────────────────┐ ┌──────────────────┐ ┌──────────────────┐
│ Increased Tension│ │ Increased Activity│ │ Increased Relative│
│  of Hyoid Muscle │ │  of Back Muscle   │ │   Weight of Head │
└────────┬─────────┘ └────────┬──────────┘ └────────┬─────────┘
```

Flow continues through: Lowered Tongue → Maxillary Arch Constriction → Maxillary Dental Crowding; Depressive and Retrusive Force to the Mandible → Mandibular Arch Constriction → Mandibular Dental Crowding; Posteriorly Displaced Condyles; Contraction of Antagonist (Elevator) Muscles → Superiorly Displaced Condyles → TMJ Dysfunction; Vertebral Compression → Cervical Spine Problems; Clenching Grinding Bracing Bruxing → Insufficient Vertical Eruption of Posterior Teeth, Occlusal Wear, Muscle Contraction Pain (Headaches); → Loss of Vertical Dimension.

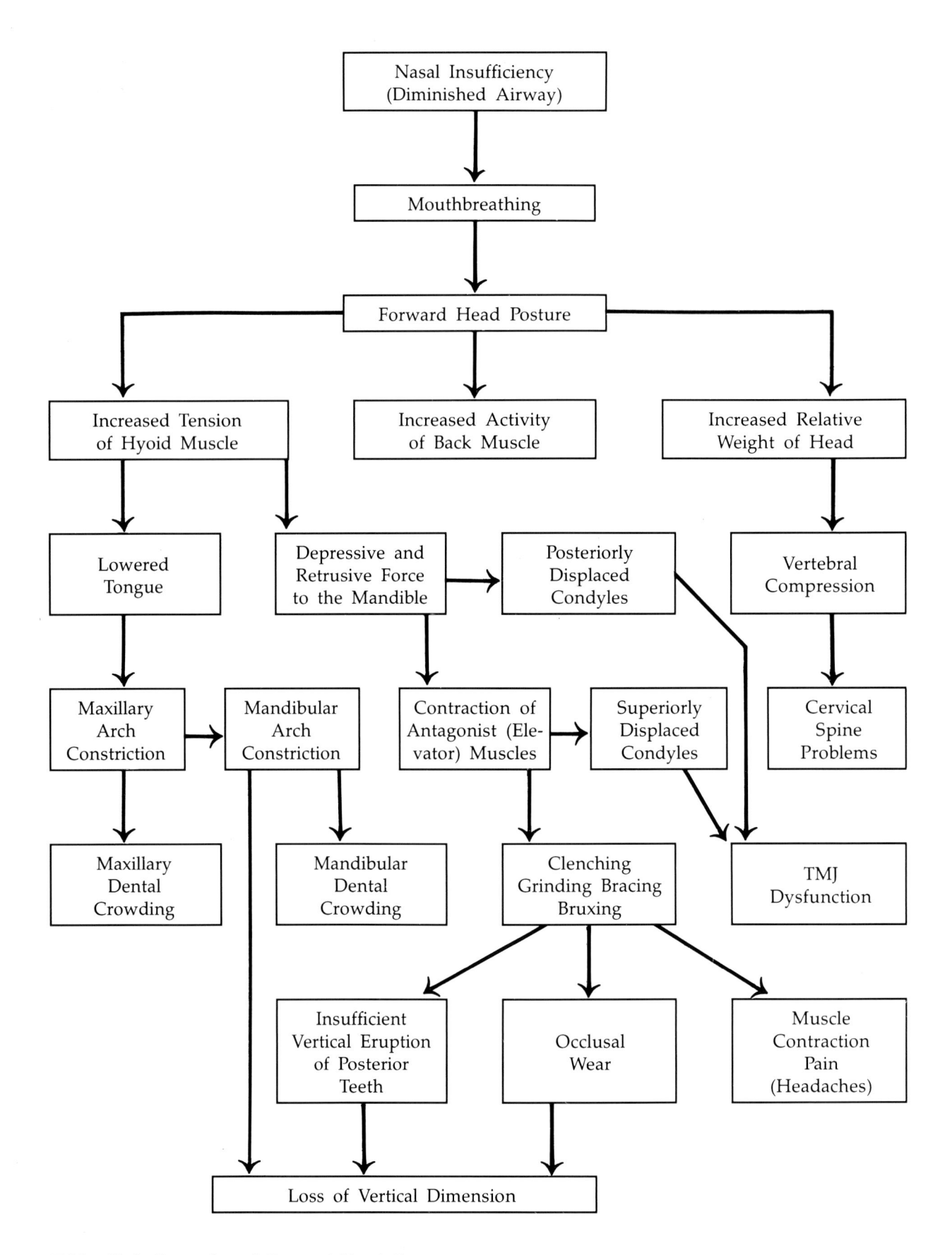

Table 13-1. Dynamics of Forward Head Posture

Cervical Spine Dysfunction

The head comprises about 10% of the body's weight when it is in a normal orthostatic position. In a situation where there is forward head posture, the relative weight of the head increases as the head comes forward. This increased leverage leads to vertebral compression, resulting in cervical spine problems.

CONCLUSION

We are entering an era of treatment in which the head, neck, and shoulders must be considered as a single functional unit. Sixty to seventy percent of all orthodontic patients who enter a practice for evaluation of dental problems exhibit signs and/or symptoms of head, neck, and shoulder dysfunction. Because of the influence of head position on the craniofacial complex, postural considerations must become a standard part of the diagnostic evaluation. It is the hope of the authors that the consideration of these factors will result in increased accuracy of diagnosis and more appropriate treatment.

SUGGESTED READING

Angel JL. Factors in temporomandibular joint form. *Am J Anat*. 1948;83:223-246.

Bjork A. Variations in the growth pattern of the human mandible: longitudinal radiographic study by the implant method. *J Dent Res*. 1963;42:400-411.

Bowbeer GRN. The five keys to facial beauty and TMJ health. *The Functional Orthodontist*. May/June 1985;2:12-29.

Bowbeer GRN. The sixth key to facial beauty and TMJ Health. *The Functional Orthodontist*. July/August 1987;4:2-35.

Cole P, Haight JS. Posture and nasal patency. *Am Rev Respir Dis*. March 1987;129:351-4.

Colquitt T. The sleep-wear syndrome. *J Prosthet Dent*. January 1987;57:33-41.

Darlow LA, Pesco J, Greenberg MS. The relationship of posture to myofascial pain dysfunction syndrome. *J Am Dent Assoc*. January 1987;114:73-75.

Fonder AC. The dental distress syndrome (DDS). *Basal Facts*. 1984;6:17-29.

Funakoshi M, Fujita N, Takehana S. Relations between occlusal interference and jaw muscle activities in response to changes in head position. *J Dent Res*. July/August 1976;55:684-690.

Gelb H. A review correlating the medical-dental relationship in the craniomandibular syndrome. New York University of Dent. 1971;41:163.

Heloe B, Heiberg AN, Krogstad BS. A multiprofessional study of patients with myofascial pain-dysfunction syndrome. I. *Acta Odontol Scand*. 1980;38:109-17.

Jarvinen S. Relation of the SNA angle to the saddle angle. *Am J Orthod*. June 1980;78:670-73.

Joseph R. The effect of airway interference on the growth and development of the face, jaws, and dentition. *Int J Orofacial Myology*. July 1982;8:4-9.

Klein JC. Nasal respiratory function and craniofacial growth. *Arch Otolaryngol Head Neck Surg*. August 1986;112:843-9.

Linder-Aronson S. Respiratory function in relation to facial morphology and the dentition. *Br J Orthod*. April 1979;6:59-71.

Linder-Aronson S, Sheikoleslam A. Changes in postural EMG activity in the neck and masticatory muscles following obstruction of the nasal airways. *Eur J Orthod*. November 1986;8:333-41.

Lowe AA, Takada K, Yamagata Y, Sakuda M. Dentoskeletal and tongue soft-tissue correlates: a cephalometric analysis of rest position. *Am J Orthod*. October 1985;88:333-41.

Luzi V. The CV value (combined variation) in the analysis of sagittal malocclusions. *Am J Orthod*. June 1982;81:478-80.

Martens DM. Tonsils, adenoids, and the airway. *Int J Orthod*. March 1979;17:8-13.

McNamara JA. Influence of respiratory pattern on craniofacial growth. *Angle Orthod*. October 1981;51:269-300.

Mews JR. Factors influencing mandibular growth. *Angle Orthod*. January 1986;56:31-48.

Mohl ND. Head posture and its role in occlusion. *NY State Dent J*. January 1976;42:17-23.

Passero PL, Wyman BS, Bell JW, Hirschey SA, Schlosser WS. Temporomandibular joint dysfunction syndrome: a clinical report. *Phys Ther*. August 1985;65:1203-7.

Preston CB. Chronic nasal obstruction and malocclusion. *Tydskr Tandheelkd Ver S Afr*. November 1981;36:759-63.

Quinn GW. Airway interference and its effect upon the growth and development of the face, jaws, dentition and associated parts "The portal of life." *NC Dent J*. Winter/Spring 1978;61:28-31.

Quinn GW, Pickrell KL. Mandibular hypoplasia and airway interference. Endangerment of life and impairment of health: laryngeal-pharyngeal obstruction. *NC Dent J*. Summer/Autumn 1978;61:19-24.

Richter HJ. Obstruction of the pediatric upper airway. *Ear Nose Throat J*. May 1987;66:209-11.

Rocabado M. Biomechanical relationship of the cranial, cervical, and hyoid regions. *J Craniomandib Prac*. June/August 1983;1.

Rubin RM. Facial deformity: a preventable disease?. *Angle Orthod*. April 1979;49:98-103.

Rubin RM. The effects of nasal airway obstruction. *J Pedod*. Fall 1983;8:3-27.

Schulhof RJ. Consideration of airway in orthodontics. *J Clin Orthod*. June 1978;12:440-4.

Shaughnessy TG. The relationship between upper airway obstruction and craniofacial growth. *J Mich Dent Assoc*. September 1983;65:431-3.

Stoll V. The importance of correct jaw relations in cervico-oro-facial orthopedia. *Basal Facts*. Spring 1977;2:34-9.

Subtelny JD. Effect of diseases of tonsils and adenoids on dentofacial morphology. *Ann Otol Rhinol Laryngol*. March/April 1975;84:50-4.

Subtelny JD. Oral respiration: facial maldevelopment and corrective dentofacial orthopedics. *Angle Orthod*. July 1980;50:147-64.

Wildman AJ. The motor system: a clinical appraisal. *Dent Clin North Am*. October 1976;20:691-705.

Williams BT. Appropriate application of therapeutic exercises. *J Am Dent Assoc*. September 1987;115:390.

Yerkes IM. Challenges in use and removal of splints. *The Functional Orthodontist*. November/December 1984;1:34-36.

Yerkes IM, Witzig J. Functional Jaw Orthopedics: Mastering More Than Technique. In: Gelb H, ed. *Management of Head, Neck, and TMJ Pain and Dysfunction*. St. Louis, Mo: Ishiyaku EuroAmerica; 1991.

Chapter 14

Foot Malfunction and Its Relationship to Craniomandibular Disorders

Howard J Dananberg, DPM

THE FOOT/BODY RELATIONSHIP

The foot has often been viewed as merely an end of the human body, and as such, the foot's functioning has often been thought to have little effect on the body as a whole. But many recent papers have described the effect of foot treatments (e.g., orthotics) on various parts of the skeletal system.[1] Since these effects are well documented, the "foot as an end structure" viewpoint must be in error.

The foot, as odd as this may initially sound, is actually at the center of the physical forces acting on the body while it is walking or running.[2] In a normal gait, the foot is planted as the heel strike phase occurs, and is then lifted from the ground at the time of toeoff. During the remainder of the single support phase of a step, the body must pivot over the planted foot, moving from a point just behind it to a point slightly ahead of it. In other words, the entire torso must revolve around the foot's fixed position. Considering the foot as the hub of a wheel, the body can be viewed much like a spoke, and the head, therefore, forms the circumference of the outermost circle. The foot is actually at the center of the rotation for movement (Fig. 14-1).

The physics of weight flow substantiates the view that the foot is the center of motion. When we are standing on any support surface, the surface must react with an equal and opposite force equivalent to our body weight in order to maintain adequate stabilization. This is in accordance with Newton's third law of motion. In other words, when the body "presses" down against the ground, the ground must "press" back with an equal force. The foot-to-ground interface is the center point where body weight and reactive ground force meet. All forces, be they initial or reactive, focus at this core location.

Placing the foot at the center of the body's ambulation machine allows for the first step in understanding its relationship to craniomandibular disorders.

THE TRUE SOURCE OF POWER FOR AMBULATION

Understanding the source of power for ambulation is critical in comprehending the effect of the foot on posture. For many years, it was assumed that the power for gait was

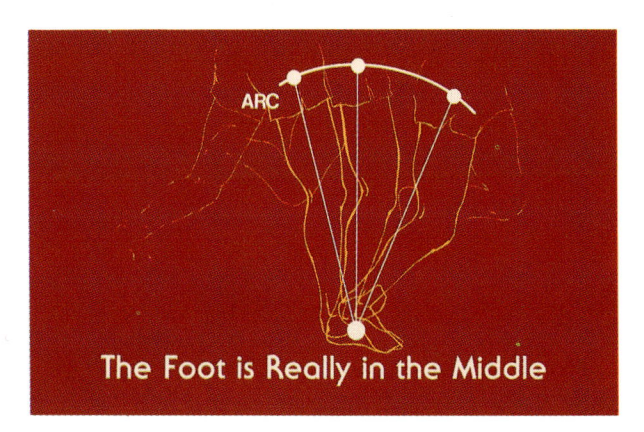

Fig. 14-1. The foot is the fixed point in the body's system for ambulation. It forms the center of all motion about its position.

located solely in the muscles of the weight-bearing limb. For instance, the calf muscles (gastrocnemius and soleus) would fire to plantarflex the ankle joint and push the body forward. This thinking, however, does not correlate with the EMG recordings of normal muscle function. In fact, the literature documents an entirely different scenario of events.

Calf muscles fire when the ankle joint dorsiflexes, and they shut off while the ankle joint plantarflexes. This is also true of the gluteals, powerful hip extensors, which fire at heel contact, while the hip flexes, and then promptly shut off for the remainder of the step, while the hip extends. The direct action of the muscles does not create the necessary motions needed for ambulation.

Taking into account the above situation, a newly published theory for understanding the kinetics of motion is presented here.[3] Four actions take place which provide the energy necessary to create a series of steps:[4]

1) Motion of the swing limb
2) Conservation of momentum
3) Gravity's action on the center of mass
4) Elastic tissue response

These four entities combine to create the power necessary to move. Each will now be briefly described.

Motion of the Swing Limb. Swing phase has also been shown to be identical in neurologically normal individuals and appears to be an instinctive motion present at birth.[5] It is "hard-wired" into the neural system. The variations are basically insignificant, regardless of age, sex, or other morphological variations. It can be considered a constant when examining gait.

The swing phase has also been called the "pull phase" of a step.[6] The action of the swing limb is to pull the center of the body forward over the stance limb. (This action is similar to the forward motion one achieves on a child's swing when pumping the legs: the body is literally pulled forward.) As the body is pulled forward, the weight-bearing limb acts as a lever against the ground, with the ball of the foot as its fulcrum point. This action essentially drives the ground backwards. Since the

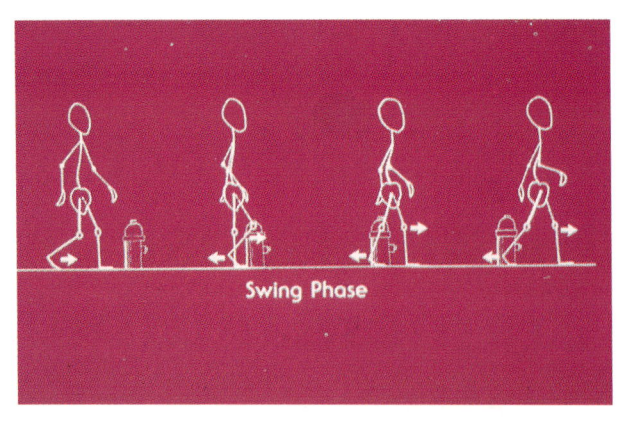

Fig. 14-2. Swing phase is in reality the pull phase. It creates the driving force and uses the stance limb as a lever, driving the ground backwards. Since the ground does not move, the body must advance.

ground is immobile, the body must advance.[7] As an analogy, imagine someone walking with crutches. The person goes forward only when they swing between the crutches. No motion occurs while the leg or legs are planted on the ground. The crutch serves as the lever, while the swinging body provides the power for motion. It is this simple principle that governs body motion. The remaining power sources assist in this basic action (Fig. 14-2).

Conservation of Momentum. A body in motion tends to stay in motion until acted upon by an outside force. The equation for momentum is as follows:

$$M = m \times a$$

M equals momentum; **m** equals the mass of the object; and **a** equals change in acceleration. According to this equation, once in motion, the body must be acted upon for it to stop.

As an aside, it can be noted at this time that heel strike creates a decelerative action upon the body. This action is overcome by the swing phase in each step. The speeding and slowing combine to create an average steady-state speed during gait. If this did not occur, then once walking began, speed would steadily increase.

Gravity's Action on the Center of Mass. The effect of gravity is always present during gait. The muscle action of the stance limb is designed to prevent it from collapsing during the single support phase of a step. That is why, during gait, muscles fire to resist motion rather than to create it.

Once the swing limb pulls the body to a vertical position over the foot, gravity will continue to pull the center of mass towards the floor. As this occurs, it acts on the stance limb, combining body weight with the action of the swing limb to drive the ground backwards. In other words, one of the essential movers for the body is its own mass.

Elastic Tissue Response. The muscles and ligaments are capable of storing and returning energy during the course of a step. R. McNeil Alexander (et al) have shown that 78% of the energy stored at heel strike can be returned later in the course of a step. This is accomplished by the stretching of structures, storing elastic energy until release is possible.

In the arch of the foot, the spring ligament courses along the apex of the underside of the dome of the arch, stretching as the arch lowers during initial contact. When the arch begins to raise (resupinate) from midstance to toeoff, this ligament assists by returning the stored energy. Many other far more complex elastic responses occur, assisting in ankle plantarflexion and hip extension during a step. The point of this chapter is not to describe all such responses, but simply to point out that they do occur.

The aggregate effect of the above actions is to efficiently drive the body forward. Note that power is created essentially extrinsic to the weight-bearing limb. The weight-bearing limb is the passive component in the system. Body weight, swing limb motion, momentum, and elastic response are the active elements. The efficiency of the system depends on the ability of the stance limb to utilize the power created by the active elements above. Failure to make use of that power, even for brief moments, leads to the accommodation, storage, and/or dissipation of the energy involved. Realizing that this failure can occur five to ten thousand times per day, several hundred million times per lifetime, the affect on the body can be seen as one of paramount importance in understanding postural imbalances.

FOOT FUNCTION

The foot serves in many capacities during the course of a single step. At initial heel strike, it must attenuate the shock of impact as well as permit adaption to the support surface. The foot must also accommodate internal rotation of the limb, which occurs immediately following heel strike. It then must be able to support the body above as the center of mass begins to pass beyond the planted foot. Last, it must provide the mechanical advantage necessary to assist in heel lift (more accurately described as body lift) prior to opposite leg contact, while accommodating external rotation of the tibia and femur brought about by pelvic response to swing phase motion.

To perform these complex tasks, the foot is provided with all the necessary mechanisms. Each aspect will be briefly explored so as to provide the background that will be needed to understand the pathological biomechanical process associated with craniomandibular disorders.

ANATOMICAL CONSIDERATIONS

The Subtalar Joint

The subtalar joint (STJ) is located beneath the ankle joint. It is formed by two bones, the talus above (the bone above the heel) and the calcaneus (heel bone) below. The STJ can be described as a screw-like differential gear which allows rotary motion occurring in one plane to be converted to triplanar rotary motion on a different axis. This all occurs during the course of every single step. It is necessary for the following reason. Since the hips connect into the hips, and not the groin, then each weight-bearing limb must undergo an externally directed rotation created by opposite swing phase. This motion is continued through toeoff, and is then redirected upon heel strike, rotating internally as part of the shock absorption mechanism. Without the STJ, each time the leg rotated inward or outward, the foot would be forced to follow suit, creating shear forces which would cause tissue damage. The STJ's ability to convert this rotary motion to actual arch raising and lowering permits stressless accommodation. These two motions are known as pronation (arch lowering) and supination (arch raising). These will be discussed in the context of their function in the chapter.

The First Metatarsophalangeal Joint

The first metatarsophalangeal joint (MTP) is located just proximal to where the great toe joins the body of the foot. It is made up of the head of the 1st metatarsal, the base of the proximal phalanx, and two small bones beneath the metatarsal head known as sesamoids. The movement of this joint is absolutely critical to normal foot function.[9] It serves many important functions with respect to the pivotal action of the body above the foot, as well as acting as a winch of sorts in assisting in the raising of the arch (supination) during the second half of the step.[10,11] Its motion is referred to as ginglymoarthrodial, meaning that the joint hinges and glides to complete its entire dorsiflexionmotion. This complex action permits the joint to flex while bearing the load of the entire body as the heel is lifted off the ground.[12]

The Plantar Aponeurosis

The plantar aponeurosis, or plantar fascia, is a structure that runs from the base of the heel to the bases of all the digits along the bottom of the arch. It is thickest at its attachment to the great toe, and thins significantly as it courses the lesser toes. It also sends slips to the skin of the ball of the foot.[13] To visualize its function, which is that of a tension band, imagine an archery bow. The string that runs from one end of the bow to the other is also a tension band. Visualize the bow being held on a table so that the concave portion faces down and the string runs across (parallel to) the table top. If force was then exerted on the top of the bow in an attempt to flatten it, the string would become taut and resist the bow's straightening. If the string were cut, the bow would then immediately flatten. The bow string would be serving as a tension band in much the same manner as the aponeurosis functions within the foot. When forces that would lower the arch present themselves during the course of a step, this structure prevents the arch ("bow") from collapsing.

FOOT FUNCTION DURING GAIT

The essence of human gait is to pass the body beyond the fixed foot. It is the foot's ability to permit this action while also completing the above mentioned tasks that makes it such a versatile structure. During the heel contact phase, the subtalar joint rotates in the direction of pronation for two distinct purposes. First, it serves to assist in shock absorption at heel strike, and second, it serves to accommodate the internal rotation taking place at that time. The shape of the underside of the heel bone also provides an additional service. Its most plantar (lower) surface is rounded, so as to serve as a rocker. This permits a rolling action and allows the body to advance from just behind the foot, at heel strike, to a point directly vertical to it when the forefoot makes ground contact. It should be noted that at this time in the step, the calcaneus reaches its peak in weight-bearing load, and then begins to gradually "unweigh" until heel lift actually occurs. This then marks the completion of the heel strike-contact phase of the gait.

From this point until weight is born by the now swinging limb (the end of the single support phase), the events which take place are critical in providing efficiency to the gait. The power segments, which were discussed earlier in the chapter, now begin to exert themselves. Their collective actions begin to "unweigh" the heel, as well as the body above, from the ground.

The line representing the center of weight passes through the foot toward the toes as the body is being pulled forward. When this imaginary line is between the great and second digits, a series of events occur which can best be described as automatic natural arch support. The following will indicate how this occurs.

As body weight flows in the direction described above, the plantar aponeurosis is called into action. It tightens significantly, causing the calcaneus and cuboid bone (just ahead of the calcaneus on the lateral side of the foot) to align in such a manner so as to "lock" the foot and prevent arch collapse.[10] This locked position is maintained while the pull of the swing limb unweighs the calcaneus from the ground. When the heel is finally bearing no more weight, heel lift occurs.

Heel lift is no simple task. Since the opposite limb is swinging and off the ground,

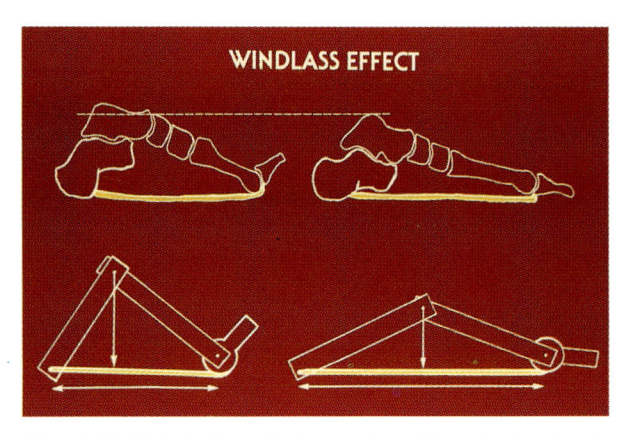

Fig. 14-3. This is the windlass effect. The plantar fascia is pulled taut by the winch-like action of the great toe, raising the arch in the process. This is a completely mechanical action, not requiring any muscle activity or other outside influence.

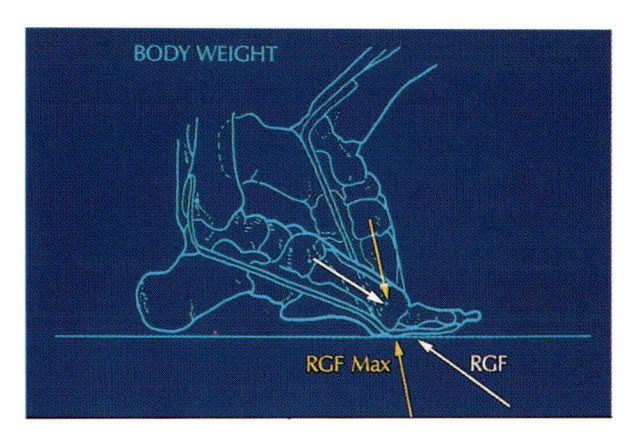

Fig. 14-4. While the heel is raised, the metatarsals move through the sagittal plane towards vertical, passing increasing weight to the support in the process. This, in turn, creates greater ground reaction force as the motion occurs.

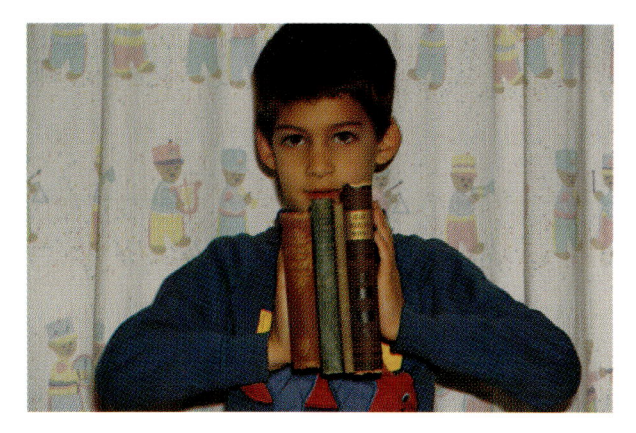

Fig. 14-5. The locking wedge effect. The books in the middle will not fall out while adequate pressure is maintained.

the stance limb is maintaining all the body's weight. Heel lift is in reality body lift, as the center of mass is raised slightly during this phase.[14] Joint mechanics within the body operate in such a manner that the center of mass does not have to be lifted a great distance, but lifting of body weight must occur.

All this time in the step, several coordinated events take place. First, the body must continue to advance forward over the planted foot. Second, the foot must supinate to accommodate external rotation of the tibia and femur. Third, the foot itself must remain stable, as the forces present during this phase can reach two to three times that of the body weight. Last, mechanically advantaged assistance in raising body weight is needed. It is at this time that the first metatarsophalangeal joint (MTP) serves all the above needs.

Just as the heel served as a rocker during a preceding phase, the head of the metatarsal now allows the body to pivot over it. As this occurs, the first MTP begins to flex or hinge backwards. This action activates the aponeurosis in two ways. The actual bending of the toe joint increases the tension being exerted on the aponeurosis, pulling the heel towards the bases of the toes. This action, known as the windlass effect, automatically raises (supinates) the arch and rotates the tibia externally[11] to synchronize it with femoral rotation (Fig. 14-3). The second action is brought about by the strands which attach to the skin of the ball. This actually tightens the skin of the ball, holding the skin firmly in place as the metatarsal head rotates within it.[13] Its stability prevents chronic tissue tearing from shear forces acting on the surface. These soft tissue injuries would be bound to occur if the skin of the ball were held flaccid.

With the skin stable and the body advancing, the metatarsal base passes forward over the planted metatarsal head. This action brings the metatarsal shaft toward a vertical attitude with respect to the ground. As this motion occurs, a particular weight transfer property is maximized: namely, the closer a solid object is to vertical, the more weight can pass to the support surface.[8] Conversely, the more parallel a solid object is to the ground, the less weight will transfer. As the heel raises and the metatarsal moves closer to vertical, increasing weight can be passed

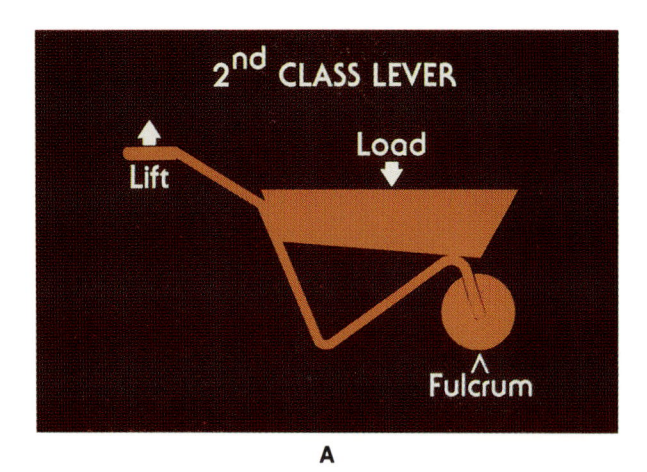

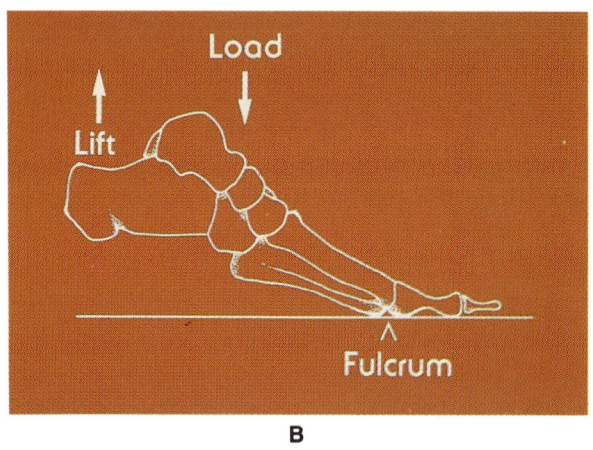

Fig. 14-6, A and B. Examining these two pictures, it can be seen how the foot provides the second class leverage which assists in raising body weight during the course of a step.

All these advantages are provided by the MTP joint. It additionally serves as a fulcrum point about which body weight is lifted at the heel off phase. The foot can be viewed as a second class lever, with the lift and load force on the same side of the fulcrum.[15] Much like a wheel on a wheelbarrow, the MTP serves to create the necessary mechanical advantage required at this time during a step (Fig. 14-6, A and B).

Summarizing, the foot provides mechanically advantaged movements for the body above it. Of paramount importance is the ability of the first MTP to dorsiflex at heel lift. This action encourages stability and efficient utilization of the pull power of the swing limb. Automatic support is created, and leverage to lift the body is provided. All actions are timed to occur simultaneously, creating a situation not unlike the gears of a clock. The ability of the normal foot to effectively make use of all these events insures normal gait and posture.

FUNCTIONAL HALLUX LIMITUS

Functional hallux limitus (FHL) has been described elsewhere.[16] It can be defined as the total inability of the first metatarsophalangeal (MTP) to hinge backwards or dorsiflex strictly during the single-support, weight-bearing phase of gait. Implied in this definition is the fact that the metatarsal base is unable to move forward through the sagittal plane while pivoting at its head. Full range of motion, however, **is present** during a non-weight-bearing examination. This range may be noted to be normal to excessive, and there may be **no complaint** of pain in and around the joint. The functional lockup of the first MTP may occur for only brief periods of time and be virtually unnoticed in gait analysis (Fig. 14-7, A and B). Other than one's clinical knowledge and/or experience, there may be no apparent reason to examine this remote joint when dealing with craniomandibular disorders.[16]

FHL is a relatively new clinical finding which has been brought to light only via computerized gait analysis. The ability to view body weight transfer via sensitive force trans-

to the ground. The ground reacts to this with an equal and opposite force directed back up the foot (Fig. 14-4). This action and reaction create what is known as the locking wedge effect, which provides the foot with sufficient force to stabilize it under the increasing strain of body weight.

The locking wedge effect can be best described as follows. Imagine removing four or five books from a library shelf. If sufficient force is exerted at either end of the stack, the books can be rotated and held parallel to the floor, and none will fall out (Fig. 14-5). It is precisely this effect that stabilizes the arch and prevents its collapse under increasing load. The bones of the feet are capable of resisting large amounts of compressive strain without fracturing. This capability is the enabling factor in a system that ingeniously develops high levels of stability as greater and greater loads are applied.

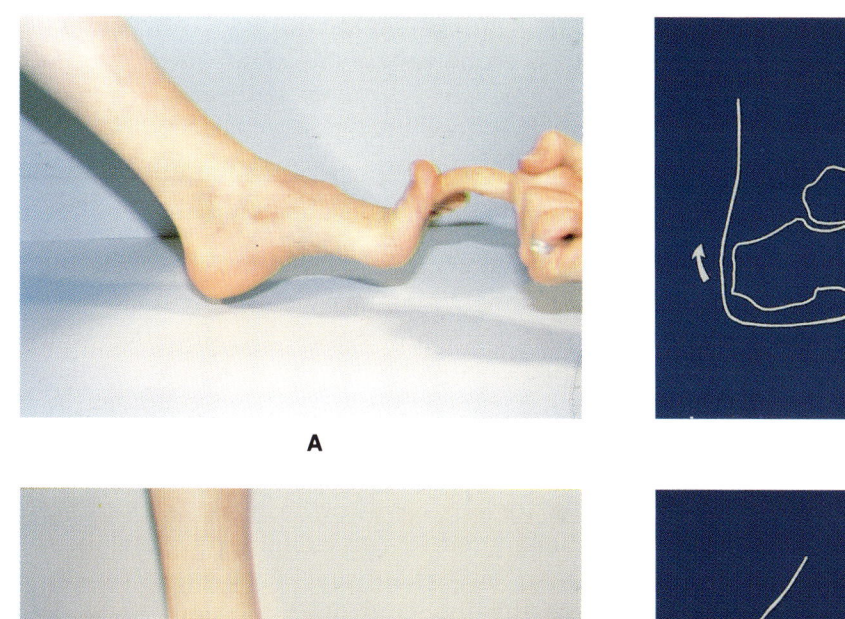

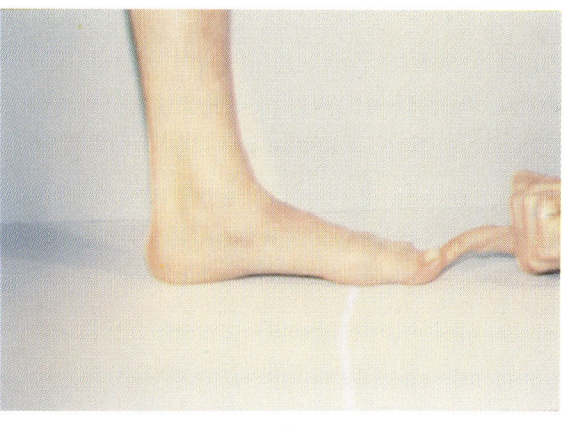

Fig. 14-7, A and B. Note the flexibility of the weight-bearing versus the locked position during stance.

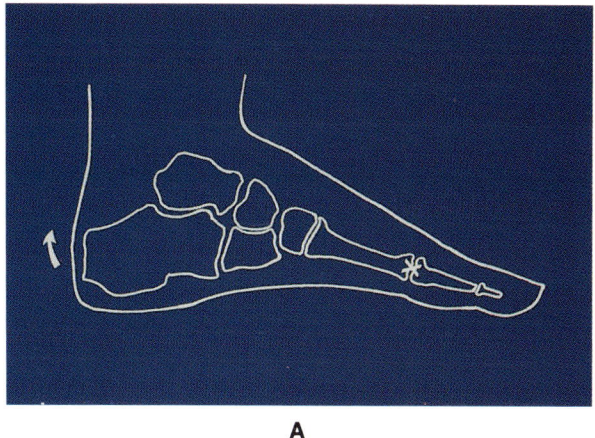

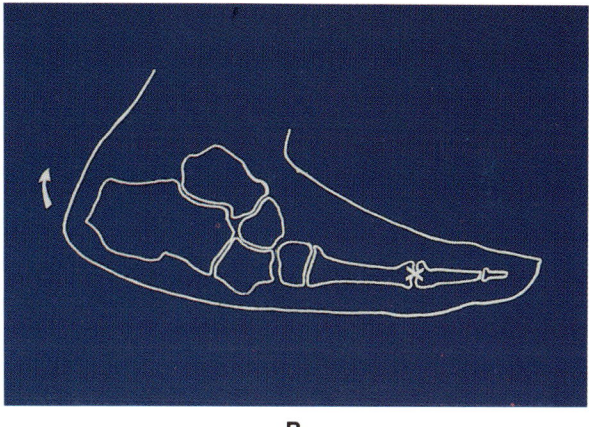

Fig. 14-8, A and B. Note the change in mid arch bones of the foot, when compensation for FHL causes arch collapse.

ducers adhered to the sole of the foot has provided the necessary clues for discovering the presence of FHL. To the naked eye, FHL is essentially invisible. Since it is the hinge effect of the 1st MTP that permits elevation of the heel from the ground, blockage of MTP motion can block heel lift from occurring.[16] The ability to see the joint bend, however, is directly related to the heel being lifted. Therefore, if FHL blocks heel lift for several moments, and the arch falls as a form of compensation, the FHL becomes hidden as the true cause of this pronation adaptation (Fig. 14-8).

The Effect of Functional Hallux Limitus on Foot Function

Earlier in this chapter, the importance of MTP hinge effect was described. Stability, supination, optimal sagittal plane motion, locking wedge effect, and efficient weight transfer were all noted. When FHL is present, all these positive movements or effects simply cannot occur. So dependent on MTP dorsiflexion are the general mechanics of the foot, that failure of motion at this joint creates havoc with efficient biomechanical process.

To truly understand the effect of FHL, it is important to recall the source of power for gait. The four factors involved are swing phase, conservation of momentum, gravity's effect on the center of mass, and elastic muscular response. What is critical to note is that all four sources are created extrinsically to any action of the weight-bearing limb. Since kinetic energy is developed to be used by the weight-bearing side, any failure in the ability to utilize this power results in the need to either store and/or somehow dissipate it.[16] It is this act of dissipation that creates the postural pathology associated with craniomandibular disorders.[17] It is important to realize that this malfunction will be repeated between five and ten thousand times on an average day. This represents the approximate number of steps taken in the course of normal daily activity. Although any single step may have no direct effect on postural alignment, when repeated day after day, year after year, the aggregate effect can create profound changes. An average person will have taken more than 87 million steps by their 30th birthday. Add athletic activity to this equation, and the number can easily reach well over 100 million steps. Ignoring the effect of foot malfunction on the erect posture can only result in partial treatment of any resulting symptomatic condition.

Compensations for Functional Hallux Limitus

Since the power to generate a step is essentially vectored straight ahead, then it would be most efficient if the body were to use this power in the same manner. The body should, in most cases, follow the path of least resistance. That would entail lifting the heel straight up and pivoting over the first and second metatarsal heads. In the presence of FHL, this is not possible. General postural alignment will then dictate the next most efficient path to follow. For example, if the hip joint, in its neutral position, is slightly externally rotated, then the foot should be slightly abducted or out toe during gait. If FHL were present in this patient, the out toe foot posture would then be exacerbated as the patient walked, rolling off the inside or medial border rather than toeing off in a straight position.

Foot posture alteration is only one way to compensate for FHL. Because gait creates a pull on the body's center mass, accommodation can take place at almost any level of the body. Also, the fact that FHL represents a sagittal plane blockade of forward motion suggests that sagittal plane accommodation is a likely sequelae.

Of the joints between the MTP and the head, many are capable of providing sagittal plane motion. What is important to remember is the element of time when considering direction of joint motion. Although the simple act of bending a joint forward through the sagittal plane is easily accomplished, doing it on the weight-bearing side during the single support phase requires a 180 degree alteration. For instance, during the late stage of the single support phase, just prior to opposite limb contact, the heel is being raised from the ground while the hip joint extends. If, however, FHL has blocked heel-off while the body is being pulled forward, the sagittal plane motion may be accommodated at the hip joint. In order for the hip to provide this necessary compensatory motion, it must flex rather than extend. This creates a slight forward lean to the waist. This can be demonstrated while watching people walk up a steep hill. The trunk must bend forward while the foot and ankle accommodate the incline of the hill. Each joint between the MTP and the head are capable of this type of adjustment to sagittal plane blockade (Fig. 14-9, A-C). The table below lists many of the major joints, followed by their normal and compensatory motions, which occur during the second half of single support.

JOINT	NORMAL MOTION	COMPENSATORY MOTION
Mid Tarsal Joint Arch	Supination	Pronation
Ankle	Plantarflexion	Dorsiflexion
Knee	Extension	Flexion
Hip	Extension	Flexion
Lumbar Spine	Lordosis	Lumbar Flexion
Cervical Spine	Lordosis	Cervical Flexion

Functional Hallux Limitus and Craniomandibular Disorders

The trigger point phenomenon within muscles of the body is a well known pathological condition.[18] The trapezius muscle, located in the upper back between the scapulae, and coursing proximally to the occipital condyles at the base of the skull, is one of the muscles most often beset by the trigger point phenomenon. Overuse of the trapezius with trigger point development has been shown to be caused by a number of different factors, including heavy overcoats, tight bra straps, whiplash from a lateral impact accident, and holding a phone by bending the neck to main-

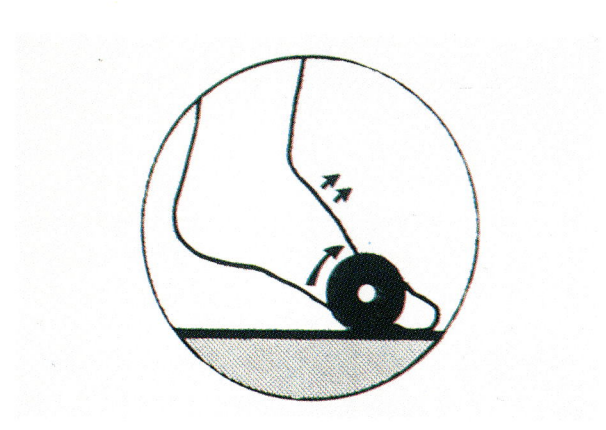

Fig. 14-9 A. The toe joint serves as a wheel, allowing the fluid movement of heel lift to occur while also allowing the digits to maintain ground contact and form the anchor point for the entire body.

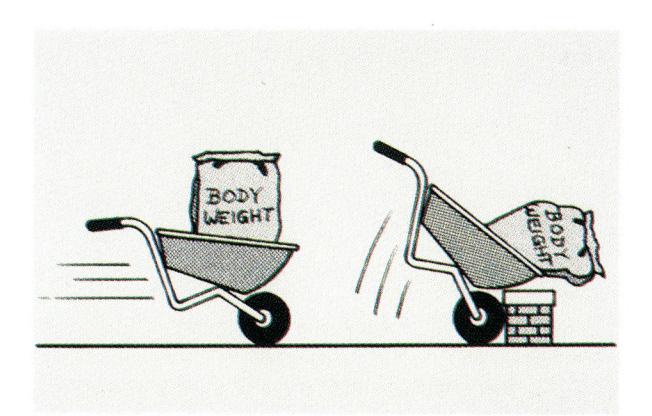

Fig. 14-9 B. Just like a wheelbarrow rolling down a path, a sudden block to forward motion will cause the contents to fall forward as momentum continues to act on the load in the wheelbarrow.

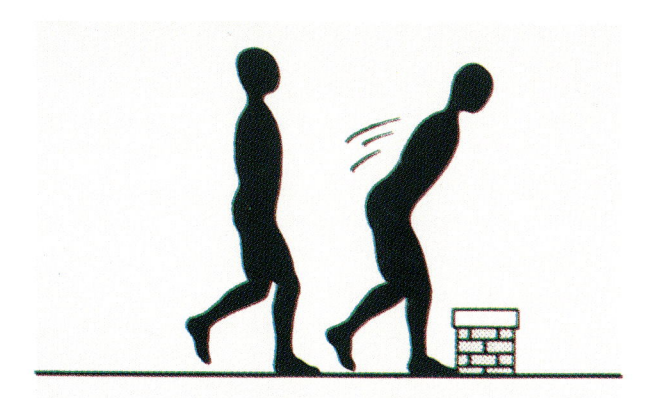

Fig. 14-9 C. When FHL is present, forward bending of the body accommodates the sagittal plane blockade it creates. When repeated a sufficient number of times, chronic injury will result.

tain it against the shoulder.[18] Walking with faulty foot mechanics has also been shown to influence the pathomechanics of trapezius overuse.[17] Trigger points within the trapezius have been shown to refer pain to areas within the lateral side of the face, angle of the jaw, neck and head.[19] These specific types of pain have been identified with the pain description associated with various craniomandibular disorders.

When compensation for FHL is created within the cervical spine, the head must drop down slightly during the single support phase. This is an abnormal motion, as the head should be maintained erect during gait, with the cervical spine increasing in lordosis during the late single support phase.

Under the above conditions, the trapezius muscle must become overly active to maintain the head in the elevated position. This form of overuse is extremely subtle and often completely overlooked. Gradually, over long periods of time, walking improperly produces continual stress to the trapezius, with the development of trigger points and the referral pain pattern described above.

Although spray and stretch techniques, massage, and other forms of therapy can all help alleviate much of the muscle tension involved,[18] it is bound to return if the etiologic agent, FHL, remains hidden and therefore untreated. It is important to remember that **NO FOOT SYMPTOMS** need to be present to create the pathomechanical stress on the trapezius.[17] This is why the problem has gone undetected for so long. It is imperative to examine the foot for this particular entity, and make appropriate referral for treatment of this asymptomatic—but causative—disorder.

EXAMINATION FOR FUNCTIONAL HALLUX LIMITUS

It is important to note that the most accurate method for detecting FHL is computerized gait analysis. There are, however, clinical tests which can also alert the treating practitioner to its presence. It is the intent of this section to provide an overview of a foot examination which can unmask the presence of FHL. Actual diagnosis and treatment of this condition should be left to to those skilled in the fabrication of foot orthotics, as this is much more complex a medical science/art than is generally believed.

In a general sense, examination of the foot consists of three distinct aspects: static non-weight bearing, static weight bearing, and gait evaluation. Each aspect will be briefly described and important highlights noted, particularly with regards to the presence of FHL. Biomechanical assessment of the foot, as well as the entire subject of gait analysis, is complex. It is not the intent of this chapter to create expertise in this practice, but rather to provide an overview so that the reader is apprised of this concept and can recognize the possibility of pathology and make the appropriate referral.

Orthotic treatment of foot malfunction only looks easy, but is, in reality, a difficult task that requires specific training and experience, as does any other medical discipline. Failed treatment that may be attributed to orthotic therapy is often the result of lack of experience and faulty device prescription rather than an actual orthotic failure. Precision is critical in device fabrication, as each step will be repeated millions of times on any given orthotic.

Static, Non-Weight Bearing Exam

In the static, non-weight bearing exam, the general range of motion of the foot joints is assessed, as well as general foot posture. The foot's general appearance should also be noted. Arch height, toe positions, and any skin lesions (callouses) are assessed. Ankle joint dorsiflexion with the knee flexed and also extended is noted. The subtalar and mid tarsal ranges are examined. It is important to note at least ten degrees of ankle joint dorsiflexion with the knee extended and at least fifteen degrees of dorsiflexion with the knee flexed. Less than those amounts indicates motion restrictions which can create significant problems.

Dorsiflexion and plantarflexion of the great toe are also checked: normal range of motion is 65 degrees. It is important to carefully examine the great toe joint in two distinct ways. First, check range of motion with the foot in the resting position. Next, with one thumb, push up on the ball of the foot, directly under the first metatarsal head, until some resistance is noted. Then, with the other thumb, attempt to flex the great toe upward while maintaining constant upward pressure on the ball. In many cases, the resistance to great toe flexion will be significant.

Static, Weight Bearing Exam

In this exam, the patient should be standing in what is known as angle and base of gait. This refers to the general direction in which the feet align during gait. To set this position, have the patient take several steps in place, then come to rest with the feet several inches apart and the toes pointing in the direction they were in while stepping. At this time, it is important for the examiner to note any difference in findings from the non-weight bearing exam.

NOTE: The patient should be standing in such a position that they can be viewed from both the front and rear. If insufficient room is available, the patient can be asked to turn. One view is not sufficient to evaluate stance position.

General assessment should be performed first. The patient's posture should be examined and general alignment noted. Change in arch height, digital contraction, and heel position should be assessed. Prominence of the medial ankle can be noted and is associated with excessive pronation, as is marked decrease in arch height as determined from the non-weight exam. Leaning toward the outside of the foot should also be noted, particularly if it occurs unilaterally. This may alert the practitioner as to foot level compensation for leg length discrepancy. An assessment of the great toe's ability to flex upwards while weight bearing should also be performed at this time. With the patient leaning slightly forward, the practitioner should squat down on one knee and attempt to raise the great toe from the ground. The patient should not assist at this time. Restriction in motion is indicative of the presence of FHL.

GAIT ANALYSIS

Gait analysis is a complex subject and several paragraphs cannot begin to describe how it is performed. Only a general overview is provided in table form to highlight some of the more important factors.

AREA OF ASSESSMENT	PURPOSE	WHAT TO WATCH FOR
Total Body	Symmetry	Sway or large amount of upper body motion. Excessive head movement.
Hip	Stability, propulsive assessment	Timing of extension as well as amount.
Knee	Stability propulsive assessment	Timing of extension and flexion, and relation of one to the other.
Feet	Alignment, Leg length	In-toe or out-toe gait. Early heel lift. Variations between feet.
Feet	FHL	Attempt to note toe bending. Watch for excessive arch collapse or delayed heel lift, especially comparing one side to the other.

TREATMENT OF FUNCTIONAL HALLUX LIMITUS

In general, the main goal in the treatment of FHL is to allow the first metatarsal to plantarflex, or move downward, during the midstance phase of gait. This action on the part of the first metatarsal permits adequate joint flexion and prevents the development of FHL.

There are three methods which can be useful in creating the maneuver: surgical, mechanical (orthotic), and shoe selection. The simplest method should be attempted first, and surgical treatment should be performed only when all else has failed. Note that surgical treatment of FHL is a new concept which involves plantarflexing the 1st metatarsal head. No significant data has been accumulated as yet regarding this method of treatment as related to the amount of plantarflexion or the best method to achieve this result.

Shoe Selection

The selection of appropriate shoes involves some simple principles. First, the shoe should fit; second, it should provide adequate support through the laces and a

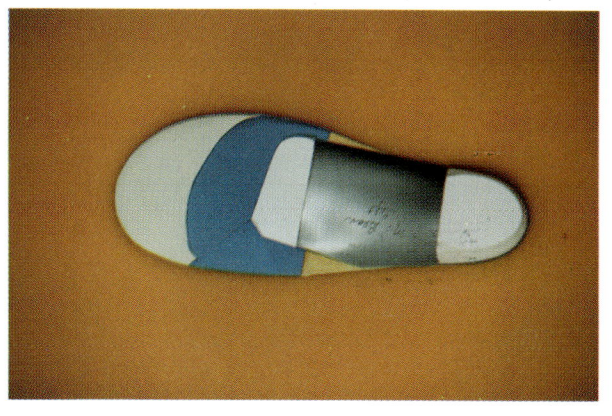

Fig. 14-10 A. Bidirectional cutout. This type is used for flexible feet with a moderate off-weight bearing arch and the suspected presence of FHL.

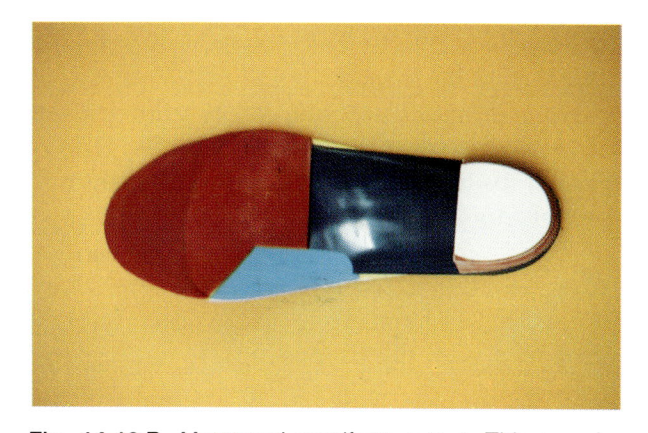

Fig. 14-10 B. Metatarsal-cuneiform cutout. This type is for flexible, flat feet. As a rule of thumb, the flatter and/or more flexible the foot, the larger the cutout.

strong heel counter; third, it should be flexible across the metatarsal break.

It is important to examine the patient's shoes to insure they are not excessively worn. This can be a major contributing factor to a gait imbalance. Check for heel counter weakness, breakdown, and excessive heel and/or forefoot wear. Next, recommend a good quality athletic shoe when appropriate, preferably a running shoe. When dress shoes are necessary, recommend the athletic shoe be carried with the patient and worn when greater than normal amounts of walking are contemplated.

One particular type of shoe made by the Brooks Athletic Shoe Co., Inc., is particularly good when the presence of FHL is suspected. These are known as Kinetic Wedge shoes. The Kinetic Wedge is a patented device designed to prevent FHL from developing. In mild cases, this will be sufficient for treating the problem, and in more moderate to severe cases, the use of this particular shoe with the appropriate orthotic device will be necessary. The kinetic wedge works by relieving the upwards pressure under the first metatarsal head, allowing it to undergo its normal range of plantarflexion motion, thus, preventing FHL (Fig. 14-10, A and B).

Orthotic Treatment and Prescription

Although space does not allow for the details necessary in prescribing an orthotic, some guidelines can be given. First, an orthotic is not an arch support. Rather, it is a device that should allow the foot to support itself. Any excessive pressure in the medial longitudinal arch by the orthotic will prevent its efficient function.

The shell of an orthotic can be constructed of a variety of materials. Generally, these should be fairly rigid in order to maintain proper foot alignment and permit natural support mechanics. Cushioning materials can be added to the device, but are generally not necessary, as pronation motion at contact is enhanced with the proper device, which provides a superior method of shock attenuation. All materials that comprise the shell of the device **MUST** end just proximal to (behind) the metatarsal heads. Any device that extends beyond this point will interfere with toe joint flexion and invariably worsen the pronation problem.

One of the most significant modifications that can be made on an orthotic is in the area of the first metatarsal head. The orthotic must permit full range of plantarflexion motion for this bone. Any restriction in this range will create or exacerbate FHL. There are three types of modifications, known as first ray cutouts, which will enhance this particular motion. These are the standard, bidirectional, and metatarsal-cuneiform cutouts. As a rule of thumb, the more pronated or flattened the foot, the larger the cutout should be (Fig. 14-11, A and B).

CASE PRESENTATION

This patient is a 32-year-old female with a four year history of a craniomandibular disorder. She has had numerous dental pro-

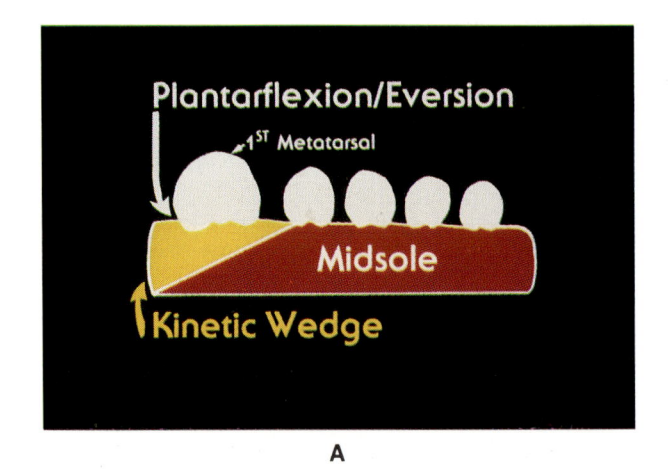

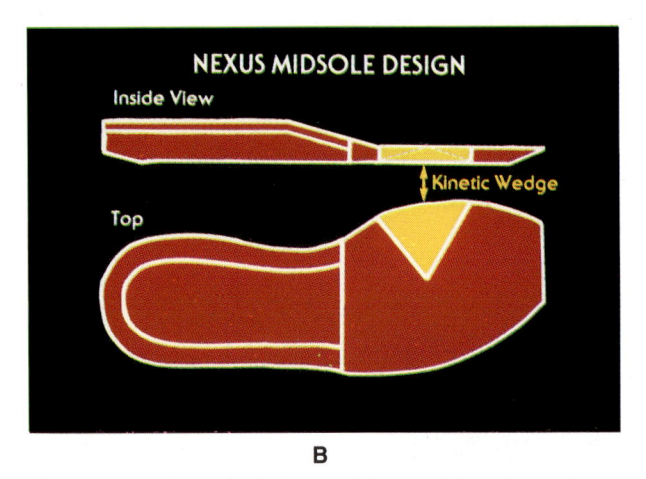

Fig. 14-11, A and B. Top, side, and head-on views of the Kinetic Wedge. The wedge area is softer and located below the head of the first metatarsal only. It permits normal motion and prevents FHL.

cedures, both conservative (bite plate) and surgical. None of these had any effect on her pain. She was referred by a physiatrist for gait analysis to determine if her problem was rooted in foot malfunction.

In Figure 14-12, the EMG recording of the left side indicates severe spasm in the trapezius muscle during gait. The right is within normal limits (symptomatic side is the left). This test was repeated and the findings confirmed. Normal trapezius function with lack of spasm was evident during relaxed posture. After an appropriate orthotic, with modifications to treat FHL as well as leg length discrepancy was prescribed, the trapezius muscle functioned normally during the gait cycle, as shown in Figure 14-13. Neck spasm was relieved with a foot orthotic, although the feet were never symptomatic.[17]

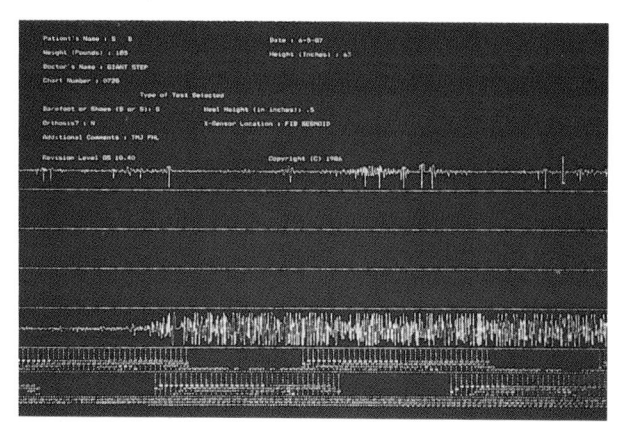

Fig. 14-12. This is an EMG recording of the trapezius muscle prior to orthotic treatment. Note the lower muscle track is in spasm (left side).

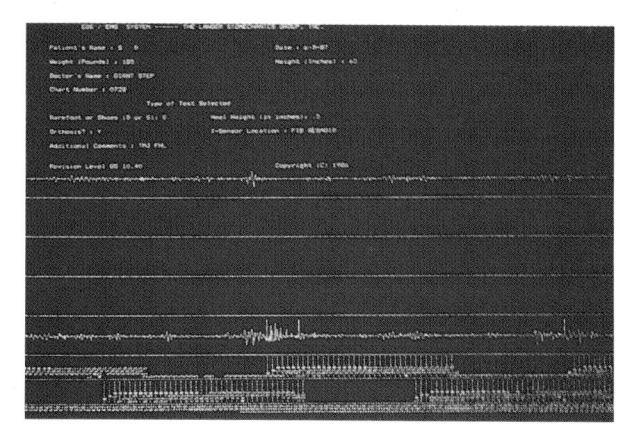

Fig. 14-13. EMG recording of the trapezius muscle after orthotic treatment. Note the similarity to the normal right side. Patient went on to become totally asymptomatic within three weeks, following four years of unsuccessful oral therapy.

CONCLUSION

Understanding that the foot lies at the center of the physics of human movement allows for the general understanding of how foot malfunction can create postural symptoms, yet remain asymptomatic and therefore disguised as the etiologic agent. Functional hallux limitus is an entity that can be totally hidden from view and yet have this profound, negative postural influence. Careful examination and diagnosis with appropriate foot treatment can have a dramatic effect on the symptomatic craniomandibular patient who otherwise would continue to live a life of constant pain. Many other chronic postural problems are rooted in foot malfunction, often FHL, and the ability to assess and treat this condition affords the practitioner a greater armamentarium with which to combat these disabling problems.

REFERENCES

1. Smith L, et al. The effects of soft and semi-rigid orthoses upon rearfoot movement in running. *J Am Podiatr Med Assoc.* April 1986;76:227-232.
2. Dananberg HJ. The foot to body perspective. *J Curr Podiatr Med.* May 1989.
3. Dananberg HJ. Functional hallux limitus and its relationship to gait efficiency. *J Am Podiatr Med Assoc.* June/July 1986.
4. Dananberg HJ. Power of movement. *J Curr Podiatr Med.* June/July 1989.
5. Cook T, Cozzens B. Human solutions for locomotion; the initiation of gait. In: Herman R, ed. *Neural Control of Locomotion.* New York, NY: Plenum Press; 1976.
6. Claeys R. The analysis of ground reaction forces in pathologic gait. *International Orthopaedics.* Spring 1983;113-119.
7. Dananberg HJ. Functional hallux limitus and its relationship to gait efficiency. *J Am Podiatr Med Assoc.* November 1986.
8. Root M, et al. *Abnormal and Normal Function of the Foot.* Los Angeles, Calif: Clinical Biomechanics Corp; 1977.
9. Inman, et al. *Human Walking.* Baltimore, Md: Williams and Wilkins; 1981.
10. Moller-Bosjen, Finn, et al. Significance of free dorsiflexion of the toes in walking. *Acta Orthop Scand.* 1979;50:471-479.
11. Hicks JH. The mechanics of the foot, II, the plantar aponeurosis and the arch. *J Anat.* London; 1954;25-30.
12. Shereff J. Kinematics of the first metatarsal joint. *J Bone Joint Surg* [Am]. March 1986;68-A:392-5.
13. Bosjen-Moller, F, et al. Plantar aponeurosis and internal architecture of the ball of the foot. *J Anat.* 1976;121:599-611.
14. Landry M, et al. Biomechanical principles in common running injuries. *J Am Podiatr Med Assoc.* January 1985;75:48-51.
15. Brachman PR. *Mechanical Foot Disorder.* Winona, Mn: The Leicht Press; 1946.
16. Dananberg HJ. Functional hallux limitus and its relationship to gait efficiency. *J Am Podiatr Med Assoc.* 1986;648-652.
17. Dananberg HJ. Functional hallux limitus and its effect on temporomandibular joint dysfunction syndrome. *J Curr Podiatr Med.* August 1988.
18. Travell G, Simons G. Myofascial pain and dysfunction. *The Trigger Point Manual.* Baltimore, Md: Williams and Wilkins;1983.
19. Travell G. Temporomandibular joint pain referred from muscles of the head and neck. *J Prosthet Dent.* July/Aug 1960;745-763.

Chapter 15

Applied Kinesiology and The Stomatognathic System

David S. Walther, DC

Applied kinesiology is a system of evaluating body function that is unique in the healing arts. It originated when Goodheart[22] began using a system of manual muscle testing[29] to examine for causes of structural imbalance and dysfunction. In the early use of this system, treatment was applied directly to the involved muscle to enhance structural function. Continued investigation found many therapeutic methods effective in returning normal muscle function. Today therapeutic effectiveness, in applied kinesiology, is found among spinal and extraspinal manipulation, various reflex techniques, cranial manipulation, acupuncture meridian balancing, and nutritional support. A wide range of therapeutic approaches exists within these groups.

One of the more unique factors of an applied kinesiology examination is how it reveals the interaction of systems and organs that takes place throughout the body. The tremendous amount of knowledge in health care today is a mixed blessing. It has caused the development of high levels of specialization. Unfortunately, a doctor's dedicated interest in a specialty may result in tunnel vision, limiting awareness of integrating factors. Many cardiologists see no further than the circulatory system; podiatrists may fail to recognize the influence of foot function on headaches and other remote health problems; and chiropractors and dentists may limit their interest to the spine and stomatognathic area, respectively.

Applied kinesiology examination enables the physician to determine 1) where correction is needed, 2) whether the corrective effort is effective, and 3) whether the correction is maintained by the patient's body. Application of examination, treatment, and re-examination in applied kinesiology has revealed that the cause of a problem is often remote from the symptomatic pattern. Similarly, the failure of a correction to hold may be due to a cause remote from the correction site. Examples of this include corrections of lower back dysfunction that are lost because of temporomandibular joint dysfunction; occlusion that continues to change because the cervical spine is unstable; and head, neck, and jaw pain resulting from foot dysfunction, even when there is no foot or ankle pain. First, we will consider the integration within the stomatognathic system.

The term "stomatognathic" is coined from the combined forms of "stomato," referring to the mouth, and "gnath," denoting relationship to the jaw;[17] thus it usually refers to the mouth and jaw, which I will call the stomatognathic area. In this discussion, we will look at a more comprehensive function referred to as the stomatognathic system. Shore[47] states that the stomatognathic system has components of "... the bones of the skull, the mandible, the hyoid, the clavicle and the sternum; the muscles and the ligaments; the dentoalveolar and the temporomandibular joints; the vascular, the lymphatic and the nerve supply systems; and the soft tissues of the head; the teeth." As support for including so much structure under the term "stomatognathic system," Shore goes on to explain that an organ —such as the heart or liver—can be dissected anatomically, but a system such as the stomatognathic must be studied as an integrated, physiologically functioning whole. We agree; it is necessary to study the interactions of the structures comprising the system, rather than

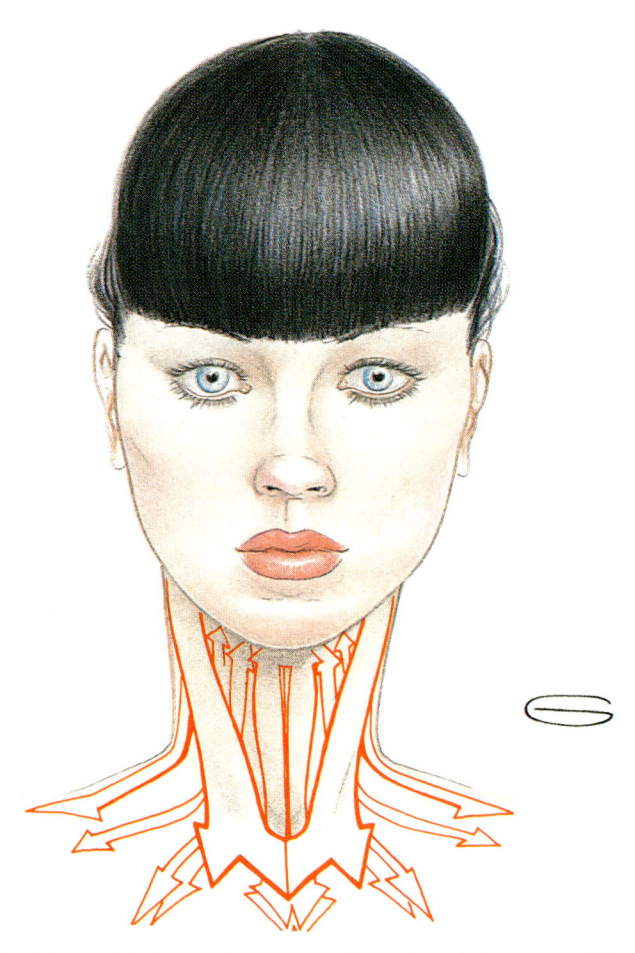

Fig. 15-1. Symmetrical muscle balance from the right to the left side.

studying individual tissues and structures as single entities.

MUSCLES OF THE STOMATOGNATHIC SYSTEM CLOSED KINEMATIC CHAIN

Head-to-Shoulder Girdle Musculature

The muscles connecting the head to the shoulder girdle are not typically thought of as a group for study. Usually these muscles are grouped as postural, deep spinal, supra- and infrahyoid muscles, and muscles of mastication. In the context of the stomatognathic system, they need to be considered as a muscle complex because they form a closed kinematic chain; when one muscle functions, other muscles must adapt because they are part of the complex. We first will consider the groups listed above, then put the interaction of the muscles into perspective to see how dysfunction of one division is capable of affecting other areas in the total complex.

Proper action of various muscles in this complex is important for normal body function. Some muscles are responsible for head balance to maintain proper equilibrium and orientation in space. Others in the closed kinematic chain are responsible for mastication, while interaction with another group is needed for swallowing. The important point is that the muscle groups of mastication, hyoid, and posture are interrelated in these activities.

The interaction of the stomatognathic system's closed kinematic muscle chain is not limited to this area; ultimately, applied kinesiology examination reveals that muscles, structures, and functions remote from the current discussion may become involved. It is adequate for now to recognize the influence of the lower body on the stomatognathic system. For example, there is rhythmic, alternate facilitation and inhibition of the sternocleidomastoid and upper trapezius muscles when

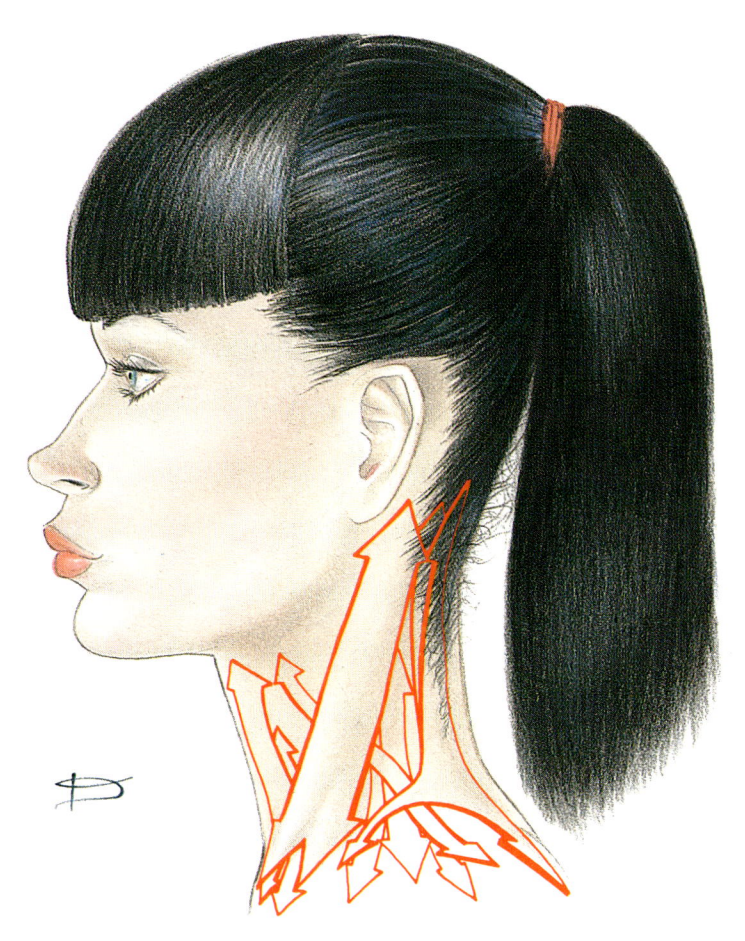

Fig. 15-2. Balance of the head-on-neck, and neck-on-body, is from regulation of muscles that are very different when compared anterior to posterior.

an individual walks or runs. These muscles pull into the cranium, influencing the cranial primary respiratory system. In addition, other activities, such as extensor muscle facilitation from the positive support mechanism of the proprioceptors of the foot and interactions of the cloacal and gait reflexes, influence posture and balance. These factors must be kept in mind, because any structural strain may disturb normal activity of the stomatognathic system. As this discussion focuses on the muscles of the head-to-shoulder girdle in their usual grouping for study, keep in mind the interactions of the total complex, which will be presented later.

Postural Muscles of the Stomatognathic System

The primary postural muscles of this area are the sternocleidomastoid and upper trapezius. These and other muscles are responsible for head leveling. If the muscles had no other responsibility than this, their importance to total body organization would be paramount. The importance of organized head leveling is emphasized by people such as Alexander,[37] Barlow,[1] Tinbergen,[52] and Dart.[7,8,9] Improper head position may be a result of poor postural habits learned early in life, or it may develop as a result of injury or habits developed later in life. A common cause of imbalanced head position is disorganization of the muscles in the stomatognathic system's closed kinematic chain.

The head and neck can be out of balance as viewed from anterior to posterior, thus comparing the right with the left side. In this instance, we are dealing with basically equal muscles since one side is the mirror image of the other (Fig. 15-1). When viewed laterally, the anterior muscles in no way parallel the posterior ones (Fig. 15-2).

A very interesting presentation on body organization is tendered by Dart.[7,8,9] He states that the principles set forth "... by Alexander (are) appropriate because (they are) based on the fundamental biological fact that the relation of the head to the neck is the primary relationship to be established in all proper positioning and movement of the body." He presents convincing evidence of the importance of this relationship. When the body is not correctly oriented to the head, the neck righting and head-on-body reflexes[26] are directly influenced. Most physicians are not concerned when they observe that a patient consistently holds his head in an abnormal position; in fact, very often it is not even noticed. Is it important?

When neck righting and head-on-body reflexes are stimulated, compensatory reactions occur throughout the body in an attempt to orient with the head position. This can be summed up with the statement, "As the head goes, so goes the body." The body is constantly trying to orient with the head position. This is problematic enough in a static standing or sitting posture; it becomes even more involved when an individual walks or runs.

The sternocleidomastoid and upper trapezius muscles are alternately facilitated and inhibited to organize the neck and head with the rest of the body during gait. They are part of the body's double-spiral muscle arrangement, as described by Dart.[8] Disorganized facilitation and inhibition of these two muscles can pull into the cranium in an imbalanced manner, causing lack of harmony between the cranial and sacral primary respiratory systems. This can cause or perpetuate cranial faults, which will be discussed later. This is particularly important because both of these muscles receive part of their innervation from cranial nerve XI. The cause of sternocleidomastoid and/or upper trapezius imbalance may be from cranial faults and/or cervical spine subluxations. These muscles have a unique nerve supply; they receive both cranial and spinal innervation.

When muscles test weak or are hypertonic, there are several treatment techniques that AK examination may indicate as appropriate for correction.[54,55,56] There may be a localized disturbance in the muscle(s) from trigger points, improperly functioning muscle proprioceptors, and/or disharmony of the muscle with its fascia. In this case, manipulation treatment to the proprioceptors, stretch and spray technique, or fascial release treatment is needed to return the muscle(s) to normal. If this is the primary problem with the muscles, the head and neck are balanced and structure returns to normal.

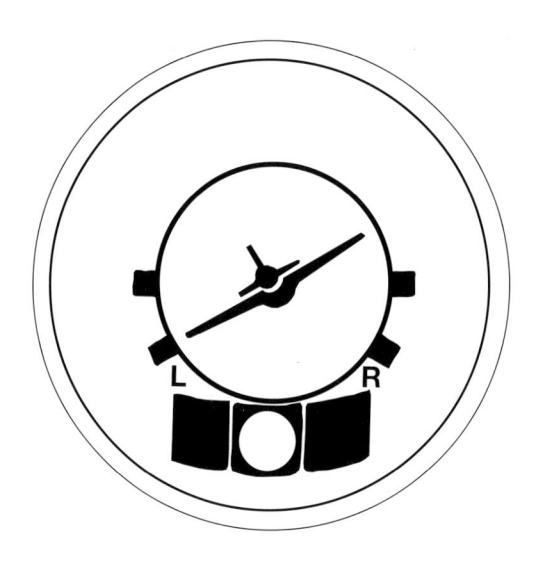

Fig. 15-3. Gyroscope indicating airplane's orientation in space.

There are additional muscles in the cervical region that need examination and if necessary, treatment. These include the scalene, longus, splenius, and semispinalis groups, as well as the smaller intrinsic muscles of the cervical-occipital region. The latter muscles are involved primarily with subluxations of the cervical spine and the occipital bone.

Spinal subluxations, malocclusion, cranial faults, and muscle imbalance can disturb the neck righting and head-on-body reflexes; any or all may cause imbalance in the closed kinematic muscle chain. If the imbalance is not caused by a primary dysfunction of these postural muscles, efforts to level the head by working with the muscles directly, changing habit patterns, or exercise, will be unsuccessful. The problem may be in some other area of the closed kinematic chain, or remote in the body. As usual, the answer is to find the primary condition and effectively treat it.

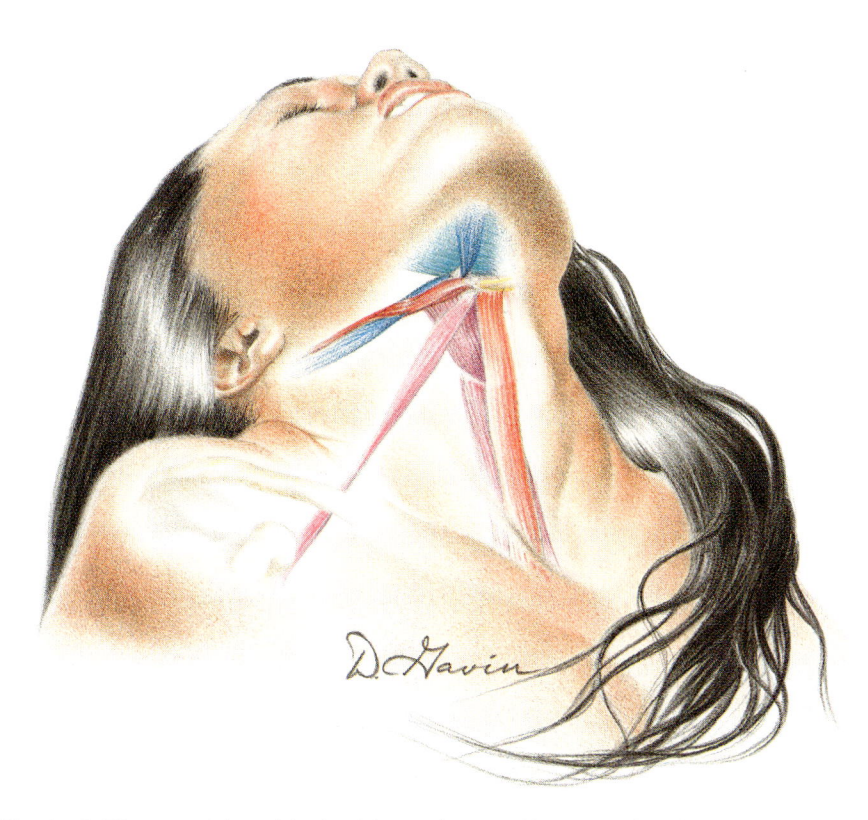

Fig. 15-4. Diverse origins of the hyoid muscles provide comprehensive proprioceptive information from the neuromuscular spindle cells of the muscles.

Hyoid Muscles

The hyoid bone is suspended from muscles much like a hammock; it has no bony communication. Its function appears to be limited to providing an attachment point for muscles. Their activity in mastication, mandibular movement, swallowing, and phonation is only briefly described in the literature. Are these activities the only contribution this neuromuscular complex makes to body organization? Goodheart[24] proposes that there is a more complex function in hyoid muscle balance. He compares the hyoid bone suspension with a gyroscope in a guidance system. A gyroscope is flexibly mounted in an object such as a missile, ship, or airplane so that it maintains its equilibrium. Sensors relay information about any change of position between the airplane and the gyroscope, providing feedback from the plane's orientation in space. If the airplane and the gyroscope are not level with each other, the instrument will show the disparity. This information is used by an autopilot or pilot to guide the vehicle (Fig. 15-3).

There are several findings in applied kinesiology examination indicating that the neuromuscular system of the hyoid provides information analogous to a gyroscope for body orientation in space, leading to proper equilibrium. The proprioceptors of the hyoid muscles appear to provide afferent information that is compared with total body position or orientation in space. The suprahyoid muscles have their origin on the skull and mandible, while the infrahyoid muscles originate from the sternum, clavicle, scapula, and thyroid cartilage. With muscles originating from such varying locations, any change of the head-neck-shoulder girdle relationship causes transmission of considerable information from the neuromuscular spindle cells of the various muscles. The central nervous system has complete information regarding the exact location of the hyoid bone at any given time (Fig. 15-4).

The stylohyoid and the posterior belly of the digastric originate on the cranium, giving specific head-to-neck information. An imbalance of these muscles may influence the cranial primary respiratory mechanism by an imbalanced pull on the structure. The sternohyoid, originating from the sternum and clavicle, relates the neck to the shoulder girdle. The omohyoid, originating clear down at the scapula, orients that structure with the neck. These origins also cause the hyoid to be part of the anterior portion of the closed kinematic chain of the head-on-shoulder girdle complex.[5,31]

Muscles of Mastication

The muscles of mastication are part of the closed kinematic chain of the stomatognathic system. Their organization is paramount for a balanced centric relation and for the teeth to accurately come into intercuspation. Perry[43] proposed a hypothesis for the neuroanatomic basis of mandibular movement that is now generally accepted and electromyographically supported. It suggests that mandibular motion is specifically guided by neuromuscular interaction to dictate the final closing position of the mandible toward intercuspation. A premature tooth contact (prematurity) can develop as a result of an ill-fitting restoration or prosthesis, or direct trauma to the tooth. Malocclusion can also develop as the result of a cranial fault, which can disturb the relationship of the right maxilla with the left.[28] Temporal bone rotation can also change the mandible's position.[35] The prematurity stimulates the periodontal ligament to send "... sensory signals into a reflex system which will guide the mandible by means of its musculature away from the areas of noxious, premature contacts. This musculature is so positioned anatomically that movements in a guiding fashion can be instituted in both the lateral or sagittal plane."[43]

Whether one opens and closes the jaw slowly or rapidly, the final tooth contact is not just by happenstance of the so-called centric relation of the mandible.[57] The closing activity is a pre-programmed, neuromuscular activity that occurs as a subconsciously learned response. The finger-to-nose neurological test is an example of the proprioceptive feedback mechanism present in the activity of the mandibular positioning reflexes. When the nervous system is functioning normally, an individual with eyes closed can easily place his finger on his nose.

In the mandibular closing reflexes, the initial information comes from the periodontal proprioceptors monitoring tooth contact. When dentition is normal, intercuspation develops with no premature or initial contacts and consequent sliding. Shore[47] states that in normal activity "... the condyles in the overwhelming majority of individuals are slightly in front of their 'most retruded' position; in other words the capsule is not in a state of unique tension but is in all its parts more or less relaxed. This in turn must be interpreted as ruling out proprioceptors of the capsule as directing the automatic closing of the jaws."

Stimulation of the periodontal proprioceptors produces a quantity of afferent information that is interpreted to cause the efferent supply to control the muscles involved in mandibular closing. This large quantity of information must be properly processed for optimal function. If there is no malocclusion, the act of stimulating the proprioceptors and the following interpretation and control of muscles is repeated over and over, and an engram develops that becomes the mandible's stable closing pattern.

With the complex interaction of the muscles of mastication, it is impressive how a normal person can snap his jaw closed from a fully opened position and have perfect coordination for complete intercuspation. Commenting on the action of the wide-open jaw snapping shut, with the muscles moving the mandible swiftly and unerringly into the centric occlusion, DuBrul[14] observes, "This is perhaps an extreme example of the nicety of coordination in all normal bodily movements." As with any other activity in the nervous system, the engram is dynamic; if there is a slight change in the occlusion over a period of time, the engram adapts to it. If, however, there is a rapid change in the occlusion from a cranial fault, dental procedure, or trauma to the tooth, the engram cannot change rapidly enough to meet the immediate demand, and malocclusion develops.

If there are many prematurities or severe malocclusion, afferent signals from the periodontal ligaments send information that can-

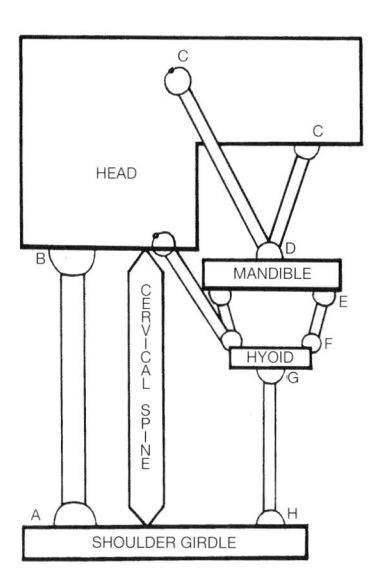

Fig. 15-5. Illustration of muscular forces in the closed kinematic chain of the head-on-shoulder girdle. The sternocleidomastoid muscle has been eliminated for clarity. (Modified from The Manual of Telephone Extension Program, Current Advances in Dentistry, University of IL, 1949.[51]

not be processed because there is no position that muscle interaction can produce for a good occlusion.[42] The resulting activity will probably be toward the optimal occlusion available under the adverse conditions.

The masticatory muscles must be routinely examined in any case of disturbed function in the stomatognathic system. Weinberg[57] lists sudden stretch, acute muscle fatigue, and acute stress syndrome as primary precipitating factors of muscle imbalance. The muscles of mastication can be secondarily involved by dysfunction of other muscles in the closed kinematic chain, or from remote factors outside the stomatognathic system.

An imbalance of the muscles of mastication, whether in deviant opening or closing of the mandible or other mandibular malposition, will influence hyoid muscle activity, thus changing the afferent information from their neuromuscular spindle cells.

MUSCLES OF HEAD-ON SHOULDER GIRDLE CORRELATION

All the muscles discussed comprise a closed kinematic chain, with each muscle interdependent on the activity of the other muscles.[3,5,20,31,41,48] The closed kinematic chain is nicely illustrated by a diagram originally presented in 1949 through the University of Illinois.[51] It is amazing that more interest and attention have not been given to improving the balance and organization of these structures and muscles (Fig. 15-5).

The activity of the posterior cervical group (A-B) must equal the activity of the anterior cervical group (C-H) for equilibrium to be present. Inhibition of the posterior group with no change in the anterior group will cause the head to tilt forward. Increased activity of the posterior group with no change in the anterior group will cause the head to tilt backward. Change in any section of the anterior group, whether it be the mandibular elevators (C-D), suprahyoid (E-F), or infrahyoid (G-H), will influence the entire group. To maintain the head in equilibrium and have mandibular elevation, there must be contraction of the mandibular elevators concurrent with inhibition of the suprahyoid muscles; otherwise, the head would bob up and down when a person chews or talks because the anterior portion of the closed kinematic chain fails to equalize the posterior division.[59]

The complex of hyoid and masticatory muscles contributes to anterior support (Fig. 15-5). Dynamic activity takes place during the process of chewing and swallowing. During trituration, the mandibular elevators are complexly activated. As the jaw closes, there must be inhibition of the suprahyoid muscles to maintain hyoid stability. While the suprahyoid muscles relax, the infrahyoid muscles stabilize the hyoid's position. The next activity is to swallow. The hyoglossus must relax to allow the tip and middle of the tongue to elevate and press against the palate. The suprahyoid muscles contract, elevating the hyoid; this is facilitated by inhibition of the infrahyoid muscles.

Postural change influences the activity of the muscles of mastication[32] and also the rest position of the mandible.[13] Even more important is the interaction of masticatory muscles with head position related to occlusion. Funakoshi et al.[20] demonstrated balanced electromyographic responses in the muscles of mastication with different head positions when the occlusion was normal; the EMG response became unbalanced in the presence of malocclusion that was artificially produced by a molar overlay, causing a premature contact. In the case of malocclusion that was equilibrated to correct occlusion, the electrical activity of the muscles changed from imbalanced to balanced.

There are many clues indicating imbalance or disorganization of the muscles in the stomatognathic closed kinematic chain. These observations are called "body language" in applied kinesiology. Dysfunction readily reveals itself if one understands the language. Obvious is the tilted, rotated, or head forward position. Limited cervical range of motion or pain on motion will usually affect other areas in the system. There should be economy of body movement, that is, a specific action should not have ancillary movement not necessary to the task at hand. Poor function is indicated when there is slight bobbing of the head with chewing. Opening the mouth should consist of simply dropping the mandible. A person who is disorganized opens his mouth by tilting the head backward while dropping the mandible. This indicates disorganization; describing this, Goodheart says they "...open their heads."

CRANIAL FAULTS

Proper movement of the cranial bones, as described by Sutherland,[50] is necessary for optimal health. The autonomous movement has been objectively measured by Frymann[18] and others. This movement also constitutes a closed kinematic chain. With normal function there is predictable movement of the cranial bones. The motion continues throughout life, cycling 10-14 times per minute, and is called "the primary respiratory mechanism."[50] The motion is separate from the heart or breathing rate; however, cranial motion is enhanced by thoracic respiration. Although this influence is always present, relaxed breathing and primary respiration do not always parallel.

Cranial motion is a combination of bending bone and suture motion. The motion between the sphenoid and the occiput is in the sagittal plane (Fig. 15-6). There is a flexion and extension at the sphenobasilar junction. Prior to the approximate age of twenty-five, the motion is at the synchondrosis between the

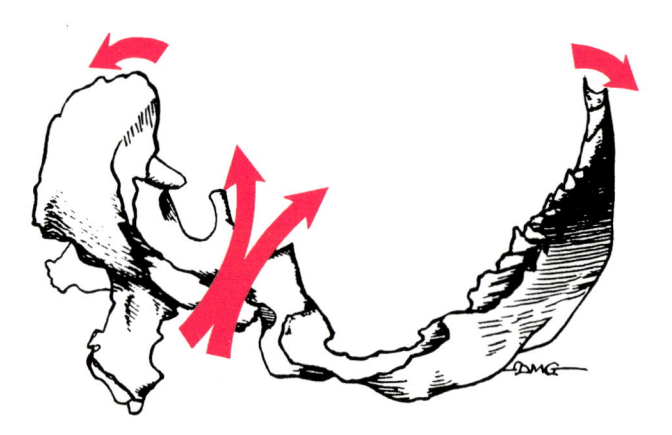

Fig. 15-6. General motion of sphenoid and occiput on inspiration.

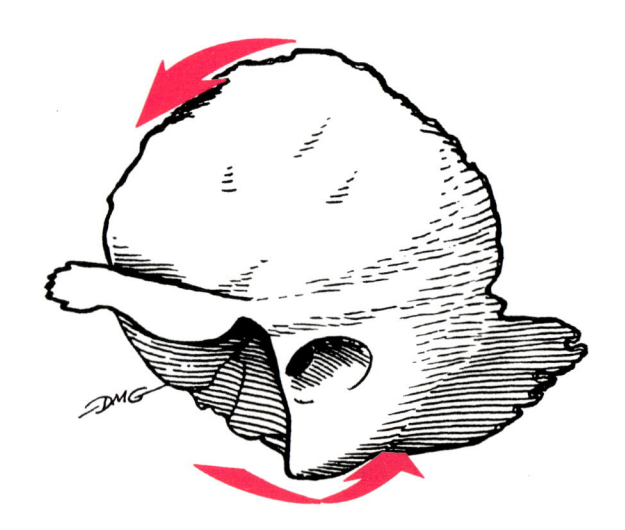

Fig. 15-7. Lateral view of temporal bone on inspiration.

bones. After ossification, the motion is flexion and extension of the cancellous bone. Sphenobasilar flexion consists of the sphenobasilar junction rising and the separation of the superior portions of the occipital squama and greater wings of the sphenoid. Sphenobasilar extension occurs with dropping of the sphenobasilar junction and approximation of the superior portion of the occipital squama and greater wings of the sphenoid. Sphenobasilar flexion is enhanced by a deep phase of thoracic inspiration; extension is enhanced by expiration. Often sphenobasilar movement is called sphenobasilar inspiration or expiration.

The general axis of temporal bone rotation is through the petrous portion, which is at approximately a 60-degree angle with the temporal bone's squamous. The apex of the petrous portion rises on inspiration with the

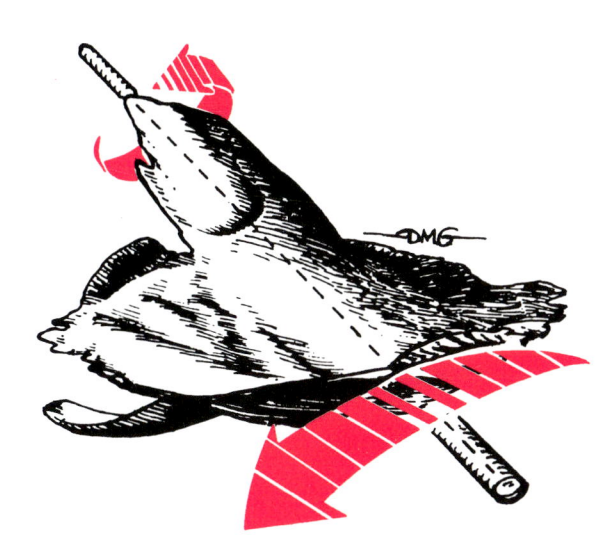

Fig. 15-8. Superior view of the axis of motion of the temporal bone on inspiration. The general axis of rotation is through the petrous portion.

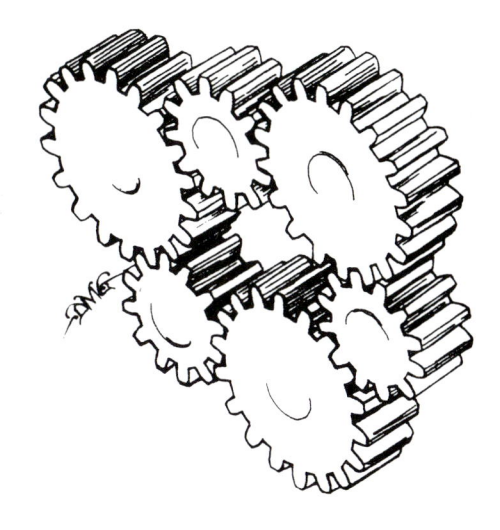

Fig. 15-10. Closed kinematic chain of gears.

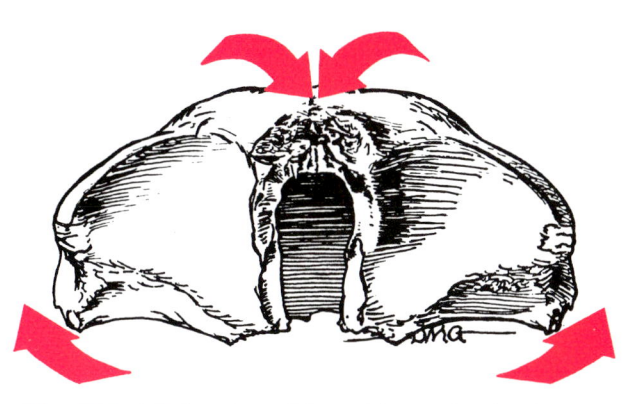

Fig. 15-9. Inferior view of frontal bone showing internal rotation on inspiration.

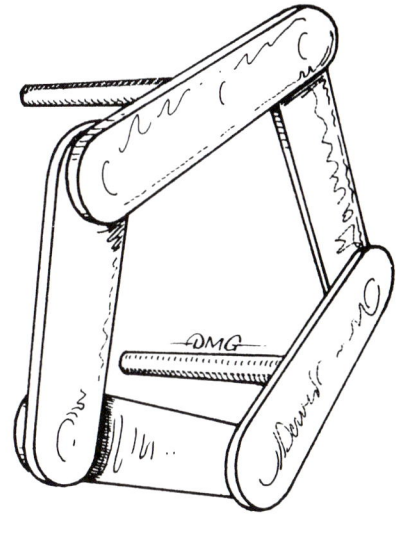

Fig. 15-11. Closed kinematic chain of levers.

sphenobasilar junction, and the petrous ridge rotates anterolaterally, causing the squamous of the temporal bone to rotate externally. The mastoid process moves posteriorly and medially with inspiration (Figs. 15-7 and 15-8).

The frontal bone, in most subjects, ossifies at the metopic suture. In some cases a remnant, or the entire suture, persists throughout life. Motion on sphenobasilar flexion (inspiration) spreads the frontal bone's squamous portion. In applied kinesiology this is called internal frontal motion, as if the metopic suture were moving internally (Fig. 15-9). On sphenobasilar extension (expiration), the squamous portions of the frontal bone move medially. In applied kinesiology and cranial osteopathy this is called external frontal rotation, as if the metopic suture area were moving externally. This can be confusing, because different terminology is used in some other techniques.[10,11]

The rest of the bones of the skull and face have specific movement in relation to sphenobasilar flexion and extension. There is continuity in this movement by way of pivot points, gear trains, sliding action, and lever mechanisms; this interaction constitutes a closed kinematic chain. In any closed kinematic chain, when one portion moves, the entire chain must move. This can be demonstrated by a system of levers or gears, both of which are present in the cranial closed kinematic chain (Figs. 15-10 and 15-11). The occipitomastoid suture acts like teeth on a gear. The vomer is a lever mechanism between the rostrum of the sphenoid and the intermaxillary and palatine sutures of the maxillary and palatine bones.

Cranial movement is an important action of the stomatognathic system; its proper function can be interfered with by malocclusion or disturbed function of the closed kinematic muscle chain of the stomatognathic system. Integral to the cranial closed kinematic chain movement is the dural mechanism.[36,53]

Cranial faults can interfere with normal health in many ways. Most often described in the osteopathic literature is interference with movement and control of the cerebrospinal fluid. It is believed that cerebrospinal fluid has a rhythmic fluctuation linked with that of the skull. This fluctuation is the movement of the cerebrospinal fluid rather than actual circulation within the system.[36] It is also hypothesized that cranial motion has a direct relation to the pressure maintained in the closed cerebrospinal fluid system. It is important to both the mechanical support and physiology of the central nervous system, and is thought to be important in carrying secretions of the pituitary gland.[34]

Nerve endings within the sutures have been described by Retzlaff et al.[44,45] If a cranial fault causes suture compression, it may result in a headache[46] or facial pain by stimulating the nerve receptors within the involved suture.

Other conditions that may be caused by cranial faults are hypertension, impaired brain circulation, disturbance in the endocrine system, vision, and hearing, and general neurologic disorganization. Many of the conditions appear to be caused by entrapment of the cranial nerves.

Nerve entrapment is considered differently by various schools of thought. Some approaches consider entrapment when there is only subtle irritation on the nerve causing functional disorders, while others limit the term to severe damage of the nerve. Entrapment neuropathy is referred to by Kopell and Thompson[30] as "... a region of localized injury and inflammation in a peripheral nerve that is caused by mechanical irritation from some impinging anatomical neighbor. It may occur at the point at which a nerve goes through a fibrous or osseofibrous tunnel, or at which the nerve changes its course over a fibrous or a muscular band. Although external force may have been applied directly to the region, in many cases there is no discernible relationship of the condition to external trauma."

There are numerous areas in which the cranial nerves traverse confining spaces. Where the nerve exits from a foramen, it is sheathed in a dural tube that can be in torsion, resulting in entrapment. It is important to recognize how a subtle pressure on a nerve can change the impulse or short circuit its route. Granit et al.[27] demonstrated subtle pressure could create an "artificial" synapse between the motor and sensory fibers of a nerve. The cross stimulation was caused by a pressure so light that it did not interfere with the original impulse. They then removed the pressure and irrigated the nerve with a saline solution; after a brief time, the nerve returned to normal function. This seems to indicate that impingement on a nerve from cranial dysfunction is a plausible explanation for disturbances observed clinically. It remains to be demonstrated electrophysiologically that this is, in reality, what occurs in cranial dysfunction.

A possible physiological explanation of peripheral nerve entrapment is presented by Gardner,[21] whose hypothesis is based on maintenance of intercellular space. He discusses the report of Weiss and Woodbridge,[58] who state that "All metazoan cells so far examined carry a negative charge at their electrokinetic surfaces." This causes the cells to have an electrostatic repulsion, since like charges repel. Their report dealt with the prevention of red blood cells from adhering to each other, and to other factors. Gardner speculated that "... in the case of brain cells, a similar repelling force would interfere with contact between adjoining cell membranes, which would explain the uniform intercellular space of 150-200 angstroms that accompanies all of the intricate meanderings of the cell processes." This electrostatic repulsion would be carried throughout the nervous system, extending into the spinal cord and peripheral nerves such as the cranial and spinal nerves. The axons then would be floating and would be acted upon by two opposing forces—those of electrostatic repulsion and of the mechanical force of the surrounding tissues. Gardner goes on to point out that the interaxonal distance would be affected by the nerve going over a sharp ridge, such as the petrous portion of the temporal bone. Other mechanical disturbances may also have an effect.

When the cross circuiting is between nerve fibers of like kind, i.e., efferent or afferent nerves, it is called "cross talk." In this case, an impulse destined for one dermatome or myotome ends up supplying another. Cross circuiting between different kinds of fibers, between efferent and afferent nerve fibers, is called "back talk."

Interference with normal transmission within the cranial nerves can cause many health problems. Within the context of this discussion, there are several cranial nerves that directly influence the structure of the stomatognathic system. Entrapment of cranial nerve V, the trigeminal nerve, changes the control of masticatory muscles; this can disrupt the engram of jaw closing and cause malocclusion. The sternocleidomastoid and upper trapezius muscles are controlled by cranial nerve XI, the spinal accessory nerve. Entrapment here can cause a failure of proper head leveling and create imbalance in the closed kinematic muscle chain of the stomatognathic system. Most of the hyoid muscles are innervated by cranial nerve XII, the hypoglossal nerve; if indeed there is contribution to orientation in space by feedback from the balance of the hyoid bone and muscles, one can certainly see how entrapment of this nerve would disturb equilibrium and general body organization.

In applied kinesiology, a cranial fault is often indicated by a muscle that tests weak but strengthens when the patient takes and holds a deep breath. This strength is maintained only while the muscle is tested with the breath being held. This shows the interrelation between thoracic respiration and cranial-sacral primary respiratory function. Although cranial respiratory motion is autonomous, it is influenced by thoracic respiration, which can be used to advantage in obtaining correction.

Interaction with Occlusion

When the muscles function in a balanced manner and the occlusion is correct, repeated contraction of the masticatory muscles activates the skull by the muscles pulling on bony levers of the skull. The activation is present with both jaw opening and closing. This can usually be demonstrated on an individual who has cranial faults. The subject is asked to repeatedly stretch his jaw open to its maximum and then close. This is done six or more times. When the skull is re-examined for cranial faults, they will be temporarily gone, in most cases. In some very rigid skulls with severely locked cranial faults, it may be necessary to have the subject stretch his jaw open as many as fifty times. There is the rare individual who has such severe, locked-in cranial faults that this procedure will not even temporarily improve function. In most cases, the apparently improved cranial function will last long enough for the examiner to re-evaluate the skull. In individuals who have only moderate cranial faults, the improvement will last longer; its duration will be shorter in those with severe faults. In some people with only minimal cranial faults, this activity may make a permanent correction. In this case, the system would probably have corrected itself anyway.

Temporarily eliminating evidence of cranial faults by stretching the jaw open several times is interesting, but what does it mean? It shows the influence of the masticatory muscles on cranial primary respiratory function. When the mandible is opened to its maximum, the mandibular closers pull strongly on the skull. The masseter pulls on the zygomatic process, providing considerable leverage on the temporal bone, and the maxilla is moved by way of the zygomatic bone. The internal pterygoid pulls on the lateral pterygoid plate and pyramidal process of the sphenoid and palatine bones. The temporalis pulls on the parietal, frontal, temporal, and sphenoid bones by way of the temporal fossa.

In addition to the traction on the bones from the muscles stretching to their maximum, there is further activity. Electromyographic evidence reveals that the masseter and temporalis become considerably active on maximal mouth opening;[33] thus they are actively pulling on what are ordinarily their origins. In addition, the major jaw opener, the external pterygoid, acts to mobilize the skull. The action of the external pterygoid at its limit of motion is to pull on the greater wing of the sphenoid and the pterygoid process. All of this activates the closed kinematic chain of the cranium, stimulating physiological motion. Often the introduction of force that creates motion in the skull is adequate for correcting minimal cranial faults. On these occasions the increased motion unlocks the mechanism, allowing it to return to its normal autonomous motion.

The philosophy of applied kinesiology recognizes that nothing occurs in the body as random activity. For every normal body action there is a purpose—improved function. Granted, sometimes the actions are compensating for some form of dysfunction. If it is true that no function taking place in the body is random, is it possible that when an individual yawns very widely it is an effort by the body to activate the cranial primary respiratory mechanism? In any event, it can readily be seen that forced mouth opening influences the mechanism.

With this mechanism the body has a self-correcting approach to return normal function after a blow on the head or the more gentle stresses that occur with everyday life. A student's cranium can be disturbed when he sits at a desk with his arm and hand propped under the zygomatic bone to hold his head. A welder's helmet or other headgear can sometimes disturb the cranial mechanism, but normal function returns with a yawn or chewing. Even walking, with the alternate contraction of the sternocleidomastoid and upper trapezius, can re-activate normal function in the skull. It is fortunate that all these auto-correction mechanisms are present, or normal health would suffer.

Unfortunately, balanced muscle action and occlusion are not always present. When they are not, chewing becomes a detrimental factor rather than an asset. When there is poor occlusion, the mandibular elevators pull into the cranium in an imbalanced manner. Appar-

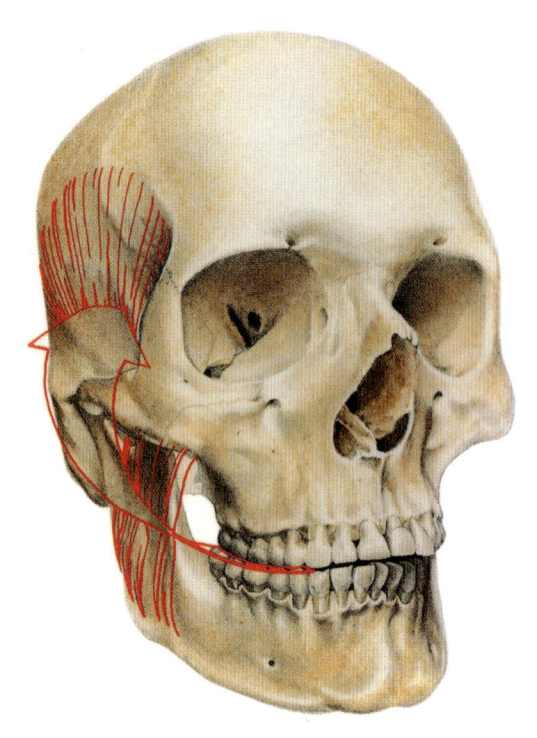

Fig. 15-12. Malocclusion can cause an imbalance of muscular pull into the cranial mechanism to cause dysfunction.

ently, it is the repetition of this mechanical stress into the cranium that causes disturbance. If an individual bites hard on a resistant object between the molars on only one side of the jaws there is obviously an imbalance present, but it is only transitory; continued chewing in a more balanced manner often returns normality to the skull. It is the continued imbalance of malocclusion that creates problems (Fig. 15-12).

The imbalanced platform from which the muscles work is not the only problem when there is malocclusion; there is considerable evidence[4,6,40,43] that malocclusion causes several changes in the action of the masticatory muscles. The muscles, as observed by electromyography, may be firing stronger on one side than on the other. There may be improper timing of the muscles in the open-close-clench cycle, and there may be disturbance in the jaw-opening reflex. The cranial primary respiratory mechanism can be corrected when these patterns are present, but as soon as an individual bites down or chews, the cranial disturbance returns. This type of recidivism is not always due to malocclusion. The muscle itself can be dysfunctioning as a

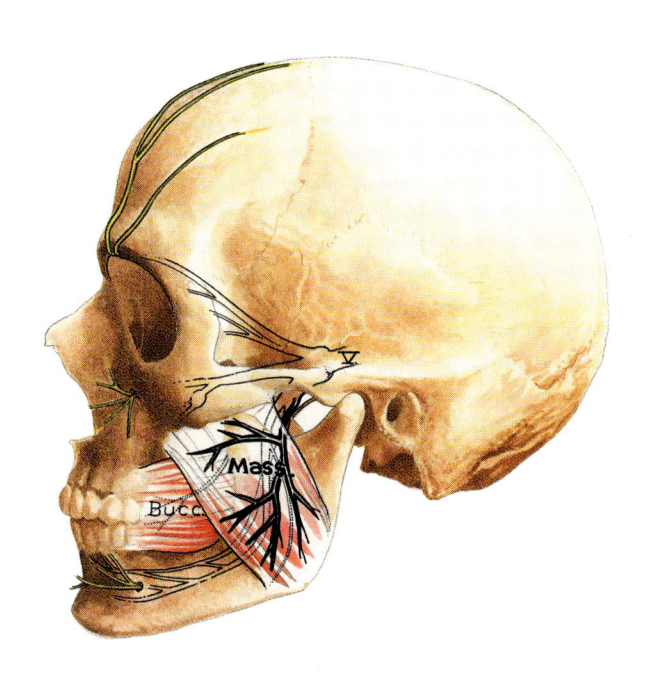

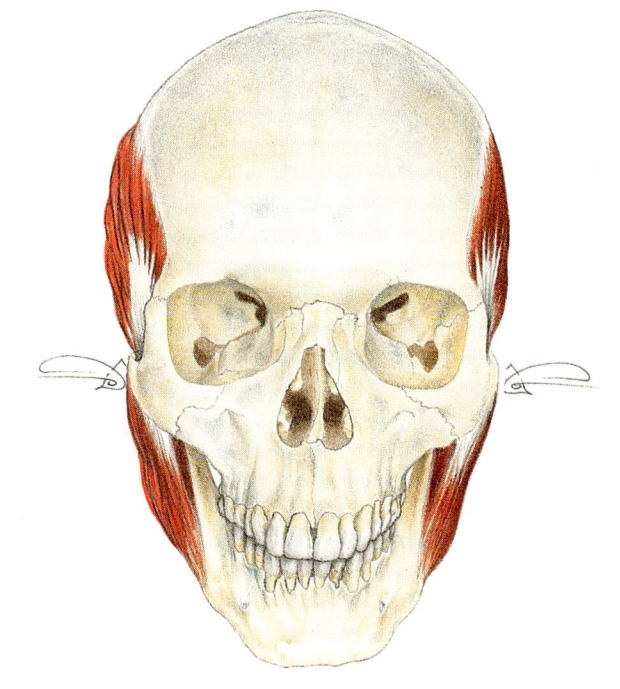

Fig. 15-13. An imbalanced nerve supply to the mandibular elevators caused by an improper engram causes strain to the cranial mechanism, possibly causing cranial faults.

Fig. 15-14. Unilateral hypertonicity or weakness of the mandibular elevators activates the skull in an imbalanced manner to possibly cause cranial faults.

result of improper neuromuscular spindle cell activity, or improper signaling from a periodontal ligament receptor could be creating the problem.

When an improper volley of nerve impulses enters into this complex picture, organization is disrupted (Fig. 15-13). It does not matter whether the improper impulses come from a periodontal ligament receptor, a neuromuscular spindle cell in a muscle of mastication, the hyoid group, muscles of the tongue, or any one of the other sources. If the temporal pattern of contraction is wrong or a muscle becomes hypo- or hypertonic, the balance within the closed kinematic chain is disturbed (Fig. 15-14). A change in the anterior affects the antagonistic posterior. If there is an imbalance from right to left, the head-leveling mechanism becomes imbalanced and equilibrium proprioceptors are improperly stimulated. This causes muscles to pull into the cranium in an imbalanced manner. Cranial faults may develop, producing cranial nerve dysfunction that may cause imbalance of the masticatory, hyoid, sternocleidomastoid, and/or upper trapezius muscles.

The stomatognathic system can be adversely influenced further by facial muscles improperly contracting, causing additional disturbance in the cranial primary respiratory mechanism. Cranial faults often affect the equilibrium proprioceptors. Entrapment of cranial nerves III, IV, and VI may cause eye movement to be disorganized, affecting the visual righting reflex. The labyrinthine reflex, innervated by cranial nerve VIII, can be affected in a similar manner. The head-on-neck equilibrium proprioceptors are located in the ligaments of the upper three cervical vertebrae.[38] They report the organization of the head-on-body or, as previously discussed, body-on-head. Disorganization in the stomatognathic system often causes poor head leveling to inappropriately stimulate these proprioceptors. The equilibrium, visual righting, labyrinthine, and head-on-neck proprioceptors must all be reporting the same information about head orientation, or else the disorganization may spread throughout the body.

How far can we go with this hypothetical example? It is amazing what long-range effects a seemingly small problem can create. Mrs. Jones' neck pain or headaches may result from something as simple as biting on a chip of bone in a salisbury steak a week ago. This may cause disturbance of the proprioceptors in the periodontal ligament, which fail to return themselves to normal and disturb the entire closed kinematic chain of the head-on-neck muscles. But the problem could be much farther reaching. If cranial faults develop and the vagus nerve becomes involved, digestive disturbances may result. The physician and patient may have no idea how the problem began. Everything in the body happens for a reason; it is the physician's challenge to find that basic underlying cause.

This comprehensive system must structurally organize with the rest of the body, including the spine, pelvis, general posture, and gait, for proper function. The nervous system is primarily responsible for the organization, but there is also contribution to organization from strictly mechanical factors such as the "core link" between the cranium and the sacrum, which are integral to overall system integration.

REMOTE INFLUENCE ON THE STOMATOGNATHIC SYSTEM

When there is obvious malocclusion or some other problem in the stomatognathic system, one should always consider whether it is primary or secondary. Certainly dysfunction of the stomatognathic system can be primary to many remote health problems, but the converse of remote dysfunction affecting the stomatognathic system is often overlooked.

Strachan and Robinson,[49] at the Chicago College of Osteopathy, were the first to observe a short leg's influence on malocclusion. Evaluating the pattern of masticatory muscles by electromyography, they removed a 3/8" heel lift from a standing subject's shoe and found an altered firing sequence of the muscles of mastication during chewing. When the lift was worn, the muscles showed the firing pattern of normal occlusion; with it removed, the firing pattern was one of a severe malocclusion. Although this is interesting, it must be put into proper perspective. An apparent short leg is only one aspect of the structural imbalance. Is the leg really short, or is there a pelvic subluxation making the leg appear short? From the foot up to the stomatognathic system there is much structure and neurologic organization which, if not balanced and functioning normally, may be manifested in secondary dysfunction of the stomatognathic system. Mintz[39] refers to this as "The Orthopedic Influence."

There is predictable neurologic control of the muscles as an individual walks and runs. Reciprocal inhibition[12] is responsible for antagonistic muscles releasing when a prime mover moves a limb. This organization in the gait mechanism can be observed with manual muscle testing by having an individual simulate a gait position. First the subject is tested standing to determine that the shoulder flexors and extensors test strong. He is then put into a simulated gait position, with the right leg forward and carrying most of the weight. In this position, a normal individual will test weak in the right shoulder flexors and left shoulder extensors; this allows the arm opposite the forward leg to readily swing forward in the cross pattern movement of the arm and leg when walking or running. It is observed in applied kinesiology that when there is inappropriate stimulation of proprioceptors as a result of foot or other subluxations, the facilitation and inhibition pattern of gait muscles is random rather than predictable. After the subluxation or other dysfunction is corrected, the predictable pattern of facilitation and inhibition returns. Very often the primary cause of a poor gait pattern is foot dysfunction that may be a result of subluxations, as mentioned, or active meridian points on the foot that have been found in applied kinesiology to affect the gait mechanism.

One type of gait evaluation in applied kinesiology is done by testing two groups of muscles at the same time—groups that function together in normal gait activity. There are six tests consisting of upper and lower muscle groups that are always contralateral.[2,23] They are shoulder and hip flexors, shoulder and hip extensors, shoulder and hip abductors, shoulder and hip adductors, gluteus medius and abdominals, and psoas major and pectoralis major. The standard AK approach to testing and correcting gait mechanism, briefly described here, is presented elsewhere.[54,56]

Activity similar to the facilitation and inhibition of the extremity muscles during gait occurs in the trunk. Activity of the psoas major and pectoralis major muscles applies torsion to the trunk, as does that of the gluteus medius and the abdominals. This torsion through the long axis of the trunk is necessary for fluid movement while walking or running; it is controlled by the same type of inhibition and facilitation of muscles as limb movement. Trunk rotation during gait extends into the relationship of the shoulder girdle, cervical spine, and head. This organization has been described by Goodheart as the "walking gait."[25]

When walking, as the right leg moves forward with hip and knee flexion, the right hemi-pelvis moves forward also; simultaneously the left shoulder flexes. In order for this to occur, there must be inhibition of the left latissimus dorsi and facilitation of the pectoralis major. Manual muscle testing of the subject in this position will confirm a normal weakening of the left latissimus dorsi, while the pectoralis major tests strong. The opposite occurs in the right shoulder; the pectoralis major tests weak because of inhibition, and the latissimus dorsi tests strong. Because of this and other muscle activity, axial torque occurs from the pelvis to the shoulder girdle, moving the right pelvis and left shoulder girdle forward. While the shoulder girdle rotates back and forth during gait, the head remains relatively free of rotation because of the role of the sternocleidomastoid and upper trapezius in the gait mechanism.

In the same gait position previously described, with the right leg and left arm and shoulder forward, the head must turn to the left in relation to the shoulder girdle to maintain a straightforward position. This is accomplished by facilitation of the upper trapezius on the right and inhibition of the sternocleidomastoid muscle on the left. When a normal subject is in this gait position, the sternocleidomastoid should test weak on the left and strong on the right. In the opposite gait position, the converse is true.

Goodheart[25] described a lack of this predictable organization, especially in individuals with disturbance in the stomatognathic system. His initial investigation included several patients suffering from chronic-clonic-tonic intermittent torticollis, which is a major debilitating condition of the stomatognathic system. Disturbance in this portion of the gait mechanism relates to recurrent cranial faults and temporomandibular joint and hyoid muscle problems. It can easily be recognized how improper actions of the sternocleidomastoid and upper trapezius on the cranium can disturb cranial function. Because of the sternocleidomastoid's insertion into the mastoid process, its inappropriate action introduces a force into the cranium's closed kinematic chain very similar to that of the therapeutic force used in applied kinesiology. This force can be detrimental as well as beneficial.

The primary problem with the sternocleidomastoid and upper trapezius muscles in relation to gait is failure of the muscles to be effectively inhibited during the appropriate phase of the gait pattern. This is tested in applied kinesiology with the patient in a gait position to determine if predictable weakening of the muscles occurs. First the sternocleidomastoid and upper trapezius muscles are tested with the patient standing in a neutral position to determine that they are strong without gait activity. If there is weakness during this test, correction must be obtained using standard applied kinesiology techniques before the gait test can be continued.

These muscles are more difficult to test in a weight-bearing position, and care must be taken that the tests are done accurately. When testing the sternocleidomastoid, the patient should be stabilized with a broad contact of the physician's hand at the upper thoracic spinal area (Fig. 15-15). The extensor test evaluates a portion of the upper trapezius and the deep extensor muscles of the cervical spine (Fig. 15-16). It appears to be a modified upper trapezius test, but in reality it is a group muscle test as done in other gait testing procedures. The patient's ear and shoulder are approximated in a manner somewhat similar to that in the standard upper trapezius test, but the patient's head is not rotated away from the side being tested. The examiner stabilizes the shoulder, as in the standard upper trapezius test; his other hand is placed over the head to separate the shoulder and

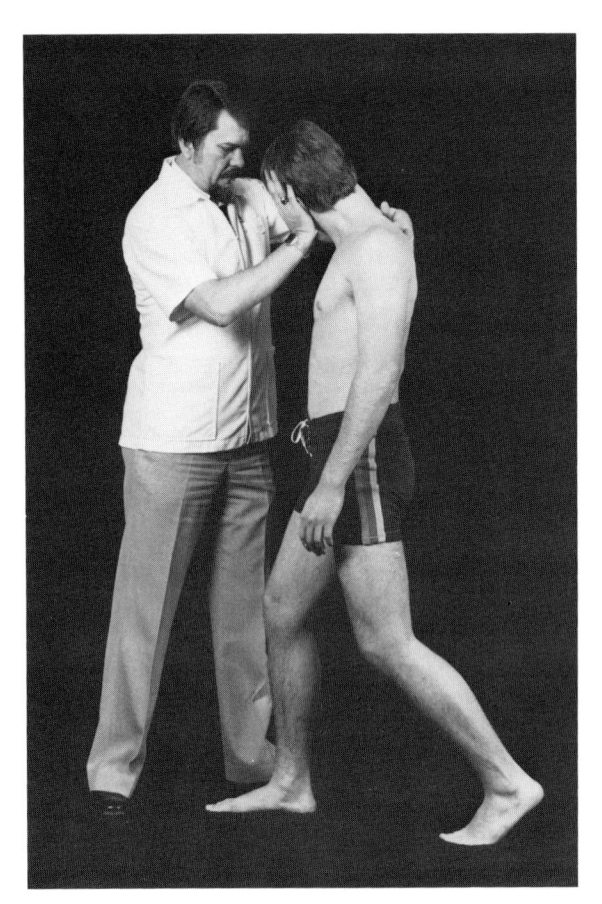

Fig. 15-15. To test the sternocleidomastoid in the gait position, the examiner must effectively stabilize the posterior thorax. The sternocleidomastoid should test weak on the trailing leg side.

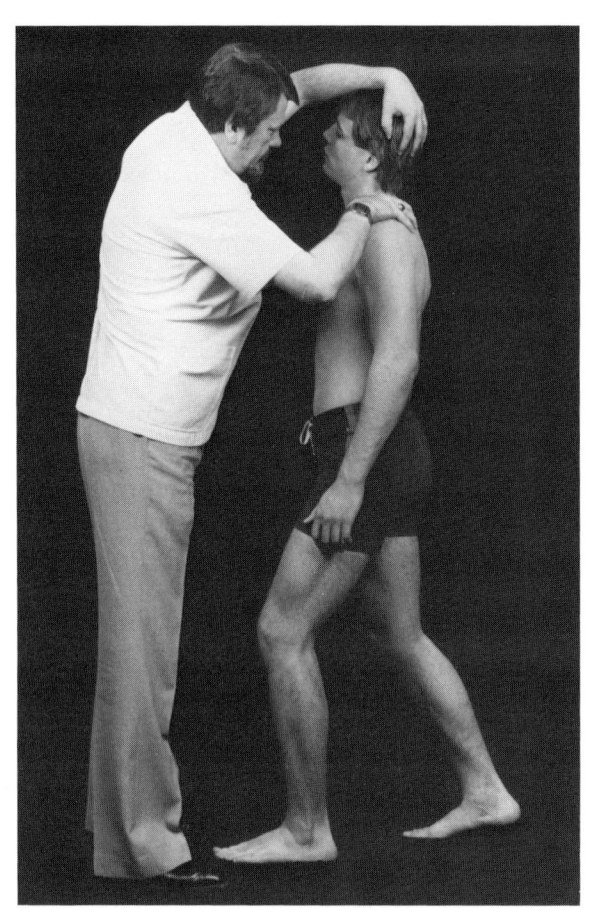

Fig. 15-16. Testing the upper trapezius and deep cervical extensors in gait activity is accomplished by the examiner contacting the head to separate it from the shoulders in lateral and anterior flexion. The patient's head is not rotated away from the side of testing as in the standard upper trapezius test. The complex of extensor muscles should test weak on the forward leg side.

head. The examiner's force is applied in such a manner that the head is brought into lateral and anterior flexion.

After first confirming the presence of strong muscles in a neutral stance, the patient is put in a gait position with one leg forward, carrying the majority of the weight. The contralateral shoulder is flexed, and the contralateral or trailing leg carries a slight amount of weight, primarily on the ball of the foot, with the toes flexed and the heel raised from the floor. When in this position, the sternocleidomastoid should test strong on the side of the forward leg, and the extensor complex should test weak. On the opposite (trailing leg) side, the extensor complex should test strong and the sternocleidomastoid weak.

When the muscles fail to weaken at the appropriate time in gait positions, there is usually disturbance in the gait mechanism from foot or ankle subluxations or other dysfunction in the foot or ankle. This may cause inappropriate stimulation to the joint proprioceptors, or it may relate with some of the nerve receptors treated in applied kinesiology. A common treatment that corrects the muscle function is applied to stress receptors. Stress receptors are cutaneous reflexes found on the head; they affect specific muscles throughout the body.[54,55] When the sternocleidomastoid temporal pattern of contraction is not appropriate, a patient may lose cranial corrections that affect the TMJ or occlusion as soon as he walks.

The muscles of mastication are also involved with the walking gait. It appears that the jaw-closer muscles are inhibited on the same side as the extensor complex during gait activity. Funakoshi and Amano,[19,20] in studying the effects of the tonic neck reflex on the jaw muscles of the rat, found that when the head was

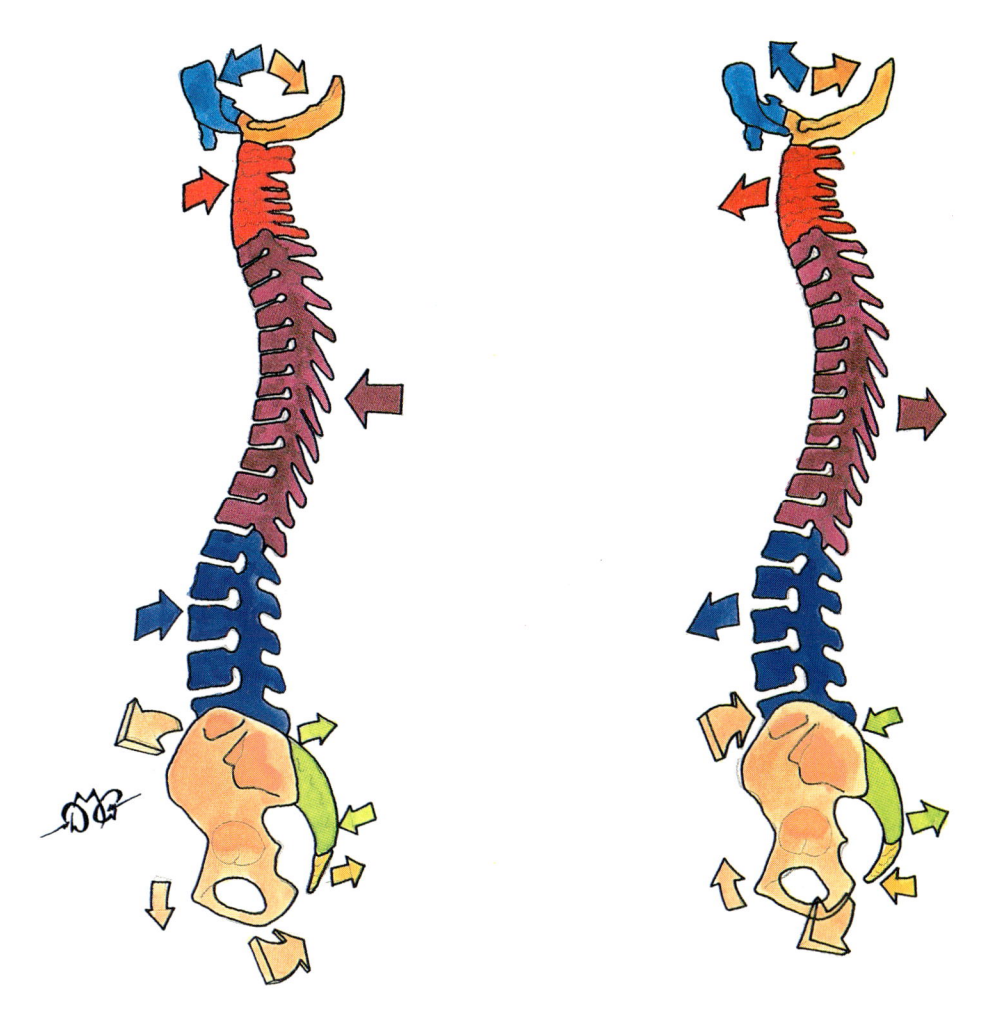

Fig. 15-17. Motion of sphenobasilar junction, spine, sacrum, coccyx, and innominate bone on sphenobasilar flexion (inspiration) and extension (expiration).

turned there was no activity of the masseter, temporal, and digastric muscles contralateral to head turn, but it increased ipsilaterally. There was also bilateral electrical activity of these muscles with forward flexion of the head, but none on tilting. Extension inhibited electrical activity of the muscles. This activity apparently came from stimulation of proprioceptors in the upper cervical ligaments, since the muscle activity was abolished when the first three cervical nerves were cut.

The criterion established by Goodheart[25] for testing this relationship is to have the patient clench his teeth on the side opposite the normally inhibited trapezius; this should not neutralize the gait-related trapezius weakness. It has been clinically found that treatment to the stress receptor for the TMJ muscles on the side opposite clenching eliminates the negation of the upper trapezius inhibition on contralateral clenching. This seems to indicate that there is a reciprocal inhibition between the right and left jaw-closing muscles during walking.

The hip flexors and extensors should have the same type of facilitation and inhibition with gait as do the shoulder and neck muscles. The pelvis and spine may be adversely affected, in turn disrupting function in the stomatognathic system. Testing and correcting this dysfunction are described elsewhere.[55]

For optimal cranial motion, there must be organization within the stomatognathic system and between the cranium and pelvis. The dural tube is the core link organizing motion between the cranium and sacrum. It has firm attachment at the foramen magnum, 2nd and 3rd cervical vertebrae, and at the 2nd sacral

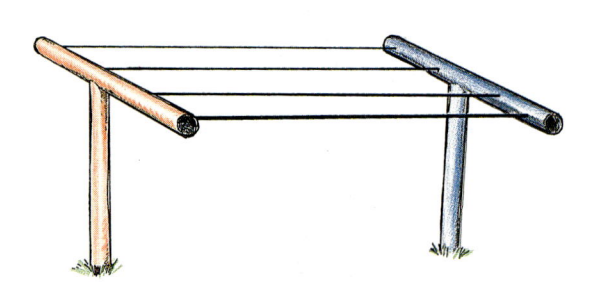

Fig. 15-18. If one pole is rotated, the other will rotate in a similar manner. This is similar to the "core-link" of the cranial-sacral primary respiratory system.

segment. Motion of the sacrum consists of lifting the anterior portion of the 2nd sacral segment as the sphenobasilar junction lifts; thus, the apex of the sacrum moves anteriorly and the base posteriorly with sphenobasilar flexion, and the opposite with extension (Fig. 15-17).

To illustrate the core link, Magoun[36] likens the dura to cables (rather than a tube) connecting the occipital bone and sacrum. With balance there will be equal tension on both sides. If the sacrum moves, it produces tension on one cable, thus pulling the occipital bone into a similar position. This model, for illustrative purposes, is further presented as clotheslines connecting two poles with crossarms. If one pole rotates, it will rotate the other pole in a similar manner since the connecting clotheslines make up a functional unit; thus organization in the cranial-sacral complex is maintained. On the other hand, distortion at either end may cause an adaptive distortion at the other end. Pelvic imbalance may develop from a fall or for some other reason. If not corrected autonomously by the body or by a physician's treatment, the cranial function may be adversely affected. This, in turn, produces imbalance in the total stomatognathic system that may be evidenced by malocclusion, TMJ dysfunction, headaches, neck pain, and/or the many other conditions that accompany dysfunction of the stomatognathic system (Fig. 15-18).

The innominate bones also have a primary movement organized with cranial function. If one compares the innominate with the temporal bone, the comparative parts move in the same direction with inspiration and expiration (Fig. 15-19). The ilium is compared with the squama of the temporal bone; it moves anterolaterally with inspiration. The ischium moves posteromedially, as does the mastoid process.

Proper foot, gait, and thoracic respiration are primary for pelvic organization. For the former two, this is obvious from the previous discussion of gait muscle facilitation and inhibition. But what about thoracic respiration? Motion of the diaphragm and abdominal muscles in respiration is integral to pelvic motion that interrelates with cranial motion.

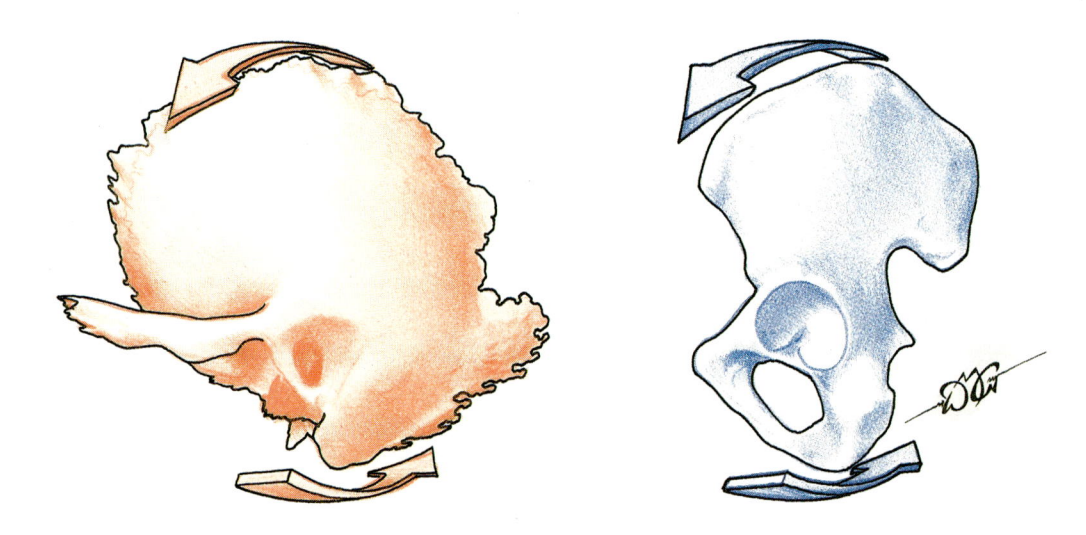

Fig. 15-19. Movement of temporal and innominate bones on inspiration (sphenobasilar flexion).

Pressure from the abdominal contents and the abdominal muscles contributes to this motion. On inspiration the abdominal contents move downward, putting pressure on the ilium to move the anterior iliac spine laterally, anteriorly, and inferiorly. Simultaneously with inspiration, the abdominal muscles relax to permit this motion. During expiration, the abdominal muscles contract, reversing the motion of the ilia.

The organization between the closed kinematic chain of the cranium, with its movement of the pelvis by the dura mater, and the abdominal muscle contribution, emphasizes how integrated the motion of the stomatognathic system is with the rest of the body.

Fonder[15] has demonstrated the influence of the stomatognathic system on body balance and the spine by changing the occlusion and mandibular position. Spinal x-rays taken before and after the equilibration and mandibular repositioning show specific postural changes.[16] Clinical changes are often seen throughout the body after making changes in the masticatory system. This shows how the structures within the stomatognathic system are integrated with each other, and how the system is related to total body activity.

All this may seem highly complicated and formidable to examine and evaluate. Certainly the interactions that take place are complex, but with a systematic method of evaluation the primary imbalance that initiates the multitude of disturbances can readily be found. It is important to understand the magnitude of these interactions, and the fact that the symptomatic area may not be the primary factor needing evaluation and treatment.

REFERENCES

1. Barlow W. *The Alexander Technique*. New York, NY: Alfred A Knopf; 1977.
2. Beardall AG. Additional gait tests. *Chiro Econ*. March/April 1977;32-33.
3. Beaudreau DE, Daugherty WF Jr, Masland W. Two types of motor pause in masticatory muscles. *Am J Physiol*. 1969;216:16-21.
4. Bessette R, Bishop B, Mohl N. Duration of masseteric silent period in patients with TMJ syndrome. *J Appl Physiol*. 1971;30:864-69.
5. Brodie AG. Anatomy and physiology of head and neck musculature. *Am J Orthod* 1950;36:831-44.
6. Carls S. Nervous coordination and mechanical function of the mandibular elevators. *Acta Odontol Scand*, 10 Supp 11. 1952;9-133.
7. Dart RA. The attainment of poise. *S African Med J*. 21; February 8, 1947;74-91
8. Dart RA. Voluntary musculature in the human body—the double-spiral arrangement. *Brit J Phys Med*. 1950;13:265-68.
9. Dart RA. The postural aspects of malocclusion (2). 1968; *Human Potential*. 1 (No. 4):
10. DeJarnette MB. *Cranial Technique 1968*. Nebraska City, NE: privately published; 1968.
11. DeJarnette MB. *Cranial Technique 1979-80*. Nebraska City, NE: privately published; 1979.
12. Denny-Brown D, ed. *Selected Writings of Sir Charles Sherrington*. New York, NY: Oxford University Press; 1979.
13. Dombrady L. Investigation into the transient instability of the rest position. *J Prosthet Dent*. 1966;16:479-90.
14. DuBrul EL. *Sicher's Oral Anatomy*. 7th ed. St. Louis, MO: The CV Mosby Co; 1980;204.
15. Fonder AC. Stress and the dental distress syndrome. *Basal Facts*. 1976; 1 (No. 3).
16. Fonder AC. *The Dental Physician*. Blacksburg, VA: University Publications; 1977.
17. Friel JP, ed. *Dorland's Illustrated Medical Dictionary*. 25th ed. Philadelphia, PA: WB Saunders Co; 1974.
18. Frymann VM. A study of the rhythmic motions of the living cranium. *JAOA*. May 1971;70:1-18.
19. Funakoshi M, Amano N. Effects of the tonic neck reflex on the jaw muscles of the rat. *J Dent Res*. July/august 1973; 52:668-73.
20. Funakoshi M, Fujita N, Takenana S. Relations between occlusal interference and jaw muscle activities in response to changes in head position. *J Dent Res*. July/August 1976;35:684-90.
21. Gardner WJ. Trigeminal neuralgia. *Clin Neurosurg*. 1967;15:1-56.
22. Goodheart GJ Jr. *Applied Kinesiology*. Detroit, MI: privately published; 1964.
23. Goodheart GJ Jr. *Applied Kinesiology 1975 Workshop Procedure Manual*. 11th ed. Detroit, MI: privately published; 1975.
24. Goodheart GJ Jr. *Applied Kinesiology 1977 Workshop Procedure Manual*. 13th ed. Detroit, MI: privately published; 1977.
25. Goodheart GJ Jr. *Applied Kinesiology 1982 Workshop Procedure Manual*. 18th ed. Detroit, MI: privately published; 1982.
26. Gowitzke BA, Milner M. *Understanding the Scientific Bases of Human Movement*. 2nd ed. Baltimore, MD: Williams & Wilkins; 1980.
27. Granit R, Leksell L, Skoglund C., Fibre interaction in injured or compressed region of nerve. *Brain*. June 1944;67:125-40.

28. Greenman PE. Roentgen findings in the craniosacral mechanism. *JAOA*. September 1970;70:23-35.
29. Kendall FP, McCreary EK. *Muscles - Testing and Function*. 3rd ed. Baltimore, MD: Williams & Wilkins; 1983.
30. Kopell HP, Thompson WAL. *Peripheral Entrapment Neuropathies*. 2nd ed. Huntington, NY: Robert E. Krieger Pub. Co; 1976.
31. Kudler GD et al. Oral orthopedics - a concept of occlusion. *J Periodontol*. April 1955;26:119-29.
32. Latif A. An electromyographic study of the temporalis muscle in normal persons during selected positions and movements of the mandible. *Am J Orthod*. 1957;43:577-91.
33. MacDougall JDB, Andrew BL. An electromyographic study of the temporalis and masseter muscles. *J Anat*. January 1953;87:37-45.
34. Magoun HI Sr. A pertinent approach to pituitary pathology. *D.O.* July 1971;11:1-9.
35. Magoun HI Sr. The temporal bone: Trouble maker in the head. *JAOA*. June 1974;73:825-35.
36. Magoun HI, ed. *Osteopathy in the Cranial Field*. 3rd ed. Belen, NM: privately published; 1976.
37. Maisel E, ed. *The Resurrection of the Body*. New York, NY: Dell Publishing Co, Inc.; 1969;5.
38. McCouch GP, Deering ID, Ling TH. Location of receptors for tonic neck reflexes. *J Neurophysiol*. May 1951;14:191-95.
39. Mintz VW. The orthopedic influence. *Diseases of the Temporomandibular Apparatus - A Multidisciplinary Approach*. Morgan D, Hall W, Vamvas SJ, ed. St. Louis, MO: The CV Mosby Co; 1977;197-201.
40. Munro RR. Electromyography of the masseter and anterior temporalis muscles in subjects with potential temporomandibular joint dysfunction. *Aust Dent J*. June 1972;17:209-18.
41. Perry C. Neuromuscular control of mandibular movements. *J Prosthet Dent*. October 1973;30:714-20.
42. Perry HT Jr. Functional electromyography of the temporal and masseter muscles in class II, division I malocclusion and excellent occlusion. *Angle Orthod*. January 1955;25:49-58.
43. Perry HT Jr. Muscular changes associated with temporomandibular joint dysfunction. *JADA*. May 1957;54:644-53.
44. Retzlaff EW, et al. The structures of cranial bone sutures. *JAOA*. February 1976;75:607,608.
45. Retzlaff EW, et al. Nerve fibers and endings in cranial sutures. *JAOA*. February 1978;77:674,675.
46. Retzlaff EW, et al. Temporalis muscle action in parietotemporal suture compression. *JAOA*. October 1978;78:141.
47. Shore NA. *Temporomandibular Joint Dysfunction and Occlusal Equilibration*. 2nd ed. Philadelphia, PA: JB Lippincott Co; 1976.
48. Stoll V. The importance of correct jaw relations in cervico-oro-facial orthopedia. *Dent Concepts*. April 18, 1950;2:5-9.
49. Strachan WF, Robinson MJ. New osteopathic research ties leg disparity to malocclusion. *Osteo News*. April 1965;6:1.
50. Sutherland WG. *The Cranial Bowl*. Mankato, MN: privately published; 1939.
51. *The Manual of Telephone Extension Program, Current Advances in Dentistry*. University of Illinois; 1949.
52. Tinbergen N. Ethology and stress diseases. *Science*. July 5, 1974;185.
53. Upledger J, Vredevoogd J. *Craniosacral Therapy*. Chicago, IL: Eastland Press; 1983.
54. Walther DS. *Applied Kinesiology, Volume I—Basic Procedures and Muscle Testing*. Pueblo, CO: Systems DC; 1981.
55. Walther DS. *Applied Kinesiology, Volume II—Head, Neck, and Jaw Pain and Dysfunction—The Stomatognathic System*. Pueblo, CO: Systems DC; 1983.
56. Walther DS. *Applied Kinesiology—Synopsis*. Pueblo, CO: Systems DC; 1988.
57. Weinberg LA. Temporomandibular dysfunctional profile: A patient-oriented approach. *J Prosthet Dent*. September 1974;32:213-25.
58. Weiss L, Woodbridge RF. Some biophysical aspects of cell contacts. *Fed Proc*. January/February 1967;26:88-94.
59. Wheeler RC. *Dental Anatomy, Physiology and Occlusion*. 5th ed. Philadelphia, PA: WB Saunders Co;1974.

CONCLUSION

This book was written to expand our knowledge in the management of the chronic pain patient, with special emphasis placed on the role of posture.

Those of us actively involved in the diagnosis and treatment of these patients realize how complex the problem is. We all know how many pain clinics there presently are as compared to ten years ago. These clinics and their staffs have attempted to address this multifactorial problem in a multidisciplinary manner.

When I first edited "Clinical Management of Head, Neck, and TMJ Pain and Dysfunction" just over ten years ago, I reported on Dr. John J. Bonica's reasons for the deficiencies in the management of chronic pain. The main topics covered were: 1) insufficient knowledge of chronic pain states; 2) improper application of knowledge, and 3) inadequate communication systems. Since that time many medical and dental schools have opened pain clinics as parts of overall health centers. However, many of the problems existing then still prevail to a great extent today. It was our hope at that time that well trained medical, dental, osteopathic and other related health professionals would be developed to staff the numerous chronic pain centers that were springing up in different parts of the country. This wish has only been partly fulfilled.

In the April 1988 edition of *Pain* the Editorial described an outline curriculum on pain for medical schools. The statement was made that the curriculum outline was presented to stimulate comments, criticisms and suggestions. It was their hope as well as ours that those individuals involved in Medical and Dental School Curriculum planning might use the Outline to draw the attention of their colleagues to the areas which should be covered if medical and dental graduates are to be adequately prepared for the management of pain.

To those of you who have read the contents of this book, I do hope we have added to your knowledge of the management of the chronic pain patient. In addition, please try to direct the attention of the proper individuals at the schools you graduated from to consider curriculum changes which will produce better health care providers for the chronic pain patient.

Harold Gelb, DMD

Index

A

abdominals, 363
abnormal posture, 97
accessory medial pterygoid muscle, 197
acupuncture meridian, 349
adaptation, 46
adaptive mechanisms, 19
adenoids, 316
aerobic exercises, 48
airway obstruction, 219, 285
Alexander, 1, 54, 177, 351
Alexander lesson, 178
Alexander technique, 54, 177
Alexander therapy, 2
alignment, 17, 26, 45
allergies, 316
allergy, 321
ambulation, 335
Amerindian skulls, 205
anatomic barrier, 27
anatomic deviation, 316
Angle's classifications, 310
anterior disc displacement, 276
anterior open bite, 114
antigonial notch, 329
aponeurosis, 339
appliance, 288
appliances, 140, 227, 317
applied kinesiology, 241, 349, 359
arch support, 346
arthritic disease, 309
Arthrosis Deformans Juvenilis (ADJ), 220
atlas, 265
atlas/axis complex, 261

B

bad posture, 26
Barre-Lieou syndrome, 112
biofeedback, 138, 317
biomechanical relationships, 94
biomechanics, 24, 202
biophysical system, 196
bite plate, 317, 346
biting force, 313
body attitude, 17
body awareness, 31
body center, 18, 50
body centering, 32
body language, 356
body mechanics, 93, 261
body use, 35
Bowbeer Nasion Vertical, 327
Bowbeer facial analysis, 326
brachyfacial, 314
breathing, 52
Bridge of the Nose Vertical, 327
bruxism, 272, 289, 315, 330
bursitis, 102

C

calcaneus, 337
center of gravity, 95
centric occlusion, 190, 242
centric position, 224
centric relation, 95, 354
cephalogram, 323
cephalometric, 164, 317
cervical, 97
cervical lordosis, 324
cervical pillows, 18
cervical spine, 104, 343
cervical spine dysfunction, 333
chewing dominance, 173
children, 271
chiropractic, 265
chiropractor, 322
chronic pain, 9, 35, 36
Class I, 309
Class I deep bite, 292
Class II, 309, 326
Class II Division 2, 292
Class III, 310
clenching, 289
clicking, 211, 272
closed kinematic chain, 350, 354, 355
closed lock, 278
comfort, 18, 44
compensation, 47
condylar displacement, 311, 317
condylar position, 274
condyle, 221, 224
contracture, 45, 49
convex facial profile, 329
cranial fault, 249, 352, 354, 356, 359
cranial motion, 356
cranial movement, 358
cranial nerve V, 359
cranial nerve VIII, 361
cranial nerve XI, 352, 359
cranial nerve XII, 359
cranial nerves III, IV, and VI, 361
cranial orientation, 321
cranial primary respiratory system, 351
cranial-sacral primary respiratory function, 359
craniocervical, 98
craniomandibular, 316
craniomandibular disorder, 335, 343, 346
craniomandibular dysfunction, 317
craniomandibular pathology, 187
craniomandibular syndrome, 309, 321
craniovertebral joints, 39
crossbite, 293, 294, 322
crowns, 318

D

deep bite, 223, 314
deep fascia, 202
deltoid, 249
dental arch, 324
dental occlusion, 261
determinants of posture, 74
diaphragm, 366
digastric groove, 197, 209
digastric muscle, 197, 323, 353
disc-capsule assembly, 187, 190
disc-condyle complex, 315
discogenic changes, 108
disotoclusion, 309
dolichofacial, 314
dorsal glides, 146
dorsal gliding, 134
dorsiflexion, 338
dynamically stabilized alignment, 26
dysplasias, 310

E

earaches, 271
elastic tissue response, 337
electromyographic, 101, 355
electromyography, 116, 211, 360
EMG, 116, 336, 346, 347
environmental factors, 310
equilibration, 318
ergonomic, 18, 35, 93, 127
ergonomic chairs, 62
exercise, 34, 51, 133
exophthalmia, 190

F

facial esthetics, 323
facial morphology, 116
facial pain, 321
facilitation, 365
fascial release, 352
feet, 19
Feldenkrais, 2
femur, 339
foot dysfunction, 349, 362
foot function, 338, 341
foot malfunction, 335
foot orthoses, 66
foot orthotics, 18
foot posture, 342
form, 17
forward head alignment, 26
Forward Head Posture (FHP), 26, 38, 97, 107, 165, 173, 221, 271, 273, 284 317, 322, 324, 328, 329, 330, 331
forward head-neck posture, 226
Frankfort Horizontal, 327
Frankfort plane, 28
Freyette's third law, 28
free-way space, 223
freeway space, 315, 317
frontalis muscle, 212
Functional Hallux Limitus (FHL), 340, 341, 345

G

gait, 338, 342, 343
gait analysis, 340, 344
gait mechanism, 362
gastrocnemius, 249, 336
Gate Control Theory, v
genetic factors, 310
glossopharyngeal nerve, 112

gluteus medius, 363
gravity, 336, 337

H

habits, 33
hand dominance, 173
head posture, 104, 113, 165, 316, 321
head retraction, 133
headache, 111, 212, 271, 366
heel, 67
heel lift, 5, 101, 337, 338, 362
heel strike, 337
hemi-pelvis, 5
high angle type, 311
hip rotation, 264
histogram, 263
hyoglossus, 355
hyoid bone, 96, 227, 323, 353
hyoid muscle, 317, 322
hyperdivergent, 311
hypermobility, 315
hypodivergent face, 311
hypoglossal nerve, 359
hypoglycemic, 212

I

ilium, 366
incisal interferences, 294
incisive position, 172
infrahyoid, 317
infrahyoid muscle, 350
infratemporal fossa, 190
inhibition, 178, 365
inhibitory technique, 179
injections, 48
innominate bones, 366
intercuspal position, 316
intercuspation, 118, 354
internal locking, 30

J

joint mechanics, 339

K

kinesthetic awareness, 14
kinetic chain, 51, 98

L

labyrinthine reflex, 361
lateral pterygoid, 190, 272
lateral pterygoid plate, 203
leg length, 4, 101, 166, 172, 261, 346
lift, 166
ligaments, 31
locking wedge effect, 340
long face syndrome, 329, 330,
long-face syndrome, 311
longus, 352
low angle type, 311
lumbar, 97
lumbar spine, 98
lumbar supports, 18

M

macroposture, 261
Magnetic Resonance Imaging (MRI), 89

malocclusion, 220, 272, 309, 352, 354, 360
mandible, 321
mandibular arch constriction, 330
Mandibular Orthopedic Repositioning Appliance (MORA), 242
mandibular plane angle, 328, 329, 330
mandibular position, 318
mandibular postural locator, 167
mandibular protrusion, 310
mandibular rest position, 163
mandibular resting position, 96
mandibular retrusion, 310, 324, 329
mandibular-capsular muscle, 196
manipulation, 34, 349
massage, 34
masseter, 272
mastication, 354
masticatory system, 261
maxillary constriction, 322
maxillary protrusion, 310
maxillary retrusion, 310
maxillofacial orthopedics, 228
mechanical pain syndromes, 45
medial pterygoid, 272
medial pterygoid muscle, 197
meridian points, 362
mesioclusion, 310
Metatarsophalangeal (MTP), 340
metatarsophalangeal joint (MTP), 338, 339
microposture, 261
mobilization, 34
momentum, 336
MORA, 242
Morton foot, 4
mouth breathing, 114, 220, 221, 271, 316, 317, 322
movement, 49
muscle deficiency, 77
muscle imbalance, 352
muscle pain, 77
muscle spasm, 80, 315
muscle testing, 363
myofascial, 190
Myofascial Pain Dysfunction (MPD), 273, 280, 315
myofascial dysfunction, 271
myofascial pain, 216
myotatic (stretch) reflex, 317

N

nasal allergies, 271
nasal obstruction, 220, 316
NBA, 28
neck pain 366
neck spasm 346
nerve entrapment, 273, 358
neuromuscular re-education, 178
neuromuscular spindle cell, 361
Neurovascular Compression Syndrome (NVCS), 103
neutral alignment, 50
neutral balanced, 17
neutral balanced alignment, 26
neutral pelvis, 30
neutral spine, 26
neutroclusion, 309
normal erect posture, 95
normal gait, 335

normal head posture, 324
nutritional, 349

O

occipitoatlantal joint, 39
Occluded Vertical Dimension (OVD), 315
Occlus-o-guide appliance, 300
occlusal equilibration, 261
occlusal interferences, 261
occlusal planes, 95
occlusion, 165, 289, 316, 321. 359, 362
omohyoid muscle, 353
on balance, 17
on balance alignment, 26
open bite, 314, 328
open mouth, 322
orbitalis muscle, 190
orders, 178
organized movement, 34
orthodontic correction, 261
orthodontics, 318
orthostatic position, 316
orthostatic posture, 95
orthotic, 344, 346
orthotics, 335
orthotic treatment, 346
osteopathic, 358
osteopathy, 357, 362
otalgia, 271
otic, 95
overbite, 292, 315, 321
overjets, 292
overlay partials, 318

P

pain, v, 35, 36
palpation, 52, 235
parafunctional activity, 322
parafunctional habits, 271, 289, 315
paraphysiologic space, 27
pectoral stretch, 136
pectoralis major, 249
pectoralis major muscles, 363
pelvic alignment, 19
pelvic asymmetry, 101
pelvic imbalance, 366
pelvic rotation, 58, 38
Pelvic-Spinal-Hip Complex (PSH-C), 37
pelvic tilt, 89
pelvis, 50, 53
periodontal ligament, 362
periodontal proprioceptors, 354
phonetics, 240
physical therapist, 322
physical therapy, 143, 173, 317
planes of orientation, 238
plantar aponeurosis, 338
plantar fascia, 338
plantarflexion, 346
plumb-line tests, 24
pose, 17
position, 17
posterior condylar position, 285
posterior nuclear migration, 139
postural alignment, 17
postural examination, 291
postural measurement, 87

Postural Vertical Dimension (PVD), 314
premature tooth contact, 354
primary respiratory mechanism, 356
principles of posture, 71
pronation, 337
proprioceptors, 352
protruded maxilla, 326
PSH-C, 37
psoas major, 363
pterygoid spasm, 190
pupilar, 95

R

radiographs, 235
reciprocal inhibition, 362
reflexes, 33
reflexes, cloacal, 351
reflexes, gait, 351
reflexes, head-on-body, 352
reflexes, mandibular, 354
reflexes, neck righting, 352
relaxation, 18, 44
repetitive, 309
retrognathic mandible, 326
retrognathic maxilla, 326
retrognathism, 116
retruded condyle, 224
retruded mandible, 328
retrusion, 330
rotator cuff, 102

S

sacral angle, 29
sagittal appliance, 296
scalene, 352
scalloped tongue, 117
Scheuermann's disease, 120
SCM, 107, 198
scoliosis, 47, 85, 89, 250, 254, 255, 285
semispinalis, 352
sensory awareness, 32
sensory reference, 65
severe overjet, 328
short-face syndrome, 311
shoulder girdle, 95, 102, 350
shoulder girdle complex, 317
shoulder retraction, 135

sidebending stretch, 136
sinusitis, 271
sitting, 57, 119
skeletal Class II, 310
skeletal Class III, 310
skeletal deep bite, 310
skeletal open bite, 310
skills, 33
sleeping, 68
slumped sitting, 59
sole, 67
soleus, 336
somatic system, 14
spasm, 31
sphenobasilar extension, 356
sphenobasilar flexion, 356
spinal accessory nerve, 359
spine, 349
splenius, 352
splenius capitus, 249
splint therapy, 276
splints, 244
Sternocleidomastoid (SCM), 109, 198, 249, 351
sternohyoid muscle, 354
stomatognathic, 234, 349, 350, 354
strabismus, 212
stress, 178
stress receptors, 364
stress-induced muscle tension, 309
stretch and spray technique, 352
stylohyoid muscle, 353
subluxation, 315, 362
subluxations, 352
suboccipital stretch, 135
suboccipitals, 249
Subtalar Joint (STJ), 337
supinate, 339
supination, 337
suprahyoid, 317
suprahyoid muscle, 350
surface reactions, 43
swing phase, 336

T

talus, 337
temporal bone, 110
temporal fossa, 190
temporal muscle, 190, 191

Temporomandibular Joints (TMJ), 271, 330, 331, 349
tendinitis, 102
tension pain, 77
the convenience bite, 190
the suboccipital spine, 109
therapeutic supports, 62
thermography, 86
thoracic, 97
thoracic kyphosis, 137
thoracic respiration, 366
thoracic spine, 101
tibia, 339
TMJ, 95, 102, 311, 314, 326, 330
TMJ dysfunction, 219, 220, 272, 273, 366
tongue-thrust, 328
tonsils, 316
trapezius, 249, 343, 351
trapezius muscle, 342, 346
trauma, 124, 309
trigeminal nerve, 111, 359
trigeminal neuralgia, 190
trigeminocervical complex, 112
trigger areas, 315
Trigger Point (TP), 3, 102, 111, 280, 342
trigger points, 31, 80, 83, 271, 273, 343

U

universal joints, 19
upper thoracic kyposis, 109
utility arch, 297

V

vagus nerve, 112
vertical dimension, 242, 243, 316, 317, 318, 322, 324, 328, 329, 330
vestibular labyrinth, 109

W

walking, 66
walking gait, 363
whiplash, 125

Z

zygomatic arch, 202